New Frontiers in Rehabilitation Medicine

New Frontiers in Rehabilitation Medicine

Edited by **Esther Henson**

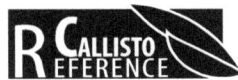

R CALLISTO REFERENCE

New York

Published by Callisto Reference,
106 Park Avenue, Suite 200,
New York, NY 10016, USA
www.callistoreference.com

New Frontiers in Rehabilitation Medicine
Edited by Esther Henson

International Standard Book Number: 978-1-63239-684-6 (Hardback)

The publisher's policy is to use permanent paper from mills that operate a sustainable forestry policy. Furthermore, the publisher ensures that the text paper and cover boards used have met acceptable environmental accreditation standards.

Trademark Notice: Registered trademark of products or corporate names are used only for explanation and identification without intent to infringe.

Printed in the United States of America.

Contents

Preface

This book aims to highlight the current researches and provides a platform to further the scope of innovations in this area. This book is a product of the combined efforts of many researchers and scientists from different parts of the world. The objective of this book is to provide the readers with the latest information in the field.

This book includes some of the vital pieces of work being conducted across the world, on various topics related to rehabilitation medicine. It explores all the important aspects of this field in the present day scenario. Rehabilitation medicine deals with restoring and enhancing the abilities and quality of life for people with physical disabilities. It includes treatment for the problems such as spinal cord injury, amputations, stroke, fibromyalgia, brain injury, etc. Extensive researches and new technologies that are required to provide human beings with a life that is not limited by physical disabilities are elaborated in this book. For all readers who are interested in this area, the case studies included in this book will serve as an excellent guide to develop a comprehensive understanding of this field. It is a vital tool for all researching and studying this field.

I would like to express my sincere thanks to the authors for their dedicated efforts in the completion of this book. I acknowledge the efforts of the publisher for providing constant support. Lastly, I would like to thank my family for their support in all academic endeavors.

Editor

Perceived Cognitive Decline in Multiple Sclerosis Impacts Quality of Life Independently of Depression

Lampros Samartzis,[1,2,3] **Efthymia Gavala,**[1] **Yiannis Zoukos,**[4]
Achilleas Aspiotis,[1] **and Thomas Thomaides**[1]

[1] Department of Neurology, General Hospital of the Greek Red Cross "Korgialeneio-Benakeio", Athens, Greece
[2] Department of Psychiatry, Athalassa Mental Health Hospital, Nicosia, Cyprus
[3] St. George's University of London Medical School, University of Nicosia, Nicosia, Cyprus
[4] Department of Neurology, St. Bartholomew's Royal London and Broomfield Hospitals, London, UK

Correspondence should be addressed to Lampros Samartzis; lampros.samartzis@gmail.com

Academic Editor: Vincent de Groot

Background/Aim. The aim of this study is to examine the effects of perceived cognitive dysfunction and of depression, on self-reported QoL, in a Greek population sample of MS patients. *Methods.* One hundred outpatients diagnosed with MS completed the Short-Form-36 Health Survey (SF-36), as well as the Perceived Deficits Questionnaire (PDQ) and the Depression subscale of the Mental Health Inventory (MHI), as part of a clinical evaluation which included the Expanded Disability Status Scale (EDSS) estimation. Multiple linear regression was conducted to determine the best linear combination of age, gender, education, EDSS, depression, attention/concentration, retrospective memory, prospective memory, and planning/organization, for predicting QoL scores. *Results.* In the multivariate regression analysis models, EDSS ($P < 0.05$), depression ($P < 0.001$), perceived planning/organization ($P < 0.05$), and perceived retrospective memory dysfunction ($P < 0.05$) independently predict quality of life scores. Age, sex, education level, and perceived attention/concentration dysfunction, as well as perceived prospective memory dysfunction, do not independently predict quality of life scores. *Conclusions.* Perceived planning/organization impairment and perceived retrospective memory impairment in MS patients predict QoL independently of the severity of disease and the severity of depression and therefore should be considered in the assessment of patient health status as well as in the design of treatment interventions and rehabilitation.

1. Introduction

Quality of life (QoL) is a useful endpoint in the study of multiple sclerosis (MS) not only as a prognostic factor but also as a quality marker of the health care provided. QoL in MS was found to be negatively affected by cognitive impairment [1] as well as by depression [2]. Depression is common in persons with MS, with a prevalence rate for major depression for MS patients in the community up to 25% [3]. Cognitive decline is also common in MS as prevalence rates in community samples of MS patients are reported around 40% [4, 5]. Cognitive impairment in MS patients could be measured with objective neuropsychological tests conducted by a clinical psychologist or measured by using self-answered questionnaires based on patients' subjective experience. Objective cognitive impairment was found to affect QoL in MS patient population [6], but subjective cognitive decline is not a well-established factor of decreased QoL in this patient group, despite the fact that it is easy to evaluate by using self-reported questionnaires. Subjective cognitive decline has also been suggested to be a consequence of depression [7, 8] and therefore should be taken into account in the treatment and rehabilitation processes. The aim of this study was to explore the hypothesis that subjective cognitive impairment affects QoL independently of depression.

2. Methods

2.1. Study Population. One hundred consecutive MS outpatients, 36 males and 64 females, took part in this study.

All patients were diagnosed according to international diagnostic criteria [9]. Concurrent drug treatments with antidepressants, anticonvulsants, mood stabilizers, or disease-modifying therapies were permitted as patients were stabilized for at least one month in a stable treatment scheme. Patients taking benzodiazepines and/or antipsychotic agents were excluded from the study as these medications may affect cognitive function. The study protocol was approved by the ethical committee of our institution and informed consent was obtained from all participants.

2.2. Clinical Evaluation. The clinical evaluation included a formal neurological examination, QoL assessment, perceived cognitive impairment evaluation, and assessment of depression, as a part of a thorough medical examination which included assessment of disability by using the Expanded Disability Status Scale (EDSS). The self-reported questionnaires were filled by the MS patients, who received help from the researcher when necessary. The researchers were neurology registrars, who were under the supervision of a consultant neurologist. The assessments were performed in the outpatient clinic, in a quite office which was available for this study purposes.

2.3. Assessment of Disability. The Expanded Disability Status Scale (EDSS) [10] was used to assess and quantify the disability of MS patients. EDSS scores between 1.0 and 4.5 refer to MS patients who are fully ambulatory, whereas EDSS scores between 5.0 to 9.5 are defined by the impairment to ambulation. Current EDSS evaluation was made by a registrar neurologist during the same visit of the patient to the MS outpatient clinic.

2.4. Assessment of QoL. The patients were asked to complete the Short-Form-36 Health Survey (SF-36) [11]. SF-36 is a psychometric tool for the quantification of health status and quality of life (QoL) which consists of eight subscales: vitality, physical functioning, bodily pain, general health perceptions, physical role functioning, emotional role functioning, social role functioning, and mental health, each of them being the weighted sum of the questions on the corresponding section.

2.5. Assessment of Perceived Cognitive Decline. Patients were asked to complete the Perceived Deficits Questionnaire (PDQ) which is a self-report disease-specific questionnaire that measures the patients' perceived degree of cognitive impairment [12]. The subscales of the PDG, namely, PDQ-attention/concentration, PDQ-retrospective memory, PDQ-prospective memory, and PDQ-planning/organization correspond to the domains of perceived cognitive decline of the patients.

2.6. Assessment of Depression. Patients were asked to complete the depression subscale of the Mental Health Inventory (MHI), that is, a self-reported questionnaire for assessing the level of depression [13].

2.7. Statistical Analysis. After descriptive statistics and correlation analysis, univariate and multivariate linear regression was conducted to determine the best linear combination of age, gender, education, EDSS, depression, attention/concentration, retrospective memory, prospective memory, and planning/organization, for predicting quality of life scores in each SF-36 subscale. All statistical procedures were performed using the SPSS Statistics version 17.0 (SPSS Inc., Chicago, Ill.).

3. Results

3.1. Baseline Characteristics. Characteristics of the total sample of 64 female and 36 male patients with MS that fulfilled the inclusion criteria therefore included in the analysis are presented in Table 1. Of the initial number of 134 MS outpatients having been assessed as eligible for taking part in the study, no more than 9 refused to take part due to personal reasons or lack of time for answering the questionnaires, and no more than 25 were excluded by the researchers mainly due to heavy use of psychotropic medication affecting current mental state (e.g., benzodiazepines and/or antipsychotics). The between-gender comparison, using independent samples t-test, revealed no significant differences between gender subgroups. The Mann-Whitney test, a nonparametric equivalent of independent samples t-test, also showed no difference between genders, in the significance level of 0.05, in any of the variables presented in Table 1.

3.2. Correlation Analysis. A correlation analysis using Pearson's r was conducted in which depression showed a low correlation with EDSS ($r = 0.256$, $P < 0.05$), but a moderate correlation with QoL ($r = 0.502$, $P < 0.001$), as well as with PDQ perceived impairment subscales: attention/concentration ($r = 0.515$, $P < 0.001$), retrospective memory ($r = 0.445$, $P < 0.001$), prospective memory ($r = 0.483$, $P < 0.001$), and planning/organization (0.601, $P < 0.001$). Figure 1 shows the relationship between depression and perceived impairment of planning/organization ability in population of patients with MS. No significant correlations, in the level of 0.05, were found between depression and gender or age of the patients.

3.3. Regression Analysis. In Table 2 the results of the multiple linear regression analysis that was conducted in order to determine the best linear combination of age, gender, education, EDSS, depression, attention/concentration, retrospective memory, prospective memory, and planning/organization are presented, for predicting quality of life scores in all SF-36 subscales. This combination of variables predicts quality of life scores, with the variables significantly contributing to the prediction.

4. Discussion

Our data showed moderate correlations between depression and perceived cognitive impairment scales. Other studies also found a relationship between cognitive impairment

TABLE 1: Characteristics of MS patients ($n = 100$).

Characteristics	Total sample	Males ($n = 36$)	Females ($n = 64$)	P value
Age, years	40.5 ± 10.3	40.9 ± 12.1	40.2 ± 9.2	NS
Education level (A/B/C) %	19/57/24	25/56/19	16/58/26	—
EDSS	3.6 ± 1.9	3.9 ± 2.2	3.4 ± 1.7	NS
MHI-depression	69.0 ± 21.0	71.7 ± 21.2	67.5 ± 20.9	NS
PDQ-attention/concentration	4.8 ± 4.0	4 ± 3.4	5.2 ± 4.3	NS
PDQ-retrospective memory	3.9 ± 4.3	3.2 ± 3.9	4.3 ± 4.5	NS
PDQ-prospective memory	2.8 ± 3.4	2.3 ± 2.9	3.1 ± 3.6	NS
PDQ-planning/organization	3.1 ± 3.8	2.4 ± 3.3	3.4 ± 4.0	NS
SF-36 physical functioning	66.0 ± 36.2	65.7 ± 42.1	66.1 ± 32.7	NS
SF-36 role physical	69.0 ± 42.4	72.2 ± 40.9	67.2 ± 43.4	NS
SF-36 general health	60.7 ± 20.1	63.9 ± 20.9	58.9 ± 19.6	NS
SF-36 vitality	55.0 ± 23.0	60.6 ± 23.8	51.9 ± 22.0	NS
SF-36 social functioning	72.4 ± 29.0	74.0 ± 30.1	71.5 ± 28.5	NS
SF-36 role emotional	75.0 ± 40.6	76.0 ± 40.3	74.5 ± 41.0	NS
SF-36 mental health	58.7 ± 17.5	62.9 ± 17.6	56.4 ± 17.2	NS

Unless specified otherwise, values are presented as means ± SD. Significance level or alpha (α) level was set at 0.05. Education level: A, primary education; B, secondary education; C, tertiary education; EDSS, Expanded Disability Status Scale; MHI, Mental Health Inventory; PDQ, Perceived Deficits Questionnaire, NS, nonsignificant.

TABLE 2: Simultaneous multiple regression analysis summary for age, education level, EDSS, depression, attention/concentration, retrospective memory, prospective memory, planning/organization, and predicting SF-36 QoL scales. Only significant factors appear in columns.

	MHI depression	PDQ-retrospective memory	PDQ-planning/organization
Physical functioning $R^2 = 0.48$, $F_{(9,86)} = 10.90$, $P < 0.001$			$B = -3.29$, SE $= 1.57$, beta $= -0.35$, $P < 0.05$
Role physical $R^2 = 0.16$, $F_{(9,86)} = 3.04$, $P < 0.05$	$B = 11.29$, SE $= 4.87$, beta $= 0.28$, $P < 0.05$		
General health $R^2 = 0.32$, $F_{(9,86)} = 5.95$, $P < 0.001$	$B = 6.70$, SE $= 2.09$, beta $= 0.35$, $P < 0.05$	$B = 2.57$, SE $= 0.95$, beta $= 0.56$, $P < 0.05$	$B = -2.17$, SE $= 1.01$, beta $= -0.42$, $P < 0.05$
Vitality $R^2 = 0.47$, $F_{(9,86)} = 10.43$, $P < 0.001$	$B = 7.72$, SE $= 2.11$, beta $= 0.349$, $P < 0.001$	$B = 2.12$, SE $= .964$, beta $= 0.40$, $P < 0.05$	$B = -3.09$, SE $= 1.02$, beta $= -0.513$, $P < 0.05$
Social functioning $R^2 = 0.543$, $F_{(9,86)} = 13.53$, $P < 0.001$	$B = 11.05$, SE $= 2.48$, beta $= 0.40$, $P < 0.001$		$B = -3.83$, SE $= 1.19$, beta $= -0.51$, $P < 0.05$
Role emotional $R^2 = 0.347$, $F_{(9,86)} = 6.61$, $P < 0.001$	$B = 17.16$, SE $= 4.16$, beta $= 0.44$, $P < 0.001$		$B = -4.11$, SE $= 2.00$, beta $= -.38$, $P < 0.05$
Mental health $R^2 = 0.69$, $F_{(9,86)} = 23.99$, $P < 0.001$	$B = 12.81$, SE $= 1.24$, beta $= 0.77$, $P < 0.001$		

EDSS, Expanded Disability Status Scale; MHI, Mental Health Inventory; SF-36, Short Form 36-item Health Survey; QoL, quality of life; PDQ, Perceived Deficits Questionnaire.

and depression in MS population [7, 8, 14–22] but there is a need for cautious interpretation of such findings [7], as cross-section studies cannot determine direction of causality. Depression could lead to cognitive decline, a phenomenon also known as pseudodementia, but also impairment of cognition could be one of the first symptoms/criteria of depression. Nevertheless, some studies reported no significant relationship between cognitive impairment and depression [23, 24], by using different psychometric tools, populations, and study design, therefore not directly comparable to our data.

Our analysis showed that specific perceived cognitive impairments affect QoL independently of depression. Specifically, perceived impairment of planning/organization affects

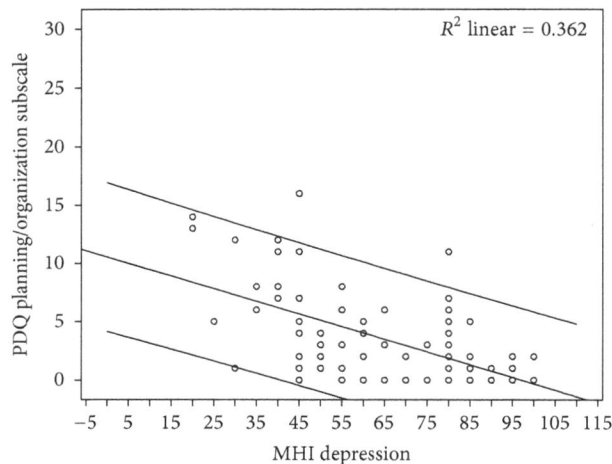

FIGURE 1: Scatter plot showing the relationship between depression and perceived impairment of planning/organization ability in population of patients with MS.

general health, vitality, social functioning, and role emotional QoL subscales independently of depression. In addition, perceived impairment of the retrospective memory affects general health and vitality subscales independently of depression. Interestingly, perceived attention/concentration dysfunction, as well as perceived prospective memory dysfunction, did not independently predict any QoL scores in our multinomial regression models. It seems that impairment in planning/organization and/or retrospective memory affects and decreases the QoL scales to a larger degree than do impairment of prospective memory and/or attention concentration.

Other studies also found self-reported cognitive impairment to correlate with impaired QoL [25], but a recent study found only weak associations between objective cognitive impairment and QoL [26]. These studies agree in the direction of the findings but differ in the degree of correlations, due to heterogeneity in the studied populations, in the fields of age, sex ratio, and the disease severity.

Depression is a well-known factor negatively affecting QoL and this is also confirmed in our data. We found evidence that depression predicts decreased QoL in the QoL scales of SF-36. Depression is a well-established QoL determinator not only in MS but also in many other medical conditions. Other studies have also demonstrated that depression affects QoL in MS population [6, 25, 27–29]. Furthermore a study reported no correlation between QoL scales and EDSS while controlling for depression and anxiety [30].

The strength of this study is that by involving a relatively large population of MS outpatients we explored associations between perceived cognitive impairment and QoL. To the knowledge of the authors this is the first evidence of this, and more extensive investigation is needed in order to delineate possible etiological factors as neurological and psychosocial correlates. A limitation of this study is that we did not include an additional objective neuropsychological assessment in

order to explore the effects of objective cognitive decline on patients QoL as well as to compare the size of correlations between subjective and objective impairment in the explored areas of cognitive function. Even if this was not the point in this study, other authors already explored this area with contradictory results [20, 22, 25, 31–35], on whether MS patients are capable of self-estimating their objective cognitive decline.

Another limitation of this study is its cross-sectional design and the lack of second measurement, something that by definition yields bidirectional results. Cross-sectional design does not make it possible to explore for causal relationships between depression, cognitive impairment, and decline of QoL, despite the moderate correlation coefficients found. A prospective longitudinal design, using a structural equation model analysis, could probably define the unidirectional or bidirectional nature of these relationships.

Some authors suggested a common effect between depression and perceived cognitive impairment [31] but this is not extracted by the findings of this study as they remain independent predictors in the regression models. This finding suggests a separate role for perceived cognitive impairment that has to be further explored. Patient concerns related to the decline of their cognition should be interpreted with caution.

Perceived cognitive dysfunctions could be taken into account in the individualized rehabilitation plan in order to maximize rehabilitation's effectiveness on patients' QoL. During the rehabilitation process, clinicians should consider the possibility that cognitive testing confirms what the patients perceive regarding organizational skill deficits as well as the possibility that cognitive testing demonstrates that these cognitive abilities are preserved.

Perceived cognitive impairment in patients with MS constitutes a constellation of symptoms that the clinician should take into consideration. This could be a secondary sign of hidden depression but could also be an independent cognitive factor that is negatively affecting patients' quality of life. Both phenomena should be taken into account in the treatment process as well as in the design of rehabilitation programs.

Highlights

(i) We examine effects of perceived cognitive impairment in QoL in a clinical sample of outpatients with MS.

(ii) We also examine if these effects are independent of MS severity and depression.

(iii) Perceived planning/organization dysfunction as well as perceived retrospective memory dysfunction independently predict QoL in MS.

(iv) Perceived attention/concentration and prospective memory dysfunctions do not.

(v) Both of these perceived cognitive dysfunctions could be taken into account in the individualized rehabilitation plan in order to maximize rehabilitation's effectiveness on patients' QoL.

Conflict of Interests

The authors declare that there is no conflict of interests.

Authors' Contribution

Lampros Samartzis, M.D., contributed to the design and conceptualization of the study, analysis, and interpretation of the data, as well as to drafting and revising the paper. Efthymia Gavala, M.D., contributed to the design and conceptualization of the study as well as to drafting and revising the paper. Yiannis Zoukos, M.D. and Ph.D., contributed to the design and conceptualization of the study and interpretation of the data, as well as to revising the paper. Achileas Aspiotis, M.D., contributed to the design and conceptualization of the study, as well as to the interpretation of the data. Thomas Thomaides, M.D. and Ph.D., contributed to the design and conceptualization of the study and interpretation of the data, as well as to revising the paper.

References

[1] R. Cutajar, E. Ferriani, C. Scandellari et al., "Cognitive function and quality of life in multiple sclerosis patients," *Journal of Neurovirology*, vol. 6, no. 2, pp. S186–S190, 2000.

[2] I. S. Lobentanz, S. Asenbaum, K. Vass et al., "Factors influencing quality of life in multiple sclerosis patients: disability, depressive mood, fatigue and sleep quality," *Acta Neurologica Scandinavica*, vol. 110, no. 1, pp. 6–13, 2004.

[3] S. B. Patten, C. A. Beck, J. V. A. Williams, C. Barbui, and L. M. Metz, "Major depression in multiple sclerosis: a population-based perspective," *Neurology*, vol. 61, no. 11, pp. 1524–1527, 2003.

[4] S. A. McIntosh-Michaelis, M. H. Roberts, S. M. Wilkinson et al., "The prevalence of cognitive impairment in a community survey of multiple sclerosis," *British Journal of Clinical Psychology*, vol. 30, part 4, pp. 333–348, 1991.

[5] S. M. Rao, G. J. Leo, L. Bernardin, and F. Unverzagt, "Cognitive dysfunction in multiple sclerosis. I. Frequency, patterns, and prediction," *Neurology*, vol. 41, no. 5, pp. 685–691, 1991.

[6] J. Benito-León, J. M. Morales, and J. Rivera-Navarro, "Health-related quality of life and its relationship to cognitive and emotional functioning in multiple sclerosis patients," *European Journal of Neurology*, vol. 9, no. 5, pp. 497–502, 2002.

[7] K. Lester, L. Stepleman, and M. Hughes, "The association of illness severity, self-reported cognitive impairment, and perceived illness management with depression and anxiety in a multiple sclerosis clinic population," *Journal of Behavioral Medicine*, vol. 30, no. 2, pp. 177–186, 2007.

[8] Y. Maor, L. Olmer, and B. Mozes, "The relation between objective and subjective impairment in cognitive function among multiple sclerosis patients—the role of depression," *Multiple Sclerosis*, vol. 7, no. 2, pp. 131–135, 2001.

[9] C. H. Polman, S. C. Reingold, G. Edan et al., "Diagnostic criteria for multiple sclerosis: 2005 revisions to the 'McDonald Criteria,'" *Annals of Neurology*, vol. 58, no. 6, pp. 840–846, 2005.

[10] J. F. Kurtzke, "Rating neurologic impairment in multiple sclerosis: an expanded disability status scale (EDSS)," *Neurology*, vol. 33, no. 11, pp. 1444–1452, 1983.

[11] E. Pappa, N. Kontodimopoulos, and D. Niakas, "Validating and norming of the Greek SF-36 Health Survey," *Quality of Life Research*, vol. 14, no. 5, pp. 1433–1438, 2005.

[12] R. A. Marrie, D. M. Miller, G. J. Chelune, and J. A. Cohen, "Validity and reliability of the MSQLI in cognitively impaired patients with multiple sclerosis," *Multiple Sclerosis*, vol. 9, no. 6, pp. 621–626, 2003.

[13] C. T. Veit and J. E. Ware, "The structure of psychological distress and well-being in general populations," *Journal of Consulting and Clinical Psychology*, vol. 51, no. 5, pp. 730–742, 1983.

[14] C. Christodoulou, P. Melville, W. F. Scherl et al., "Negative affect predicts subsequent cognitive change in multiple sclerosis," *Journal of the International Neuropsychological Society*, vol. 15, no. 1, pp. 53–61, 2009.

[15] F. H. Barwick and P. A. Arnett, "Relationship between global cognitive decline and depressive symptoms in multiple sclerosis," *Clinical Neuropsychologist*, vol. 25, no. 2, pp. 193–209, 2011.

[16] A. C. Gilchrist and F. H. Creed, "Depression, cognitive impairment and social stress in multiple sclerosis," *Journal of Psychosomatic Research*, vol. 38, no. 3, pp. 193–201, 1994.

[17] D. C. Mohr, L. P. Dick, D. Russo et al., "The psychosocial impact of multiple sclerosis: exploring the patient's perspective," *Health Psychology*, vol. 18, no. 4, pp. 376–382, 1999.

[18] D. C. Mohr, D. E. Goodkin, N. Gatto, and J. van der Wende, "Depression, coping and level of neurological impairment in multiple sclerosis," *Multiple Sclerosis*, vol. 3, no. 4, pp. 254–258, 1997.

[19] P. A. Arnett, C. I. Higginson, W. D. Voss, W. I. Bender, J. M. Wurst, and J. M. Tippin, "Depression in multiple sclerosis: relationship to working memory capacity," *Neuropsychology*, vol. 13, no. 4, pp. 546–556, 1999.

[20] J. M. Bruce and P. A. Arnett, "Self-reported everyday memory and depression in patients with multiple sclerosis," *Journal of Clinical and Experimental Neuropsychology*, vol. 26, no. 2, pp. 200–214, 2004.

[21] J. M. Bruce, A. S. Bruce, L. Hancock, and S. Lynch, "Self-reported memory problems in multiple sclerosis: influence of psychiatric status and normative dissociative experiences," *Archives of Clinical Neuropsychology*, vol. 25, no. 1, pp. 39–48, 2010.

[22] R. H. Benedict, D. Cox, L. L. Thompson, F. Foley, B. Weinstock-Guttman, and F. Munschauer, "Reliable screening for neuropsychological impairment in multiple sclerosis," *Multiple Sclerosis*, vol. 10, no. 6, pp. 675–678, 2004.

[23] A. Moller, G. Wiedemann, U. Rohde, H. Backmund, and A. Sonntag, "Correlates of cognitive impairment and depressive mood disorder in multiple sclerosis," *Acta Psychiatrica Scandinavica*, vol. 89, no. 2, pp. 117–121, 1994.

[24] J. DeLuca, S. K. Johnson, D. Beldowicz, and B. H. Natelson, "Neuropsychological impairments in chronic fatigue syndrome, multiple sclerosis, and depression," *Journal of Neurology Neurosurgery and Psychiatry*, vol. 58, no. 1, pp. 38–43, 1995.

[25] S. M. Gold, H. Schulz, A. Mönch, K. Schulz, and C. Heesen, "Cognitive impairment in multiple sclerosis does not affect reliability and validity of self-report health measures," *Multiple Sclerosis*, vol. 9, no. 4, pp. 404–410, 2003.

[26] K. Baumstarck-Barrau, M. Simeoni, F. Reuter et al., "Cognitive function and quality of life in multiple sclerosis patients: a cross-sectional study," *BMC Neurology*, vol. 11, article 17, 2011.

[27] S. Hart, I. Fonareva, N. Merluzzi, and D. C. Mohr, "Treatment for depression and its relationship to improvement in quality of life and psychological well-being in multiple sclerosis patients," *Quality of Life Research*, vol. 14, no. 3, pp. 695–703, 2005.

[28] M. P. Amato, V. Zipoli, and E. Portaccio, "Multiple sclerosis-related cognitive changes: a review of cross-sectional and longitudinal studies," *Journal of the Neurological Sciences*, vol. 245, no. 1-2, pp. 41–46, 2006.

[29] S. Fruewald, H. Loeffler-Stastka, R. Eher, B. Saletu, and U. Baumhacki, "Depression and quality of life in multiple sclerosis," *Acta Neurologica Scandinavica*, vol. 104, no. 5, pp. 257–261, 2001.

[30] A. C. J. W. Janssens, P. A. van Doorn, J. B. de Boer et al., "Anxiety and depression influence the relation between disability status and quality of life in multiple sclerosis," *Multiple Sclerosis*, vol. 9, no. 4, pp. 397–403, 2003.

[31] J. Lovera, B. Bagert, K. H. Smoot et al., "Correlations of Perceived Deficits Questionnaire of multiple sclerosis quality of life inventory with Beck Depression Inventory and neuropsychological tests," *Journal of Rehabilitation Research and Development*, vol. 43, no. 1, pp. 73–82, 2006.

[32] L. S. Middleton, D. R. Denney, S. G. Lynch, and B. Parmenter, "The relationship between perceived and objective cognitive functioning in multiple sclerosis," *Archives of Clinical Neuropsychology*, vol. 21, no. 5, pp. 487–494, 2006.

[33] R. A. Marrie, G. J. Chelune, D. M. Miller, and J. A. Cohen, "Subjective cognitive complaints relate to mild impairment of cognition in multiple sclerosis," *Multiple Sclerosis*, vol. 11, no. 1, pp. 69–75, 2005.

[34] C. Christodoulou, P. Melville, W. F. Scherl et al., "Perceived cognitive dysfunction and observed neuropsychological performance: longitudinal relation in persons with multiple sclerosis," *Journal of the International Neuropsychological Society*, vol. 11, no. 5, pp. 614–619, 2005.

[35] P. A. Arnett, "Longitudinal consistency of the relationship between depression symptoms and cognitive functioning in multiple sclerosis," *CNS Spectrums*, vol. 10, no. 5, pp. 372–382, 2005.

Clinical Understanding of Spasticity: Implications for Practice

Rozina Bhimani[1] **and Lisa Anderson**[2]

[1] Department of Nursing, St. Catherine University, St. Paul, MN 55105, USA
[2] Department of Integrative Biology and Physiology, University of Minnesota, Minneapolis, MN 55455, USA

Correspondence should be addressed to Rozina Bhimani; rhbhimani@stkate.edu

Academic Editor: Jeffrey Jutai

Spasticity is a poorly understood phenomenon. The aim of this paper is to understand the effect of spasticity on daily life and identify bedside strategies that enhance patient's function and improve comfort. Spasticity and clonus result from an upper motor neuron lesion that disinhibits the tendon stretch reflex; however, they are differentiated in the fact that spasticity results in a velocity dependent tightness of muscle whereas clonus results in uncontrollable jerks of the muscle. Clinical strategies that address function and comfort are paramount. This is a secondary content analysis using a qualitative research design. Adults experiencing spasticity associated with neuromuscular disorder were asked to participate during inpatient acute rehabilitation. They were asked to complete a semistructured interview to explain and describe the nature of their experienced spasticity on daily basis. Spasticity affects activities of daily living, function, and mobility. Undertreated spasticity can lead to pain, immobility, and risk of falls. There were missed opportunities to adequately care for patients with spasticity. Bedside care strategies identified by patients with spasticity are outlined. Uses of alternative therapies in conjunction with medications are needed to better manage spasticity. Patient reports on spasticity are important and should be part of clinical evaluation and practice.

1. Introduction

Disability can have devastating effects on people's lives. It is estimated that about 15% of people in the world live with different types of disabilities [1]. Among these disabilities, physical disability due to neuromuscular dysfunctions (such as spinal cord injury, multiple sclerosis, stroke, and traumatic brain injury) is particularly devastating because neuromuscular dysfunction can lead to immobility, social isolation, pressure ulcers, increased urinary tract infections, and other sequelae due to primary disability [1]. Spasticity is one of the sequelae of neuromuscular disability [2]. Martin et al. [3] estimate prevalence of lower limb spasticity for stroke (40–600 per 100,000), multiple sclerosis (2–350 per 100,000), cerebral palsy (260–340 per 100,000), and spinal cord injury (22–90 per 100,000). They estimate annual incidence of lower limb spasticity for stroke to be 30–485 per 100,000, traumatic brain injury 100–235 per 100,000, and spinal cord injury 0.2–8 per 100,000.

The most common understanding of spasticity has roots in Lance's study [4]. In this study, spread of phasic reflexes in four normal subjects and sixteen patients experiencing spasticity was evaluated through electromyography. Later this study provided the basis for the spasticity definition [5], which is now commonly available in the literature. There is plenty of research available on spasticity; however, patients' feedback on their understanding of spasticity is missing from the literature. Spasticity symptom experiences can be devastating and patients' spasticity interpretation may differ. Ethical clinical practices require clinicians to incorporate patients' understanding of this phenomenon in their plan of care. Bhimani et al.'s [6] original study reports on the patient understanding of spasticity and their results indicate that there is a discrepancy between patients and clinicians understanding of spasticity. Therefore, omitting patient reports from clinical decision making can have grave and serious consequences on their lives manifesting as side-effects of spasticity therapy, administration of invasive and inappropriate therapies, unnecessary pain, and suffering.

2. Background

2.1. Movement and Posture Physiology. One of the essential functions of the human motor system is to determine the correct joint positions and movements, specifically, a motor program, required to carry out the daily activities of life. In addition, a motor system must integrate the motor intention of the individual with the muscle tone and body position information from the musculoskeletal system to determine that motor program. Muscle tone refers to continuous partial resistance that prevents full relaxation of voluntary muscles. This resistance is felt due to the elasticity and compliance of the tissue when a limb is moved through passive range of motion [7]. This partial tension in the muscle is needed for a muscle to act quickly and smoothly to carry out a future task. For example, an act of throwing a ball contracts the bicep muscles while the triceps muscles also cocontract to stabilize the elbow joint during this movement. On the other hand, the act of tapping the bicep tendon causes the bicep muscles to contract (increase in muscle tone: an agonist act) while the triceps muscle relaxes (decrease in muscle tone: an antagonist act) at the same time to maintain muscle length. This change in muscle action is mediated by a monosynaptic reflex arc through spinal cord of the central nervous system (CNS). This type of normal reflex function is known as the tonic stretch reflex (TSR). The connection of the CNS with muscles further provides reflex activity to maintain balance and posture in the body. The stretch reflex is a negative feedback mechanism that maintains muscle length; compliance is an intrinsic property of the muscle and connective tissue [8].

Homeostasis of normal muscle tone is disrupted for many reasons. In some instances, pathways to maintain muscle tone are disrupted due to injury-producing lesions in motor neurons. Neurons that connect the brain to the spinal cord are known as upper motor neurons (UMNs), whereas neurons that connect the spinal cord to muscles are called lower motor neurons (LMNs). From the brain, upper motor neurons provide the movement instructions transmitted through the lower motor neuron to the muscles. When the lower motor neurons are damaged, the result is twitching of contiguous fibers (fasciculation), muscle weakness, and atrophy [9]. When the UMNs are impaired, information needed to maintain a normal TSR is disrupted, leading to the pathologies of muscle tone that create spasticity, which can be permanent (see Figure 1). The consequences of these pathologies may result in dependency in activities of daily living (ADL) and mobility, create pressure ulcers, and increase caregiver burden [10].

3. Review of the Literature

This is a critical review of the literature that clarifies neurological disorder of spasticity, hypertonia, and related terms. Following types of hypertonia are clarified by outlining the pathophysiology for spasticity and clonus. Neurological terms such as spasticity and hypertonia and associated terms require clear understanding and interpretation in clinical practice for safe patient care.

4. Hypertonia

Hypertonia is an "umbrella term" that describes any condition leading to tight or stiff muscles. Many clinicians use the term hypertonia interchangeably with spasticity; however, spasticity is a type of hypertonia that is velocity dependent or in other words is increased with movement, though spasticity can be present at rest. In clinical practice, spasticity is often confused with other conditions such as clonus and rigidity. The velocity dependent aspect of spasticity distinguishes it from rigidity, which is not velocity dependent. Rigidity is a symptom seen with basal nuclei lesions, such as Parkinson's disease. With rigidity, muscles exhibit the same degree of tightness regardless of the amount of movement or sensory input [11]. Spasticity as a sensory-motor disorder acknowledges that sensory stimuli are an influence on the experience of worsening spasticity. Clonus is also distinguished from spasticity; clonus is involuntary jerks and tremors of the limb. It can concurrently be present with spasticity and rigidity.

4.1. Upper Motor Neuron. The tight, stiff muscle experienced with hypertonia is a symptom of upper motor neuron dysfunction. Nerve impulses are normally relayed from the UMN to interneurons in the spinal cord and then through the LMN to muscles [8]; UMN damage and the loss of this relay information can impact functions such as walking, breathing, and swallowing. Disruptions in these functional movements can compromise activities of daily living and even can be life threatening. Tight muscles can cause pain and disrupt sleep at night. The increased muscle tone can have a devastating effect on the quality of life. Tight and rigid muscles can result in contractures that affect ambulation, ADLs, comfort, and sleep [10, 12]. Therefore, upper motor neuron dysfunctions demand the full array of therapeutic treatments and interventions [13].

5. Pathophysiology of Spasticity

Spasticity is a part of a disabling UMN syndrome. The UMN lesions decrease the inhibitory drive in the corticospinal tract to produce spasticity. Spasticity is generated through local activation of muscle spindles, but the propagation and manifestation of spasticity require involvement of the central nervous system [2, 14]. The UMN lesion disrupts communication between the brain and the spinal cord, producing a state of net disinhibition of the spinal reflexes. In spasticity, when a limb muscle is stretched muscle spindles respond by sending action potentials to the spinal cord via sensory neurons. However, the negative feedback system between muscle spindles and alpha-motor neurons is disrupted because of the UMN lesion, and abnormal muscle activation occurs. There are many interrelated feedback mechanisms that can account for spasticity [15, 16]. For example, the UMN lesions decrease the inhibitory drive in the corticospinal tract, which can affect alpha-motor neuron excitability causing increased muscle contraction, particularly in flexor muscles. Furthermore, motor tract that originates in the brainstem can increase excitation of spinal neurons [15, 16] (see Figure 2). Also disruption of interneuron mediated inhibition of the antagonist muscle or increased action potentials in the sensory neurons from the muscle spindle can lead to hypertonia [15, 16].

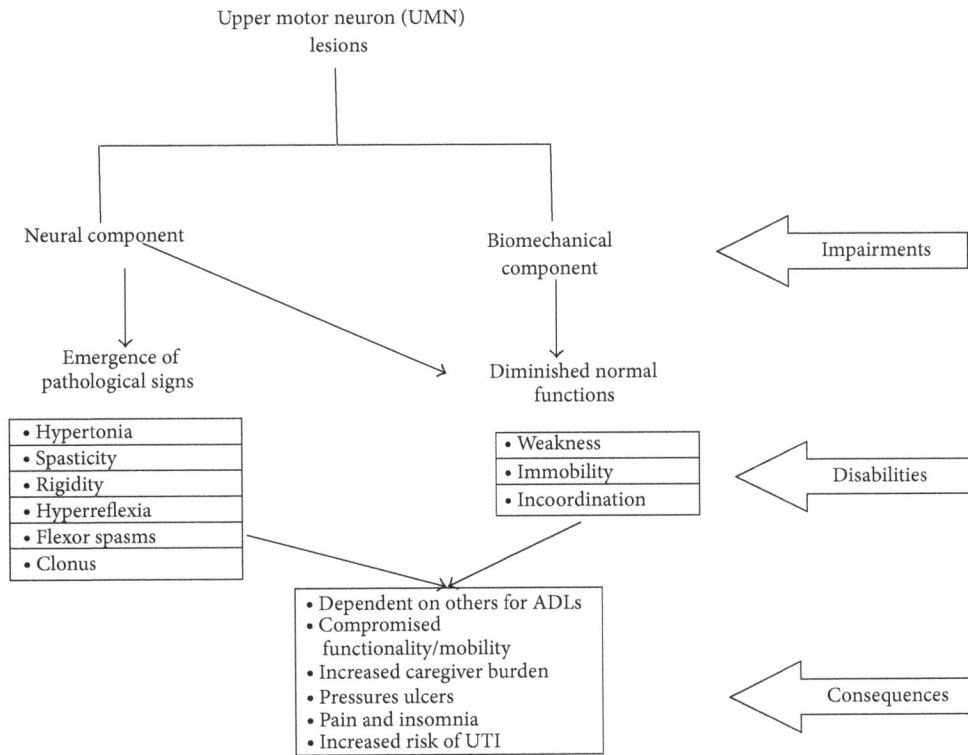

FIGURE 1: Upper motor neuron (UMN) syndrome impairment, disabilities, and its consequences.

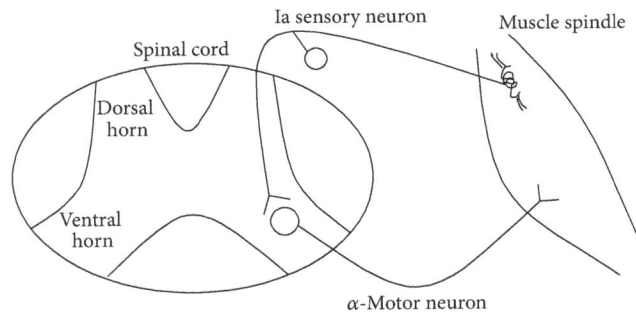

FIGURE 2: Basic monosynaptic stretch reflex.

5.1. Sensory Experiences. Spasticity is a sensory-motor phenomenon. The new definition from the Support Program for Assembly of a Database for Spasticity Measurement (SPASM) project defines spasticity as "disordered sensory-motor control, resulting from an upper motor neuron lesion" [17, page 72]. Involvements of both the sensory input and motor outputs are identified in producing spasticity. Currently clinical practice is still based on the narrow Lance [5] definition of spasticity. Lance [5] defined spasticity as a "motor disorder characterized by a velocity-dependent increase in tonic stretch reflexes (muscle tone) with exaggerated tendon jerks, resulting from hyperexcitability of the stretch reflex" (page 485). This definition is useful in clinical practice, because, by providing the guideline of "velocity-dependent increase in tonic stretch reflexes," it delineates

spasticity from other similar movement disorders such as hypertonia, rigidity, and hyperreflexia. Unfortunately, this ignores the important aspect of sensory input in the experience of spasticity. Lance's [5] definition is therefore limiting and somewhat misleading [6]. Therefore, it is imperative that clinical practice incorporates the new 21st century definition to operationalize the management of spasticity.

6. Pathophysiology of Clonus

The pathophysiology of spasticity and clonus is separate but interrelated. Clonus is generally more easily induced in the ankles and feet. When the ankle is dorsiflexed, muscle spindles are stretched in the gastrocnemius muscle which is sensed by sensory receptor Ia and impulses are sent to the spinal cord where it synapses on the alpha-motor neurons leading to more activation of alpha neurons to the gastrocnemius and soleus. Contraction of the gastrocnemius and soleus leads to plantarflexion. Cycles of plantarflexion and dorsiflexion follow as the gastrocnemius and soleus contract quickly and then relax and stretch in a repeating loop [18]. Competing explanations for the ankle clonus are found in the literature. Though initially ankle clonus was thought to be the oscillations of antagonistic muscles, later EMG studies show that this is not the case. During ankle clonus, strong EMG activity is observed in the gastrocnemius and soleus but not in the anterior tibialis, the antagonistic dorsiflexor [18]. Ankle clonus was therefore hypothesized to be an exaggerated stretch reflex of the gastrocnemius and soleus only. Other investigators have observed EMG activity in the anterior tibialis, occurring simultaneously with EMG activity in the plantarflexors [19, 20], leading to the hypothesis that a central pattern generator mechanism in the spinal cord was at least jointly responsible for clonus. The observation that cold therapy significantly decreases clonus, whereas the central alpha2 antagonist, tizanidine, does not, suggests that peripheral mechanism is more important [21], though the mechanism is still being debated.

With an UMN lesion leading to spasticity and clonus, alpha neurons are activated too much with the loss of inhibition from corticospinal and dorsal reticulospinal corticobulbar pathway and excitation from vestibulospinal and medial reticulospinal pathways [16]. Highly activated alpha neurons increase the sensitivity of muscle spindles, making hypertonic spasticity and the repeating contractions of clonus possible [16]. Furthermore, interneuron mediated relaxation of antagonist muscles is prevented, adding to more contraction and oscillation of impulses [16, 22].

7. Quality of Life Issues

Spasticity and its consequences negatively influence quality of life. Management of spasticity is an important care issue in neuroscience because it can affect quality of life. Very few first-person accounts of spasticity are available. Most literature has focused on the quantification of symptoms but patient's input is lacking [13, 23, 24].

Despite the fact that spasticity is a lived experience, there are very few studies on patient accounts and perception of spasticity. Bhimani et al. [6] and Mahoney et al. [25] have explored overall understanding of spasticity. Both report similar findings that patients understanding of spasticity was based on the individual interpretations and meaning assigned to the experience. Symptom experiences of spasticity were either accepted or managed medically or with use of alternative therapies. Social consequences of spasticity experiences were embarrassment and social stigma, which led to self-isolation. In addition, participants reported sensory experiences and found themselves unable to articulate these sensations. Patients often used word spasm to report both clonus and spasticity.

Spasticity is a fertile area for research. Clinical outcome measures to assess spasticity at the bedside cannot completely account for the myriads of spasticity experiences. Understanding of spasticity and clonus from patient perspective and how it affects daily life is needed for clinical understanding and bedside practice.

8. Method

The purpose of this study is to understand the effect of spasticity and clonus on daily life and identify bedside strategies that enhance patient's function and improve comfort.

8.1. Research Question. What are spastic patient experiences of activities of daily living, function, mobility, comfort, and pain?
Specific aims were

(1) to identify missed opportunities for care during inpatient rehabilitation stay;

(2) to identify bedside strategies for care in practice.

8.2. Design. This is a secondary analysis of the original longitudinal qualitative study to identify strategies that impact spastic patient's activities of daily living, mobility, and comfort.

8.3. Sample. The study setting was a 31-bed acute rehabilitation unit in a large nonprofit tertiary-care hospital and a stand-alone rehabilitation center with 56 beds both located in a metropolitan area of the Midwestern United States. Both settings were at Commission on Accreditation of Rehabilitation Facilities (CARF) certified for spinal cord injury (SCI). Administrative and institutional review board permissions were obtained from both facilities. A total of 23 participants were recruited with neurological disorders associated with spasticity. Out of 23 participants, the first 10 participants were recruited from the hospital-based rehabilitation unit. The remaining 13 participants were recruited from the stand-alone center. The majority of patients were Caucasian (83%), with the diagnoses of spinal cord injury (61%), stroke (17%), cerebral palsy (13%), and multiple sclerosis (9%). About equal number of men (48%) and women (52%) were recruited, with a majority of participants (57%) under the age of 45 and the rest were under the age of 65. Neurological deficits included inability to perform ADLs independently (100%) and mobility impairments where 22% needed some assistive device while 78% were wheelchair bound, of which 13% could not move upper or lower extremities. All participants' hearing, vision, and speech were preserved.

8.4. Procedure and Data Analysis. The original research study focused on understanding spasticity over time. Subjective understanding of spasticity was extracted from responses to a daily open-ended question about spasticity. The purpose was to allow patients to freely express their spasticity experiences nested in daily routines. In addition to daily open-ended question, twice a week patients were asked in-depth questions to capture changes in spasticity through words during their routines of daily living. Participants were followed up for seven days in the inpatient rehabilitation setting.

During data analysis for the original study, it was apparent that the participants provided large amounts of data. Therefore, a secondary data analysis was undertaken guided by the current research question. Colaizzi's method [26, 27] guided the secondary analysis. Initially, transcripts were read in their entirety to get the sense of the content. During this phase, interesting areas of the content for patient daily routines, mobility, comfort, and nursing interventions were noted using memos. These were emerging codes. Careful attempt was made to assure that the context was carried through these emerging codes. Refinement of this organized data led to categories reflecting the most descriptive topics in all or most of the data. Then these categories were viewed for their content to make sure that they captured the category. Here, similarities and uniqueness in content along with confusion and contraindications were identified. Content analysis for this data continued until discrepancies were resolved and themes emerged.

Lincoln and Guba's [28] criteria for qualitative paradigm guided the rigor in the study. Keeping in mind the rigor for qualitative inquiry, the researcher kept reflective journaling to identify her preconceived notions and biases. Audit trails for content analysis were reviewed several times to enhance credibility. Conformability was achieved by evaluating separate data chunks at different times. These steps further enhanced dependability, transformability, and authenticity.

9. Results

9.1. Activities of Daily Living. Experiences of spasticity were embedded in the circadian rhythm. Spasticity experiences were not bounded by the days or hours. Instead, the best clues for understanding spasticity may be understood through rhythms of one's biological clocks and daily activities of life habits based on the institutional routine during acute rehabilitation. At a glance, spasticity may appear to be unreliable and unpredictable; however, closer look reveals that experiences of spasticity appear to be linked with activities of daily rhythm, as these participants become cognizant of how certain things affect their symptoms of spasticity.

> *In the morning when the aides are turning me over, when they turn me, they have to turn me so many hours every night. Those are when I'm going through my worst spasms then in the middle of the night and late in the afternoon. #101*

Patients' spasticity fluctuated throughout the day. Individual participants reported that their life revolved around activities of daily living (ADL). Most of them spent considerable amount of time dealing with their routines. ADL routines either in the morning or at bedtime require considerable energy and participants often felt frustrated because the body did not respond on command.

> *Spasticity should be, I think be termed as anything that any involuntary muscle movement that interferes with a person's daily living and that is the*

> *exact opposite of what they tell their body to do. #201*

> *It made it difficult for dressing, getting up and all that stuff, that's all I know, that's the big change. I can't go anywhere I want, because I just can't get up and go, that's my change area. I can't normally do what I normally do. #141*

Since increase in clonus and spasticity activity may be triggered by simple touch, patients felt helpless and troubled. Some participants in the study reported being afraid that their condition might cause an injury to their caregivers during ADL.

> *I'm always afraid I will kick whoever getting me up and stuff. #151*

> *Like last night I told the RA (assistant) to get out of the way and zap I was kicking and waving on my bed and she was out of the way. She said you almost kicked me. I replied, Yes, but I gave you lead time, you know not to come close to me when I'm having a spasm (clonus). I don't think anybody is ever going to understand that unless, well maybe in 500 years. # 181*

Missed Opportunity. Most participants wanted their caregivers to slow down while assisting them with ADLs. Often they felt that caregivers were so engaged in "tasks" that they lack patience with them. They felt rushed in their care which compromised their sense of control over ADLs.

> *A little more patience. I think they lack a lot of patience. Some of them, not all of them. You have some who come in that just lack patience with the patients that are here. #191*

> *A lot of times they seem like they're in a rush and a lot of them like say, for shaving, cleaning their ears out or whatever it is, you know stuff like that that is an every-day thing. #171*

9.2. Function and Mobility. Physical cost of spasticity is paramount as mobility limitations and limb impairments reduce their chances to fully engage in their lives. Spasticity patients struggle with mobility, function, and transfer issues. Although some participants had families and jobs, they were dependent on others for their daily routine care. This dependency on others can diminish their quality of life. Mobility impairments leading to possible falls are a genuine concern. Gait instability or violent tremors can contribute to the risk of fall. Fear of falling is a genuine worry because muscles do not respond on command.

> *Just that it's an out of control feeling. Things kind of jerk up and tighten up a little bit. If I didn't have seat on my chair, I'd probably be laying on the ground. #151*

Use of a wheelchair did not always make them feel secure; often issues with body positioning relative to the chair were a concern as participants reported.

> I also think that the way that your chair is made effects that. Because if you can move around and put your legs in a different position when you're feeling tense, I think that would help a lot. #161

> I don't know, because I'm sitting upright all the time and I'm not laying back. The more lay back the more my spasms kick in. If I'm sitting up, they're not bad, if I lay back, they're bad. #131

Missed Opportunity. Common concerns reported by patient participants were that their caregiver did not understand their mobility restrictions. Just because they were in a wheelchair, they did not perceive themselves mobile as given that spasticity affected their entire body.

> I think they either should, like say like somebody ain't got the use of their hands and that they should after the aide get done with you, they should help you down to the elevator you got to go down. Like me, I can't push the buttons or stuff like that I think they should follow them down. Right now what I'm doing I'm going myself and then just seeing if there's somebody there to, I'm asking people walking by to turn the elevator on. #191

9.3. Pain, Comfort, Insomnia, and Fatigue: A Vicious Cycle. Pain and insomnia are intricately linked in this population due to muscle tightness. The patients experiencing clonus may have sleep issues as constant jerking motion may not allow them to fall asleep easily. On the other hand, spasticity patients simply cannot relax due to tight muscles. Therefore, aggressive management of the troubling symptoms is needed to improve quality of life. This uncomfortable symptom experience of insomnia can lead to fatigue, which in turn creates stress and further increases spasticity. Therefore, caregivers must be cognizant of all these interrelated clusters of symptoms and address these issues in a comprehensive manner.

> During later in the day they (clonus) too get more frequent so I guess that's about all on that one… Oh, sometimes they wake me up. Then I have to get repositioned and get some ice. #131

> There's nothing else you can think about but the pain that's going through your arms and through your legs, there's not too much you can do about it. # 191

> If muscles are incredibly tight and I haven't stretched at all, I do experience quite a bit of pain… I'm always tired so I have to really concentrate in order to get my body to do anything that I want it to do. #201

> Right now I'm in a real bad sharp pain radius and it's really killing me. It's really testing me and I just want to go somewhere and bark I'm in pain right now. #141

> We were sitting by the parking lot in the shade and I had quite a few (clonus). I decided to go in because I was drained, I couldn't even drive (wheelchair) I was drained so much. Like I'd run a marathon. #181

The most prominent finding of this study relates to the impact of daily stressors on the spasticity experiences. Most patients were very vocal about the negative impact of stress from emotions such as being angry, feeling rushed, and experiencing anxiety. To combat this, some participants took refuge in meditation, acupuncture, and prayers.

> Once I get stressed or if there is a lot of stuff going on, my tone will automatically increase. #81

> I like to talk on the phone, it relaxes me… usually I talk to my parents and my friends, like today I'm going to talk to this friend of mine that I haven't talked to in a long time. #161

> Where they have this little Chinese herbal medicines or needles in different parts of your body this is an energy movement or guided imagery or things like that. #151

Missed Opportunity. Most spastic patients require stretching throughout the day to manage spasticity. If not done with frequent intervals, it led to suffering and pain.

> So if you don't move then you come out and try to move it ain't going to work. I mean the muscles are all this cramped up. That's why they had a hard time trying to stretch me out I was screaming a lot, because all the muscles were all the way you left me lay bent up so try to straighten something when you're bent, laying in there like that, that's all I can say on that. #141

9.4. Other Factors. Comorbidities also seemed to affect spasticity. One participant was experiencing urinary tract infection and a kidney stone. There was an increase in clonus activity where spontaneous series of uncontrollable tremors were noted without provocation. Spasticity was noted to increase as well.

> I started realizing I had good days and I had bad days and when I really noticed it is when I would get a UTI and then my spasticity would be terrible and I would be so uncomfortable. #81

> I do have a UTI now, an upper urinary tract infection and that, in me, can set off spasms (clonus). I'm prone to colonizing if they put me on antibiotics. I was worried about that on the

last week because my UTI wasn't clearing up. But they're managing it with something else and I drank a couple of full water bottles during the day, which makes me have to go and I think it's clearing it out is what's happening. #181

Missed Opportunity. Clinician often used vocabularies that patient did not understand. One participant did not know that the "complete" and "incomplete" spinal cord injury have different connotation in medical jargon.

I was thinking it meant that the nerves is there (partial and incomplete SCI) and they going to connect, if you strong enough, they going to start connecting to each other, that was what I was thinking it was, connecting to each other and if I got the strength to do it, it will come together and you will be ok, I got to have the strength and the willpower and I got to make it happen and I can't make it happen...That ain't true, it don't work that way, it do not work that way. #111

9.5. Bedside Care Strategies

9.5.1. Medications and Other Modalities. Spasticity is managed by physical therapy, drugs, and surgery. Oral antispasmodic medications such as baclofen, tizanidine, and dantrium are used for initial management of spasticity and clonus while intrathecal baclofen may be used for severe symptom management [29, 30]. Usefulness of oral medications may be limited due to the side-effects such as hepatic toxicity, fatigue, drowsiness, weakness, and nausea. Our participants provided some guidance to clinicians. Although most felt medications were needed, they felt that approach to spasticity management must be holistic.

To sum it all up, I think doctors should give their patients options and strategies for coping with spasticity based on what the patient says versus what is happening clinically. #201

I think there should also be a more holistic approach like deep breathing and stuff like that seems to help me and like being in warm water. Right now it's more of a clinical, what can we do with drugs to treat this condition mindset. I think a lot more can be done with natural medicine and that's what I'm hoping anyway. #71

9.5.2. Stretching. Range of motion and stretching is a corner stone of spasticity management. Since muscle tightness causes pain and contractures, most participants were on scheduled physical therapy and stretching routines. Some stretching was done as a part of activities of daily living while intentional stretching was embedded throughout the day. Participants felt that this care strategy was particularly important to maintain comfort and function.

They are laying there, my left leg I can feel more in that leg than in the right leg. It feels so stiff so when they move them I can feel the pain in it when they start doing the exercises. They are supposed to do it every so often when I'm lying down, especially early in the morning and before I go to bed at night but I don't know what kind of schedule they have here. Every schedule is always different, you know when the aide comes in so this morning she did a little bit of it, but I don't think she did enough of it.

Especially in the morning I like to stretch and it takes me a while to get up or feel like I want to get up and get moving because I like to stretch. #151

It's a lot different when I'm going to physical therapy that they stretch a lot better than the aides do it. My leg feels a lot better, I can feel the tightness going away, which the aides do it, they don't, the tightness is still there when I get down to therapy and I can feel it in my legs as I'm going down there. #91

9.5.3. Comfort Strategies. Over time participants had figured how to self-manage their symptoms of spasticity and clonus. They shared the fact that keeping sudden noise and touch to minimum is important in preventing inducement of clonus and spasticity. Pool therapy with warm water was desired and seen as a good relaxation therapy.

I think the water just holds you up so you don't have to concentrate. They have had things that hold your head up so you barely have to do anything so the muscles completely relax, that's when I would say I am the least spastic or when I am in any type of water, I'm a lot more relaxed than normally. #161

"What makes it better is generally environmental factors that just hot and cold and not having too much going on." #31

Most participants identified warm temperature helpful in management of spasticity; however, one participant reported use of ice at night time to facilitate sleep.

Lately, I've been waking up in the morning with severely cramped arms to the point I couldn't move again. Not this morning, every morning for about a week prior, I've been waking up with arms just clenched to my chest and I couldn't move them until I got range in the morning and then they seemed to loosen up a little bit. One thing I did different last night when I didn't wake up this morning with the cramped arms, was I wore a sweatshirt to bed. I was hot sleeping, the room is cool, air conditioned, it was cold outside last night and I wore my sweatshirt to bed and it kept my upper torso warm and I woke up with basically no cramping this morning so I'm going to keep doing that from now on. #181

The cold pack does help at night. #121

A loud noise you know something like that...I'm going to jump now, I think that would change if I didn't have so much spasticity. #30

9.5.4. Mood and Alternative Medicine. Feeling negative or depressed was reported to increase spasticity. Most participants acknowledge mind-body connections and felt that their care strategies should include more than "western medicine" approach. Participants shared utilization of alternative medicine in conjunction with western medications.

If I'm relaxed, I'm happy, if I'm upset, I'm more tense, at least for me. Mood really changes it for me. I think when you're more relaxed, it's different. I think more people should, or the doctors should recommend acupuncture or something for relaxation, I don't know if I would do it but if I had a doctor's order, I might. My roommate does it and she really likes it, she's like you should try it. #161

We're going to waste a lot of money by going backwards instead of trying to go forward and try some of their natural herbs and the way they do the acupuncture, it's been helping a lot of other people. And, they've been doing it a long time before we even thought about it. #20

My mother-in-law is teaching me meditation and I'm going hypnotism too at the same time. Those two things with the medication is kind of keeping me in save. That's where I am right now. Those three things is going on and my family. My family is a big help. #111

9.5.5. Individualize Care. Most patients considered their understanding to be unique and individual, as the essence of spasticity was learned through personal accumulated experiences over time. There was a strong sense that, to understand spasticity, one must live it to understand the pain and suffering.

I don't think anybody is ever going to understand that unless, well maybe in 500 years, you can't live inside another person's body, you don't know what you're going through and it's very difficult to explain to other people... The only to experience it is to have to happen to you, I think. #181

Someone who hasn't experienced severe spasticity has no frame of reference so their perception of their spasticity may be more severe than the clinician thinks... in my opinion, it would be very important for doctors to look at a patient based on what their baseline is as far as spasticity. #201

10. Discussion

Research provides the guidance for clinical issues in practice. Qualitative researchers are required to understand human meaning associated with a phenomenon to provide better health care experiences. As Van Manen [31] pointed,

to establish a strong relation with a certain question, phenomenon, or notion, the researcher cannot afford to adopt an attitude of so-called scientific disinterestedness. To be oriented to an object means that we are animated by the object in a full and human sense. To be strong in our orientation means that we will not settle for superficialities and falsities (Page 33).

The understanding of a phenomenon is socially, temporally, and contextually bound and dependent on the individual's realities. The essence of a phenomenon may be universal but its varied interpretation provides some degree of depth and richness of those experiences. Interpretation is fluid, based on context and temporal nature of the experiences. Van Manen [31] further adds,

the "data" of human science research are human experiences. It seems natural, therefore, that if we wish to investigate the nature of a certain experience or phenomenon, the most straight forward way to go about our research is to ask selected individuals to write their experiences down (Page 63).

The results of this study indicate that spasticity is a lived experience. The richness of this lived experience captures its essence in the context of health. The lived experience of spasticity calls for the eudemonistic approach of well-being. This incorporation of patient accounts captures the essence of their symptom experiences, which in turn assists clinicians in matching their practice with patient experiences. This clarity and congruency have implications for the quality of life for patients who suffer from spasticity. Therefore, this study provides glimpses into the lives of spastic patients through their own lived experiences. Although researchers and clinicians want accurate definitions, precise measurement tools, and state-of-the-art interventions to help human suffering, individuals who are suffering from spasticity, their input is critical for evidence-based practice. The clinicians face many challenges when caring for spasticity patients as this population experiences myriad of sensations due to neurological deficits. Some patients may be experiencing L'Hermittes sign, which could be part of the multiple sclerosis or spinal cord injury experience, where patients describe a sensation of electric shock going through their body [32]. Others may describe sensation of pain with spasticity. In this population, most clinicians associate pain with neuropathic pain from neurological disorders [16]. However, if the patient is experiencing spasticity, one must take the time to assess the entirety of the situation to understand whether pain is due to spasticity, development of neuropathic pain, or something else. Correct evaluation of spasticity symptoms is imperative in providing safe, effective, and individualized care with compassion.

10.1. Implication for Practice. Spasticity is often accompanied by uncomfortable pain, which may be due to the nerve entrapment in the muscles. Untreated spasticity can lead to contractures. Subsequently, pain, pain-induced insomnia, contractures, mobility impairment, potential for falls, and development of pressure ulcers due to tight muscles over bony prominences can impact quality of life.

Bedside interventions such as avoiding inactivity and utilizing warm pool therapy may be helpful. Our findings support Boyraz et al. [21] that cold temperature may be helpful for some patients experiencing clonus. Most of these patients may benefit from stretching and range of motion exercises in maintaining comfort, posture, and movement. Medications are important in managing their symptoms on a daily basis as it provides comfort and relaxes their muscles enough so that they remain functional. The other important interventions are the use of physical and occupational therapies [6]. The participants in our study reported use of alternative therapies such as acupuncture, meditation, and prayers being helpful in decreasing spasticity. Their feedback and suggestions provide opportunity to explore the role of alternative therapies in managing spasticity.

Mobility impairments leading to possible falls are a genuine concern. Even though risk of falls is an obvious issue, fall risk assessments are not routinely employed in an outpatient clinical practice. Since it is clear that an inherent risk for falls is present in this population, routine formal assessment of this risk should be done so that clinicians can assess patients status and their environment to minimize this hazard.

The experience of spasticity is a quality of life issue, as its effects are pervasive in all domains of life. Therefore, clinicians must be cognizant of the consequences of this experience and mobilize appropriate resources based on individual needs. Individuals not only need medical intervention but also may require psychological counseling and strong spiritual connections to find an acceptable quality of life.

11. Conclusion

Spasticity is a consequence of neuromuscular disorders, which affects quality of life in those who experience this phenomenon. Confusion regarding spasticity and related phenomenon in clinical practice warrants a pragmatic approach to this issue. Similar terminologies for hypertonia must be evaluated in the context of pathophysiology, impact on functioning, symptom consequences, and treatment options. The goals of rehabilitation are to improve function, comfort, and ADLs, decrease caregiver burden, and prevent pressure ulcers. Clinicians working in the field of rehabilitation strive to help people make their own lives work. This requires careful assessment and intervention of spasticity related symptoms.

What Does this Paper Contribute to the Wider Global Clinical Community?

(i) This paper clarifies spasticity and related disorders pathophysiology and terminologies for clinical practice.

(ii) This secondary analysis highlights understandings of spasticity on daily life and bedside strategies that enhance patients' function and improve comfort.

Conflict of Interests

The authors declare that there is no conflict of interests regarding the publication of this paper.

References

[1] World Health Organization, "Disability and rehabilitation: World report on disability," http://www.who.int/disabilities/world_report/2011/report/en/index.html.

[2] National Institute of Neurological Disorders and Stroke, NINDS Spasticity Information Page, http://www.ninds.nih.gov/disorders/spasticity/spasticity.htm.

[3] A. Martin, S. Abogunrin, H. Kurth, and J. Dinet, "Epidemiological, humanistic, and economic burden of illness of lower limb spasticity," Neuropsychiatric Disease and Treatment, vol. 10, pp. 111–122, 2014.

[4] J. W. Lance and P. de Gail, "Spread of phasic reflexes in normal and spastic subjects," Journal of Neurology, Neurosurgery, and Psychiatry, vol. 28, pp. 328–334, 1965.

[5] J. W. Lance, "The control of muscle tone, reflexes, and movement: Robert Wartenberg lecture," Neurology, vol. 30, no. 12, pp. 1303–1313, 1980.

[6] R. H. Bhimani, C. P. McAlpine, and S. J. Henly, "Understanding spasticity from patients' perspectives over time," Journal of Advanced Nursing, vol. 68, no. 11, pp. 2504–2514, 2012.

[7] R. N. Boyd and L. Ada, "Physiotherapy management of spasticity," in Upper Motor Neurone Syndrome and Spasticity : Clinical Management and Neurophysiology, M. P. Barnes and G. R. Johnson, Eds., pp. 79–81, Cambridge University Press, Cambridge, UK, 2008.

[8] E. Widmaier, H. Raff, and K. Strang, Vanders Human Physiology: The Mechanism of Body Function, McGraw Hill, New York, NY, USA, 2014.

[9] A. B. Sanderson, W. D. Arnold, B. Elsheikh, and J. T. Kissal, "The clinical spectrum of isolated peripheral motor dysfunction," Muscle & Nerve, 2014.

[10] R. Bhimani, "Intrathecal baclofen therapy in adults and guideline for clinical nursing care," Journal of Rehabilitation Nursing, vol. 33, no. 3, pp. 110–116, 2008.

[11] A. A. Mullick, N. K. Musampa, A. G. Feldman, and M. F. Levin, "Stretch reflex spatial threshold measure discriminates between spasticity and rigidity," Clinical Neurophysiology, vol. 124, no. 4, pp. 740–751, 2013.

[12] F. Pati and C. Vila, "Symptoms, prevalence and impact of multiple sclerosis in younger patients: a multinational survey," Neuroepidemiology, vol. 42, pp. 211–218, 2014.

[13] A. Jušić, "Differential diagnosis and treatment of muscle hypertonia as practiced in Zagreb's Centre/Institute for Neuromuscular Diseases," Acta Myologica, vol. 32, pp. 170–173, 2013.

[14] G. Sheean and J. R. McGuire, "Spastic hypertonia and movement disorders: pathophysiology, clinical presentation, and quantification," Physical Medicine & Rehabilitation, vol. 1, no. 9, pp. 827–833, 2009.

[15] J. B. Nielsen, C. Crone, and H. Hultborn, "The spinal pathophysiology of spasticity—from a basic science point of view," Acta Physiologica, vol. 189, no. 2, pp. 171–180, 2007.

[16] A. Muhkerjee and A. Chakravarty, "Spasticity mechanism-for the clinicians," *Frontiers in Neurology*, vol. 2010, p. 149, 2010.

[17] J. H. Burridge, D. E. Wood, H. J. Hermens et al., "Theoretical and methodological considerations in the measurement of spasticity," *Disability and Rehabilitation*, vol. 27, no. 1-2, pp. 69–80, 2005.

[18] W. A. Cook Jr., "Antagonistic muscles in the production of clonus in man," *Neurology*, vol. 17, no. 8, pp. 779–780, 1967.

[19] J. A. Beres-Jones, T. D. Johnson, and S. J. Harkema, "Clonus after human spinal cord injury cannot be attributed solely to recurrent muscle-tendon stretch," *Experimental Brain Research*, vol. 149, no. 2, pp. 222–236, 2003.

[20] D. M. Wallace, B. H. Ross, and C. K. Thomas, "Motor unit behavior during clonus," *Journal of Applied Physiology*, vol. 99, no. 6, pp. 2166–2172, 2005.

[21] I. Boyraz, F. Oktay, C. Celik, M. Akyuz, and H. Uysal, "Effect of cold application and tizanidine on clonus: clinical and electrophysiological assessment," *Journal of Spinal Cord Medicine*, vol. 32, no. 2, pp. 132–139, 2009.

[22] R. H. Bhimani, L. C. Anderson, S. J. Henly, and S. A. Stoddard, "Clinical measurement of limb spasticity in adults: state of the science," *Journal of Neuroscience Nursing*, vol. 43, no. 2, pp. 104–115, 2011.

[23] E. Bravo-Esteban, J. Taylor, J. Abián-Vicén et al., "Impact of specific symptoms of spasticity on voluntary lower limb muscle function, gait and daily activities during subacute and chronic spinal cord injury," *NeuroRehabilitation*, vol. 33, no. 4, pp. 531–543, 2013.

[24] B. Silver and S. R. Wulf, "Stroke: posthospital management and recurrence prevention," *Family Practice Essentials*, vol. 40, pp. 28–38, 2014.

[25] J. S. Mahoney, J. C. Engebretson, K. F. Cook, K. A. Hart, S. Robinson-Whelen, and A. M. Sherwood, "Spasticity experience domains in persons with spinal cord injury," *Archives of Physical Medicine and Rehabilitation*, vol. 88, no. 3, pp. 287–294, 2007.

[26] C. Sanders, "Application of Colaizzi's method: interpretation of an auditable decision trail by a novice researcher," *Contemporary Nurse*, vol. 14, no. 3, pp. 292–302, 2003.

[27] G. A. Sosha, "Employment of Colaizzis strategy in descriptive phenomenology: a reflection of a researcher," *European Scientific Journal*, vol. 7, pp. 31–43, 2012.

[28] Y. S. Lincoln and E. G. Guba, *Naturalistic Inquiry*, Sage, Beverly Hills, Calif, USA, 1985.

[29] E. M. Delhaas, N. Beersen, W. K. Redekop, and N. S. Klazinga, "Long-term outcomes of continuous intrathecal baclofen infusion for treatment of spasticity: a prospective multicenter follow-up study," *Neuromodulation*, vol. 11, no. 3, pp. 227–236, 2008.

[30] S. McGuinness, J. Hillan, and S. B. Caldwell, "Botulinum toxin in gait dysfunction due to ankle clonus: a case series," *NeuroRehabilitation*, vol. 32, no. 3, pp. 635–647, 2013.

[31] M. Van Manen, *Researching Lived Experience: Human Science for an Action Sensitive Pedagogy*, State University of New York Press, Albany, NY, USA, 1990.

[32] A. H. Al-Araji and J. Oger, "Reappraisal of Lhermitte's sign in multiple sclerosis," *Multiple Sclerosis*, vol. 11, no. 4, pp. 398–402, 2005.

3

Balance, Falls-Related Self-Efficacy, and Psychological Factors amongst Older Women with Chronic Low Back Pain: A Preliminary Case-Control Study

Annick Champagne,[1] François Prince,[1] Vicky Bouffard,[1] and Danik Lafond[1,2]

[1] *Department of Kinesiology, University of Montreal, Montreal, QC, Canada H3T 1J4*
[2] *Department of Physical Activity Sciences, University of Quebec, Trois-Rivières, QC, Canada G9A 5H7*

Correspondence should be addressed to Danik Lafond, danik.lafond@umontreal.ca

Academic Editor: Maureen Simmonds

Objective. To investigate balance functions in older women and evaluate the association of the fear-avoidance beliefs model (FABM) factors with balance and mobility performance. *Participants*. Fifteen older women with CLBP was compared with age-matched pain-free controls ($n = 15$). *Main Outcome Measures*. Pain intensity, falls-related self-efficacy and intrinsic constructs in the FABM were evaluated. Postural steadiness (centre of pressure (COP)) and mobility functions were assessed. Linear relationships of FABM variables with COP and mobility score were estimated. *Results*. CLBP showed lower mobility score compared to controls. CLBP presented lower falls-related self-efficacy and it was associated with reduced mobility scores. FABM variables and falls-related self-efficacy were correlated with postural steadiness. Physical activity was reduced in CLBP, but no between-group difference was evident for knee extensor strength. No systematic linkages were observed between FABM variables with mobility score or postural steadiness. *Conclusions*. Back pain status affects balance and mobility functions in older women. Falls-related self-efficacy is lower in CLBP and is associated with reduced mobility. Disuse syndrome in CLBP elderly is partly supported by the results of this preliminary study.

1. Introduction

Back pain is among the most important factors affecting health status and functional capacity in elderly people [1], with a prevalence of 12 to 42% in subjects over 65 years of age [1]. It is more common in older women than in men [2], and women are more likely to have pain for prolonged periods [3]. Leveille et al. [1] determined that severe back pain increases the likelihood of disability by 3- to 4-fold, whereas mild or moderate back pain is not associated with reduced functional activities of daily living. Low back pain (LBP) was found to be related to 2-fold greater difficulty in daily living activities and the risk of falling [4]. Episodic chronic low back pain (CLBP) with advancing in age may cause neurophysiological changes that could further impact age-related deterioration of postural control [5].

According to the FABM [6], pain-related behaviours such as avoidance of physical activity and hypervigilance are consequences of catastrophizing misinterpretations or thoughts/beliefs triggered by pain experience. In young adults with CLBP, elevation of pain-related fear leads to heighten disability [7]. However, there is increasing evidence that pain-related fear does not systematically influence physical activity reduction or the emergence of the disuse syndrome [8–10]. In young adults with LBP, it seems plausible that pain-related fear provokes avoidance behaviours related to specific movements, that are believed to be potentially painful or at risk of reinjury, instead of impacting on general physical activity participation [8].

Nevertheless, constructs of the fear-avoidance beliefs model have not been studied extensively in older adults with LBP as in young adults. For example, Kovacs et al. [11] found that disability was not influenced by fear-avoidance beliefs related to physical activity in Spanish older adults. LBP elderly subjects reported more fear-avoidance and perceived less functional capacity, but did not show decreased physical activity compared to controls [12]. Moreover, fear-avoidance beliefs established using a specific-movement approach were found to predict functional capacity but was not a good predictor of physical activity participation [12]. High level of fear-avoidance beliefs was associated with falling [13, 14], whereas falling experience often contribute to decrease confidence in movement and in balance [15] in community-dwelling elderly individuals. Reduction of activities triggered by fear-avoidance beliefs also have an impact on physical abilities [13]. Despite the high prevalence of LBP in older adults and its influence on health-related outcomes, little information is available regarding the influence of LBP and fear-avoidance beliefs on balance and mobility functions as well as disuse syndrome in community-dwelling older persons. Important information could be gathered from direct measurement of balance and mobility functions in this population. In fact, pain-related fear has been associated with decreased physical function like reduced walking speed and lower-limb strength [16] in young adults with LBP.

Therefore, the aims of this preliminary study are twofold: (1) to evaluate balance and mobility functions by direct measurements in a sample of older women compared with controls and (2) to examine if falls-related self-efficacy and constructs of fear-avoidance beliefs model are linked with poorer balance and mobility functions. We expect the following outcomes: (1) older adults with CLBP will have lower falls-related self-efficacy and (2) they will present lower balance and mobility functions. Although disuse syndrome has not been conclusively observed in elderly people with spinal pain [12], we maintain the following assumptions: (1) CLBP subjects will be less physically active and (2) falls-related self-efficacy, fear of movement, disability, and disuse outcomes will be linearly associated with balance and mobility functions in older adults with CLBP.

2. Materials and Methods

2.1. Participants. Fifteen CLBP women and 15 female controls without reporting pain, aged over 60 years, were recruited from the local community (Table 1). The controls were free of musculoskeletal pain during the last year and reported never having experienced disabling LBP. CLBP participants were included if they incurred LBP for at least 6 months, consecutively or episodically, and presented tension, soreness, and/or stiffness in the lower back region with radiating pain limited to the buttocks. The exclusion criteria were known causes of LBP, neurological or vestibular disease, dizziness, severe visual or hearing impairment, acute illness or pain, cognitive impairment, and medical conditions that could make testing potentially unsafe. Chronic health conditions and medications were screened from participant responses to interviewer-administered questionnaire, an extended version of the physical activity readiness questionnaire. Subjects answered "yes (1)" or "no (0)" when asked if they were presently suffering from health conditions or taking medications, and positive answers were summed. All subjects gave their informed, written consent according to the protocol approved by the University Ethics Committee (CER-10-156-04-02.01).

2.2. Falls-Related Self-Efficacy. Participants were instructed to complete the Activities-specific Balance Confidence (ABC) Scale to assess falls-related self-efficacy [17]. They were also asked to recall their falls in the last 6 months. A fall was defined as any event that led to unplanned, unexpected contact with a supporting surface.

2.3. Back Pain Outcomes. On the day of testing, participants were told to rate back pain intensity on a quadruple numerical pain scale (QNPS) [18]. Functional disability related to LBP was evaluated with a modified French version of the Oswestry Disability Index (ODI) [19] calculated on 9 items without replacing the question about sexual activity by employment/homemaking ability [20]. Pain-related fear of movement was evaluated with the French version of the Tampa Scale for Kinesiophobia (TSK) [21].

The Baecke questionnaire (BPAQ) estimated physical activity level [22]. Only physical activity during sports and leisure time indexes were calculated; their summation provided an index of physical activity participation (PASL). The maximal isometric knee extensor (KE) force of each leg was estimated with a load cell in the seated position and the knee at 90°. Two 5-s trials of maximum isometric effort were conducted, and peak value was expressed as a relative strength index—a ratio of strength to body composition (body mass index, BMI) measurement. KE strength was averaged because no between-sides difference was found. PASL and KE strength were used to infer on disuse syndrome.

2.4. Sensorimotor Functions and Balance Functions. Several aspects of sensorimotor functions that affect balance, such as visual acuity, tactile sensitivity, and kinesthetic sense were studied [23]. Visual acuity was examined with a Snellen chart, and a Semmes-Weinstein-type pressure aesthesiometer assessed tactile sensitivity at the lateral malleolus of both ankles. Reposition error at the knees (extension) and trunk (flexion) were calculated during 5 trials. For each segment, subjects had to start in a neutral position, reach a target angle of approximately 15°, hold the position for 10 s, and return to the initial position. Absolute differences in degrees between the target angle and position reached (absolute error) were averaged. Variable error was considered to measure inconsistency. Segmental angles were calculated with an optoelectronic system (Optotrak Certus, NDI, Waterloo, Ontario, Canada).

Postural steadiness was evaluated by instructing the subjects to stand upright as still as possible, with eyes opened, on a force plate (OR6-2000, AMTI, Watertown, MA, USA) according to a procedure described elsewhere [24]. Center of pressure (COP) speed and frequencies were used to infer on postural steadiness. Cumulative power was calculated from consecutive frequency windows of 0.1-Hz width and expressed as percentages of total power between 0 and 4 Hz. It has been shown that visual, vestibular, and proprioceptive contributions on balance control are related to specific frequency bands of COP signals [25]. Total power at the 3 frequency bands was calculated: B1 = [0–0.1 Hz] for visual; B2 = [0.1–0.5 Hz] for vestibular; B3 = [0.5–1.0 Hz] for proprioception.

TABLE 1: Subject characteristics.

	Controls n = 15	CLBP n = 15	P value
Age	69.4 (6.4)	68.9 (6.6)	.846
Body mass (kg)	67.5 (13.2)	72.2 (10.7)	.289
Height (m)	1.60 (0.06)	1.62 (0.08)	.447
BMI (kg/m^2)	26.1 (4.4)	27.4 (3.7)	.390
ODI (%)	0 [0]	15.6 [13.3–24.4]	.000
TSK	33.4 (9.5)	43.8 (5.9)	.001
ABC	93.5 (4.6)	79.5 (17.2)	.005
Pain—low back region			
NPS-A	0 [0-0]	2 [1–4]	.000
NPS-W	0 [0-0]	7 [5–7]	.005
Chronic conditions	0.80 (0.77)	1.53 (1.19)	.055
Medications			
<4	11	11	.999
≥4	4	4	
Visual acuity	5.9 (1.0)	6.3 (0.9)	.262
Tactile sensitivity	4.1 (0.3)	4.0 (0.5)	.394
Repositioning sense (°)			
Trunk AE	1.4 [1.2–3.1]	1.5 [0.9–2.9]	.976
Trunk VE	0.6 [0.5–1.2]	0.4 [0.3–1.8]	.698
Knee AE	3.6 [2.5–5.6]	5.3 [2.9–8.1]	.403
Knee VE	2.6 [0.8–3.8]	2.4 [1.7–5.1]	.283

Data are mean (SD) or median [Inter-quartile range]. ODI: Oswestry disability index; TSK: fear of movement/reinjury; ABC: falls-related self-efficacy; NPS-A: averaged pain level; NPS-W: pain level at its worst; NPS-B: pain level at its best; BMI: body mass index; AE: absolute error; VE: variable error.

The Timed up and go (TUG) [26] and One-leg stance test (OLS) [27] were also administered. A practice trial was allowed, and 2 subsequent trials were averaged. Maximal walking speed was estimated by the incremental shuttle walk test [28]. Each of these tests (TUG, OLS, and walking speed) was attributed a score of 1 to 4 using quartiles of performance (1st quartile = 1 and 4th quartile = 4) from values proposed by Choquette et al. [29] and summed to generate mobility scores (0–12). TUG scores were reversed, with lower scores reflecting better performance.

2.5. *Statistical Analysis.* Data were explored for normal distribution and homogeneity of variances. Data that showed skewed distributions were log-10-transformed prior to inferential analysis and presented as median values with 25th–75th percentiles. Subject characteristics, psycho-behavioural variables, sensorimotor function measures, and disuse-related variables were compared among groups by independent *t*-test. We undertook one-way repeated-measures analysis of variance with directions as within-subject factors to compare groups for COP measures. Post hoc Tukey-HSD analyses were performed for significant *F*-tests. We considered confounding variables, such as age, BMI, medication, and number of chronic conditions. Age and sum of comorbidities were not retained as confounding variables because they were not correlated with any COP measures and mobility score. Analysis of covariance with LBP status as a between-subjects factor and BMI as covariate compared

PASL. Univariate comparisons were made with Pearson correlation coefficients to determine the strength of associations between FABM-related variables with mobility score in the CLBP group. Partial correlations, correcting for medication, quantified linear relationships between pain level at its worst, and dependent variables. Statistical significance was set at $P < 0.05$, and all statistical analyses were conducted with STATISTICA software (Statsoft Inc., Tulsa, OK, USA).

3. Results

Subject characteristics are presented in Table 1. No significant between-group differences were observed for anthropometric characteristics and sensorimotor functions (visual acuity, tactile sensitivity, and repositioning errors at the trunk and knees).

CLBP subjects perceived lower falls-related self-efficacy than the controls (79.5 versus 93.5%) and showed more fear of movement/re-injury (43.8 versus 33.4). The level of perceived disability is relatively low (median = 15.4%).

Table 2 reports performance on 3 tests of mobility, the mobility score and disuse-related variables. Controls performed better on TUG and walked faster than CLBP subjects. No between-group difference was found for OLS time. The controls' mobility score was significantly higher than that of CLBP subjects. They were significantly more active than their CLBP counterparts but no significant between-group difference was apparent for KE strength. Table 3 discloses

TABLE 2: Mobility functions and disuse-related variables.

	Controls (n = 15)	CLBP (n = 15)	P value
Timed up and go (s)	9.2 (2.0)	12.0 (3.6)	.012
One-leg stance (s)	12.0 (8.8)	10.9 (8.3)	.740
Walking speed (m/s)	1.66 (0.17)	1.43 (0.16)	.001
Mobility score (0–12)	8.9 (1.5)	6.9 (2.2)	.009
PASL	17.5 (4.9)	12.4 (5.3)	.012*
F/BMI (N·kg^{-1}/m^2)	9.3 [7.6–11.2]	8.8 [7.3–10.8]	.611

PASL: physical activity participation; F/BMI: relative knee extensor strength index. *adjusted for BMI.

TABLE 3: Intercorrelations among psychobehavioural and disuse variables in the CLBP group.

	ODI	TSK	NPS-W	NPS-A	PASL	F/BMI
ABC	−0.60*	−0.22	0.48†	−0.07	0.44	−0.12
ODI		0.34	−0.01†	0.34	−0.44	−0.21
TSK			−0.40†	0.35	0.12	0.35
NPS-W				0.26†	−0.18†	0.08†
NPS-A					−0.11	0.03
PASL						0.41

ODI: Oswestry disability index; TSK: fear of movement/reinjury; ABC: falls-related self-efficacy; NPS-W: pain level at its worst; NPS-A: averaged pain level; PASL: physical activity participation; *P < 0.05; †partial correlation controlling for medication.

the level of association between psychobehavioural variables in CLBP. ABC scores were linked with increased ODI scores. Falls-related self-efficacy showed slight nonsignificant correlations with pain level at its worst and PASL.

No significant between-group difference was evident for COP speed, a measure of postural steadiness (Figure 1(a)). Figure 1(b) illustrates the power of frequency bands (B1 to B3) for each group. CLBP manifested significantly decreased power at the B3 frequency band compared to the controls (P = 0.005). After correcting for BMI, B3 remained significantly different between groups in both anteroposterior (A/P) and M/L directions

Table 4 reports levels of association between psychobehavioural outcomes and disuse-related variables with COP speed and mobility score in the CLBP group. Mobility score was not correlated with any psychobehavioural outcomes and disuse-related variables (0.04 < r < 0.47). Pain level was significantly linked with COP speed. Falls-related self-efficacy was also related to COP speed in the M/L direction. No significant linkage was found between disuse-related variables and mobility score or COP speed.

4. Discussion

This preliminary study demonstrated that elderly CLBP displayed reductions in mobility performance and changes in postural control. It also highlighted associations of FABM outcomes and falls-related self-efficacy with balance functions after accounting for key covariates. Older women with low to mild back pain had lower falls-related self-efficacy linked with reduced mobility functions. Lower falls-related self-efficacy, decreased mobility functions, and diminished physical activity participation, observed in this

study, could be important predictors of higher risk of falling and functional declines in CLBP women [1, 4].

The fear-avoidance belief model has been proposed to explain the development of CLBP [6]. Pain experiences are assumed to initiate fear of pain and fear of movement/reinjury that eventually lead to avoidance behaviours. Consequently, pain- and movement-related fear has been linked with decreased performance of physical tasks in young CLBP adults [16]. Reduction of physical capacities and activities as a result of avoidance behaviours is referred to as disuse syndrome [30]. However, disuse syndrome in young CLBP adults is a controversial issue [31]. Recently, Basler et al. [12] investigated the validity of the fear-avoidance belief model in a large sample of elderly CLBP and found no decline in PASL compared to the controls. They reported that fear-avoidance beliefs predicted physical disability but not PASL. In contrast, our results showed decreased PASL in elderly CLBP without a concomitant reduction of KE strength, as an indicator of physical deconditioning, compared to controls. Accordingly, Bousema et al. [32] noted a decline in physical activity without signs of physical deconditioning in young CLBP adults. We observed a significant correlation between perceived disability due to back pain and movement-related fear. However, in contrast to Basler et al. [12], PASL reduction was not associated with movement-related fear in the present study. This divergence in regards to decreased PASL in elderly CLBP could be explained by the fact that PASL was assessed with the Baecke questionnaire previously validated in CLBP subjects [22].

Fear-avoidance beliefs have been related to specific components of physical functions, such as knee extensors strength and COP displacements, in a sample of frail, elderly subjects, including fallers and multiple fallers [13]. Our sample of elderly CLBP did not experience frequent falls,

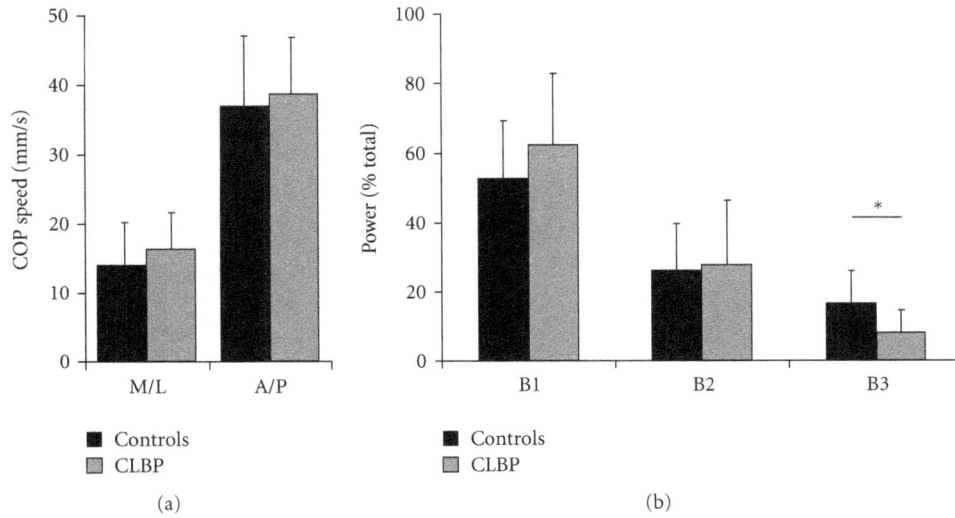

FIGURE 1: Comparison of postural steadiness between older CLBP women (grey) and controls (black). (a) Center of pressure (COP), speed in anteroposterior (A/P), and mediolateral (M/L) directions; (b) Power frequency bands (B1 to B3) for each group, expressed as a percentage of total power of COP signals. Data are mean ± SD; *$P < 0.05$.

TABLE 4: Pearson correlation coefficients and partial correlations with mobility scores and COP measures (eyes open condition) for the CLBP group.

Mobility score	COP speed	
	A/P	M/L
NPS-W		−0.77
NPS-A		−0.75[†]
ODI		
TSK		
ABC		−0.63
F/BMI		
PASL		

Only significant correlations are shown ($P < 0.05$). ODI: Oswestry disability index; TSK: fear of movement/reinjury; ABC: falls-related self-efficacy; NPS-W: pain level at its worst; NPS-A: averaged pain level; F/BMI: relative quadriceps strength index; PASL: physical activity participation; COP: center of pressure; A/P: anteroposterior direction; M/L: mediolateral direction; [†] partial correlation coefficients adjusted for medication.

which could explain why our data did not show a significant association between TSK with knee extensors strength and COP speed, respectively. Fear-avoidance beliefs in elderly CLBP may be correlated with greater disability, as seen in LBP young adults [33]. Our results did not disclose a significant association between fear-avoidance beliefs and back pain disability. Kovacs et al. [34] also discerned that fear-avoidance beliefs concerning physical activities were not related to back pain disability in elderly CLBP. In a larger sample of older Americans, Sions, and Hicks [35] established that fear-avoidance beliefs accounted for only 3% of variance of ODI scores, but high fear-avoidance beliefs were linked with greater falls experienced in the past year.

Self-efficacy, which is important in the maintenance of mobility in healthy ageing, is an independent factor of physical capacities [36]. The present study demonstrated a reduction of falls-related self-efficacy in elderly CLBP but no association was noted between falls-related self-efficacy and disuse-related variables. Balance impairments combined with weak muscular strength are assumed to be independent risk factors for falls or fractures [37], and knee extensors strength discriminates the ability to recover from gait perturbations to prevent falls [38]. In our study, knee extensors strength was not influenced by back pain status and was not correlated with COP speed or mobility score. Indeed, we did not see an association between falls-related self-efficacy and knee extensors strength. However, neither back extensor strength [39] nor endurance [40] were evaluated. Falls-related self-efficacy in elderly CLBP may be influenced by perceived capability concerning physical activities involving back movements. In support of this hypothesis, we observed a significant correlation ($r = −0.60$) between falls-related self-efficacy and perceived back disability.

Some researchers have suggested that greater M/L sway increases the risk of falls [41]. We did not observe changes of postural steadiness in the M/L direction in elderly CLBP. Interestingly, falls-related self-efficacy was correlated with COP speed in the M/L direction. We noted a global decline of COP power spectral frequencies between 0.5 and 1.0 Hz that could be inferred to be a deficit in somatosensory input or integration for postural control [25]. Some authors have argued that pain may interfere in the somatosensory integration process or alter proprioceptive input acuity. This pain adaptation phenomenon is hypothesized to affect postural control [42]. Brumagne et al. [43] reported that LBP young people have reduced lumbosacral position sense that could be related to altered paraspinal muscle spindle afference or central integration problems. They also concluded that LBP elderly individuals may mostly rely on distal somatosensory input for postural control [44]. Consequently, we initially expected to find a systematic increase of postural sway and a significant decline of trunk and knee kinesthesia in elderly CLBP. In our study, however, back pain status does not influence joint repositioning senses and does not explain the COP frequency results. Goldberg et al. [45] witnessed an increase in trunk repositioning errors in elderly balance-impaired subjects. Those in the balance-impaired group were classified on the basis of One-leg stance time (<5 s). In our study, 4 CLBP and 2 controls had One-leg stance time <5 s. Trunk repositioning errors were assessed in upright stance by Goldberg et al. [45], whereas we have isolated trunk repositioning errors from postural control constraints. These differences in protocols may explain divergence of the results.

Higher fear of falling has been shown to be associated with activity restrictions and the increased likelihood of falling [46]. We saw a slight, nonsignificant correlation ($r = 0.44$) between falls-related self-efficacy and PASL. Sample size in this study and the retrospective design of falls assessment limited the detection of any linkage between falls occurrence and falls-related self-efficacy or activity restriction. Very few CLBP subjects had fallen during the previous 6 months of study entry. The use of retrospective self-reported falls might have led to underreporting [47]. However, declining physical activities cannot only be explained by a greater rate of falling because higher fear of falling and activity restriction have been encountered in older subjects who never experienced falls [48]. Another limitation is that pain duration was not assessed. However, having LBP with advancing age does not seem to be a cumulative phenomenon, and is more likely to be a disorder that originates from adulthood with persistence over 60 years [3]. Consequently, estimating pain duration may be difficult in elderly CLBP. Although the possible contribution of osteoporosis in back pain outcomes and falls-related self-efficacy cannot be excluded, vertebral fracture status could be a contributing factor in pain status rather than in balance and functional deficits [49]. We excluded clinically-relevant disease-related factors, such as diagnosed vertebral fracture, osteoporosis, and lumbar spinal stenosis. Depressive symptoms were not examined and could be a confounding factor for disabling LBP or falls-related self-efficacy.

In conclusion, our work, conducted among CLBP elderly women, highlights that falls-related self-efficacy is lower than in controls and is associated with reduced mobility functions. Postural control is affected by LBP status in older women and could be explained by alteration of somatosensory integration. These results may help clinicians to better manage CLBP in older patients and further highlight potential physical and psychobehavioural predictors of falls and functional decline in this population.

Acknowledgments

This work was supported in part by Fonds institutionnel de la recherche (UQTR no. 3071081). A. Champagne is funded by a scholarship from Fonds de la recherche en santé du Québec.

References

[1] S. G. Leveille, J. M. Guralnik, M. Hochberg et al., "Low back pain and disability in older women: independent association with difficulty but not inability to perform daily activities," *Journals of Gerontology Series A*, vol. 54, no. 10, pp. M487–M493, 1999.

[2] J. Hartvigsen, K. Christensen, and H. Frederiksen, "Back and neck pain exhibit many common features in old age: a population-based study of 4,486 danish twins 70–102 years of age," *Spine*, vol. 29, no. 5, pp. 576–580, 2004.

[3] C. Leboeuf-Yde, J. Nielsen, K. O. Kyvik, R. Fejer, and J. Hartvigsen, "Pain in the lumbar, thoracic or cervical regions: do age and gender matter? A population-based study of 34,902 Danish twins 20–71 years of age," *BMC Musculoskeletal Disorders*, vol. 10, article 39, 2009.

[4] G. E. Hicks, J. M. Gaines, M. Shardell, and E. M. Simonsick, "Status and functional capacity of older adults: findings from the retirement community back pain study," *Arthritis and rheumatism*, vol. 59, no. 9, pp. 1306–1313, 2008.

[5] D. K. Weiner, T. E. Rudy, L. Morrow, J. Slaboda, and S. Lieber, "The relationship between pain, neuropsychological performance, and physical function in community-dwelling older adults with chronic low back pain," *Pain Medicine*, vol. 7, no. 1, pp. 60–70, 2006.

[6] J. W. S. Vlaeyen and S. J. Linton, "Fear-avoidance and its consequences in chronic musculoskeletal pain: a state of the art," *Pain*, vol. 85, no. 3, pp. 317–332, 2000.

[7] J. Rainville, R. J. Smeets, T. Bendix, T. H. Tveit, S. Poiraudeau, and A. J. Indahl, "Fear-avoidance beliefs and pain avodance in low back pain-translating research into clinical practice," *Spine Journal*, vol. 11, no. 9, pp. 895–903, 2011.

[8] M. Leeuw, M. E. J. B. Goossens, S. J. Linton, G. Crombez, K. Boersma, and J. W. S. Vlaeyen, "The fear-avoidance model of musculoskeletal pain: current state of scientific evidence," *Journal of Behavioral Medicine*, vol. 30, no. 1, pp. 77–94, 2007.

[9] R. J. E. M. Smeets, H. Wittink, A. Hidding, and J. A. Knottnerus, "Do patients with chronic low back pain have a lower level of aerobic fitness than healthy controls? Are pain, disability, fear of injury, working status, or level of leisure time activity associated with the difference in aerobic fitness level?" *Spine*, vol. 31, no. 1, pp. 90–97, 2006.

[10] C. Leonhart, D. Ledhr, J. F. Chenot, S. Keller, J. Luckmann, and H. D. Basler, "Are fear-avoidance beliefs in low back pain patients a risk factor for low physical activity or vice versa? A cross-lagged panel analysis," *Psycho-Social Medicine*, vol. 29, no. 6, 2009.

[11] F. Kovacs, V. Abraira, A. Cano et al., "Fear avoidance beliefs do not influence disability and quality of life in Spanish elderly subjects with low back pain," *Spine*, vol. 32, no. 19, pp. 2133–2138, 2007.

[12] H. D. Basler, J. Luckmann, U. Wolf, and S. Quint, "Fear-avoidance beliefs, physical activity, and disability in elderly individuals with chronic low back pain and healthy controls," *Clinical Journal of Pain*, vol. 24, no. 7, pp. 604–610, 2008.

[13] K. Delbaere, G. Crombez, G. Vanderstraeten, T. Willems, and D. Cambier, "Fear-related avoidance of activities, falls and physical frailty. A prospective community-based cohort study," *Age and Ageing*, vol. 33, no. 4, pp. 368–373, 2004.

[14] J. M. Sions and G. E. Hicks, "Fear-avoidance beliefs are associated with disability in older American adults with low back pain," *Physical Therapy*, vol. 91, no. 4, pp. 525–534, 2011.

[15] C. J. Büla, S. Monod, C. Hoskovec, and S. Rochat, "Interventions aiming at balance confidence improvement in older

adults: an updated review," *Gerontology*, vol. 57, no. 3, pp. 276–286, 2011.

[16] S. M. Al-Obaidi, R. M. Nelson, S. Al-Awadhi, and N. Al-Shuwaie, "The role of anticipation and fear of pain in the persistence of avoidance behavior in patients with chronic low back pain," *Spine*, vol. 25, no. 9, pp. 1126–1131, 2000.

[17] A. M. Myers, P. C. Fletcher, A. H. Myers, and W. Sherk, "Discriminative and evaluative properties of the activities-specific balance confidence (ABC) scale," *Journals of Gerontology Series A*, vol. 53, no. 4, pp. M287–M294, 1998.

[18] M. Von Korff, R. A. Deyo, D. Cherkin, and W. Barlow, "Back pain in primary care: outcomes at 1 year," *Spine*, vol. 18, no. 7, pp. 855–862, 1993.

[19] D. Vogler, R. Paillex, M. Norberg, P. de Goumoëns, and J. Cabri, "Cross-cultural validation of the Oswestry disability index in French," *Annales de Readaptation et de Medecine Physique*, vol. 51, no. 5, pp. 379–385, 2008.

[20] J. M. Fritz and J. J. Irrgang, "A comparison of a modified oswestry low back pain disability questionnaire and the Quebec back pain disability scale," *Physical Therapy*, vol. 81, no. 2, pp. 776–788, 2001.

[21] D. J. French, P. J. Roach, and S. Mayes, "Peur du mouvement chez des accidentés du travail: L'échelle de kinésiophobie de Tampa (EKT)," *Canadian Journal of Behavioural Science*, vol. 34, no. 1, pp. 28–33, 2002.

[22] T. Jacob, M. Baras, A. Zeev, and L. Epstein, "Physical activities and low back pain: a community-based study," *Medicine and Science in Sports and Exercise*, vol. 36, no. 1, pp. 9–15, 2004.

[23] S. R. Lord and J. A. Ward, "Age-associated differences in sensori-motor function and balance in community dwelling women," *Age and Ageing*, vol. 23, no. 6, pp. 452–460, 1994.

[24] D. Lafond, H. Corriveau, R. Hébert, and F. Prince, "Intrasession reliability of center of pressure measures of postural steadiness in healthy elderly people," *Archives of Physical Medicine and Rehabilitation*, vol. 85, no. 6, pp. 896–901, 2004.

[25] U. Oppenheim, R. Kohen-Raz, D. Alex, A. Kohen-Raz, and M. Azarya, "Postural characteristics of diabetic neuropathy," *Diabetes Care*, vol. 22, no. 2, pp. 328–332, 1999.

[26] D. Podsiadlo and S. Richardson, "The timed "Up and Go": a test of basic functional mobility for frail elderly persons," *Journal of the American Geriatrics Society*, vol. 39, no. 2, pp. 142–148, 1991.

[27] P. A. Goldie, O. M. Evans, and T. M. Bach, "Steadiness in one-legged stance: development of a reliable force-platform testing procedure," *Archives of Physical Medicine and Rehabilitation*, vol. 73, no. 4, pp. 348–354, 1992.

[28] A. MacSween, N. J. L. Johnson, G. Armstrong, and J. Bonn, "A validation of the 10-meter incremental shuttle walk test as a measure of aerobic power in cardiac and rheumatoid arthritis patients," *Archives of Physical Medicine and Rehabilitation*, vol. 82, no. 6, pp. 807–810, 2001.

[29] S. Choquette, D. R. Bouchard, C. Y. Doyon, M. Sénéchal, M. Brochu, and I. J. Dionne, "Relative strength as a determinant of mobility in elders 67-84 years of age. A nuage study: nutrition as a determinant of successful aging," *Journal of Nutrition, Health and Aging*, vol. 14, no. 3, pp. 190–195, 2010.

[30] J. A. Verbunt, H. A. Seelen, J. W. Vlaeyen et al., "Disuse and deconditioning in chronic low back pain: concepts and hypotheses on contributing mechanisms," *European Journal of Pain*, vol. 7, no. 1, pp. 9–21, 2003.

[31] P. Hendrick, S. Milosavljevic, L. Hale et al., "The relationship between physical activity and low back pain outcomes: a systematic review of observational studies," *European Spine Journal*, vol. 20, no. 3, pp. 464–474, 2011.

[32] E. J. Bousema, J. A. Verbunt, H. A. M. Seelen, J. W. S. Vlaeyen, and J. André Knottnerus, "Disuse and physical deconditioning in the first year after the onset of back pain," *Pain*, vol. 130, no. 3, pp. 279–286, 2007.

[33] M. Grotle, N. K. Vøllestad, and J. I. Brox, "Clinical course and impact of fear-avoidance beliefs in low back pain—prospective cohort study of acute and chronic low back pain—II," *Spine*, vol. 31, no. 9, pp. 1038–1046, 2006.

[34] F. Kovacs, J. Noguera, V. Abraira et al., "The influence of psychological factors on low back pain-related disability in community dwelling older persons," *Pain Medicine*, vol. 9, no. 7, pp. 871–880, 2008.

[35] J. M. Sions and G. E. Hicks, "Fear-avoidance beliefs are associated with disability in older American adults with low back pain," *Physical Therapy*, vol. 4, no. 4, pp. 1–10, 2004.

[36] T. E. Seeman, J. B. Unger, G. McAvay, and C. F. Mendes De Leon, "Self-efficacy beliefs and perceived declines in functional ability: MacArthur studies of successful aging," *Journals of Gerontology Series B*, vol. 54, no. 4, pp. P214–P222, 1999.

[37] A. M. Tromp, S. M. F. Pluijm, J. H. Smit, D. J. H. Deeg, L. M. Bouter, and P. Lips, "Fall-risk screening test: a prospective study on predictors for falls in community-dwelling elderly," *Journal of Clinical Epidemiology*, vol. 54, no. 8, pp. 837–844, 2001.

[38] M. Pijnappels, J. C. E. van der Burg, N. D. Reeves, and J. H. van Dieën, "Identification of elderly fallers by muscle strength measures," *European Journal of Applied Physiology*, vol. 102, no. 5, pp. 585–592, 2008.

[39] B. Holmes, S. Leggett, V. Mooney, J. Nichols, S. Negri, and A. Hoeyberghs, "Comparison of female geriatric lumbar-extension strength: asymptotic versus chronic low back pain patients and their response to active rehabilitation," *Journal of Spinal Disorders*, vol. 9, no. 1, pp. 17–22, 1996.

[40] P. Suri, D. K. Kiely, S. G. Leveille, W. R. Frontera, and J. F. Bean, "Increased trunk extension endurance is associated with meaningful improvement in balance among older adults with mobility problems," *Archives of Physical Medicine and Rehabilitation*, vol. 92, no. 7, pp. 1038–1043, 2011.

[41] B. E. Maki, P. J. Holliday, and A. K. Topper, "A prospective study of postural balance and risk of falling in an ambulatory and independent elderly population," *Journals of Gerontology*, vol. 49, no. 2, pp. M72–M84, 1994.

[42] G. L. Moseley and P. W. Hodges, "Are the changes in postural control associated with low back pain caused by pain interference?" *Clinical Journal of Pain*, vol. 21, no. 4, pp. 323–329, 2005.

[43] S. Brumagne, P. Cordo, R. Lysens, S. Verschueren, and S. Swinnen, "The role of paraspinal muscle spindles in lumbosacral position sense in individuals with and without low back pain," *Spine*, vol. 25, no. 8, pp. 989–994, 2000.

[44] S. Brumagne, P. Cordo, and S. Verschueren, "Proprioceptive weighting changes in persons with low back pain and elderly persons during upright standing," *Neuroscience Letters*, vol. 366, no. 1, pp. 63–66, 2004.

[45] A. Goldberg, M. E. Hernandez, and N. B. Alexander, "Trunk repositioning errors are increased in balance-impaired older adults," *Journals of Gerontology Series A*, vol. 60, no. 10, pp. 1310–1314, 2005.

[46] A. C. Scheffer, M. J. Schuurmans, N. Van dijk, T. Van der hooft, and S. E. De rooij, "Fear of falling: measurement strategy, prevalence, risk factors and consequences among older persons," *Age and Ageing*, vol. 37, no. 1, pp. 19–24, 2008.

[47] L. Mackenzie, J. Byles, and C. D'Este, "Validation of self-reported fall events in intervention studies," *Clinical Rehabilitation*, vol. 20, no. 4, pp. 331–339, 2006.

[48] B. E. Maki, P. J. Holliday, and A. K. Topper, "Fear of falling and postural performance in the elderly," *Journals of Gerontology*, vol. 46, no. 4, pp. M123–M131, 1991.

[49] M. Hübscher, L. Vogt, K. Schmidt, M. Fink, and W. Banzer, "Perceived pain, fear of falling and physical function in women with osteoporosis," *Gait and Posture*, vol. 32, no. 3, pp. 383–385, 2010.

4

Cognitive Impairment Affects Physical Recovery of Patients with Heart Failure Undergoing Intensive Cardiac Rehabilitation

Giuseppe Caminiti, Francesca Ranghi, Sara De Benedetti, Daniela Battaglia, Arianna Arisi, Alessio Franchini, Fabiana Facchini, Veronica Cioffi, and Maurizio Volterrani

Cardiovascular Research Unit, Department of Medical Sciences, IRCCS San Raffaele, Via della Pisana 235, 00163 Rome, Italy

Correspondence should be addressed to Giuseppe Caminiti, giuseppe.caminiti@sanraffaele.it

Academic Editor: Jeffrey Jutai

Purpose. To determine whether the presence of cognitive impairment (CI) affects physical recovery of patients with chronic heart failure (CHF) undergoing a cardiac rehabilitation program (CRP). *Methods*. We enrolled 80 CHF patients (M/F = 53/27). CI was evaluated by means of the Mini-Mental State Examination (MMSE), exercise tolerance was evaluated by six-minute walking test (6 mwt). All patients underwent a 6-week CRP program at 50–70% of maximal V_{O2}. Patients were divided into two groups according to their MMSE (group 1: 16–23; group 2: 24–30). *Results*. MMSE resulted directly related to ejection fraction ($r = 0.42$; $P = 0.03$), and it was inversely related to creatinine ($r = -0.36$; $P = 0.04$). At 6 week group 1 had a lower increase in distance walked at 6 MWT than group 2 ($P = 0.008$). At multivariate logistic regression MMSE 16–23 predicted a reduced exercise recovery in the overall population (OR = 1.84; 95% CI = 1.50–2.18) and in women (OR = 1.42; 95% CI = 1.22–1.75), while it was not predicted in males. *Conclusions*. CI is a marker of advanced CHF and is an independent predictor of lower exercise recovery after CRP.

1. Introduction

Lack of physical fitness is a strong predictor of poor prognosis in patients with chronic heart failure (CHF). Conversely exercise training, often performed in the contest of a cardiac rehabilitation program (CRP), is established as adjuvant therapy for these patients [1]. However, not all CHF subjects have the same benefits from CRP. It has been demonstrated that lack of significant improvement in exercise capacity after a CRP worsens the prognosis of CHF independently of other already known predictive factors [2]. To identify factors related to a lower response to CRP program is of remarkable interest for physicians in order to optimize the rehabilitative intervention. However, reasons for an unfavourable response to CRP are still partially known [3].

Cognitive impairment (CI) has been reported in patients who suffer from a variety of cardiovascular disorders [4] and it has been recognized to affect over one-third of older patients with CHF [5]. Several factors contribute to the high prevalence of CI among CHF subjects, the most important being the cerebral hypoperfusion due to a reduced cardiac output [6, 7]. Conversely CHF is associated with changes in brain regions that are important for demanding cognitive processing [8]. From a clinical point of view, the presence of CI in CHF patients has a negative impact on the course of the disease. At first CI may negatively influence self-management of CHF by reduced medication adherence and their failure to recognize early symptoms awareness. Moreover, CI seems to be related to a more complex clinical profile of CHF patients and to a worst outcome [9, 10].

Recently it has been hypothesized that CI could be also related to lack of improvement with exercise training in patients undergoing CRP [11].

The prevalence of CI among patients with CHF undergoing CRP and its impact on exercise recovery have not well investigated. Because of its potential deleterious effects on CHF management we postulated that CI could determine lack of response to exercise training performed by CHF patients in the context of CRP.

The aim of the study was to determine whether the presence of CI affects physical recovery of patients with CHF undergoing a cardiac rehabilitation program after a recent episode of acute decompensation.

2. Methods

We evaluated 126 consecutive patients admitted to Cardiac Rehabilitation Unit of IRCCS San Raffaele in Rome evaluated for undergoing an aerobic cardiac rehabilitation program as in-hospital patients, between May 2009 and November 2010. Inclusion criteria were left ventricular ejection fraction (LVEF) < 40%, history of CHF (at least 6 months), and a recent cardiac decompensation (<2 months). Exclusion criteria were inability to exercise, history of claudicatio, clinical instability, ventricular arrhythmias, primary valve disease, congenital heart disease, hypertrophic or restrictive cardiomyopathy, acute coronary syndrome within the past 2 weeks, or patients with planned coronary revascularization or cardiac surgery, active myocarditis, severe COPD, and pericardial effusion. Moreover, in order to exclude subjects with more advanced CI or dementia patients with MMSE score < 16/30 were not admitted to the study.

At entry baseline, anthropometric, clinical, morphological, and biochemical variables were collected by the medical and nonmedical staff. In the first 48 h after admission all eligible patients underwent fasting blood sample collection, evaluation of cognitive function though the administration of the Mini-Mental State Evaluation (MMSE). Glomerular filtration rate was calculated through the Modification of Diet in Renal Disease (MDRD) formula [12]. Exercise tolerance was evaluated by the six-Minute Walking Test (6 MWT). Patients enrolled were divided in two groups according to the MMSE score obtained; group 1 with MMSE between 16 and 23 (43 patients); group 2 with MMSE between 24 and 30 (37 patients). Then all patients underwent an intensive 6-week program of aerobic CRP.

Assessment of Exercise Tolerance. Exercise tolerance was evaluated by 6 MWT that was performed at admission and before discharge. The test was performed according to the standardized procedure [13] and was supervised by a physical therapist. Patients were asked to walk at their own maximal pace a 100 m long hospital corridor with 10-meter signs on the floor. Every minute a standard phrase of encouragement was told. Patients were allowed to stop if signs or symptoms of significant distress occurred (dyspnoea, angina), though they were instructed to resume walking as soon as possible. Results of 6 MWT were expressed in distance walked (metres). Functional recovery was defined as the increase of the distance walked at 6 MWT performed at the end of CRP with respect to the 6 MWT performed at baseline (Δ6 MWT).

Assessment of Cognitive Impairment. CI was investigated through the Mini-Mental State Examination (MMSE) [14], which is the most commonly administered psychometric screening assessment of cognitive functioning. The MMSE scale ranges from 0 to 30 and includes 10 domain items, which measure orientation to time, orientation to place, registration, attention and calculation, recall, naming and repetition, comprehension, reading ability, writing ability, and design copy.

According to the literature published on the MMSE, it is a relatively sensitive marker of CI [15]. MMSE was administered at admission by a trained psychologist.

Physical Rehabilitation Program. It was performed according to the AHA guidelines [16]. Every exercise session included warm-up, cooling down and flexibility exercises, and 30–60 minutes of submaximal aerobic exercise with cycling or treadmill at 50–70% of their maximal theoretical V_{O_2}. Patients underwent two exercise sessions every day for 6 days/week over a six-week period.

2.1. Statistical Analysis. Results are expressed as median ± standard deviation (SD) or percentages where appropriate. Baseline characteristics of patients with and without CI were compared with t-tests for continuous variables that were normally distributed, Wilcoxon Mann-Whitney test for continuous variables that were not normally distributed, and Chi-square tests for dichotomous variables. Relations between variables were assessed by Pearson correlation or Spearman's rank test for nonnormally distributed data. Prediction power of CI on functional recovery was evaluated through logistic regression analysis. The difference of distance walked at 6 MWT between baseline and the the end of the CRP (Δ6 MWT) was dichotomized according to its median value (105.3 m). We considered as having a good exercise recovery subjects with Δ6 MWT over 105.3 meters and weak exercise recovery those with Δ6 MWT below 105.3 meters. This categorical variable was used as dependent variable in the logistic regression analysis. The regression model was applied to the overall population, to the male and female genders. A value of $P < 0.05$ was considered significant. All analyses were performed using a commercially available statistical package (SPSS for Windows 12.0, Chicago, IL, USA).

3. Result

Out of 126 patients screened 85 patients (age 72.6 ± 10.6; M/F 53/27) met the inclusion criteria. Forty-one patients were not included because they were not able to perform a 6 MWT at admission because of their poor clinical conditions. Another five patients out of 85 were not included in the study. Two patients (2.3%) died during the hospitalization for acute decompensation, before starting CRP, and both had MMSE 16–23. Three patients with MMSE 16–23 and one with MMSE 24–30 were not included because they did not start the CRP; the reason for noninclusion was in every case worsening clinical status needed management in acute care. 80 patients completed the CRP and final evaluations and their data were considered for the study.

MMSE 16–23 was found in 54.4% of the overall population. 29 (55.2%) male and 14 (52.7%) female patients had MMSE 16–23. Overall females had a lower MMSE score than males (22.3 ± 4 versus 24.9 ± 5, $P = 0.07$).

TABLE 1: Statistical comparison among baseline variables of subjects of group 1 and group 2.

	Group 1 (MMSE 16–23) N = 43	Group 2 (MMSE 24–30) N = 37
Age, y	73.5 ± 13	70.7 ± 11*
M/F	29/14	24/13
BMI (kg/m^2)	27 ± 8	26 ± 4
NYHA class	2.7 ± 0.5	2.2 ± 0.4*
Resting HR, bpm	88 ± 7	76 ± 7*
Systolic BP, mmHg	108 ± 19	107 ± 21
Diastolic BP, mmHg	82 ± 10	80 ± 14
Echography		
LVEF	27.4 ± 7	34.9 ± 6*
LVDD	63.1 ± 11	62.6 ± 8
E/A	1.4 ± 0.7	1.4 ± 0.8
E deceleration time	171 ± 23	180 ± 17
Laboratory tests		
NT proBNP, pg/mL	302.7 ± 51	223.4 ± 34*
Creatinine, mg/dL	1.9 ± 0.3	1.4 ± 0.5*
GFR, mL/min	34.9 ± 9	50.1 ± 7*
Haemoglobin, g/dL	10.4 ± 3	11.1 ± 4
Comorbidities		
Hypertension	29 (67)	24 (65)
Diabetes	21 (48)	12 (32)*
Dislipidemia	17 (39)	15 (40)
COPD	16 (37)	11 (30)
Atrial fibrillation	15 (35)	10 (27)*
Therapy		
Beta-blockers	36 (84)	30 (81)
ACE-i/ARBs	39 (91)	36 (97)
Diuretics	34 (79)	27 (73)
Digoxin	9 (21)	6 (28)

*Intergroup differences $P < 0.05$.
GFR: glomerular filtration rate.
LVDD: left ventricular diastolic diameter.
LVEF: left ventricular ejection fraction.

Baseline clinical features of our patient population are reported in Table 1. Patients of group 1 were older, had an higher resting heart rate, and had more often diabetes and atrial fibrillation than patients of group 2. Moreover, patients of group 1 had a lower LVEF and higher levels of NT-pro-BNP and NYHA class than patients of group 2.

The score obtained at MMSE resulted directly related to EF ($r = 0.42$; $P = 0.03$) and it was inversely related to creatinine levels ($r = -0.36$; $P = 0.04$).

At the end of the study the distance walked at 6 MWT increased in both groups compared to baseline (group 1: from 155.4 ± 36 m to 253.1 ± 47 m; group 2 from 182.6 ± 42 m to 313.7 ± 69 m) with a significant greater increase in group 1 compared to group 2 ($P = 0.004$). Among patients of group 1 males had a greater increase of distance walked at 6 MWT compared to females (males: from 168.4 ± 56 m to 275.5 ± 45 m; females: from 131.7 ± 26 m to 213.1 ± 34 m;

TABLE 2: Logistic regression analysis evaluating the independent predictor power of CI (MMSE < 24) in the overall population, and according to gender.

MMSE 16–23 versus MMSE 24–30	Odds ratio (95% CI)	P value
Overall population		
Unadjusted model	2.21 (1.62–2.55)	<0.001
Adjusted model	1.84 (1.50–2.18)	0.024
Males		
Unadjusted model	1.5 (0.98–1.91)	0.036
Adjusted model	1.20 (0.87–1.52)	0.354
Females		
Unadjusted model	1.76 (1.30–2.07)	0.031
Adjusted model	1.42 (1.22–1.75)	0.047

Adjusted for LV ejection fraction, diabetes, age, atrial fibrillation, creatinine, and haemoglobin.

between-gender $P = 0.03$). In group 2 males and females had a similar increase of distance walked at 6 MWT (males: from 208.4 ± 49 m to 360.8 ± 61 m; females: from 178.4 ± 57 m to 284.3 ± 61 m; between-gender $P = 0.09$).

The independent prediction power of CI on functional recovery was evaluated through a logistic regression analysis in which we included as covariates some confounding variables such as diabetes, creatinine, haemoglobin, age, ejection fraction, and atrial fibrillation (Table 2). After adjusting for these covariates the presence of lower CI resulted significantly is related to a lower functional recovery in the overall population (adjusted OR = 1.84; 95% CI = 1.50–2.18, $P = 0.024$). Repeating the regression in each gender analysis and adjusting for the same covariates, CI maintained its significant predictor power only in the female gender (OR = 1.42; 95% CI = 1.22–1.75, $P = 0.047$), while there was not independent association between CI and functional recovery among males.

4. Discussion

The present study shows three important findings. First, CI has a high prevalence rate among patients with CHF undergoing a cardiac rehabilitation program after an acute cardiac event. Second, our data suggest that the presence of CI could be a marker of clinical complexity of patients and of a more advanced stage of CHF. Third, CI in these patients is associated with a reduced response to the exercise training program.

In our cohort 54% of CHF subjects had a MMSE 16–23 corresponding to a moderate-to-severe CI. There is a great variability in the literature concerning the prevalence of CI among CHF patients. In the review of Almeida and Flicker [5], it ranges from 25% to 74%. This variability observed can probably be explained by diverse study designs, CHF severity, age of patients, sample sizes, instruments used to assess cognitive impairment, and diagnostic criteria between different studies. However, our results are in line with previous studies considering similar population of elderly

CHF patients hospitalized or recently discharged from acute care facilities [17, 18]. In the cross-sectional study of Zuccalà et al. [17] on 57 consecutive CHF inpatients with no prior history of dementia, with a mean age of 76.7 years, 53% scored below 24/30 on the MMSE.

Several factors contribute to the high prevalence of CI among CHF, the most important being the cerebral hypoperfusion due to a reduced cardiac output [3, 4]. This is demonstrated by an increasing body of evidence suggesting that a decreased heart function is independently associated with impairment in various cognitive domains [5, 6]. Alternatively, a multiple-cardiogenic emboli hypothesis has been advanced and this hypothesis is in agreement with the higher rate of atrial fibrillation among patients of group 1 we observed.

In our study patients with CHF and CI had a more severe clinical profile with a higher number of comorbidities than patients without CI. Patients of group 1 were older, with an higher resting heart rate, a higher rate of diabetes, and atrial fibrillation than patients of group 2. Moreover, group 1 had a more advanced stage of heart disease as demonstrated by the higher NYHA stage, lover LVEF, and higher levels of NT-proBNP. Our observations are widely confirmed in the literature; Zuccalà et al. [18] demonstrated that CI among patients with CHF is associated with several comorbid conditions, some of which are potentially treatable. Moreover, a strong association between the severity of CI from a side to the severity of LV systolic dysfunction and severity of NYHA symptoms from the other side has been observed by other authors [19, 20]. Taken together these data seem to indicate that CI is a marker, easy to assess, and of clinical complexity of CHF patients who adhere to a CRP after an acute clinical event. Our data are also in agreement with other studies demonstrating that CI has an adverse impact on disease course by influencing the burden of disease, survival rates, and resource consumption. In a study investigating the in-hospital mortality among CHF patients, CI was found to increase the mortality by five times [9]. Recently O'Donnel et al. [21] found in a large population of patients with prior cardiovascular disease an inverse association between baseline MMSE score and risk of stroke, hospitalization for CHF, and death. That association was independent of all other prognostic factors. In a 5-year follow-up study, McLennan et al. [22] found that even patients who had mildly impaired cognition at baseline experienced significantly reduced event-free survival and overall life expectancy.

Comparing the results of the two 6 MWTs performed before and after CRP, we observed a significant improvement in the distance walked for both group 1 and group 2 subjects. However, group 2 reached an almost complete functional recovery after CR while group 1 subjects seem to have less benefits from CRP. In our cohort an MMSE score 16–23 was predictive of a lower exercise recovery as demonstrated by the multivariate logistical regression analysis also after adjusting for several confounding variables. It is well known that the response to CRP among CHF patients is variable. Lack of improvement of exercise capacity after training may be due to clinical parameters related to heart failure or to several other factors such as intercurrent illness, exacerbation of disease (e.g., acute coronary syndrome), injury (e.g., orthopedic complications), inadequate adherence to the exercise prescription, and poor patient compliance. The possibility to predict a poor response to CRP appears as a relevant information for physicians who plan the rehabilitative intervention. Tabet et al. [2] have shown that the absence of improvement in exercise capacity after an exercise training programme is a predictor of poor prognosis in patients with CHF. The concept that patients with CI may experience reduced benefit from an exercise-based cardiac rehabilitation program has been recently proposed. Kakos et al. [23] analyzed a cohort of forty-four older adults enrolled in a 12-week exercise-based CRP. Cognitive function was investigated through the Trail Making Test Part B, a measure of executive functions, and MMSE. Authors demonstrated that patients with poorer executive functions at baseline derived less benefit from their course of rehabilitative treatment. Our results suggest that the exercise recovery is reduced mostly in female patients. In our study male patients with CI showed a similar improvement of functional capacity than those without CI, while women with CI had the poorest functional recovery. There are no data for gender differences on the relation between CI and exercise capacity and the underlying mechanisms remain unclear [11]. We speculate that it could depend on a higher degree of CI among females in our cohort as demonstrated by the lower MMSE score they obtained at baseline evaluation. However, because of the limited sample size this data needs further confirmation in larger studies.

Limitations. The most important limitation of this study is the small sample size and our data, especially with regard to gender differences, need further confirmation in larger studies. In order to asses CI in this study we used the MMSE. Brief screening instruments such as the MMSE can be easily administered by health professionals in the clinical practice to confirm the presence of cognitive impairment. MMSE, however, may be insufficient in identifying subtle cognitive deficits and more detailed neuropsychological assessment is required. The real number of patients with CI in this study, particularly mild CI, could be underestimated due to the low sensibility of the MMSE for this less severe condition as reported by other authors [24]. During the study, we measured cognitive function only once and we do not know whether cognitive function improved or declined at the end of the study after CRP. At least in this study informations on instrumental social support were not taken into account and this could affect our results and limit our conclusions.

In conclusion, CI is a marker of advanced CHF and reduced physical performance. CHF patients with CI have lower exercise recovery than patients without CI after CRP. Because it is an independent correlation with lower exercise recovery, we suggest that CI should be investigated in every patients with CHF undergoing a cardiac rehabilitation program. The assessment of CI at the admission, together with other baseline evaluations, could help physicians in order to determine patients' risk profile, to predict the response to CRP, and planning an individual tailored rehabilitative intervention.

Authors' Contribution

The authors confirm that all authors have contributed to this work and the final version of this paper has been accepted by all of them.

References

[1] I. L. Piña, C. S. Apstein, G. J. Balady et al., "Exercise and heart failure: a statement from the American Heart Association Committee on Exercise, Rehabilitation, and Prevention," *Circulation*, vol. 107, no. 8, pp. 1210–1225, 2003.

[2] J. Y. Tabet, P. Meurin, F. Beauvais et al., "Absence of exercise capacity improvement after exercise training program: a strong prognostic factor in patients with chronic heart failure," *Circulation*, vol. 1, no. 4, pp. 220–226, 2008.

[3] J. P. Schmid, M. Zurek, and H. Saner, "Chronotropic incompetence predicts impaired response to exercise training in heart failure patients with sinus rhythm," *European Journal of Preventive Cardiology*. In press.

[4] L. H. P. Eggermont, K. De Boer, M. Muller, A. C. Jaschke, O. Kamp, and E. J. A. Scherder, "Cardiac disease and cognitive impairment: a systematic review," *Heart*, vol. 98, pp. 1334–1340, 2012.

[5] O. P. Almeida and L. Flicker, "The mind of a failing heart: a systematic review of the association between congestive heart failure and cognitive functioning," *Internal Medicine Journal*, vol. 31, no. 5, pp. 290–295, 2001.

[6] T. C. T. F. Alves, J. Rays, R. Fráguas et al., "Localized cerebral blood glow reductions in patients with heart failure: a study using 99mTc-HMPAO SPECT," *Journal Neuroimaging*, vol. 15, pp. 150–156, 2005.

[7] N. Gruhn, F. S. Larsen, S. Boesgaard et al., "Cerebral blood flow in patients with chronic heart failure before and after heart transplantation," *Stroke*, vol. 32, no. 11, pp. 2530–2533, 2001.

[8] O. P. Almeida, G. J. Garrido, C. Beer, N. T. Lautenschlager, L. Arnolda, and L. Flicker, "Cognitive and brain changes associated with ischaemic heart disease and heart failure," *European Heart Journal*, vol. 33, pp. 1769–1776, 2012.

[9] G. Zuccalà, C. Pedone, M. Cesari et al., "The effects of cognitive impairment on mortality among hospitalized patients with heart failure," *American Journal of Medicine*, vol. 115, pp. 97–103, 2003.

[10] R. Rozzini, T. Sabatini, and M. Trabucchi, "Cognitive impairment and mortality in elderly patients with heart failure," *American Journal of Medicine*, vol. 116, no. 2, pp. 137–138, 2004.

[11] B. A. Franklin, "Cognitive impairment: a new predictor of exercise trainability and outcomes in cardiac rehabilitation?" *Preventive Cardiology*, vol. 13, no. 3, pp. 97–99, 2010.

[12] A. S. Levey, J. P. Bosch, J. B. Lewis, T. Greene, N. Rogers, and D. Roth, "A more accurate method to estimate glomerular filtration rate from serum creatinine: a new prediction equation," *Annals of Internal Medicine*, vol. 130, no. 6, pp. 461–470, 1999.

[13] American Thoracic Society, "ATS statement: guidelines for the sixminute walk test," *American Journal of Respiratory and Critical Care Medicine*, vol. 166, pp. 111–117, 2002.

[14] M. F. Folstein, S. E. Folstein, and P. R. McHugh, "'Mini mental state'. A practical method for grading the cognitive state of patients for the clinician," *Journal of Psychiatric Research*, vol. 12, no. 3, pp. 189–198, 1975.

[15] J. R. Harvan and V. Cotter, "An evaluation of dementia screening in the primary care setting," *Journal of the American Academy of Nurse Practitioners*, vol. 18, no. 8, pp. 351–360, 2006.

[16] G. J. Balady, P. A. Ades, P. Comoss et al., "Core components of cardiac rehabilitation/secondary prevention programs: a statement for healthcare professionals from the American Heart Association and the American Association of Cardiovascular and Pulmonary Rehabilitation," *Circulation*, vol. 102, no. 9, pp. 1069–1073, 2000.

[17] G. Zuccalà, C. Cattel, E. Manes-Gravina, M. G. Di Niro, A. Cocchi, and R. Bernabei, "Left ventricular dysfunction: a clue to cognitive impairment in older patients with heart failure," *Journal of Neurology Neurosurgery and Psychiatry*, vol. 63, no. 4, pp. 509–512, 1997.

[18] G. Zuccalà, E. Marzetti, M. Cesari et al., "Correlates of cognitive impairment among patients with heart failure: results of a multicenter survey," *American Journal of Medicine*, vol. 118, no. 5, pp. 496–502, 2005.

[19] O. P. Almeida and S. Tamai, "Congestive heart failure and cognitive functioning amongst older adults," *Arquivos de Neuro-Psiquiatria*, vol. 59, no. 2, pp. 324–329, 2001.

[20] A. L. Jefferson, J. J. Himali, R. Au, S. Seshadri, C. De Carli, C. J. O'Donnel et al., "Relation of left ventricular ejection fraction to cognitive aging (from the Framingham Heart Study)," *American Journal of Cardiology*, vol. 108, no. 9, pp. 1346–1351, 2011.

[21] M. O'Donnel, K. Teo, P. Gao et al., "Cognitive impairment and risk of cardiovascular events and mortality," *European Heart Journal*, vol. 33, no. 14, pp. 1777–1786, 2012.

[22] S. N. McLennan, S. A. Pearson, J. Cameron, and S. Stewart, "Prognostic importance of cognitive impairment in chronic heart failure patients: does specialist management make a difference?" *European Journal of Heart Failure*, vol. 8, no. 5, pp. 494–501, 2006.

[23] L. S. Kakos, A. J. Szabo, J. Gunstad et al., "Reduced executive functioning is associated with poorer outcome in cardiac rehabilitation," *Preventive Cardiology*, vol. 13, no. 3, pp. 100–103, 2010.

[24] J. Cameron, L. Worrall-Carter, K. Page, S. Stewart, and C. F. Ski, "Screening for mild cognitive impairment in patients with heart failure: montreal Cognitive Assessment versus Mini Mental State Exam," *European Journal Cardiovascular Nursing*. In press.

5

Impact of "Sick" and "Recovery" Roles on Brain Injury Rehabilitation Outcomes

David A. Barclay

Department of Social Work, Gallaudet University, 800 Florida Avenue NE, Washington, DC 20008, USA

Correspondence should be addressed to David A. Barclay, david.barclay@gallaudet.edu

Academic Editor: K. S. Sunnerhagen

This study utilizes a multivariate, correlational, expost facto research design to examine Parsons' "sick role" as a dynamic, time-sensitive process of "sick role" and "recovery role" and the impact of this process on goal attainment (H1) and psychosocial distress (H2) of adult survivors of acquired brain injury. Measures used include the Brief Symptom Inventory-18 , a Goal Attainment Scale, and an original instrument to measure sick role process. 60 survivors of ABI enrolled in community reentry rehabilitation participated. Stepwise regression analyses did not fully support the multivariate hypotheses. Two models emerged from the stepwise analyses. Goal attainment, gender, and postrehab responsibilities accounted for 40% of the shared variance of psychosocial distress. Anxiety and depression accounted for 22% of the shared variance of goal attainment with anxiety contributing to the majority of the explained variance. Bivariate analysis found sick role variables, anxiety, somatization, depression, gender, and goal attainment as significant. The study has implications for ABI rehabilitation in placing greater emphasis on sick role processes, anxiety, gender, and goal attainment in guiding program planning and future research with survivors of ABI.

1. Introduction

Based on nonmilitary hospital, emergency room, and death records, an estimated 1.7 million Americans suffer a traumatic brain injury (TBI) each year [1]. Additional US military cases of TBI total over 20,000 annually [2]. Add to that number the additional annual 700,000 stroke victims [3], and the prevalence of people suffering any type of acquired brain injury (ABI) totals over 2.5 million Americans annually. For purposes of perspective, each year 12,000 people suffer a traumatic spinal cord injury [4], 50,000 are diagnosed with AIDS, and 176,000 are diagnosed with breast cancer [5]. Following medical treatment for acquired brain injury (ABI), many persons continue treatment in outpatient community reentry rehabilitation programs. Upon discharge, however, many survivors of ABI fail to demonstrate optimal goal attainment [6] and suffer heightened psychosocial distress as demonstrated by increased depression and anxiety [7–11]. Although there is not a consensus in the literature related to the prevalence of depression and anxiety, the number of brain injury survivors

who suffer from depression can be as high as 77% and those who suffer from anxiety can be as high as 66% of the brain injury survivors studied [7–11]. Two recent studies emphasize the amount and longevity of depression in brain injury survivors. Jorge et al. [12] found that over one-third of their sample survivors met the criteria for major depressive disorder and over two thirds met the criteria for an anxiety disorder. According to Konrad et al. [13], depression and anxiety continue to be an issue many years postinjury. Their study sample of 33 mild TBI survivors 6 years postinjury had significantly higher depression scores as measured by the Beck Depression Inventory than the general population.

Social and community integration can be severely hampered if individual rehabilitation goals are not met [14] and if the survivor continues to experience psychosocial distress, specifically anxiety and depression. Much of the current literature suggests that a brain injury survivor's quality of life suffers if he/she does not achieve optimal goal attainment at time of discharge and if he/she continues to experience anxiety and depressive symptoms at time of discharge. Often, social and emotional behavior impairments are considered by the survivor as more disabling than the physical residuals of the injury [15]. These psychosocial behavioral impairments can negatively impact neuropsychological functioning [16] and can impede psychosocial adjustment following rehabilitation [17, 18]. Increases in depression and anxiety are a common residual problem for the brain injury survivor [19, 20] and have been shown to impact cognitive recovery, return to work/school and the family system [21–26].

In understanding human behavior, both the structure of a role and the process of the assumption of a role are important [27]. In examining possible explanations for poor goal attainment and continued psychosocial distress after rehabilitation, Talcott Parsons' sick role theory can be applied as a framework for understanding illness behavior and outcome pathways. Sick role is conceptually defined as one's acceptance of certain rights and responsibilities associated with the role of being sick. Parsons [26] emphasized the impact that society has on the structure of roles. Societal and self-generated expectations and legitimations of the role, in particular, are important to the understanding and to the role-taking process. Thus part of the process of experimentation with and acceptance of new roles is whether the self and/or society accepts that role and in what condition [26, 27]. Environmental elements and both self and society can reinforce the structure and process of a role by either the nurturing or rejection of a role. Thus, the physical rehabilitation environment can directly control role assumption through availability of resources, and the ABI survivor's social environment can control role assumption through direct commands or interpersonal behaviors [27].

Parson's original blueprint of the sick role [26, 28] was restricted to societal norms that influenced a person's role during temporary, acute physical illness. The four major tenets of his sick role concept are (1) the sick person is exempt from social responsibility, (2) the sick person is exempt from self-blame for being sick, (3) the sick person should want to get well, and (4) the sick person should seek medical advice and cooperate with medical experts [26]. Parsons combined these rights and responsibilities to form a one-dimensional set of societal expectations called the "sick role." Sociologically, his main concern was how the sick role prevented individuals from performing their tasks in society and whether certain parts of society had more or less of a tendency to assume and/or condone assumption of the sick role.

Early research on assumption of the sick role focused on societal perceptions of sick people; in particular people who had an acute illness [29]. The research focused on whether they, from the perception of others, had a legitimate right to assume the sick role. However, during the decades that followed, Parsons' model has been extended beyond perceptions of those who had temporary, acute illness to include patterns in the actual ill person's assumption and relinquishment of the sick role. In addition, studies were expanded to include persons with chronic illness and psychiatric illness. Several studies focused on variables impacting a person's willingness to adopt the sick role, rather than on the expectations that society holds towards those people [30–33].

This current study investigates the sick role as a process of assumption and relinquishment of rights and responsibilities. If the sick role is framed as a process of rights and responsibilities, then a person may take one of three common paths with regards to the sick role: (1) he or she may accept the sick role rights when appropriate and then assume the necessary responsibilities of therapy and recovery, and then relinquish the sick role, or (2) he or she may reject the sick role rights and responsibilities in denial of his/her illness and thus be in denial of any limitations or requirements for therapy, or (3) he or she may overidentify with the rights of the sick role, exemption from responsibility, and dependence on others, without desiring to get well and without seeking and cooperating with therapies.

Currently, no studies directly apply sick role concepts to the ABI survivor rehabilitation process. However, several articles apply the sick role to other populations (e.g., cardiac patients) who follow a similar path of ABI survivors in terms of the seriousness and suddenness of their change in abilities. In the cardiac population, age and gender were significant predictors of sick role tendencies [30–33]. In particular, men tended to relinquish the sick role more readily than women and younger people tended to relinquish the sick role more readily than older people [32, 33]. Because the literature indicates the variables of age and gender affect assumption of the sick role, they are taken into account as possible external sources of variance in the present research project.

2. Methods

2.1. Design. This study utilized a multivariate, correlational, expost facto research design. Control variables were age, gender, and level of functioning. The study sought to answer the following question. What is the relationship between the independent variables of survivor sick role process and the dependent variables of goal attainment and psychosocial distress in adults with acquired brain injuries involved in the rehabilitation process? The following two hypotheses were developed to help answer this question.

Hypothesis 1. Controlling for age and gender, those survivors of ABI with higher levels of acceptance of their sick role rights at the beginning of rehabilitation and higher levels of acceptance of their sick role responsibilities upon discharge will have lower levels of psychosocial distress.

Hypothesis 2. Controlling for age and gender, those survivors of ABI with higher levels of acceptance of their sick role rights at the beginning of rehabilitation and higher levels of acceptance of their sick role responsibilities upon discharge will have higher levels of goal attainment.

2.2. Participants. Participants were 60 adult survivors of acquired brain injury (ABI) who attended outpatient community reentry rehabilitation at one of two programs located in the Washington, DC, metropolitan area in the USA. For the purposes of this study, an ABI survivor was defined as someone who had experienced any insult to the brain which resulted in impairment of cognitive abilities and/or physical functioning [34].

The study utilized a convenience sample of adult (18 years of age or over) survivors of ABI. Candidates were referred and screened by their primary therapists in their rehabilitation program. Candidates were not eligible if there was evidence of severe memory deficits or an unmanaged mood or substance abuse disorder. To further control for possible memory impairments impacting the validity of this study, after referral to the study, participants were asked to self-report on their ability to recall events and feelings that they experienced at the beginning of their rehabilitation in retrospect. Participation was voluntary, although a $10 compensation was given to all participants. A written informed consent form was reviewed with all candidates. Prior to participating, all participants signed the informed consent forms which were preapproved by two separate Institutional Review Boards (The Catholic University of America and Gallaudet University, Washington, DC).

2.3. Data Collection. This research was part of a larger research study conducted as part of the dissertation process for completion of doctoral studies. Questionnaires were administered to the participants over a 15-month period. Individual survivor goals were established for each survivor by the rehabilitation agency based on agency assessment. The 54-item study instrument for this research study consisted of demographic questions, two previously published instruments, and one original instrument. The demographic questionnaire contained 13 closed-ended questions about the control variables of age and gender and included additional questions about marital status, injury, income, education, and spiritual support.

2.4. Barclay Sick Role Process Inventory (BSRPI). The independent variable of level of sick role is conceptualized as the survivor's process of acceptance of sick role rights and responsibilities from the beginning to the end of the period of rehabilitation. No published measures specifically addressed the sick role rights and responsibilities in adult ABI survivors, so the researcher developed one for the study. The study uses a new scale, named the Barclay Sick Role Process Inventory (BSRPI) (see Appendix (A)) to measure these levels of acceptance of sick role rights and responsibilities over time. This new sick role process scale was adapted from Myers and Grasmick's [35] instrument measuring the static concept of sick role in pregnancy.

The BSRPI is a 24-item instrument. The completed scale has 12 items phrased in the past, "When I first started in this rehabilitation program ...," and 12 items phrased in the present, "Now ...," in order to identify the rights and responsibilities acceptance process. Item responses are rated on a 4-point scale ranging from (1) strongly disagree to (4) strongly agree. Data from this inventory can be analyzed to reflect individual and total rights and responsibilities both before and after rehabilitation and to reflect the change in acceptance of rights and responsibilities over time.

Content validity was determined using a review of the literature and a panel of experts in the field of brain injury and mental health. In addition, internal consistency of items on the BSRPI was analyzed using Cronbach's alpha. The reliability alpha in the sample (n = 60) for the entire instrument was .70. However, the instrument actually measures four distinct concepts. The reliability alpha in the sample (n = 60) for each concept is as follows: .69 for individual rights at time of intake; .88 for individual responsibilities at time of intake; .58 for individual rights at time of discharge; .79 for individual responsibilities at time of discharge.

One concern of the use of collecting retrospective data from ABI survivors is the fact that memory problems are a common issue with this population. As a control for this validity concern, participants were accepted only upon referral by their primary therapists in the rehabilitation agencies. The therapists were instructed not to refer anyone with evidence of severe memory deficits or an unmanaged mood or substance abuse disorder. As an additional control, participants were asked the following two screening questions. (1) Do you remember how you were feeling when you were first admitted to this rehabilitation program? (2) Do you remember how you felt when you first met your rehabilitation therapists? They were also asked to identify and clarify a few of their identified feelings to further validate their answers. If they answered "no" to either question, they were screened out of the participant pool.

2.5. Rating Scale for Functional Independence (RSFI). Level of functioning was measured by the Rating Scale for Functional Independence (RSFI) to control for the impact of level of functioning at time of intake on the participants' goal attainment and psychosocial distress. Level of functioning is conceptually defined as a subject's overall physical, cognitive, psychosocial, and behavioral ability to function. Both agencies where participants were recruited from utilized the RSFI. The RSFI is a way for the therapist to rate the functional independence of their client on a 7-point scale as follows: 1 = total assistance, 2 = maximal assistance, 3 = moderate assistance, 4 = minimal assistance, 5 = supervision, 6 = modified independence, and 7 = complete independence. There is a rubric with details on the measurable differences between each level of independence. The RSFI has not been studied related to reliability or validity. The participants' level of functioning at intake and discharge was assessed by the primary therapists with responses ranging from 1 to 7 with the ability to assess levels at .5 increments.

2.6. Brief Symptom Inventory-18 (BSI). Psychosocial distress, specifically depression and/or anxiety, was measured by the Brief Symptom Inventory-18 (BSI). This tool measures depression and anxiety and has alpha coefficients of greater than .90 [36]. The BSI is an 18-item instrument designed to measure psychological distress both during and at the end of treatment based on the three dimensions of depression, anxiety, and somatization. Individual scores are provided for each dimension along with a Global Severity Index (GSI) score which represents the overall level of psychological distress.

2.7. Goal Attainment Scale (GAS).

Goal attainment is conceptually defined as the level of success in meeting individualized goals upon discharge that were established at the beginning of the ABI survivor's rehabilitation program. Operationally, this was measured by a Goal Attainment Scale [37] generated by the primary therapists (see Appendix (B)) for the participants' cognitive, psychosocial, occupational, and physical rehabilitation. Overall goal attainment was recorded on a 5-point scale from most unfavorable outcome (1) to most favorable outcome (5). The primary therapists at the agency responsible for establishing and monitoring various goals were asked to give a numerical rating of each subject's goal attainment in each therapy discipline. These scores were then averaged across the number of individual rehabilitation goal areas for each participant.

3. Results

3.1. Sociodemographic Findings.

Forty-seven of the 60 participants, or 78% of the sample, self-identified as males and 13, or 22% of the sample, self-identified as females. Participants ranged in age from 18 to 83 years of age, with the mean age being 43.6 years old. The reported racial/ethnic composition was as follows: 61% self-identified as Caucasian/White (non-Hispanic), 31.7% self-identified as African American/Black, 5% self-identified as Hispanic, and 1.7% self-identified as Asian/Pacific Islander. The participants had sustained the following type of injuries: 35% were due to stroke, 43% were due to acceleration/deceleration injury, and 22% were due to an "other" category which included alcoholic seizure, tumor, surgery, and encephalitis. Table 1 illustrates the sociodemographic data described above.

3.2. Descriptive Statistics for the Study Instruments.

Table 1 shows the descriptive statistics for the Barclay Sick Role Process Inventory (BSRPI), Brief Symptom Inventory-18 (BSI-18), and Goal Attainment Scale (GAS). Norms are not available for the BSRPI scales. However, the BSRPI responsibility at discharge actual range is smaller than the potential range and the mean score is fairly high. This signifies that the study sample scored at the high end of the scale which would be expected in the sick role process. This is conceptually significant because, according to sick role theory, the majority of the sample tended to assume high levels of sick role responsibilities at discharge. The BSRPI reliability is good with an alpha of .69 for measuring rights and an alpha of .79 for measuring responsibilities.

Participants had a BSI-18 mean raw score of 7.52 which is only slightly higher than both the community and oncology raw score norms published by the author of the BSI-18 [38]. This signifies that the study sample reported slightly higher levels of psychosocial distress than samples in the general community and the cancer community. This could be explained by the added potential for psychosocial distress

in the ABI community. The BSI-18 reliability for the study sample is very good with an alpha of .84.

The participants had a mean score of 3.04 on the GAS. Norms are not available for the GAS. However, a mean score of 3.04 signifies that the primary therapists reported that the study sample generally achieved their predicted level of goal attainment at an expected level. As shown in Table 2, the potential range (1–5) and the actual range (1.25–4.6) are very similar, signifying the therapists did indeed assign goal attainment ratings all along the achievement continuum. Among all of the variable measures, the GAS had the lowest reliability coefficient (.67).

3.3. Bivariate Analysis.

Pearson's product-moment correlation was used to investigate bivariate relationships among variables. Table 2 depicts the bivariate correlations among goal attainment (Goal), psychosocial distress total (Psy-Tot), somatization (Som), depression (Dep), anxiety (Anx), assumption of sick role rights before (PreRig) and after (PostRig) rehabilitation, assumption of sick role responsibilities before (PreRes) and after (PostRes) rehabilitation, level of functioning (LOF), time after injury in months (Time), age (Age), and gender (Gen). As can be seen in Table 2, goal attainment was significantly negatively correlated with total psychosocial distress ($r = -.518$, $P < .01$) and also with all three subscales of somatization ($r = -.277$, $P < .01$), depression ($r = -.386$, $P < .01$), and anxiety ($r = -.439$, $P < .01$). However, the analysis suggests that there is no significant relationship between goal attainment and any other variable, including sick role process variables.

Total psychosocial distress was significantly positively correlated with postrehab sick role rights ($r = .310$, $P < .05$) and gender ($r = .428$, $P < .01$). Anxiety was significantly positively correlated with goal attainment ($r = -.439$, $P < .01$) and gender ($r = .570$, $P < .01$) and postrehab sick role rights ($r = .443$, $P < .01$) and significantly negatively correlated with postrehab sick role responsibilities ($r = -.388$, $P < .01$). Somatization was significantly positively correlated with both pre- and postrehab sick role rights ($r = .298$, $P < .05$); ($r = .315$, $P < .05$) and gender ($r = .430$, $P < .01$). Depression was only significantly correlated with prerehab sick role responsibilities ($r = -.338$, $P < .05$). The assumption of sick role responsibilities at time of discharge is negatively correlated with both age ($r = -.37$, $P < .01$) and level of functioning ($r = -.32$, $P < .05$).

3.4. Multivariate Analysis.

Controlling for age and gender, higher levels of acceptance of sick role rights at the beginning of rehabilitation and higher levels of acceptance of sick role responsibilities upon discharge were hypothesized to predict lower levels of psychosocial distress in H1 and higher levels of goal attainment in H2. In order to examine the relative predictive contribution of the independent variables on the dependent variables, two stepwise regression analyses were conducted based on the hypotheses and significant relationships found in the bivariate analyses. Related to H1, the first stepwise regression analysis examined the contribution of the hypothesized sick role process variables, the control variables

TABLE 1: Summary statistics of the study scales.

	Mean	SD	Alpha	Potential range	Actual range
BSRPI*—rights at intake	12.65	2.82	.69	5–20	7–20
BSRPI—responsibility at discharge	21.80	2.54	.79	6–24	15–24
Brief Symptom Inventory: SI-18	7.52	7.08	.84	0–72	0–32
Goal Attainment Scale	3.04	0.84	.67	1–5	1.25–4.60

* Barclay Sick Role Process Inventory.

TABLE 2: Bivariate correlations of independent variables, control variables, and dependent variables.

Variable	1	2	3	4	5	6	7	8	9	10	11	12
(1) Goal	—											
(2) PsyTot	−518**	—										
(3) Som	−.277*	.478**	—									
(4) Dep	−386**	.754**	−.026	—								
(5) Anx	−439**	.865**	.453*	.389**	—							
(6) PreRig	.196	.036	.298*	−.189	.122	—						
(7) PreRes	.221	−.169	.020	−.308*	−.007	.145	—					
(8) PostRig	−.220	.310*	.315*	−.012	.443**	.431**	−.293*	—				
(9) PosRes	.224	−.367**	−.157	−.216	−.388**	.142	.380**	−.415**	—			
(10) LOF	−.042	.028	−.085	.076	.014	−.153	−.232	.010	−.318*	—		
(11) Time	−.010	.137	.166	.006	.102	.011	.088	.136	.015	−.044	—	
(12) Age	−.125	.070	−.003	.056	.075	−.292*	−.125	.139	−.368**	.222	−.120	—
(13) Gen	−.191	.428**	.430**	.026	.570**	.284*	.170	.350**	−.135	−.037	.049	.120

* $P < .05$.
** $P < .01$.

of age and gender, and the significant variable of goal attainment as predictor variables for psychosocial distress. Tests for multicollinearity indicated that a very low level of multicollinearity was present (VIF numbers for all variables were less than 1.5). As can be seen in Table 3, the model summary included goal attainment, gender, and postrehab responsibilities accounting for 40% of the shared variance of psychosocial distress with goal attainment contributing the majority of the explained variance. Pre-rehab sick role rights and responsibilities, postrehab rights, and age were excluded from the model. The observed power for this multiple regression model, given an alpha of.05, n of 60, and 6 predictor variables, is .99. H1 was not fully supported by the analysis, with only postrehab responsibilities being a significant predictor variable for psychosocial distress in this model.

The second stepwise regression analysis examined the contribution of the hypothesized sick role process variables, the control variables of age and gender, and the significant variables of depression, anxiety, and somatization. Tests for multicollinearity indicated that a very low level of multicollinearity was present (VIF numbers for all variables were less than 1.2). As can be seen in Table 4, the model summary included anxiety and depression accounting for 22% of the shared variance of goal attainment with anxiety contributing to the majority of the explained variance. All sick role variables, gender, and age were excluded from the model. The observed power for this multiple regression model, given an alpha of .05, n of 60, and 9 predictor

variables, is .80. H2 was not supported by the analysis; no variable of sick role process was found to be a significant predictor of goal attainment in this model.

4. Discussion

This study pioneers the application of sick role theory and expansion of role theory on brain injury rehabilitation. Theoretically, this study expanded upon Parsons' static sick role and applied it as a more dynamic process of assumption and relinquishment of sick role rights and responsibilities. An instrument was developed to help measure this sick role process. However, using stepwise regression analysis, the data did not fully support either research hypothesis related to sick role process. Consequently, controlling for age and gender, survivors of ABI with higher levels of acceptance of their sick role rights at the beginning of rehabilitation and higher levels of acceptance of their sick role responsibilities upon discharge did not significantly demonstrate lower levels of psychosocial distress nor higher levels of goal attainment. Although the data did not support the full hypotheses related to sick role process, several important significant relationships were uncovered related to sick role variables and other variables that can be used to better understand and improve rehabilitation with survivors of ABI. The most interesting relationships uncovered have to do with those between goal attainment and psychosocial distress, especially when examined as being potentially both independent and

TABLE 3: Significant variables using stepwise regression analysis to predict psychosocial distress*.

Predictor	Beta	t	Significance level	Adjusted R^2
Goal attainment	−3.42	−3.87	.000	.256
Gender**	5.4	3.10	.003	.359
Postrehab response	−.651	−2.25	.029	.402

*$F = 14.2$, $R^2 = .402$.
**Lower score (1) = male; higher score (2) = female.

TABLE 4: Significant variables using stepwise regression analysis to predict goal attainment*.

Predictor	Beta	t	Significance level	Adjusted R^2
Anxiety	−.340	−2.73	.008	.179
Depression	−.254	−2.04	.046	.221

*$F = 9.3$.

dependent variables in the rehabilitation process. Bivariate analysis showed a moderate significant negative relationship between psychosocial distress and goal attainment, but what is not clear is if the survivor was not achieving their goals due to their psychosocial distress or if the lack of goal achievement was increasing their psychosocial distress, or both. If psychosocial distress is identified as the dependent variable, goal attainment explained the majority of the variance in psychosocial distress, followed by gender and then assumption of postrehab rights. The literature supports the findings of goal attainment on psychosocial distress [19, 21] and emphasizes the need for establishing achievable goals and monitoring psychological and emotional status of the survivors, especially for those who have not achieved their rehabilitation goals.

To more accurately understand how psychosocial distress factors into the rehabilitation process and outcomes, it can be broken down into its three measurable components of depression, anxiety, and somatization and then the various relationships examined. In the regression model in Table 4, anxiety explained the majority of variance in goal attainment, followed by depression. In the bivariate analysis, participants who reported higher levels of anxiety not only had lower levels of goal attainment, they also had higher levels of sick role rights both before and after rehab, lower levels of postrehab sick role responsibilities, and tended to be female. Related to sick role process, these correlations support a profile of more anxious survivors who stay in the dependent role of "sick person" and who are not moving into the role of "recovering person." The majority of the literature reviewed focus on the role of depression in the rehabilitation outcomes, but the results of the present study point to anxiety as a more important factor. Depression had a significant negative correlation only with goal attainment and prerehab sick role responsibilities, suggesting a relationship between higher levels of depression and lower levels of sick role "recovery" responsibilities at the beginning of rehabilitation.

Similar to anxiety, somatization was significantly positively correlated with both pre- and postrehab sick role rights and gender. Those survivors who reported high levels of somatic symptoms tended also to enter rehab and exit rehab with high levels of dependent "sick role" rights and be female. Although the somatization subscale is designed to collect data on somatic symptoms associated with psychological stress (i.e., sleep problems, nausea), the instrument does not differentiate nor expand on the causes of the somatic symptoms. Brain injury survivors often have somatic symptoms that are due to their physical injuries and not to their psychological issues. So the subscale results cannot be unilaterally categorized nor analyzed as being "psycho-somatic." However, what is clear is that there is a relationship between a survivors somatic symptoms and their initial and continued acceptance of sick role rights. Related to ABI rehabilitation, health care providers should be focusing on the reduction of somatic symptoms and consider them in relation to survivors moving from dependence towards recovery.

In the study, gender was positively correlated with assumption of sick role rights both before and after rehab, psychosocial distress, somatization, and anxiety, meaning that women tended to assume sick role rights and have higher levels of various psychosocial distress than men. The literature supports that women tend to assume the static sick role of both rights [32]; however, the literature does not support that female ABI survivors tend to have higher levels of psychosocial distress than male ABI survivors. This correlation would need to be addressed in further research due to the small number of women in the study sample ($n = 13$). However, if the correlation that women tend to have greater psychosocial distress, anxiety, or somatization at time of discharge is further supported, then that would increase support for consideration of gender during intake and for program planning and discharge.

In the study, age had a significant negative correlation with sick role responsibilities at time of discharge ($r = −.37$, $P < .01$) and a significant positive correlation with assumption of sick role rights at time of intake ($r = .34$, $P < .01$). The literature suggests that younger people tend to accept the static sick role at the beginning of rehabilitation and tend to relinquish the static sick role at the end of rehabilitation more than older people [32].

Examined as a process, the data for this study suggests that older people tended to assume more sick role rights than younger people but then did not relinquish those rights and move onto accepting the sick role responsibilities. These correlations support the need for program planning that encourages older adults' assumption of sick role responsibilities.

Future research in the area of community reentry rehabilitation for adults survivors of ABI is needed to improve their short-term rehabilitation outcomes and long-term community reentry outcomes. This research should be used in conjunction with other empirical and theoretical literature to ultimately improve the quality of life of adult survivors of traumatic brain injury. Future research can use the results of this study as a foundation to build upon the idea of the sick role as a process. Sick role process was defined in the current study by measuring only two of the four sick role variables, prerehab sick role rights, and postrehab sick role responsibilities. Future research can utilize the four sick role variables which all had significant bivariate relationships with other variables, especially anxiety, goal attainment, depression, age, and gender. Operationally, the concept of sick role rights at the beginning of the rehabilitation should be examined further in future research due to the moderate reliability of the instrument that measured that specific concept. In addition, the instrument was memory dependent and this should be a consideration in future research.

4.1. Limitations of the Study. The present study has some methodological limitations that weaken the ability to generalize findings beyond the scope of this particular sample group. Sampling technique, sample size, instrumentation, control of independent, and human error are all variables which limit this study's generalizability.

The technique of convenience sampling was utilized due to limitations of resources. Randomization was not used which is a main quantitative tool for control of extraneous variables. The small sample size ($n = 60$) also weakened the power of the analysis when multiple variables were analyzed within the sample. Related to instrumentation, although the BSRPI was developed with consultation from brain injury experts, validity would have been increased if the experts were also experts on the concept of sick role. Reliability would have been increased if the BSRPI had been pilot tested several times prior to its use. ABI survivors sometimes have limited insight into their own problems due to cognitive processing which is a threat to internal validity, although screening methods were used to attempt to control for this threat.

Control variables that were derived from the prior literature were utilized to reduce the possibility of external sources of variance. However, there are possibly other independent variables that were not considered that were not in prior literature. Lastly, this researcher was the only person who collected data, which increased interrater reliability. However, human error is always a possibility when collecting data and inputting and analyzing data.

Appendix

A. Barclay Sick Role Process Inventory

Instructions:

Please answer the following statements with (a)Strongly Disagree, (b)Disagree, (c)Agree, or (d)Strongly Agree.

Statements in Part I will focus on your beliefs and feelings you had at the beginning of your rehabilitation.

Statements in Part II will focus on your beliefs and feelings now.

Part I: Please Answer All of Questions in Part I Based on How You Felt at the Beginning of Your Rehabilitation

(1) When I first started in this program, I had a right to be excused from all my daily responsibilities.

    (a) Strongly Disagree
    (b) Disagree
    (c) Agree
    (d) Strongly Agree

(2) When I first started in this program, my family and friends should not have expected me to do as much for them as I did before my brain injury.

    (a) Strongly Disagree
    (b) Disagree
    (c) Agree
    (d) Strongly Agree

(3) When I first started in this program, I expected that others care for and protect me.

    (a) Strongly Disagree
    (b) Disagree
    (c) Agree
    (d) Strongly Agree

(4) When I first started in this program, I believed it was not my fault that I had a brain injury.

    (a) Strongly Disagree
    (b) Disagree
    (c) Agree
    (d) Strongly Agree

(5) When I first started in this program, I deserved any disability benefits for which I was qualified (for example: time off from work or school or disability checks).

    (a) Strongly Disagree
    (b) Disagree

(c) Agree

(d) Strongly Agree

(6) When I first started in this program, I thought my injury was a punishment for past sins.

   (a) Strongly Disagree

   (b) Disagree

   (c) Agree

   (d) Strongly Agree

(7) When I first started in this program, my priority was to get back to work or school and my normal routine.

   (a) Strongly Disagree

   (b) Disagree

   (c) Agree

   (d) Strongly Agree

(8) When I first started in this program, I was looking forward to getting back to work and my normal routine.

   (a) Strongly Disagree

   (b) Disagree

   (c) Agree

   (d) Strongly Agree

(9) When I first started in this program, I wanted to get better than I was.

   (a) Strongly Disagree

   (b) Disagree

   (c) Agree

   (d) Strongly Agree

(10) When I first started in this program, I believed it was important to get expert rehabilitation care.

   (a) Strongly Disagree

   (b) Disagree

   (c) Agree

   (d) Strongly Agree

(11) When I first started in this program, it was important to me to regularly attend all rehabilitation and medical appointments.

   (a) Strongly Disagree

   (b) Disagree

   (c) Agree

   (d) Strongly Agree

(12) When I first started in this program, it was important to me to follow all of my therapists' suggestions and apply those suggestions in my home life.

   (a) Strongly Disagree

   (b) Disagree

   (c) Agree

   (d) Strongly Agree

Part II: Please answer all of questions in Part II based on how you feel now

(1) Now, I have the right to be excused from all my daily responsibilities.

   (a) Strongly Disagree

   (b) Disagree

   (c) Agree

   (d) Strongly Agree

(2) Now, my family and friends should not expect me to do as much for them as I did before my brain injury.

   (a) Strongly Disagree

   (b) Disagree

   (c) Agree

   (d) Strongly Agree

(3) Now, I expect others to care for and protect me.

   (a) Strongly Disagree

   (b) Disagree

   (c) Agree

   (d) Strongly Agree

(4) Now, I believe it is not my fault that I have a brain injury.

   (a) Strongly Disagree

   (b) Disagree

   (c) Agree

   (d) Strongly Agree

(5) Now, I deserve any disability benefits for which I am qualified (for example: time off from work or school or disability checks).

   (a) Strongly Disagree

   (b) Disagree

   (c) Agree

   (d) Strongly Agree

(6) Now, I think my injury is a punishment for past sins.

   (a) Strongly Disagree

   (b) Disagree

   (c) Agree

   (d) Strongly Agree

(7) Now, my priority is to get back to work or school and my normal routine.

   (a) Strongly Disagree

   (b) Disagree

   (c) Agree

   (d) Strongly Agree

(8) Now, I am looking forward to getting back to work and my normal routine.

   (a) Strongly Disagree
   (b) Disagree
   (c) Agree
   (d) Strongly Agree

(9) Now, I want to get better than I am.

   (a) Strongly Disagree
   (b) Disagree
   (c) Agree
   (d) Strongly Agree

(10) Now, it is important that I get expert rehabilitation care.

   (a) Strongly Disagree
   (b) Disagree
   (c) Agree
   (d) Strongly Agree

(11) Now, it is important to me to regularly attend all rehabilitation and medical appointments.

   (a) Strongly Disagree
   (b) Disagree
   (c) Agree
   (d) Strongly Agree

(12) Now, it is important to me to follow all of my therapists' suggestions and apply those suggestions in my home life.

   (a) Strongly Disagree
   (b) Disagree
   (c) Agree
   (d) Strongly Agree

B. Goal Attainment Scale

Primary therapist "Goal attainment scale" Name of client: Based on your prediction when the client first entered the rehabilitation program, for your specific discipline, please mark the outcome for this client

Level of Predicted Attainment

(1) Most unfavorable outcome thought likely

   (a) Psychosocial —
   (b) Occupational —
   (c) Physical —
   (d) Cognitive —

(2) Less than expected success

   (a) Psychosocial —
   (b) Occupational —
   (c) Physical —
   (d) Cognitive —

(3) Expected level of success

   (a) Psychosocial —
   (b) Occupational —
   (c) Physical —
   (d) Cognitive —

(4) More than expected success

   (a) Psychosocial —
   (b) Occupational —
   (c) Physical —
   (d) Cognitive —

(5) Most favorable outcome thought

   (a) Psychosocial —
   (b) Occupational —
   (c) Physical —
   (d) Cognitive —

References

[1] M. Faul, L. Xu, M. M. Wald, and V. Coronado, *Traumatic Brain Injury in the United States: Emergency Department Visits, Hospitalizations and Deaths, 2002–2006*, Centers for Disease Control and Prevention, National Center for Injury Prevention and Control, Atlanta, Ga, USA, 2010.

[2] H. Fischer, "U.S. Military casualty statistics: operation new dawn, operation Iraqi freedom, and operation enduring freedom," Congressional Research Service 7-5700, RS22452, September 2010, http://www.fas.org/sgp/crs/natsec/RS22452.pdf.

[3] J. Prejean, R. Song, A. Hernandez et al., "Estimated HIV incidence in the United States, 2006–2009," *PLoS ONE*, vol. 6, no. 8, Article ID e17502, 2011.

[4] W. Rosamond, K. Flegal, G. Friday et al., "Heart disease and stroke statistics—2007 Update: a report from the American Heart Association Statistics Committee and Stroke Statistics Subcommittee," *Circulation*, vol. 115, no. 5, pp. e69–e171, 2007.

[5] National Spinal CordInjury Statistical Center (NSCISC), https://www.nscisc.uab.edu/PublicDocuments/fact_figures_docs/Facts%202012%20Feb%20Final.pdf.

[6] M. D. Van Den Broek, "Why does neurorehabilitation fail?" *Journal of Head Trauma Rehabilitation*, vol. 20, no. 5, pp. 464–473, 2005.

[7] J. R. Fann, W. J. Katon, J. M. Uomoto, and P. C. Esselman, "Psychiatric disorders and functional disability in outpatients with traumatic brain injuries," *American Journal of Psychiatry*, vol. 152, no. 10, pp. 1493–1499, 1996.

[8] G. J. Demakis, F. M. Hammond, and A. Knotts, "Prediction of depression and anxiety 1 year after moderate-severe traumatic brain injury," *Applied Neuropsychology*, vol. 17, no. 3, pp. 183–189, 2010.

[9] R. E. Jorge, R. G. Robinson, S. E. Starkstein, and S. V. Arndt, "Influence of major depression on 1-year outcome in patients with traumatic brain injury," *Journal of Neurosurgery*, vol. 81, no. 5, pp. 726–733, 1994.

[10] E. M. S. Sherman, E. Strauss, D. J. Slick, and F. Spellacy, "Effect of depression on neuropsychological functioning in head injury: measurable but minimal," *Brain Injury*, vol. 14, no. 7, pp. 621–632, 2000.

[11] R. Van Reekum, I. Bolago, M. A. J. Finlayson, S. Garner, and P. S. Links, "Psychiatric disorders after traumatic brain injury," *Brain Injury*, vol. 10, no. 5, pp. 319–327, 1996.

[12] R. E. Jorge, R. G. Robinson, D. Moser, A. Tateno, B. Crespo-Facorro, and S. Arndt, "Major depression following traumatic brain injury," *Archives of General Psychiatry*, vol. 61, no. 1, pp. 42–50, 2004.

[13] C. Konrad, A. J. Geburek, F. Rist et al., "Long-term cognitive and emotional consequences of mild traumatic brain injury," *Psychological Medicine*, vol. 41, no. 6, pp. 1197–1211, 2011.

[14] K. Baker, C. Tandy, and D. Dixon, "Traumatic brain injury: a social worker primer with implications for practice," *Journal of Social Work in Disability & Rehabilitation*, vol. 1, pp. 25–42, 2002.

[15] D. X. Cifu, L. Keyser-Marcus, E. Lopez et al., "Acute predictors of successful return to work 1 year after traumatic brain injury: a multicenter analysis," *Archives of Physical Medicine and Rehabilitation*, vol. 78, no. 2, pp. 125–131, 1997.

[16] K. M. Hall, P. Karzmark, M. Stevens, J. Englander, P. O'Hare, and J. Wright, "Family stressors in traumatic brain injury: a two-year follow-up," *Archives of Physical Medicine and Rehabilitation*, vol. 75, no. 8, pp. 876–884, 1994.

[17] B. A. Moore and J. Donders, "Predictors of invalid neuropsychological test performance after traumatic brain injury," *Brain Injury*, vol. 18, no. 10, pp. 975–984, 2004.

[18] M. A. Keiski, D. L. Shore, and J. M. Hamilton, "The role of depression in verbal memory following traumatic brain injury," *Clinical Neuropsychologist*, vol. 21, no. 5, pp. 744–761, 2007.

[19] C. Stephens, *Personality and emotional coping in traumatic brain injured adults undergoing rehabilitation [Ph.D. thesis]*, University of North Carolina at Chapel Hill, 1999.

[20] M. Stratton and R. J. Gregory, "Examining perspective-taking in the severely head injured," *Brain Injury*, vol. 8, pp. 631–645, 1994.

[21] D. Dawson, *The determinants and correlates of outcome following traumatic brain injury: a prospective study [Ph.D. thesis]*, University of Toronto, 1999.

[22] A. A. Lubusko, A. D. Moore, M. Stambrook, and D. D. Gill, "Cognitive beliefs following severe traumatic brain injury: association with post-injury employment status," *Brain Injury*, vol. 8, no. 1, pp. 265–276, 1994.

[23] K. Meredith and G. Rassa, "Aligning the levels of awareness with the stages of grieving," *Journal of Cognitive Rehabilitation*, vol. 17, pp. 10–14, 1999.

[24] M. Oddy, T. Coughlan, A. Tyerman, and D. Jenkins, "Social adjustment after closed head injury: a further follow-up seven years after injury," *Journal of Neurology Neurosurgery and Psychiatry*, vol. 48, no. 6, pp. 564–568, 1985.

[25] C. A. Wallace, J. Bogner, J. D. Corrigan, D. Clinchot, W. J. Mysiw, and L. P. Fugate, "Primary caregivers of persons with brain injury: Life change 1 year after injury," *Brain Injury*, vol. 12, no. 6, pp. 483–493, 1998.

[26] T. Parsons, *The Social System*, Free Press, Glencoe, Ill, USA, 1951.

[27] B. J. Biddle and E. J. Thomas, "Role Theory: Concepts and Research," pp. John Wiley & Sons–New York, NY, USA, 1966.

[28] T. Parsons, "Definitions of health and illness in the light of American values and social structure," in *Social Structure and Personality*, T. Parsons, Ed., pp. 257–291, The Free Press of Glencoe, New York, NY, USA, 1964.

[29] G. Gordon, *Role Theory and Illness: A Sociological Perspective*, College and University Press, New Haven, Conn, USA, 1966.

[30] A. Arluke, L. Kennedy, and R. C. Kessler, "Reexamining the sick-role concept: an empirical assessment," *Journal of Health and Social Behavior*, vol. 20, no. 1, pp. 30–36, 1979.

[31] J. S. Brown and M. Rawlinson, "Relinquishing the sick role following open heart surgery," *Journal of Health and Social Behavior*, vol. 16, no. 1, pp. 12–27, 1975.

[32] J. S. Brown and M. E. Rawlinson, "Sex differences in sick role rejection and in work performance following cardiac surgery," *Journal of Health and Social Behavior*, vol. 18, no. 3, pp. 276–292, 1977.

[33] G. G. Kassebaum and B. O. Baumann, "Dimensions of the sick role in chronic illness," *Journal of Health and Human Behavior*, vol. 106, pp. 16–27, 1965.

[34] Centers for Disease Control, "Traumatic brain injury in the United States: a report to Congress," Centers for Disease Control, January 2001, http://www.cdc.gov/ncipc/pubres/tbi_congress/.

[35] S. T. Myers and H. G. Grasmick, "The social rights and responsibilities of pregnant women: an application of Parsons' sick role model," *Journal of Applied Behavioral Science*, vol. 26, pp. 157–172, 1992.

[36] L. R. Derogatis and N. Melisaratos, "The Brief Symptom Inventory: an introductory report," *Psychological Medicine*, vol. 13, no. 3, pp. 595–605, 1983.

[37] D. Landy and H. Wechsler, "Rehabilitation, socialization and pathway organizations," in *Role Theory: Concepts and Research*, B. Biddle and E. Thomas, Eds., pp. 376–382, John Wiley & Sons, New York, NY, USA, 1966.

[38] L. Derogatis, *Brief Symptom Inventory 18: Administration, Scoring, and Procedures Manual*, NCS Pearson, Bloomington, Minn, USA, 2001.

6

Reliability of Measuring the Cervical Sagittal Translation Mobility with a Simple Method in a Clinical Setting

Yvonne Severinsson,[1] Lena Elisson,[2] and Olle Bunketorp[2]

[1] Department of Stomatognathic Physiology, Institute of Odontology, The Sahlgrenska Academy,
  University of Gothenburg, Gothenburg, Sweden
[2] Department of Orthopaedics, The Institute of Clinical Sciences, The Sahlgrenska Academy,
  University of Gothenburg, Gothenburg, Sweden

Correspondence should be addressed to Yvonne Severinsson, yvonne.severinsson@gmail.com

Academic Editor: Nicola Smania

Introduction. The cervical sagittal translation mobility is related to neck pain. A practical method for measuring the specific cervical mobility is needed. The aim was to describe a simple method for measuring the cervical sagittal translation mobility and to evaluate its reliability in a clinical setting. *Method.* The head protraction and retraction ranges of thirty healthy seated subjects were measured from a dorsal reference plane by two physiotherapists utilizing a tape measure. A standard inclinometer/goniometer was used to minimize angular movements of the head during the translational movements. The measurements were made twice for each subject with a two-hours interval between each measurement. The inter-rater and intra-rater agreements were evaluated with intraclass correlation coefficients (ICCs) and with the distribution of the difference of the measurements. The systematic differences were analysed with the Wilcoxon signed rank test. *Results.* The intra-rater agreement was good. The inter-rater agreement was moderate in the first measurement and good in the second. A systematic difference was noted between raters in the first measurement but not in the second, possibly indicating a learning effect. *Discussion.* The method used in the study is simple and reliable and can be recommended for clinical use.

1. Introduction

The biomechanics of the cervical spine is complex. Symptoms arising from the cervical spine vary, and researchers suggest that neck pain should be subdivided into upper cervical spinal pain and lower cervical spinal pain, above or below an imaginary transverse plane through C4 [1]. The cervical sagittal translation movements consist of protraction and retraction; protraction causing a flexion of the lower cervical spine and an extension of the upper cervical spine, and retraction the opposite [2, 3]. It has been suggested that these cervical movements are important in the rehabilitation of the neck [4–7]. Head posture is related to the natural configuration of the cervical spine [8]. Forward head posture can be defined when the center of gravity of the head is displaced ventral to the gravity line through the body of C7.

Neck pain is often associated with a restricted range of motion in the cervical spine [9–11], and several authors have studied the significance of head posture in subjects with neck pain [12–15]. Static forward head posture, such as having the head in a protracted position for long periods of time, causes posterior neck pain to develop in healthy subjects, according to Harms-Ringdahl and Ekholm [16]. There is also evidence that neck patients have significantly less range of the cervical sagittal translation mobility than normal subjects [13]. Cervical sagittal translation mobility has been studied in WAD (Whiplash Associated Disorders) patients and appears to be especially related to neck distortion in rear-end car impacts [17].

Clearly the mobility of the cervical spine is an important parameter in the physiotherapist's clinical work. An objective assessment of the active cervical range of motion (ACROM) requires a good measurement accuracy. Different measurement instruments have been tested for validity and reliability for ACROM, including flexion, extension, rotation, and side bending [18–25], and an inclinometer/goniometer is considered to be practical to use [22]. A practical method for measuring head posture [26, 27] and the total head excursion has also been presented [12, 13]. The range of cervical sagittal translation mobility has been assessed in radiographic studies [28–31]. However, to our knowledge, a simple and reliable method to accurately make such measurements in a clinical setting has been neither described nor tested. The aim of this study was to describe a simple method for the measurement of the cervical sagittal translation mobility and to evaluate its reliability in a clinical setting.

2. Method

The study was conducted by two physiotherapists (A and B); both specialized in issues of the cervical spine, well trained for this purpose, and with extensive experience in the use of the measurement device.

2.1. Subjects and Data Collection. Thirty healthy subjects, 21 women (mean age 44, range 26–64) and nine men (mean age 33, range 25–54), were included. Eleven women and three men, all physiotherapists, were recruited from the Department of Physiotherapy at Sahlgrenska University Hospital in Gothenburg. Six male dental students were recruited from the Institute of Odontology at The Sahlgrenska Academy in Gothenburg. Ten female dental nurses were recruited from a specialist clinic at the Public Dental Service in Gothenburg. All subjects were verbally informed of the purpose of the study and invited to participate. The only exclusion criterion was ongoing neck problems. The data collection was carried out during February and March 2009.

2.2. Measurement Equipment. A Myrin's inclinometer/goniometer (Art. Nr. 711432, Bålsta, Sweden) was used. The instrument has an inclination needle, affected by gravity, that is used to measure side bending, flexion, and extension. It also has a compass needle that is used to measure horizontal rotation. The instrument was attached to the head by means of a Velcro strip. A metal tape measure was used to measure, in millimeters, the sagittal translation mobility during head protraction and retraction.

2.3. Procedure. The subjects were measured in random order, using identical equipment, arranged in the same way. Independently of each other, the raters A and B measured one subject each in the same room and on the same occasion, and the two subjects changed places immediately after the measurements. Each rater filled in their own protocol after testing each subject. All protocols were separated from each other and not checked between the measurements. Each subject was examined four times. The first two measurements of each subject were made before noon (12.00 P.M.) by A and B and were made within 30 minutes of each other. After two hours elapsed, the measurements were then repeated using the identical method and instrument as had been used for the first measurement.

The translation mobility of each subject was measured with the subject sitting on a stool close to a wall while maintaining good upright balanced posture, with both feet on the floor, with normal lumbar lordosis, hands on thighs, and with 90 degrees in the hip and knee joints. The subject was requested to assume a neutral head position, with the purpose of positioning the head's center of mass in a vertical plane through the atlantooccipital joints with the nose pointing forward in line with the sternum and bellybutton. A wedge-formed pad was fixed between the upper thoracic spine and the wall in an attempt to minimize the thoracic spine motions. The pad was placed with its upper edge at the spinous processes of C7-TH1. The inclinometer was placed above the right ear with its needle pointing vertically towards the centre of the external ear channel. The inclinometer was calibrated and held at zero in order to avoid head flexion/extension during these movements.

The distance between the wall and the vertical line of the inclinometer needle was measured with the metal tape measure with the subject's head in the neutral position. The end of the tape measure was placed so that it extended from the wall at a 90 degree angle and laid horizontally close to the needle (Figure 1). After measuring the neutral position, the subject was asked to protract the head maximally while the rater checked the inclinometer. In order to achieve a pure translation, divergences from the vertical line were corrected, in case a head flexion or extension occurred. If so, the needle indicated this movement and the rater guided the subject into the right position. At the maximum protraction, the distance between the needle and the wall was measured again (Figure 1). The subject then moved the head backwards to the neutral position. A similar procedure was used for retraction (Figure 1). The movements were performed once, and the values of the measurements were added to the protocol in centimeters carried to one decimal point. The difference between the maximum protraction and the maximum retraction ranges—the sagittal mobility (SM)—was calculated for each subject and then analyzed statistically.

2.4. Ethical Considerations. Approval from the ethical committee was not applied for the study.

2.5. Calculations and Statistical Analyses. All data were compiled and analyzed with the standard version of SPSS 17.0 (Statistics Package for the Social Sciences, Chicago, IL, USA), except for the within-rater standard deviation (WRSD), which was calculated by use of the following formula [32]:

$$\text{WRSD} = \sqrt{\left[\frac{\text{SMdiff}_n^2}{2 * N} \right]}, \qquad (1)$$

where SMdiff_n = difference for the sagittal mobility between the first and second measurement for case n; $n = 1, 2, \ldots, N$; $N = 30$.

Systematic differences between the two measurements of the sagittal mobility made by each rater and between the measurements made by the two raters were both analyzed

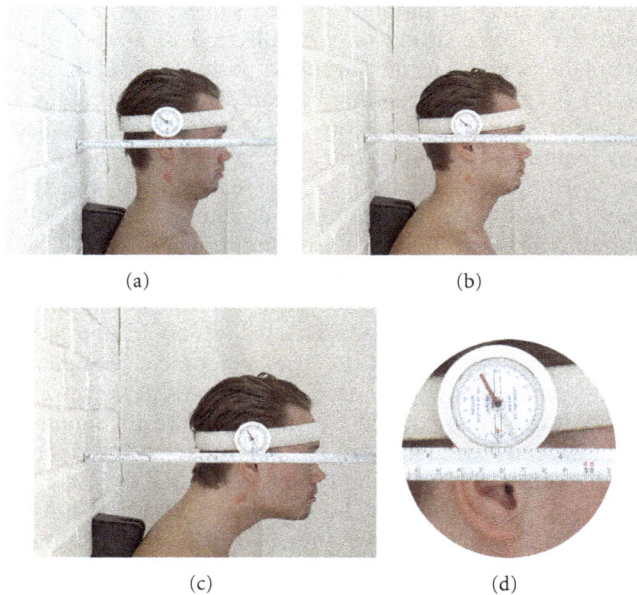

FIGURE 1: Measuring in the retracted, neutral, and protracted position of the head with the inclinometer and metal tape measure.

with Wilcoxon Signed Rank Test for related samples. All significance tests were two-tailed and conducted at the 5% significance level.

The intra-rater and the inter-rater reliability were both described with the intraclass correlation coefficient (ICC), using the SPSS alfa two-way mixed model and consistency type. ICC values ≥0.81 were considered very good, 0.61–0.80 good, 0.41–0.60 moderate, and ≤0.40 fair or poor [33].

The 95% limits of the inter-rater agreements were calculated as the mean value of the differences between the raters ± 1.96 times the standard deviation of these differences. Bland-Altman plots and scatter plots of the differences between the measurements versus the means are given both for the inter-rater and the intra-rater analysis.

3. Results

The measurement data for protraction, neutral position, and retraction are presented in Table 1.

The statistical data for estimation of the intra-rater and the inter-rater agreement are presented in Table 2 and Table 3, respectively.

The mean value of the sagittal mobility (SM; protraction minus retraction) for all measurements was 9.1 cm (range 4.4–14.0; SD = 1.9). The differences for SM measured by A on the two occasions, versus the mean values of SM, are shown in Figure 2(a) (intra-rater comparison). The differences were not correlated to the mean values for A (Pearson correlation coefficient = 0.26; P = 0.16). Figure 2(b) shows the corresponding data for B, and in this case such a correlation was found (Pearson correlation coefficient = −0,48; P = 0.007).

The differences for SM measured by A and B on the first occasion versus the mean values are shown in Figure 3(a) (inter-rater comparison). These differences were significantly correlated to the mean values (Pearson correlation coefficient = 0.74; P < 0.001). The corresponding values for the second measurement are shown in Figure 3(b). No correlation was found between the differences and the mean values for the second measurements (Pearson correlation coefficient = 0.28; P = 0.14).

4. Discussion

This study describes a simple method for measuring the cervical sagittal translation mobility in a clinical setting, using an existing measuring device for cervical angular movements, combined with a metal tape measure. The instrument used for cervical angular movements in the study is well known and has been used since many years in Sweden. Similar instruments may exist on the market. We cannot see why these would give less accuracy using the same method, but this should be confirmed.

The intra-rater agreement was good. The systematic difference was not statistically significant for either of the raters, and the intraclass correlation coefficient (ICC) was 0.7 for both of them (Table 2). The differences for A showed a somewhat greater variation (SD 1.72, range −3.3 : 4.2 cm) than for B (SD 1.07, range −2.0 : 2.5 cm). However, the differences for A were not correlated to the mean values (Figure 2(a)). Such a correlation was found for B (Figure 2(b)). The within-rater standard deviation was 1.2 cm for A and 0.8 cm for B (Table 2). The mean of these values (1.0 cm) is eleven percent of the mean value (9.1 cm) of the sagittal mobility. For A, the differences were less or equal to 1.5 cm in seventeen of the thirty cases (57%) and less or equal to 1 cm in fourteen cases (47%). For B, the differences between the measurements were less or equal to 1.5 cm in twenty-six of the thirty cases (87%) and less or equal to 1 cm in twenty-four cases (80%).

The inter-rater agreement was moderate and showed a systematic difference at the first examination (ICC = 0.53; P = 0.036; Table 3; Figure 3(a)). However, the differences between the raters varied widely (SD: 1.88 cm; 95% limits of agreement: −2.91; 4.47), and A recorded greater differences than B in most cases, especially at greater mobility (Figure 3(a)). The differences were less or equal to 1.5 cm in sixteen of the thirty cases (53%). The inter-rater agreement was good and without systematic difference at the second measurement (ICC = 0.67; P = 0.412; Table 3; Figure 3(b)). The SD for the difference was 1.5 cm (95% limits of agreement −2.7; 3.3). The differences were less or equal to 1.5 cm in twenty of the thirty cases (67%). A better agreement during the second measurements compared with the first ones may be an effect of what was learned by the raters during the first series of measurements.

Various circumstances may affect the reliability of the methodology employed in this study. Variations in the measurements taken by the raters, both inter-rater and intra-rater reliability, are due to factors relating to the subjects

TABLE 1: Horizontal distance (cm) between the reference plane (the wall) and the measuring point (the Myrin inclinometer needle) during maximum active protraction, neutral position, and maximum active retraction for the two raters and the two measurements.

Case	Sex	Age	Rater A						Rater B					
			Measurement 1			Measurement 2			Measurement 1			Measurement 2		
			Protraction	Neutral	Retraction	Protraction	Neutral	Retraction	Protraction	Neutral	Retraction	Protraction	Neutral	Retraction
1	f	26	25.3	17.5	16.0	25.0	18.0	15.6	24.5	18.0	15.3	24.5	18.5	15.5
2	f	24	22.5	16.5	14.5	25.3	18.0	14.0	24.5	17.7	15.0	23.0	17.5	14.5
3	f	50	23.8	18.5	14.0	23.3	18.2	13.5	23.0	18.6	15.0	22.0	18.0	16.0
4	f	37	23.2	17.0	11.7	22.8	18.0	13.0	23.0	17.0	14.0	22.0	16.0	12.0
5	f	25	21.7	17.0	11.9	21.2	16.3	11.9	22.0	17.0	14.0	21.5	16.5	12.5
6	f	53	26.8	18.8	16.0	25.5	18.0	16.2	26.0	18.5	16.5	24.5	19.0	14.5
7	f	61	23.6	18.2	15.3	21.5	17.6	14.0	23.5	18.3	15.5	24.5	18.5	17.0
8	f	44	19.0	15.0	12.0	21.5	16.5	12.8	20.5	16.0	12.0	22.5	17.0	12.0
9	f	39	21.8	16.5	14.8	22.0	17.0	14.5	21.5	15.0	12.5	22.0	17.0	14.0
10	f	34	24.5	17.0	13.5	24.5	18.0	14.0	23.0	16.5	14.0	24.0	18.0	15.5
11	f	56	23.5	17.0	13.5	22.8	17.4	13.5	23.0	17.0	13.5	24.0	18.0	14.5
12	m	39	19.5	15.3	10.9	21.5	17.2	13.0	20.5	17.0	13.0	21.5	17.0	14.5
13	m	27	26.0	16.0	12.2	26.0	16.0	12.8	24.0	16.8	14.0	25.0	17.5	14.0
14	m	32	24.5	15.7	13.5	25.0	16.0	13.0	24.0	17.0	15.5	25.0	17.5	15.0
15	m	25	33.2	27.3	26.2	22.0	17.0	13.5	23.0	16.5	14.5	21.0	16.0	12.5
16	m	29	25.8	16.8	12.2	25.2	18.5	13.4	24.0	16.3	14.0	24.0	17.0	12.0
17	m	31	27.5	17.3	13.8	26.0	17.3	14.0	26.5	19.2	16.5	27.0	20.0	16.5
18	m	25	28.5	18.5	14.5	25.7	17.5	14.0	27.0	18.0	16.0	26.0	18.0	14.5
19	m	33	24.5	16.5	11.3	21.5	16.5	12.5	23.5	17.5	12.5	23.0	17.0	13.0
20	m	25	25.5	19.5	15.5	29.0	20.5	17.0	28.0	19.6	18.0	27.0	20.0	16.0
21	f	46	22.5	16.5	14.5	24.3	17.0	13.5	22.5	17.2	15.0	23.5	18.0	15.0
22	f	63	20.0	16.0	13.0	20.6	16.0	13.7	23.5	17.2	15.0	22.5	17.5	14.0
23	f	45	18.2	15.5	12.8	21.7	16.6	14.3	22.0	15.5	13.0	20.5	16.0	14.0
24	f	56	19.8	15.3	13.2	18.2	15.5	13.8	21.0	16.5	14.8	20.0	15.5	13.8
25	f	39	22.4	17.5	14.2	20.0	15.3	11.6	22.3	18.5	14.5	21.0	16.0	13.0
26	f	40	22.4	17.2	12.5	21.0	15.2	14.0	21.5	16.2	12.5	23.0	16.5	13.0
27	f	56	21.0	18.0	15.2	19.5	16.0	12.3	23.0	18.2	15.0	22.2	18.5	14.0
28	f	41	22.3	15.8	11.6	23.2	17.2	13.2	22.5	16.5	13.0	24.0	18.0	13.0
29	f	46	19.7	14.5	10.2	20.2	15.9	12.3	19.5	16.3	12.0	20.5	16.2	12.3
30	f	45	20.7	16.5	13.5	22.7	19.0	16.5	23.2	19.0	17.0	24.0	20.5	18.0

TABLE 2: Assessment of the intra-rater agreement for the cervical translation mobility in the sagittal plane for rater A and B. The mean values for the differences between the two measurements made by A and the two measurements made by B are presented together with its SD, medians, and ranges, as well as the P values for the systematic difference, the within-rater standard deviation, and the intraclass correlation coefficient (ICC).

Rater	N	Difference between the first and second measurements on each subject made by each of the raters (cm)					Systematic difference P value	Within-rater standard deviation (cm)	ICC
		Mean	SD	Median	Range				
					Min	Max			
A	30	0.29	1.72	0.50	−3.30	4.2	0.32	1.22	0.71
B	30	−0.22	1.07	−0.20	−2.00	2.5	0.20	0.76	0.72

TABLE 3: The inter-rater agreement for the total cervical translation mobility in the sagittal plane. Mean values, standard deviations (SD), medians, minimum and maximum ranges of motion for rater A and B and for the differences between A and B are presented, as well as the limits of agreement (individual reference interval (mean ± 1.96 ∗ SD)), the P values for the systematic differences, and the intraclass correlation coefficients (ICC).

Measurement nr	N	Rater A					Rater B					Difference between rater A and B						95% Limits of agreement		Systematic difference	ICC
					Range					Range						Range				P value	
		Mean	SD	Median	Min	Max	Mean	SD	Median	Min	Max	Mean	SD	Median	Min	Max	Lower	Higher		
1	30	9.5	2.5	9.7	5.4	14.0	8.8	1.2	9.0	6.2	11.0	0.8	1.9	1.0	−3.6	3.8	−2.9	4.5	0.036	0.53
2	30	9.2	2.1	9.3	4.4	13.2	9.0	1.7	8.8	6.0	12.0	0.3	1.5	0.1	−3.0	3.8	−2.7	3.3	0.412	0.67

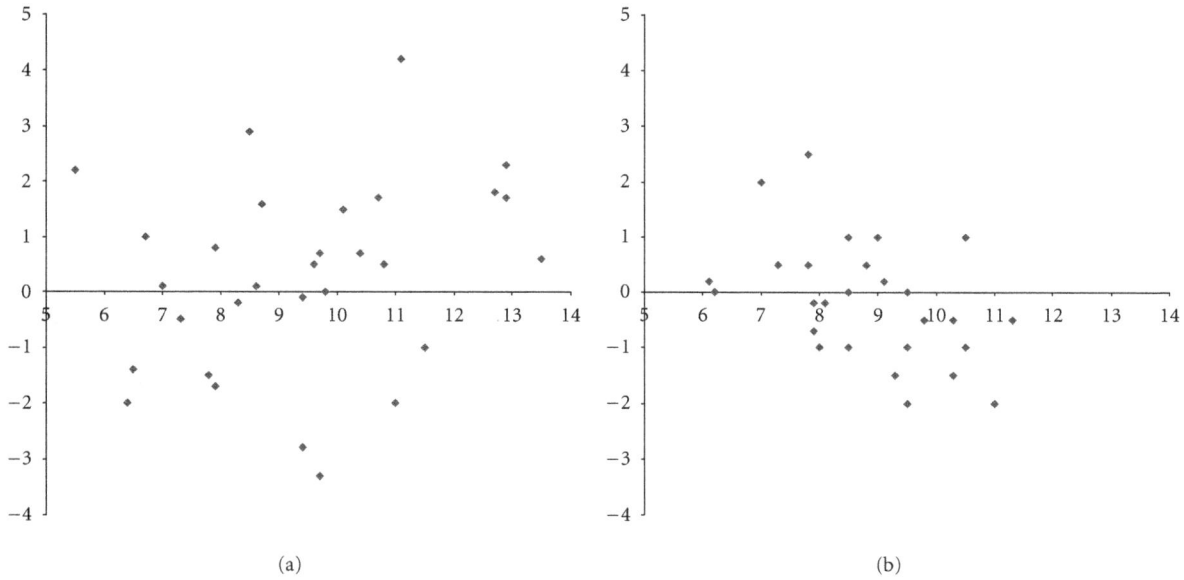

FIGURE 2: (a) Bland-Altman plot showing differences for the sagittal mobility (cm) at the two measurements (Y-axis) made by rater A versus the mean values of these measurements (X-axis). Every dot represents one subject. (b) Bland-Altman plot showing differences for the sagittal mobility (cm) at the two measurements (Y-axis) made by rater B versus the mean values of these measurements (X-axis). Every dot represents one subject.

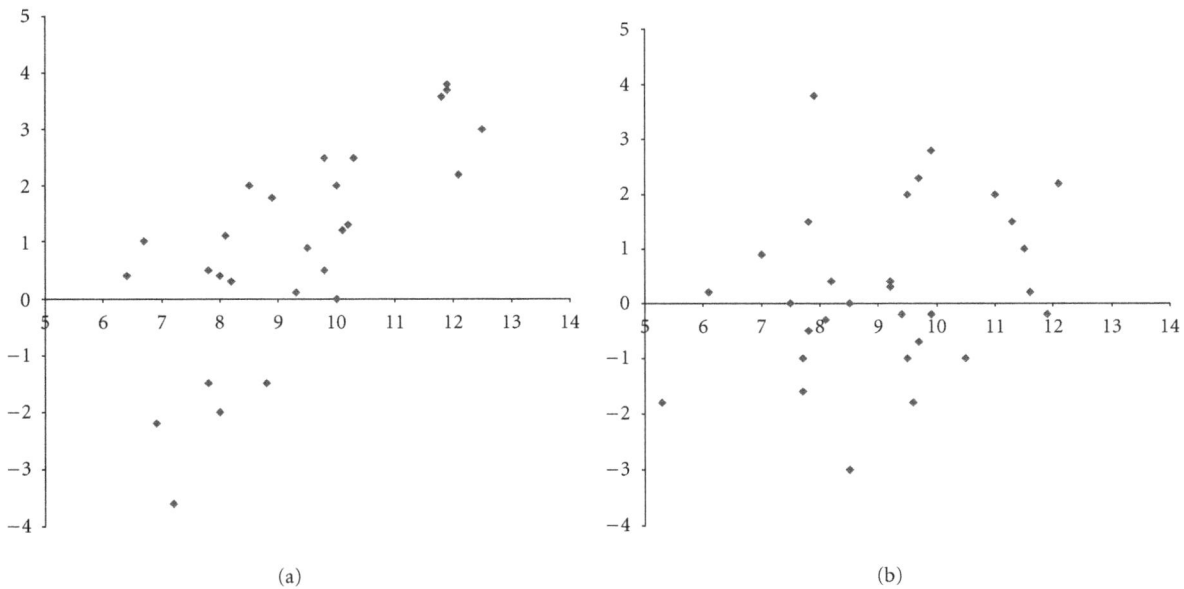

FIGURE 3: (a) Bland-Altman plot showing differences for the sagittal mobility (cm) at the first measurements (Y-axis) made by rater A and rater B versus the mean values of these differences (X-axis). Every dot represents one subject. (b) Bland-Altman plot showing differences for the sagittal mobility (cm) at the second measurements (Y-axis) made by rater A and rater B versus the mean values of these differences (X-axis). Every dot represents one subject.

individually, the measurement instruments and the measurement process. The subject may differ in range of motion for various reasons. Some subjects may have had more neck or back stiffness in the morning because of pathological changes or muscle tension. Some subjects complained about neck pain after the first measurements, which could inhibit

movements during the second measurements. Other factors are the motivation of the subjects, their ability to understand the instructions, and the raters' behaviour, that is, to inspire and instruct the subjects, or the subject's ability to make and repeat the movement in the same way [19, 21]. It is also important to standardize the position of the instrument on the head, to check the vertical pointer in order to adjust the head inclination during the horizontal movements when necessary, and to the place wedge correctly at C7-Th1 in order to avoid thoracic movements. Variation also depends on the sitting position, how the head is moved during the translation as well as during measurement of the distance between the wall and neutral position, which may vary each time a subject changes positions. A critical point was to keep the tape measure horizontal during the measurements. The use of a metal tape measure made this easier, and the authors do not think that small deviations from the horizontal position will influence the measurements so much.

Penning [2] demonstrated ten degrees greater extension during protraction in the upper cervical segments than in the other segments compared with normal full-length extension. He has also shown that the flexion ability in the upper cervical was ten degrees greater during retraction than during normal full-length flexion. Head translation in the sagittal plane also produces displacements in cervical-thoracic motion segments. Persson et al. [34] measured the total head excursion and found that approximately ten percent of the total head excursion originated from the thoracic regions in the sitting position. The authors tried to control for this bias by stabilizing the upper thoracic segments using a wedge for the subject to lean against. Thoracic movements may still have contributed to the measure differences between the raters in our study. This technical error was not observed by Hanten et al. [12, 13], who measured the total head excursion using a simple measurement method in normal and patient comparisons.

The reliability of nonradiological measurements of the cervical translation mobility has not been investigated sufficiently, and to our knowledge there is no reference for normative values, which have been estimated with a simple instrument in a clinical setting. The method presented in this study has been used for WAD patients [17]. Hanten et al. [12, 13] measured the total head excursion in the sagittal plane, and they concluded that the mean distance from the fully retracted to the fully protracted position was 7 cm for subjects with neck pain and 10.9 cm for subjects without neck pain; however, they did not test the reliability of their methodology. Hanten et al. [12, 13] also found that women had different head posture than men. In our study we investigated only healthy subjects without regard to age or gender and found that the mean distance from the fully retracted to the fully protracted position was 9.1 cm. Age and asymptomatic degenerative changes affect the cervical range of motion [20, 22]. The total cervical sagittal translation mobility has been measured on sagittal flexion radiographs and the authors found that women differed significantly from men [28, 30, 31]. Also a nonradiological study has shown that women have greater cervical translation mobility in the sagittal plane than men [34].

The authors consider that the cervical sagittal translation mobility is important when treating neck patients [4–7, 11–17, 27, 34]. A static protracted head posture for long periods is stressful to the anatomical structures of the cervical spine and causes pain and other symptoms, which may be related to the neck [16]. Clinical studies have shown that impaired neck rotation, extension, and neck retraction predict high disability [5, 6]. To unload the cervical spine from a static protracted position (forward head posture) and in that way improve other cervical movements and decrease neck pain, retraction exercise is a common treatment method used by physiotherapists [4–6]. Professionals dealing with these issues have been seeking a reliable instrument for measuring all cervical motions [35]. The authors can recommend the method used in the present study for the assessment of the cervical sagittal translation mobility in a clinical setting. However, there are limitations of the study. The number of subjects was quite small, and so was the number of measurements. Measurements were performed at different times and at different places. Further, recruiting subjects for the study was prolonged due to the scheduling conflicts of both the raters and those being recruited. Moreover, the short period of time available to complete the study possibly diminished the overall reliability. The reliability might be improved by employing a better standardized procedure and by ensuring that the same instructions were given to the study subjects. The reliability for this measurement method should also be confirmed with a greater number of subjects and raters.

5. Conclusions

The method used in the study is simple and can be recommended for clinical use. The intra-rater agreement was good. The inter-rater agreement was moderate at the first measurement and good at the second one, indicating a learning effect. Further investigations with similar devices, used in clinical settings, are recommended in order to confirm the results.

Conflict of Interests

The authors declare no conflict of interest.

Acknowledgments

The authors want to thank all physiotherapists at Sahlgrenska University Hospital, all dental students at The Sahlgrenska Academy, and the dental nurses at Public Dental in Gothenburg who have contributed to this paper. They also want to thank Nils-Gunnar Pehrsson for statistical advice. The authors want to thank Robert and Gun Casey for the linguistic review.

References

[1] N. Bogduk and S. Mercer, "Biomechanics of the cervical spine. I: normal kinematics," *Clinical Biomechanics*, vol. 15, no. 9, pp. 633–648, 2000.

[2] L. Penning, "Normal movements of the cervical spine," *American Journal of Roentgenology*, vol. 130, no. 2, pp. 317–326, 1978.

[3] N. R. Ordway, R. J. Seymour, R. G. Donelson, L. S. Hojnowski, and W. Thomas Edwards, "Cervical flexion, extension, protrusion, and retraction a radiographic segmental analysis," *Spine*, vol. 24, no. 3, pp. 240–247, 1999.

[4] R. McKenzie and S. May, *The Cervical & Thoracic Spine: Mechanical Diagnosis & Therapy*, vol. 1, Spinal Publications New Zealand, Raumati Beach, New Zealand, 2nd edition, 2006.

[5] S. L. Olson, D. P. O'Connor, G. Birmingham, P. Broman, and L. Herrera, "Tender point sensitivity, range of motion, and perceived disability in subjects with neck pain," *Journal of Orthopaedic and Sports Physical Therapy*, vol. 30, no. 1, pp. 13–20, 2000.

[6] M. E. Rosenfeld, A. Seferiadis, J. Carlsson, and R. Gunnarsson, "Active intervention in patients with whiplash-associated disorders improves long-term prognosis: a randomized controlled clinical trial," *Spine*, vol. 28, no. 22, pp. 2491–2498, 2003.

[7] H. Takasaki, T. Hall, S. Kaneko, Y. Ikemoto, and G. Jull, "A radiographic analysis of the influence of initial neck posture on cervical segmental movement at end-range extension in asymptomatic subjects," *Manual Therapy*, vol. 16, no. 1, pp. 74–79, 2011.

[8] C. M. Visscher, W. de Boer, and M. Naeije, "The relationship between posture and curvature of the cervical spine," *Journal of Manipulative and Physiological Therapeutics*, vol. 21, no. 6, pp. 388–391, 1998.

[9] H. Lee, L. L. Nicholson, and R. D. Adams, "Cervical range of motion associations with subclinical neck pain," *Spine*, vol. 29, no. 1, pp. 33–40, 2004.

[10] T. Prushansky, E. Pevzner, C. Gordon, and Z. Dvir, "Performance of cervical motion in chronic whiplash patients and healthy subjects: the case of atypical patients," *Spine*, vol. 31, no. 1, pp. 37–43, 2006.

[11] T. Rudolfsson, M. Björklund, and M. Djupsjöbacka, "Range of motion in the upper and lower cervical spine in people with chronic neck pain," *Manual Therapy*, vol. 17, no. 1, pp. 53–59, 2012.

[12] W. P. Hanten, R. M. Lucio, J. L. Russell, and D. Brunt, "Assessment of total head excursion and resting head posture," *Archives of Physical Medicine and Rehabilitation*, vol. 72, no. 11, pp. 877–880, 1991.

[13] W. P. Hanten, S. L. Olson, J. L. Russell, R. M. Lucio, and A. H. Campbell, "Total head excursion and resting head posture: normal and patient comparisons," *Archives of Physical Medicine and Rehabilitation*, vol. 81, no. 1, pp. 62–66, 2000.

[14] C. Fernández-De-Las-Peñas, C. Alonso-Blanco, M. L. Cuadrado, and J. A. Pareja, "Forward head posture and neck mobility in chronic tension-type headache: a blinded, controlled study," *Cephalalgia*, vol. 26, no. 3, pp. 314–319, 2006.

[15] C. H. T. Yip, T. T. W. Chiu, and A. T. K. Poon, "The relationship between head posture and severity and disability of patients with neck pain," *Manual Therapy*, vol. 13, no. 2, pp. 148–154, 2008.

[16] K. Harms-Ringdahl and J. Ekholm, "Intensity and character of pain and muscular activity levels elicited by maintained extreme flexion position of the lower-cervical-upper-thoracic spine," *Scandinavian Journal of Rehabilitation Medicine*, vol. 18, no. 3, pp. 117–126, 1986.

[17] O. B. Bunketorp and L. K. Elisson, "Cervical status after neck sprains in frontal and rear-end car impacts," *Injury*, vol. 43, no. 4, pp. 423–430, 2012.

[18] T. Mayer, S. Brady, E. Bovasso, P. Pope, and R. J. Gatchel, "Noninvasive measurement of cervical tri-planar motion in normal subjects," *Spine*, vol. 18, no. 15, pp. 2191–2195, 1993.

[19] D. E. Hole, J. M. Cook, and J. E. Bolton, "Reliability and concurrent validity of two instruments for measuring cervical range of motion: effects of age and gender," *Manual Therapy*, vol. 1, no. 1, pp. 36–42, 1995.

[20] M. Tousignant, L. De Bellefeuille, S. O'Donoughue, and S. Grahovac, "Criterion validity of the Cervical Range of Motion (CROM) goniometer for cervical flexion and extension," *Spine*, vol. 25, no. 3, pp. 324–330, 2000.

[21] A. Peolsson, *Functional analyses of the cervical spine: reliability, reference data and outcome after anterior cervical decompression and fusion [Ph.D. dissertation]*, Linköping, Sweden, 2002.

[22] E. M. Malmström, M. Karlberg, A. Melander, and M. Magnusson, "Zebris versus Myrin: a comparative study between a three-dimensional ultrasound movement analysis and an inclinometer/compass method: intradevice reliability, concurrent validity, intertester comparison, intratester reliability, and intraindividual variability," *Spine*, vol. 28, no. 21, pp. E433–E440, 2003.

[23] C. H. P. De Koning, S. P. Van Den Heuvel, J. B. Staal, B. C. M. Smits-Engelsman, and E. J. M. Hendriks, "Clinimetric evaluation of active range of motion measures in patients with non-specific neck pain: a systematic review," *European Spine Journal*, vol. 17, no. 7, pp. 905–921, 2008.

[24] M. A. Williams, C. J. McCarthy, A. Chorti, M. W. Cooke, and S. Gates, "A Systematic review of reliability and validity studies of methods for measuring active and passive cervical range of motion," *Journal of Manipulative and Physiological Therapeutics*, vol. 33, no. 2, pp. 138–155, 2010.

[25] I. Audette, J. P. Dumas, J. N. Côté, and S. J. De Serres, "Validity and between-day reliability of the cervical range of motion (CROM) device," *Journal of Orthopaedic and Sports Physical Therapy*, vol. 40, no. 5, pp. 318–323, 2010.

[26] T. R. Garrett, J. W. Youdas, and T. J. Madson, "Reliability of measuring forward head posture in a clinical setting," *Journal of Orthopaedic and Sports Physical Therapy*, vol. 17, no. 3, pp. 155–160, 1993.

[27] B. M. Nilsson and A. Söderlund, "Head posture in patients with whiplash-associated disorders and the measurement method's reliability—a comparison to healthy subjects," *Advances in Physiotherapy*, vol. 7, no. 1, pp. 13–19, 2005.

[28] H. V. Mameren, J. Drukker, H. Sanches, and J. Beursgens, "Cervical spine motion in the sagittal plane (I) range of motion of actually performed movements, an X-ray cinematographic study," *European Journal of Morphology*, vol. 28, no. 1, pp. 47–68, 1990.

[29] N. R. Ordway, R. Seymour, R. G. Donelson, L. Hojnowski, E. Lee, and W. T. Edwards, "Cervical sagittal range-of-motion analysis using three methods: cervical range-of-motion device, 3 space, and radiography," *Spine*, vol. 22, no. 5, pp. 501–508, 1997.

[30] W. Frobin, G. Leivseth, M. Biggemann, and P. Brinckmann, "Sagittal plane segmental motion of the cervical spine. A new precision measurement protocol and normal motion data of healthy adults," *Clinical Biomechanics*, vol. 17, no. 1, pp. 21–31, 2002.

[31] C. J. Centeno, W. Elkins, M. Freeman, J. Elliot, M. Sterling, and E. Katz, "Total cervical translation as a function of impact vector as measured by flexion-extension radiography," *Pain Physician*, vol. 10, no. 5, pp. 667–671, 2007.

[32] J. M. Bland and D. G. Altman, "Measurement error," *British Medical Journal*, vol. 313, no. 7059, pp. 744–753, 1996.

[33] M. Gellerstedt and B. Furberg, *D12: Diagnostik—En Tolkningsfråga?* E. Merck AB, Stockholm, Sweden, 2007.

[34] P. R. Persson, H. Hirschfeld, and L. Nilsson-Wikmar, "Associated sagittal spinal movements in performance of head pro- and retraction in healthy women: a kinematic analysis," *Manual Therapy*, vol. 12, no. 2, pp. 119–125, 2007.

[35] J. Chen, A. B. Solinger, J. F. Poncet, and C. A. Lantz, "Meta-analysis of normative cervical motion," *Spine*, vol. 24, no. 15, pp. 1571–1578, 1999.

7

Preoperative Strength Training for Elderly Patients Awaiting Total Knee Arthroplasty

D. M. van Leeuwen,[1,2] C. J. de Ruiter,[1] P. A. Nolte,[3] and A. de Haan[1,2]

[1] *MOVE Research Institute Amsterdam, Faculty of Human Movement Sciences, VU University Amsterdam,*
 Van der Boechorststraat 9, 1081 BT, Amsterdam, The Netherlands
[2] *Institute for Biomedical Research into Human Movement and Health, Manchester Metropolitan University, Manchester M1 5GD, UK*
[3] *Department of Orthopedics, Spaarne Hospital, Spaarnepoort 1, 2134 TM Hoofddorp, The Netherlands*

Correspondence should be addressed to A. de Haan; a.de.haan@vu.nl

Academic Editor: Jiu-jenq Lin

Objective. To investigate the feasibility and effects of additional preoperative high intensity strength training for patients awaiting total knee arthroplasty (TKA). *Design*. Clinical controlled trial. *Patients*. Twenty-two patients awaiting TKA. *Methods*. Patients were allocated to a standard training group or a group receiving standard training with additional progressive strength training for 6 weeks. Isometric knee extensor strength, voluntary activation, chair stand, 6-minute walk test (6MWT), and stair climbing were assessed before and after 6 weeks of training and 6 and 12 weeks after TKA. *Results*. For 3 of the 11 patients in the intensive strength group, training load had to be adjusted because of pain. For both groups combined, improvements in chair stand and 6MWT were observed before surgery, but intensive strength training was not more effective than standard training. Voluntary activation did not change before and after surgery, and postoperative recovery was not different between groups ($P > 0.05$). Knee extensor strength of the affected leg before surgery was significantly associated with 6-minute walk ($r = 0.50$) and the stair climb ($r- = 0.58$, $P < 0.05$). *Conclusion*. Intensive strength training was feasible for the majority of patients, but there were no indications that it is more effective than standard training to increase preoperative physical performance. This trial was registered with NTR2278.

1. Introduction

Knee osteoarthritis (OA) is a degenerative joint disease which is characterized by a gradual loss of cartilage [1] and can result in pain, limited physical performance, and lower quality of life [2]. If conservative treatment is ineffective, patients may decide to undergo a total knee arthroplasty (TKA), which can significantly reduce knee pain and can increase physical performance in patients with severe OA [1]. For patients undergoing TKA, the isometric strength of the knee extensors was shown to decrease by up to 60% four weeks after surgery, and this decrease was accompanied by decreases in the ability to voluntarily activate the knee extensor muscles [3]. Even after six months to thirteen years following TKA, the strength of the knee extensor muscles at involved side remains 12–30% lower than the uninvolved side, and strength almost never matched values for healthy

controls [4]. This postoperative weakness has important consequences for activities of daily life, because knee extensor strength is strongly related to functional performance, such as walking and stair climbing [5] especially after TKA [6]. There are indications that preoperative strength is related to postoperative abilities [7, 8]. Intensive strength training *after* TKA has shown to be beneficial for decreasing pain and improving strength and physical performance when compared to usual care [2]. Multiple studies have investigated the effect of preoperative strength training on postoperative recovery [9–15]. However, few of these studies reported significant increases in preoperative strength following the training. Reviewing these studies, it is clear that the intensity of training, when documented, was either rather low [10, 13–15] or not progressively increased [13] or the number of sessions was too small to produce significant training effects [9]. Progressive, high intensity strength training is recommended to increase muscle strength [16]. Because the preoperative training period is typically rather short (the time between the decision for TKA and the actual surgery is typically 4 to 8 weeks), a high intensity and progressive loading may be needed to increase preoperative strength and performance and therefore promote postoperative recovery. However, it is unclear if this type of training is feasible in this patient group, since pain may be a limiting factor.

The aims of the present study were to investigate the feasibility and the effects of additional preoperative high intensity strength training for elderly patients awaiting TKA compared to standard preoperative training in a pilot study. We hypothesised that preoperative intensive strength training would lead to increases in strength and performance before surgery. We hypothesised that increases in strength were primarily caused by improved voluntary activation, because the first adaptations to strength training are primarily neural [17] and training time is limited.

2. Methods

2.1. Participants. All patients above 55 years awaiting TKA in the Spaarne Hospital in Hoofddorp were considered candidates for the present study and were asked to participate. Patients were excluded if they had (1) American Society of Anesthesiologists (ASA) score >2 [18], (2) contraindications for training the lower limbs, or (3) contraindications for electrical stimulation (unstable epilepsy, cancer, skin abnormalities, or having a pacemaker).

All patients had at least 1 year symptoms of severe osteoarthritis of the knee (Kellgren and Lawrence [19] grades 3 and 4). For additional exercise, patients were asked about their physical activity at each measurement occasion. The patients did not perform strength training before inclusion in this study. No severe coexisting diseases were present. Therefore, we do not expect a limiting effect on function or exercise responses of our participants.

2.2. Sample Size. Isometric knee extension strength of the surgical leg before TKA was defined as the primary outcome variable for the power analysis. The effect size for strength training with patients having osteoarthritis has been reported to be 0.35 [20] and 0.30 for preoperative training [14]. Because the control group also received therapy, we used an effect size of 0.20. For 0.8 power, $\alpha = 0.05$ and assuming a correlation of 0.85 between repeated measurements, a total of 18 participants was needed to assess significant differences between groups over time. Because 4 participants dropped out before the second measurement, four additional patients were included and in total 22 patients were enrolled in the study.

2.3. Randomization and Blinding. Participants were randomized in a 1:1 ratio (parallel design) to either the standard treatment or standard treatment with additional strength training. A research nurse approached potential candidates by phone, generated the random allocation sequence with use of custom software, enrolled patients, and assigned them to the interventions. Randomization was done by minimization of gender and age (median age of patients on the waiting list). After the inclusion of 15 patients, 2 participants had dropped out and two patients received the intervention instead of standard training and the ratio between strength training and standard training was 10/3. To increase comparability between groups, the remaining 7 patients were allocated to the standard training group. The principal investigator (DL) was blinded during measurements, but not during analyses of the results. The participants and therapists were not blinded.

2.4. Surgical Procedure. Patients underwent an uncemented TKA (mobile bearing total knee prosthesis, LCS Complete, Depuy, Warsaw, Indiana, United States) with standardized perioperative protocol and the same surgical technique. The surgical technique consisted of a midline incision with a flexed knee, medial arthrotomy, and bone cuts with Milestone instruments without the use of tourniquet or drains. Perioperative antibiotics (Kefzol 1 gram i.v.) and antithrombotics (Fraxiparine 0.3 mL i.m.) were used. The patients were mobilized the first day postoperatively. On average the patients left the hospital the 4th postoperative day. The surgeries were performed by experienced orthopedic surgeons (>50 TKA per year) and patients received protocolized inpatient physical therapy. The VU Medical Centre Medical Ethics Committee and the local ethics committee of the Spaarne Hospital approved the study, and all participants signed informed consent and the rights of the subjects were protected.

2.5. Intervention. Patients were allocated to standard treatment or received standard treatment with additional strength training (Figure 1). The standard training group received treatment according to guidelines from the Dutch association of orthopaedics [21] and the Dutch physiotherapy association (KNGF) [22] for training patients with OA. Therapy included information and advice, exercise of activities of daily life, training of walking with aids, maintenance of mobility, and aerobic training (walking, cycling), but the patients in this group were not allowed to perform resistance training. The intensive strength training group received the same treatment as the standard training group, with additional intensive strength training, consisting of a progressive strength program targeting the lower limbs. Table 1 shows exercises, sets, and repetitions. We abstained from 1 RM testing to minimize pain sensations, because pain could lead to premature ending of the training. Instead, the training weights were adjusted to the abilities of the patients in relation to the number of repetitions. For the first training (3 × 15 repetition), patients were asked to perform the maximum number of repetitions with the selected weight. If either more or less than 15 repetitions were performed, the weight for the next set was adjusted with ~3% per repetition. For example, if a patient could perform 22 repetitions with 30 kg, the weight was increased with 7 (22 − 15 repetitions) ∗ 3% to 36.6 kg. Dumbbells or plates were used for small increments. To ensure progressive overload, repetitions decreased during the program, and the weights were increased when the number of repetitions decreased (~3% per repetition). For the squat

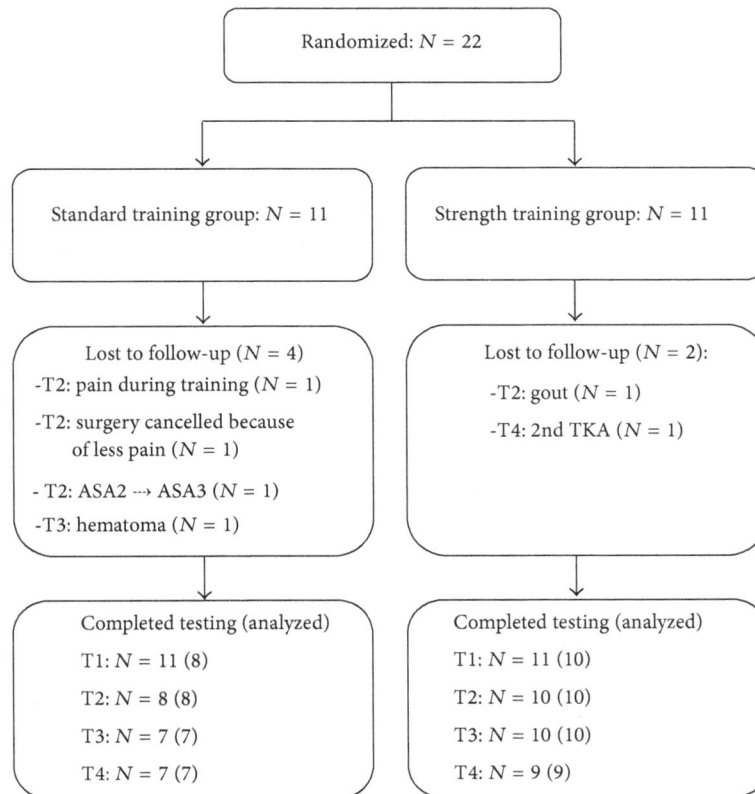

FIGURE 1: Flowchart of inclusion and follow-up in the two training groups.

TABLE 1: Exercises, sets and repetitions for the strength training group.

	Week 1	Week 2	Week 3	Week 4	Week 5	Week 6
Leg press 1-leg	3×15	3×12	4×12	3×10	4×10	4×8
Step up 1-leg	3×15	3×12	4×12	3×10	4×10	4×8
Squat	3×15	3×12	4×12	3×10	4×10	4×8
Leg extension 1-leg	3×15	3×12	4×12	3×10	4×10	4×8

exercise, intensity was increased by the increasing the range of motion before using dumbbells. Both the uninvolved and the involved limb were trained, and the weight was adjusted to abilities. The patients trained two to three times per week. In addition, a home program consisting of step-up and squat exercises was performed two to three times per week by the strength training group. In case of pain or other discomfort, the program was modified, but the intensity stayed as high as possible. After surgery, no interventions were applied; both groups received standard care including strength training. 13 physiotherapy centres participated by complying with the training program. 22 patients entered the study. Figure 1 shows allocation and follow-up.

2.6. Measures. All measurements were performed at the Spaarne Hospital before training (T1), after 6 weeks of training (T2, the week before TKA), 6 weeks after surgery (T3), and 12 weeks after surgery (T4).

2.6.1. Feasibility. The feasibility was evaluated by checking training logs for adherence. Physiotherapists were instructed to note alterations of the training program. If training intensity was progressively increased and all exercises were executed, the program was considered feasible. The number and contents of the training sessions for the control group were also monitored by checking training logs.

2.6.2. Torque Measurements. Measurement of the contractile properties of the knee extensor and flexor muscles took place on a custom-made adjustable dynamometer. The lower leg was tightly strapped to a force transducer (KAP-E, 2 kN, A.S.T., Dresden, Germany), mounted to the frame of the chair about 25 cm distally of the knee joint. Participants sat in the dynamometer with a hip angle of 80° (0° is full extension), firmly attached to the seat with straps at the pelvis to prevent extension of the hip during contraction and a strap at the chest. All measurements were performed on both legs at a knee angle of 60° (0° is full extension), during isometric contraction. The nonsurgical leg was measured first to get accustomed to the procedures and electrical stimulation (see below). Force data were digitized (1 kHz), filtered with a 4th order bidirectional 150 Hz Butterworth low-pass filter, and stored on a PC for offline analysis. Force signals were corrected for gravity: the average force applied by the weight of the limb was set at zero. Torque was calculated by multiplying force with the distance between the force transducer and the knee joint. After 3 submaximal attempts, participants were asked to perform at least 3 maximal isometric knee extensions and flexions, and more if torque increased more than 10%, with at least two minutes of rest in between attempts. Maximal Voluntary Torque was defined as the highest torque recorded.

2.6.3. Electrical Stimulation. Constant current electrical stimulation (pulse width 200 μs) was applied through self-adhesive surface electrodes (Schwa-Medico, Leusden, The Netherlands) by a computer-controlled stimulator (model DS7A, Digitimer Ltd., Welwyn Garden City, UK). The distal electrode (8 × 13 cm) was placed over the medial part of the quadriceps muscle just above the patella and the proximal electrode (8 × 13 cm) over the lateral portion of the muscle to prevent inadvertent stimulation of the adductors. Before placing the electrodes the skin in the area of the electrodes was shaved. The stimulation current was increased until force in response to doublet stimulation (two pulses at 100 Hz) levelled off. After assessing maximal doublet force, the stimulation intensity was lowered and set to produce 50% of the maximal doublet force. This stimulation intensity ensured that a substantial amount of muscle mass was stimulated but significantly reduced discomfort at the same time [23]. Voluntary activation was calculated with use of the superimposed twitch technique. In short, upon a maximal voluntary contraction, a superimposed doublet was delivered to the muscle. Two seconds after each contraction, a (potentiated) doublet was delivered to the relaxed muscle to calculate voluntary activation with use of the following equation:

$$\text{Voluntary activation (\%)} = 1 - \left(\frac{\text{superimposed force}}{\text{potentiated resting doublet}} \right) * 100\% \quad (1)$$

(see [23, 24]).

2.6.4. Functional Tasks. A 5-time sit-to stand test was performed with the arms folded in front of the chest. Patients were instructed to stand up and sit down as quickly as possible. The six-minute walk test (6MWT) was used to quantify walking ability. Participants walked back and forth over 30 meters as many times as possible for a period of 6 minutes at their own pace, in a 60-meter-long corridor. The score recorded was the total distance travelled during 6 minutes. Participants were instructed to "walk as quickly and safely as you can for 6 minutes."

To investigate stair-climbing, the time required to ascend 9 steps, turn around, and descend 9 steps was used. Participants were allowed to use the handrail and instructed to "walk as quickly and safely". All tests except the 6MWT were

repeated twice, and the fastest time was used for analysis. The 6MWT and the stair climb test are widely used as specific tests to quantify functional performance in patients [6, 25–28].

2.6.5. Quality of Life and Physical Activity. Quality of life was assessed with the Western Ontario and McMaster Universities Osteoarthritis Index (WOMAC). The WOMAC questionnaire is used to obtain pain, stiffness, and functioning specifically for patients with OA. Scores were transformed to a 0 to 100 scale, where a 100 score signifies the best quality of life.

2.7. Statistics. Data are presented as mean ± SD. An ANOVA repeated measure was used to assess differences between the patient groups over time with a Bonferroni post-hoc correction. Two separate analyses were performed. The first analysis was done with preoperative data of patients with data on T1 and T2 (N = 18, T1 and T2) because the primary aim was to study effects of training on preoperative strength and performance. A second analysis was done on all complete data sets (T1–T4; N = 16) to investigate postoperative recovery (T3 and T4). Because not all patients were randomized, a per-protocol analysis was performed. A chi-square test was used to investigate differences in gender at baseline. Other baseline characteristics were analysed using the Kruskal-Wallis Test.

Effect size was calculated by subtracting the mean pre-post (T1-T2) change in the standard group from the mean pre-post change in the intensive training group, divided by the pooled pre-test standard deviation [29].

Pearson's correlation coefficient was used to investigate relationships between normally distributed variables. The level of significance for all tests was set at 0.05 and all analyses were performed with SPSS (version 16.0, SPSS Inc.).

3. Results

3.1. Feasibility. Twenty-two patients were recruited between October 2010 and December 2011. Figure 1 shows a flowchart of allocation and follow-up. All participants in the strength training group completed preoperative training, and there was one dropout in the standard training group. Four participants did not complete the 2nd preoperative test due to various reasons (Figure 1). Only data were analysed from patients who completed testing at T2.

Eight out of 11 patients in the strength training group completed training without adaptations. For 3 patients, small adjustments were made in intensity due to pain, to prevent premature ending of the training. Patients in the strength training group completed 12 ± 2 training sessions (range 11–17), and patients in the standard training group completed 11 ± 4 sessions (range 4–16).

In a pilot study, split squats were included in the training program, but too many patients reported pain during this exercise. Also reduction in range of motion in knee extensions and leg press showed to be an effective way to reduce pain, while maintaining a high training intensity.

TABLE 2: Characteristics of patients of the two training groups and drop-outs.

	Strength training (N = 10)	Standard training (N = 8)	Drop-outs (N = 4)	P
Sex (men/women)[a]	7/3	4/4	1/3	0.30
Age (years)[b]	71.8 (7.5)	69.5 (7.1)	73.3 (3.4)	0.33
BMI (kg/m²)[b]	27.9 (4.6)	27.9 (3.1)	26.3 (2.1)	0.71

[a]Differences tested using χ^2 test.
[b]Presented as mean (standard deviation), differences tested using Kruskall-Wallis Test.

Table 2 shows baseline characteristics for the patients in the strength training group, the standard training group who completed testing at T2, and the patients that dropped out. There were no significant differences between the groups.

3.2. Pre-Surgery Effects

3.2.1. Strength Measures.
Table 3 shows average values for strength measures. Before surgery there were no main effects of group or time: at baseline and T2, there were no significant differences in strength measures between groups and no changes in time for the total group. The effect size of maximal voluntary knee extension strength was 0.11. The post-hoc power was 0.87. There were also no significant interactions between group and time for any strength measure during this six-week preoperative training period. Strength training did not lead to increases in maximal knee extension torque (Table 3), voluntary activation, or doublet torque compared to the standard training group. At T1 and T2, the affected leg was not weaker than the unaffected leg and also voluntary activation was not different between both legs. The patients who dropped out before T2 did not have a significantly lower knee extension strength of the affected leg than the patients who completed testing at T2 (98 Nm versus 113 Nm, $P = 0.61$). The percentage of men and women in the two groups differed. Therefore, we also compared knee extension torque between the two groups at baseline with correction for gender. Both without ($P = 0.929$) and with correction for gender ($P = 0.769$), there was no difference in maximal knee extension torque at baseline.

3.2.2. Functional Tasks.
Before surgery (from T1 to T2) there were no main effects of "group," but there were main effects of "time" for chair stand and 6MWT. For both groups combined chair stand (-1.1 s, $P = 0.003$) and 6MWT (25 m, $P = 0.013$) significantly improved before surgery (Table 3) and there was a trend for improvement in voluntary knee flexion strength of the affected side (3.4 Nm, $P = 0.090$). There were no significant interactions between "time" and "group," indicating that any changes over time were similar between groups.

3.3. Post-Surgery Effects

3.3.1. Strength Measures.
After surgery there were no main effects of "group". There was a main effect of "time" for maximal knee extension torque, doublet torque, and maximal knee flexion torque of the affected knee. Maximal torque of the knee extensors and doublet torque significantly decreased from T2 to T3 (6 weeks after surgery) and subsequently significantly increased from T3 to T4 (12 weeks after surgery, $P < 0.05$, Table 3). Knee flexor torque significantly increased from T3 to T4. At T4, maximal torque for knee extension and doublet torque were still between 20 and 30% lower compared with their preoperative values at T2, whereas maximal torque for knee flexion was back to baseline levels.

An unexpected finding was that there was a significant interaction between maximal torque of the knee flexors and group. Post-hoc testing indicated that maximal torque of the knee flexors decreased in the standard training compared to the intensive training groups between T2 and T3. As expected, doublet torque and knee extensor torque were lower for the affected side compared to the unaffected side on T3 and T4 and knee flexor torque was lower at T3 only ($P < 0.05$) compared to the unaffected side. Voluntary activation did not change after surgery.

3.3.2. Functional Tasks.
After surgery, there were no main effects of "group", but there were main effects of "time" for several variables. Six weeks after surgery (T3), stair climbing time increased compared to T2 for both groups combined. From T3 to T4, significant main effects of time were present for chair stand, stair climb, 6MWT, and WOMAC score ($P < 0.05$, Table 3), without any significant interaction between group and time, again indicating that any changes over time were similar between groups.

3.4. Relationships between Quadriceps Strength and Physical Performance.
Table 4 shows Pearson's correlation coefficients between maximal knee extension strength and chair, stair climb, and 6MWT performance at the four moments of testing. Only after surgery, maximal knee extension strength was related to chair stand ($r^2 = 0.27$ and $r = 0.31$, $P < 0.05$). Stair climb performance was related to maximal torque of both legs on all occasions (r^2 between 0.28 and 0.55, $P < 0.05$) and 6MWT was significantly related to strength on T2, T3, and T4 ($r^2 > 0.25$, $P < 0.05$). In general, relationships between voluntary knee extensor strength and the functional tests became stronger over time.

4. Discussion

The main findings of the present study were that intensive strength training is feasible for the majority of the patients awaiting TKA, but that there are no indications that this intensive strength training is more effective than a standard training. The feasibility and pre- and postoperative effects will be separately discussed.

TABLE 3: Strength measures, functional tasks, and WOMAC scores before (T1, T2) and after (T3, T4) surgery.

			T1 (N = 10/8)	T2 (N = 10/8)		T3 (N = 10/7)		T4 (N = 9/7)
MVT extension (Nm)	Affected side	STR	106 ± 45	111 ± 50	*	63 ± 30	*	76 ± 34
		STAND	121 ± 52	121 ± 50		70 ± 35		97 ± 40
	Unaffected side	STR	116 ± 47	123 ± 47		116 ± 44		118 ± 43
		STAND	137 ± 59	139 ± 57		128 ± 65		138 ± 56
Doublet Torque (Nm)	Affected side	STR	49 ± 13	50 ± 16	*	34 ± 10	*	39 ± 12
		STAND	51 ± 19	48 ± 17		35 ± 13		39 ± 14
	Unaffected side	STR	53 ± 12	52 ± 14		50 ± 14		51 ± 16
		STAND	50 ± 15	50 ± 16		50 ± 17		50 ± 13
VA (%)	Affected side	STR	79 ± 13	78 ± 15		79 ± 9		80 ± 10
		STAND	80 ± 13	85 ± 8		84 ± 4		90 ± 8
	Unaffected side	STR	75 ± 19	78 ± 15		80 ± 13		83 ± 11
		STAND	84 ± 12	85 ± 10		88 ± 6		91 ± 6
MVT flexion (Nm)	Affected side	STR	40 ± 22	43 ± 19	†	37 ± 18	*	42 ± 17
		STAND	46 ± 25	50 ± 24		36 ± 16		50 ± 23
	Unaffected side	STR	43 ± 29	47 ± 26		47 ± 27		47 ± 26
		STAND	57 ± 33	55 ± 30		55 ± 30		55 ± 26
Chair stand test (s)		STR	12.6 ± 2.6	11.3 ± 2.1	*	13.3 ± 3.4	*	11.8 ± 1.8
		STAND	12.3 ± 2.7	11.4 ± 1.8		12.5 ± 2.5		10.8 ± 1.5
Stair climb test (s)		STR	12.4 ± 3.1	11.6 ± 3.4	*	20.9 ± 10.8	*	12.8 ± 3.4
		STAND	12.9 ± 3.8	12.4 ± 3.3		17.6 ± 7.5		14.1 ± 0
6MWT (m)		STR	453 ± 81	471 ± 92	*	380 ± 109	*	456 ± 62
		STAND	460 ± 52	493 ± 55		440 ± 87		513 ± 97
WOMAC score (points)		STR	64 ± 11	65 ± 20		70 ± 16	*	83 ± 15
		STAND	67 ± 11	67 ± 8		79 ± 11		93 ± 4

MVT: Maximal voluntary torque; VA: voluntary activation; 6MWT: six-minute walk test; WOMAC: McMaster Universities Osteoarthritis Index; STR: strength training group; STAND: standard training group. The numbers of patients in the intervention and standard training groups are displayed at the different times. Values represent mean ± standard deviation. *Significantly different compared to previous measurement for both groups combined ($P < 0.05$). †Significant difference for groups between T3 and T2 ($P = 0.043$).

TABLE 4: Pearson correlation coefficients between maximal knee extension strength and functional tests.

		Chair stand test	Stair climb test	6-minute walk test
Affected side	T1	−0.03	−0.53*	0.41
	T2	−0.32	−0.58*	0.50*
	T3	−0.56*	−0.68*	0.76*
	T4	−0.56*	−0.74*	0.86*
Unaffected side	T1	−0.17	−0.59*	0.46
	T2	−0.32	−0.64*	0.54*
	T3	−0.47	−0.59*	0.66*
	T4	−0.52*	−0.73*	0.77*

*$P < 0.05$.

4.1. Feasibility. One of the aims of the present study was to investigate the feasibility of additional preoperative high intensity strength training for elderly patients awaiting TKA. In this training group, no patients dropped out because of the intervention. For 3 out of 11 patients, changes in the program had to be made because of pain or discomfort, but for the other 8 patients the training program could be performed without alterations. Although the groups were of limited size, intensive strength training seems feasible, at least for patients with ASA 1 or 2.

4.2. Pre-Surgery Effects. The effect size of the training on strength was small, 0.11, and not significant. This was not in line with our expectations, but it might be explained by the relatively short training time. Six weeks of training two times per week might not be enough to significantly increase strength in patients with end-stage OA, even if a high training intensity is used. In a systematic review investigating effects of strength training in OA patients, positive effects have been reported on strength, performance, and pain compared to control groups [30]. The average duration of the studies in this review was 9 months. Longer interventions may be needed to significantly increase preoperative strength and physical performance.

There were no differences in strength between the affected and the unaffected leg before surgery, although a difference in strength is often observed [14, 31, 32]. This might be explained by the fact that 2 patients were having a second TKA at a later stage and 4 patients already had an earlier TKA. This indicates that the nonsurgical leg was not "unaffected" in all patients.

The finding that strength training did not increase preoperative strength or promote postoperative outcome is in line with the majority of earlier studies [9, 10, 12–14]. In the present study, there were improvements in chair stand and the 6MWT for the entire group before surgery. It is important to note that both groups in the current study received training. In the absence of training, strength and performance often decline in the preoperative period [9, 14, 15], which was not the case in the current study. The standard training group in the present study underwent aerobic training (walking and cycling), balance training, and training of activities of daily life, such as chair rises and basic step training. In many other studies no exercise is prescribed during the preoperative period for a control group [9–15]. Because both groups trained, this may not only have prevented the decline as is seen in many other studies during the preoperative phase, but it also seems to suggest that the exact content of the training program is less relevant during a short preoperative phase. This finding is in line with the results of a recent study in which a control group improved walking and stair climbing after 6 weeks of nonspecific upper-body strength training [33]. There are no indications in the present study that additional heavy resistance training is superior to a program of more general aerobic training including some functional (strength demanding) tasks.

4.3. Post-Surgery Effects. The recovery of voluntary torque, stair climb, and walking ability at T4 was comparable to two earlier studies [34, 35], but somewhat lower than reported by others [14, 32]. There was a significant interaction ($P = 0.043$) between group and time for maximal torque of the knee flexors from T2 to T3. This interaction was probably not caused by the intensive strength training, because no interaction was present before surgery, and the preoperative training program was primarily focused on the knee extensors. Therefore, we consider this to be a sporadic finding. There were no other significant interactions between group and time after surgery.

4.4. Voluntary Activation. Before surgery, there were no differences in voluntary activation between the surgical and nonsurgical leg. As stated before, the lack of changes might be caused by an earlier or a future TKA of the nonsurgical leg. There were also no changes in voluntary activation after training and after surgery. The absence of changes in voluntary activation is not in line with two earlier studies [3, 36] that measured lower activation 4 weeks after surgery, but in accordance with two other studies in which no changes were found 12 weeks after surgery [37, 38]. The different findings regarding changes in voluntary activation may be explained by differences in timing of the measurements after surgery among studies. Thirty three months after surgery, significant increases in voluntary activation have been observed compared to before surgery [31]. Voluntary activation may decrease the first weeks after surgery and improve on a longer term.

4.5. Relationships between Quadriceps Strength and Physical Performance. The relationships between strength and physical performance and the observation that relationships are stronger later after surgery are in line with other studies [6, 32]. This may indicate that knee extension strength is an important factor for performance, especially in later stages of recovery. Consequently, postoperative strength training may improve functional recovery, which is in line with earlier research [2].

4.6. Clinical Relevance and Limitations. A major strength of the current study compared to other studies is that preoperative training had a relative high intensity and loads were progressively increased. For patients, the results of the present study indicate that it is unnecessary to subject patients to intensive training before TKA. A limitation is the low sample size in this study. Especially when studying postoperative effects, a larger sample size would be needed. It is, however, unlikely that preoperative strength training would be effective to promote recovery *after* surgery compared to standard preoperative training, because neither significant effects nor trends for superior effects of strength training were observed *before* surgery. Another limitation of the present study is a lack of randomization and the lack of blinding for therapists and patients.

5. Conclusion

We conclude that intensive strength training is feasible for the majority of the patients awaiting TKA. There were no indications that this intensive strength training is more effective than a standard training with respect to maximal knee extensor strength, voluntary activation, and performance in functional tests.

Conflict of Interests

The authors declare that there is no conflict of interests regarding the publication of this paper.

Acknowledgment

The authors would like to thank Jeanette Verhart for her efforts including the participants.

References

[1] S. M. Seed, K. C. Dunican, and A. M. Lynch, "Osteoarthritis: a review of treatment options," *Geriatrics*, vol. 64, no. 10, pp. 20–29, 2009.

[2] S. C. Petterson, R. L. Mizner, J. E. Stevens et al., "Improved function from progressive strengthening interventions after total knee arthroplasty: a randomized clinical trial with an imbedded prospective cohort," *Arthritis Care and Research*, vol. 61, no. 2, pp. 174–183, 2009.

[3] J. E. Stevens, R. L. Mizner, and L. Snyder-Mackler, "Quadriceps strength and volitional activation before and after total knee arthroplasty for osteoarthritis," *Journal of Orthopaedic Research*, vol. 21, no. 5, pp. 775–779, 2003.

[4] W. Meier, R. Mizner, R. Marcus, L. Dibble, C. Peters, and P. C. Lastayo, "Total knee arthroplasty: muscle impairments, functional limitations, and recommended rehabilitation approaches," *Journal of Orthopaedic and Sports Physical Therapy*, vol. 38, no. 5, pp. 246–256, 2008.

[5] M. R. Maly, P. A. Costigan, and S. J. Olney, "Determinants of self-report outcome measures in people with knee osteoarthritis," *Archives of Physical Medicine and Rehabilitation*, vol. 87, no. 1, pp. 96–104, 2006.

[6] Y. Yoshida, R. L. Mizner, D. K. Ramsey, and L. Snyder-Mackler, "Examining outcomes from total knee arthroplasty and the relationship between quadriceps strength and knee function over time," *Clinical Biomechanics*, vol. 23, no. 3, pp. 320–328, 2008.

[7] J. R. Jaggers, C. D. Simpson, K. L. Frost et al., "Prehabilitation before knee arthroplasty increases postsurgical function: a case study," *Journal of Strength and Conditioning Research*, vol. 21, no. 2, pp. 632–634, 2007.

[8] R. L. Mizner, S. C. Petterson, J. E. Stevens, M. J. Axe, and L. Snyder-Mackler, "Preoperative quadriceps strength predicts functional ability one year after total knee arthroplasty," *Journal of Rheumatology*, vol. 32, no. 8, pp. 1533–1539, 2005.

[9] D. S. Rooks, J. Huang, B. E. Bierbaum et al., "Effect of preoperative exercise on measures of functional status in men and women undergoing total hip and knee arthroplasty," *Arthritis Care and Research*, vol. 55, no. 5, pp. 700–708, 2006.

[10] J. A. Rodgers, K. L. Garvin, C. W. Walker, D. Morford, J. Urban, and J. Bedard, "Preoperative physical therapy in primary total knee arthroplasty," *Journal of Arthroplasty*, vol. 13, no. 4, pp. 414–421, 1998.

[11] J. Crowe and J. Henderson, "Pre-arthroplasty rehabilitation is effective in reducing hospital stay," *Canadian Journal of Occupational Therapy*, vol. 70, no. 2, pp. 88–96, 2003.

[12] D. D. D'Lima, C. W. Colwell Jr., B. A. Morris, M. E. Hardwick, and F. Kozin, "The effect of preoperative exercise on total knee replacement outcomes," *Clinical Orthopaedics and Related Research*, no. 326, pp. 174–182, 1996.

[13] L. A. Beaupre, D. Lier, D. M. Davies, and D. B. C. Johnston, "The effect of a preoperative exercise and education program on functional recovery, health related quality of life, and health service utilization following primary total knee arthroplasty," *Journal of Rheumatology*, vol. 31, no. 6, pp. 1166–1173, 2004.

[14] R. Topp, A. M. Swank, P. M. Quesada, J. Nyland, and A. Malkani, "The effect of prehabilitation exercise on strength and functioning after total knee arthroplasty," *PM and R*, vol. 1, no. 8, pp. 729–735, 2009.

[15] A. M. Swank, J. B. K. Kachelman, B. Wendy et al., "Prehabilitation before total knee arthroplasty increases strength and function in older adults with severe osteoarthritis," *Journal of Strength and Conditioning Research*, vol. 25, no. 2, pp. 318–325, 2011.

[16] American College of Sports Medicine position stand, "Progression models in resistance training for healthy adults," *Medicine & Science in Sports & Exercise*, vol. 41, no. 3, pp. 687–708, 2009.

[17] D. A. Gabriel, G. Kamen, and G. Frost, "Neural adaptations to resistive exercise: mechanisms and recommendations for training practices," *Sports Medicine*, vol. 36, no. 2, pp. 133–149, 2006.

[18] A. S. O. Anesthesiologists, "New classification of physical status," *Anesthesiology*, vol. 24, p. 111, 1963.

[19] J. H. Kellgren and J. S. Lawrence, "Radiological assessment of osteo-arthrosis," *Annals of the rheumatic diseases*, vol. 16, no. 4, pp. 494–502, 1957.

[20] M. Fransen and S. McConnell, "Exercise for osteoarthritis of the knee," *Cochrane Database of Systematic Reviews*, no. 4, 2008.

[21] NOV, Richtlijn diagnostiek en behandeling van heup-en knieartrose, 2007.

[22] E. M. H. M. Vogels, "KNGF-richtlijn Atrose heup-knie," *Nederlands Tijdschrift Voor Fysiotherapie*, vol. 115, no. 1, 2005.

[23] D. M. van Leeuwen, C. J. de Ruiter, and A. de Haan, "Effect of stimulation intensity on assessment of voluntary activation," *Muscle Nerve*, vol. 45, no. 6, pp. 841–848, 2012.

[24] J. P. Folland and A. G. Williams, "Methodological issues with the interpolated twitch technique," *Journal of Electromyography and Kinesiology*, vol. 17, no. 3, pp. 317–327, 2007.

[25] R. L. Mizner and L. Snyder-Mackler, "Altered loading during walking and sit-to-stand is affected by quadriceps weakness after total knee arthroplasty," *Journal of Orthopaedic Research*, vol. 23, no. 5, pp. 1083–1090, 2005.

[26] A. de Haan, C. J. de Ruiter, L. H. van Der Woude et al., "Contractile properties and fatigue of quadriceps muscles in multiple sclerosis," *Muscle Nerve*, vol. 23, no. 10, pp. 1534–1541, 2000.

[27] C. J. De Ruiter, B. G. M. Van Engelen, R. A. Wevers, and A. De Haan, "Muscle function during fatigue in myoadenylate deaminase-deficient Dutch subjects," *Clinical Science*, vol. 98, no. 5, pp. 579–585, 2000.

[28] K. H. Gerrits, M. J. Beltman, P. A. Koppe et al., "Isometric muscle function of knee extensors and the relation with functional performance in patients with stroke," *Archives of Physical Medicine and Rehabilitation*, vol. 90, no. 3, pp. 480–487, 2009.

[29] S. B. Morris, "Estimating effect sizes from pretest-posttest-control group designs," *Organizational Research Methods*, vol. 11, no. 2, pp. 364–386, 2008.

[30] A. K. Lange, B. Vanwanseele, and M. A. Fiatarone Singh, "Strength training for treatment of osteoarthritis of the knee: a systematic review," *Arthritis Care and Research*, vol. 59, no. 10, pp. 1488–1494, 2008.

[31] A. Berth, D. Urbach, and F. Awiszus, "Improvement of voluntary quadriceps muscle activation after total knee arthroplasty," *Archives of Physical Medicine and Rehabilitation*, vol. 83, no. 10, pp. 1432–1436, 2002.

[32] R. L. Mizner, S. C. Petterson, and L. Snyder-Mackler, "Quadriceps strength and the time course of functional recovery after total knee arthroplasty," *Journal of Orthopaedic and Sports Physical Therapy*, vol. 35, no. 7, pp. 424–436, 2005.

[33] C. McKay, H. Prapavessis, and T. Doherty, "The effect of a prehabilitation exercise program on quadriceps strength for patients undergoing total knee arthroplasty: a randomized controlled pilot study," *PM & R*, vol. 4, no. 9, pp. 647–656, 2012.

[34] M. J. Bade, W. M. Kohrt, and J. E. Stevens-Lapsley, "Outcomes before and after total knee arthroplasty compared to healthy adults," *Journal of Orthopaedic and Sports Physical Therapy*, vol. 40, no. 9, pp. 559–567, 2010.

[35] D. Ouellet and H. Moffet, "Locomotor deficits before and two months after knee arthroplasty," *Arthritis Care and Research*, vol. 47, no. 5, pp. 484–493, 2002.

[36] R. L. Mizner, S. C. Petterson, J. E. Stevens, K. Vandenborne, and L. Snyder-Mackler, "Early quadriceps strength loss after total knee arthroplasty: the contributions of muscle atrophy and failure of voluntary muscle activation," *Journal of Bone and Joint Surgery A*, vol. 87, no. 5, pp. 1047–1053, 2005.

[37] D. Vahtrik, H. Gapeyeva, H. Aibast et al., "Quadriceps femoris muscle function prior and after total knee arthroplasty in women with knee osteoarthritis," *Knee Surgery, Sports Traumatology, Arthroscopy*, vol. 20, no. 10, pp. 2017–2025, 2011.

[38] A. Berth, D. Urbach, W. Neumann, and F. Awiszus, "Strength and voluntary activation of quadriceps femoris muscle in total knee arthroplasty with midvastus and subvastus approaches," *Journal of Arthroplasty*, vol. 22, no. 1, pp. 83–88, 2007.

8

Barriers and Facilitators to Community Mobility for Assistive Technology Users

Natasha Layton

School of Health and Social Development, Deakin University, 221 Burwood Highway, Burwood, VIC 3125, Australia

Correspondence should be addressed to Natasha Layton, natasha@footy.com.au

Academic Editor: K. S. Sunnerhagen

Mobility is frequently described in terms of individual body function and structures however contemporary views of disability also recognise the role of environment in creating disability. *Aim*. To identify consumer perspectives regarding barriers and facilitators to optimal mobility for a heterogeneous population of impaired Victorians who use assistive technology in their daily lives. *Method*. An accessible survey investigated the impact of supports or facilitators upon actual and desired life outcomes and health-related quality of life, from 100 AT users in Victoria, Australia. This paper reports upon data pertaining to community mobility. *Results*. A range of barriers and enablers to community mobility were identified including access to AT devices, environmental interventions, public transport, and inclusive community environs. Substantial levels of unmet need result in limited personal mobility and community participation. Outcomes fall short of many principles enshrined in current policy and human rights frameworks. *Conclusion*. AT devices as well as accessible and inclusive home and community environs are essential to maximizing mobility for many. Given the impact of the environment upon the capacity of individuals to realise community mobility, this raises the question as to whether rehabilitation practitioners, as well as prescribing AT devices, should work to build accessible communities via systemic advocacy.

1. Introduction

Getting around at the home and in the community is a core activity, central to much human participation and therefore of key interest to rehabilitation practitioners. Identifying the constraints and supports which consumers perceive as impacting their current and desired life outcomes will both inform the work of rehabilitation practitioners and identify any barriers usually beyond the gaze of rehabilitation practice [1].

1.1. Mobility. Mobility, defined by the Oxford Dictionary of English [2] as the capacity to move, is a core element of human capacity. Independent mobility, preferably without the need for assistive technology (AT), is viewed as a key outcome measure, alongside communication and self-care, in the rehabilitation literature [3]. Health-related quality-of-life measures also regard the capacity to independently mobilize as a key indicator for quality of life [4, 5].

The extent of mobility will depend upon both the capacity of the person and the nature of the environments in which the person operates. A tension exists in considering the relationship between the person and the environment in which mobility takes place. The rehabilitation approach typically addresses the capacities and deficits within the individual and therefore predominantly locates the mobility issue with the person [6]. This is at odds with social models of disability where barriers present in the environment are seen as disabling, and the dismantling of these barriers will minimize disablement [7, 8]. Recent disability theorists acknowledge the influence of both individual impairment effects and barriers within the environment which may need addressing [9–11]. To some extent such contemporary conceptualizations of disability are realized in the biopsychosocial model put forward by the International Classification of Functioning, Disability and Health (ICF) [12]. Mobility is classified as one complete ICF activity and participation chapter (chapter 4 page 138) and underpins performance in

TABLE 1: Description of Research methods.

Research question	Research methods	Administration and tools
Oversight and triangulation	a. Stakeholder reference committee	Face to face meetings (4)
	Ethics Approval	Deakin University
	Survey pilot	n-9
Survey sample (n-100)		
Demographics of respondents	Demographic questions	Survey section 3: 12 questions
How are AT, EI and PC used in relation to each other and what else is enabling?	Use of supports and improvement over life domains	Survey section 1: 80 questions
How does the presence or absence of enablers effect life for people with disabilities? Costs aside, what would improve life?	Health-related Quality of Life measure	Survey section 2: AQoL 6D (20 questions)

a number of other chapters, for example, Other Life Areas (chapter 8 page 164) and Community, Social & Civic Life (chapter 9: 168). A third section of the ICF framework is that of Environmental Factors, which "make up the physical, social and attitudinal environment in which people live and conduct their lives" (page 171) [12]. In line with the social model of disability then, the ICF acknowledges barriers and facilitators which may impact human performance, beyond body structures and functions [13].

1.2. Mobility within Health and Human Rights Frameworks. In Australia as with other countries, the importance of mobility is enshrined in policy goals at various levels of government [14, 15]. Australia is a signatory to the Convention on the Rights of Persons with Disabilities (CRPD) [16] and mobility is identified as a key right within this. "General principles" (Article 3) describes "full and effective participation and inclusion in society" and "equality of opportunity and accessibility", while Article 19 addresses "Living independently and being included in the community" and Article 20 "Personal mobility". "Accessibility" (Article 9) directs signatories to

> "take appropriate measures to ensure to persons with disabilities access, on an equal basis with others, to the physical environment, to transportation, to information and communications, including information and communications technologies and systems, and to other facilities and services open or provided to the public, both in urban and in rural areas" [16].

These frameworks open the way for a more multilayered response to the complexities involved in mobilizing, including the nature of the environment(s) in which mobilization occurs [13].

1.3. What Interventions Enable Mobility? Enablers and AT Solutions. AT devices, environmental interventions (EI), and personal care or support are key interventions which can be used throughout the lifespan, across occupational roles and at various stages of the disease trajectory [17]. Most effective when used in combination, they represent the key means by

which people living with disabilities maximize their capacity for participation [18]. These interventions and supports have been termed "enablers", in that they enable performance in life domains of importance [19]. While these enablers have generally been researched separately, relationships between them are emerging, for example, the impact of assistive technology upon personal care use [20, 21] and the relationship of assistive technologies and environmental interventions [22, 23]. Evidence for the interrelationship of these three enablers is found in the Equipping Inclusion Studies [24], from which data for this paper is drawn. Here, two-thirds of participants utilized an individualised combination of all three enablers in their daily lives [24]. This study provides empirical evidence to support the notion of the Assistive Technology Solution (AT solution), defined as follows:

> "as an individually tailored combination of hard (actual devices) and soft (assessment, trial and other human factors) assistive technologies, environmental interventions and paid and/or unpaid care" [25].

The concept of an "AT solution" is useful in describing the suites of facilitators or enablers used to engage in community mobility elicited in the study described below.

2. Method

Victoria's Aids and Equipment Action Alliance (AEAA) [26] is a nonprofit, multimember group consisting of people with disabilities, advocates, health professionals, and service providers. In 2008 the AEAA commissioned *The Equipping Inclusion Studies* [24], a series of mixed methods studies intended to investigate the impact of AT solutions upon the lives of adults with a disability. Deakin University ethics approval was gained to sample 100 users of assistive technology devices, from the population of those 18 years and over with disabilities in Victoria, Australia. In line with participatory research principles, AEAA provided a stakeholder reference group to advise the researchers particularly in the areas of recruitment, data analysis, and dissemination. Table 1 outlines the research questions and methods pertaining to The Equipment Survey which is one aspect of

The Equipping Inclusion Studies and is the source of the data presented in this paper.

2.1. Survey Tool and Pilot. A 60-question survey was devised to identify the range of AT devices and other enablers (the elements of each persons' AT solution) used by participants. Open-ended responses describing the nature and extent of activities and participation enabled by AT use were prompted for a range of life areas [27]. Additionally, information was sought regarding potential improvements envisioned by participants and the impact of current and potential AT solutions upon difficulty levels and time use. These questions formed the first section of the survey, with a health-related quality-of-life measure (AQoL 6D) [5] forming the second section, and demographic questions as a final section. The survey was piloted with a sample of 9 individuals with disabilities and underwent minor edits prior to distribution. A key methodological challenge with the extensive question-set related to survey completion. The pilot process validated the decision to allow questions to be left incomplete, in order to enable participants to complete sections of meaning to them, despite the potential disadvantage of missing data. Responses were therefore included in analysis if they contained one or more responses in section one.

2.2. Sample and Recruitment. The survey intended to capture a diverse sample in order to elicit a wide range of AT user experience. Invitations to participate in the survey were issued through the AEAA networks and through a range of Victorian health, community, and disability publications and alerts. Paper copies of the survey were also made available at disability support services and community health centres. To participate, participants sent in completed surveys, contacted the researcher to obtain a copy of the paper survey, or went to the advertised web link to fill in the accessible online survey. This could be completed and saved in stages due to its length. In order to elicit the responses of AT users themselves, as opposed to carers who may have additional or conflicting perspectives upon valued outcomes, proxy reporting was not used. Strategies to include AT users with a wide range of abilities included the offer of gift vouchers to the value of $20 in recognition for time spent in survey completion and the availability of personal assistance with scribing to complete the survey. The survey was available in a paper version as well as a fully accessible online survey format (see [28] for a comparative effectiveness report on accessible online surveys and description of this bespoke online survey tool devised for this study).

The survey produced quantitative and qualitative data, which was analysed using WHO International Classification of Functioning, Disability and Health [12], ISO 9999 Assistive Products for People with Disabilities [29], and UN Convention on the Rights of Persons with Disabilities [16].

3. Results

A wide cross-section of people with a disability responded to advertisements and snowball sampling methods via health and disability organizations, and word of mouth within the disability community. The decision to allow partial completion of the survey resulted in gaps including the demographic data; hence the data below identifies the proportion of participants who provided information on the demographic indices.

3.1. Study Population. Eighty of the 100 respondents provided demographic information, identifying nearly 60 separate diagnoses, including 60% with physical disabilities, 14% with multiple conditions, and 13% with sensory disabilities. The remaining 13% did not complete this question. Most common conditions were neurological (stroke, polio, cerebral palsy, and spinal cord injury) followed by musculoskeletal (amputation, arthritic conditions). Fifty-nine percent were female and 41% male. Most were aged 45–64 years (39%) or 25–44 years (20%), with 13% over the age of 65 (28% did not complete this question). Sixty-two percent lived independently either alone or with a partner, 14% lived in the family home, and 2% resided in a specialist residential care facility (22% did not complete this question). Seventy-eight responded to questions regarding employment, and of these, 25% were employed and 20% identified substantial volunteering roles. Annual incomes were low, with 75% of participants receiving government pensions or allowances, 19% receiving part-time wages, and 6% in receipt of other income (not defined). Sixty-seven participants completed the health-related quality-of-life (HRQOL) measure. Analysis of this data showed the HRQOL of the study population to be less than half that of the norm for the Australian population (0.32 compared to 0.80) as measured by the Assessment of Quality of Life Measure (AQoL-6D) [30].

A substantial dataset emerged from the survey related to community mobility. These findings have been reanalysed here with a particular focus on the interface between individuals, their AT solutions, and the wider community in which mobility occurs.

3.2. Participation in Life Areas Enabled by AT Solutions. Participants reported high utilization of three elements of an AT solution: devices; environmental interventions (including home modifications and the community environs), and personal care. Participants currently utilize an average of 13 items or elements within their AT solution (AT devices, environmental modifications, and personal care), averaging 9 AT devices each. In most cases (66%), all three elements were used by participants. Only 2% of participants relied on AT devices alone, while 16% used AT devices and personal care in combination and 15% used AT devices and environmental interventions together.

All 100 participants utilized individualised AT solutions to participate in multiple life areas, describing over 900 instances of engagement across the ICF activity and participation chapters [12]. Figure 1 contains overall-usage figures for AT devices (including mobility devices) and personal care. Figure 1 also contains a breakdown of environmental interventions into home modifications and inclusive community environs—a theme which will be explored further in this paper and reflects enablers beyond the garden gate.

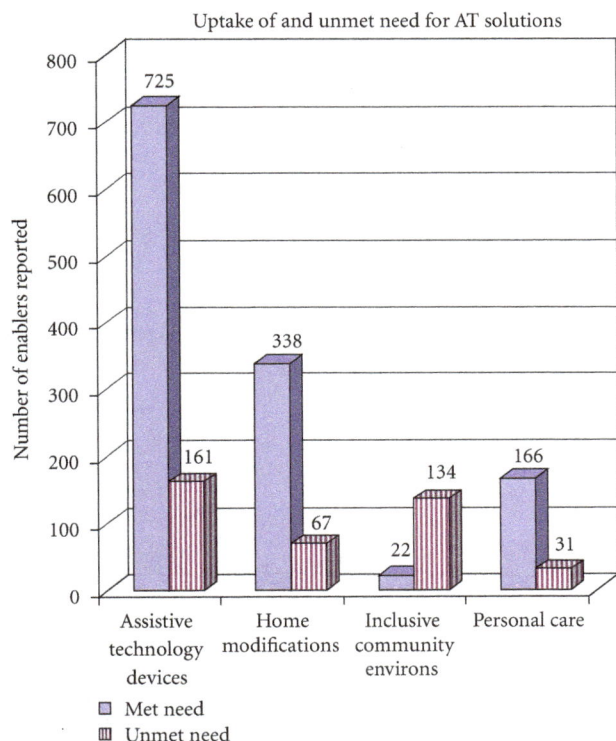

FIGURE 1: Uptake of and unmet need for AT solutions.

Also shown in Figure 1 are total reported items of unmet need. As can be seen from the ratios pictured, provision was a major issue with significant undermet and unmet need reported by the study population. The figures shown in Figure 1 translate into unmet need of 6.5% for home modification, in comparison to 85.9% unmet need for inclusive community environs, which in part reflects the focus of government funding programs as discussed below. A critique of the Victorian government equipment funding scheme can be found in the full publication of *The Equipping Inclusion Studies* [24]. Of relevance to this paper was evidence of the lack of coverage of environmental interventions, despite their central importance to the effectiveness of other enablers and to the survey participants overall. As well as funding shortfalls and lack of response to life changes in the need for alterations to the home, the data evidenced substantial barriers in the wider community. As shown in Figure 1, these themes are reported separately as either home modifications or inclusive community environs.

3.3. Facilitators and Barriers to Community Mobility: Interrelated Enablers. Elements of AT solutions were repeatedly seen to be effective in more than one area of activity. A number of respondents described making tradeoffs between activities. This involved rationing their participation based on insufficient enablers. Participants identified interdependent and overlapping enablers, describing situations where barriers in one area led to a need for more supports or

enablers in other contexts leading to a decreased need for other supports.

> "If the environment was more accessible I wouldn't need any carer help. I do not use any now but sometimes it is difficult and I rely on friends to drag me up steps etc."

> "[I need] street changes—I use a chin-controlled chair and when I try to move the chair along street paths and cross the road, poorly constructed bumpy and steep crossovers are extremely difficult to navigate with my chin. When paths are not flat and smooth, my head moves too much for my chin to remain on the chin control, it makes it nearly impossible for me to get out in most areas locally like to the park or shop. The use of blue stones for crossovers is appalling for wheelchair users. [I need] better access into some buildings, venues and shops that haven't provided access for the disabled in wheelchairs".

3.4. Facilitators and Barriers to Community Mobility: The Experience of Constructing Individualised AT Solutions. Most respondents identified current difficulty levels of "moderate" to "moderate to severe" (3-4 on a 6-point scale) across life areas, and qualitative data showed dissatisfaction and frustration with current participation levels. Many participants described constructing an AT solution that worked for them as an ongoing process as their impairments, their life stages, and their occupational roles changed over time. Over 90% of participants identified ways in which their enablers could or should change in future, related either to ageing equipment, their own changing needs, or the desire for more effective participation:

> "I work full time, drive my own modified car. As I age, getting in and out of the car is getting more difficult. I may need further modification to the car to make it easier to get into… (I need) provision of an electric wheelchair so that I can go out as it is getting harder with age to wheel myself distances".

Frequently, participants felt unable to action needed changes due to a lack of resources and lack of responsiveness in the government equipment funder or lack of control over the external environment. For example, a maximum of $4,400 is allocated for home modifications once per lifetime, by the state government equipment funder. This covers less than 25% of the cost of a standard modification (e.g., modifying one entrance and one bathroom), and was reported to cause significant stress and difficulty in planning around life transitions or as physical needs alter,

> "As I get older my needs change. As my house is heritage listed it is difficult to change things inside, I would love to have wider doors, some rooms I cannot enter and the others I have a 2 cm leeway".

Another issue concerns the fact that the enablers identified were often mainstream products and services and

TABLE 2: Mobility device useage and unmet need (N-100).

AT used for mobility categorised by ISO 9999 Chapters	Useage	Unmet need
12 03 & 12 06 Assistive products for walking		
(i) Walking sticks	11	
(ii) Walking frames	17	1
(iii) Crutches	2	
12 12 Car adaptations		
(i) Vehicle modifications	36	6
(ii) Vehicle transfer aids	2	1
(iii) Vehicle seating & restraints	6	
12 18 Cycles		1
12 22 Human-driven wheelchairs	48	11
12 22 Powered wheelchairs (including scooters)	50	7
12 24 Wheelchair accessories (includes conversion kits, trays, postural supports)	14	9
24 36 Assistive products for carrying and transporting		
(i) Lifters, carriers & trailers	13	4
(ii) Scooter/wheelchair hoists	3	3

therefore unfunded by government equipment funding schemes,

> "As I mainly use public transport I spend time planning on internet the route and means of transport (timetables) and how they connect. Often 1 Bus and 2 trains or 2 buses and 1 train to get somewhere; can be limited by access and the time of day/night travelling. (I use) a hand held GPS for navigating my way around the streets and electronic diary for planning, organising and remembering; telephone and mobile phone; computer with accessible technology [such as] screen reader".

In the above example, this participant with a degenerative condition is enabled by current mainstream technologies (GPS, internet access) which would require self-funding as they are not disability specific items available under the government equipment funding scheme. He is, however, limited by community enablers (timetables and public transport availability).

3.5. Classification and Provision of Enablers: AT Devices. The International Standards Organisation (ISO) provides an internationally accepted classification system for assistive products for persons with disability [29]. Products of specific relevance to mobility and access are covered in Chapter 12 (assistive products for personal mobility), and Chapter 18 (furnishings and adaptations to homes and other premises) [29]. Study participants used 243 mobility devices and identified unmet need for 55 mobility devices (see Table 2). Significantly, 18.6% of the AT device categories listed in the ISO are present on the State funding equipment list. The implications of this more than 80% shortfall is that, where users cannot self-fund, prescribers are substantially limited in the AT devices they can provide [31].

3.6. Classification of and Provision of Enablers: Environments. While ISO 9999 includes a section covering many environmental modification products in Chapter 18 Furnishings and adaptations to homes and other premises [29]; the WHO ICF was found to offer the most useful taxonomies for classifying environmental factors, in that all enablers fitted within either Chapter 1: Products and Technology; Chapter 2: Natural environment and human-made changes to environment; Chapter 3: Support and Relationships; Chapter 4: Attitudes; or Chapter 5: Services, systems and policies [12].

3.6.1. Environment: Home Modifications. Ninety-six participants reported on home modifications. Modifications to the home were utilised by 39 of these respondents (43%) who described having a total of 332 home modifications. Forty-three respondents (45%) named 64 instances of unmet need for home modifications. While many home adaptations were desired as a result of changing circumstances such as ageing or a change in lifestyle and health, some were required as a result of poor architectural planning and regulation.

3.6.2. Classification of Enablers beyond the Garden Gate: Inclusive Community Environs. A diversity of factors in the community were described which related to, but moved beyond, the built environment alone. This emergent theme was termed "inclusive community environs" and sits alongside environmental interventions as a subset of the environment component of an AT solution (see Table 3). Twenty percent of participants explicitly named enabling community elements while over half of all participants (52%) identified barriers. This was the only category in which the level of unmet need exceeded current instances of provision. In total, 134 barriers were described within the environment beyond the garden gate. Of these, 48 concerned the need for universal design and physical access to environs and buildings (36% of unmet

TABLE 3: Unmet need for accessible community environs.

ICF Chapter; Issues and Examples	Supporting quotes (verbatim)
ICF Chapter 2 Public buildings Issue: "Universal design in all public buildings, and private buildings designed for the public for example, hotels, restaurants" Examples: Stepless entry; Easy open doors; Accessible toilets; Appropriate height reception/sales desks at shops and other venues; Seating; Accessible swimming pools/gyms	"When buildings are renovated or first built of they should have ramps, easy opening doors, access to upper floors and counters that are accessible to people in wheelchairs" "easy access to buildings would save huge amounts of time and stress" (I want to) "Have a choice about what cafes and shops I go to. Freedom not to plan my every move." "If more workplaces were wheelchair friendly then maybe people with disabilities would be more easily included in work!" "a bad access example is when i go to vote. I have trouble getting into the building and I need a lot of help as access is through a very steep temporary ramp... i need to go with a carer"
Instances of unmet need reported: 48 Percentage of unmet need (36%)	
ICF Ch 2 &5 Public transport Issue: "Travel more freely" Examples: More low floor buses Accessible tram stops Large print and talking timetables	"A change to disabled parking would be most beneficial—as I cannot park in ordinary parking bays, I have to wait sometimes up to two hours for a disabled parking bay" [I need] "plenty of places to sit and rest, public transport stops closer together" "My church is in Melbourne and no trams there yet—got the stops but no accessible trams on that line!" (I need) "A nearby low floor bus. Closest bus is not accessible. 2.5 Km to nearest accessible bus. Many places unable to go to directly by bus as no low floor bus"
Instances of unmet need reported: 31 Percentage of unmet need 23%	
ICF Chapter 2 Public Space Issue: "Get out and about... get to things" Examples: Continuous paths of travel Footpaths Kerb access	"CBD parking in Melbourne not one on steet (sic) park meets the requirements in regards to the width, as my car is fitted with a wheel chair hoist on the roof and i find it difficult to find a park where I'm not lowering my chair into oncoming traffic." "Accessible milk bar nearby—the three I could use (in different directions) all have steps. Improved footpath crossings at intersections" (I need) "a cut in path in my nature strip near my front door as the nearest cut in the gutter is up the road which when getting a maxitaxi I get rather wet, council will not let me do it even though I was willing to pay"

TABLE 3: Continued.

ICF Chapter; Issues and Examples	Supporting quotes (verbatim)
Tactile street signage	"Ongoing need for improvements in footpaths and crossovers everywhere."
Street crossings	
Accessible parking	

Instances of unmet need reported: 32
Percentage of unmet need: 24%

| ICF Ch 3,4,5 Public information and support Issues: Accessible information

Examples:

Accessible websites

Venue access info

Helpful trained staff | "An impossible change—peoples attitudes, just because I am in a chair I am not stupid!!!!"<br>"Accessible hotels/holiday venues: this area needs a huge change to accommodate people with disabilities. Accommodation venues state that they are accessible but they are not or do not meet the Standards. In my case, I will not now go to a venue unless I see photographs of the toilet and shower to ascertain if I will be able to manage when I get there" |

requirements), while 31 barriers related to lack of accessible public transport (23%) and 23 related to inaccessible public space (24%). Frequently, a lack of seamless infrastructure meant some accessibility initiatives did not translate into a realistic solution.

3.7. Compliance with the UN Convention on the Rights of Persons with Disabilities. The CRPD [16] framework was used during analysis to code the qualitative examples of activities and participations described by participants. Data was coded as instances of failing to realise CRPD principles in two ways. Firstly, the activity or participation event was recorded if it was experienced as difficult to the extent that participants were subjected to undue effort to participate or relinquished the task altogether. For example, an adult with a spinal cord injury described her difficulties with banking due to access, as follows:

> "Effort in running around finding accessible banks or embarrassing myself by yelling from the front door and having to be a dependent disabled person, reliant on people's good will."

Secondly, data was included in the CRPD analysis if the activities being described mapped directly to human rights expectations as expressed in the CRPD. The article with the highest level of noncompliance related to lack of AT provision was that of Accessibility (Article 9) with 32 instances of failure to realise reported; for example,

> "My rented flat has steps to get in the main entrance, so have to drive into downstairs car park, or come in the car entrance on the wheelchair. Ensuring all new apartment blocks with lifts have an entrance with no steps would be a big bonus! Also the apartment has a huge (20 cm) lip to get onto the balcony, so need to build a ramp."

Overall, 34 instances of participation consistent with the CRPD were explicitly named in the study data; however 134 instances of unsuccessful attainment relating to articles from the CRPD were also reported. Thus, the ratio of achievement to nonachievement against CRPD articles for the 100 participants in this study was approximately 1 : 4. This indicates that Australia has a substantial way to go in ensuring its obligations are met under the Convention.

4. Discussion

The right to engage in a full life despite the presence of impairment is enshrined within human rights documents such as CRPD [16] and operationalised within health and disability frameworks such as WHO ICF [12]. Survey participants represented a small but varied cohort of adults with disability and provided evidence of the efficacy of AT devices, environmental interventions, and personal care. The voices of these participants demonstrated the capacity of many "user experts" to name barriers, identify plausible facilitators, and identify likely impacts and outcomes. These impacts and outcomes align well with broad conceptualizations of life such as those provided by ICF Activities and Participation Chapters [12]. Mobility is not seen as an end in itself, rather a necessary capacity in order to participate in occupations of meaning, as the following statement by a retired physicist living with postpolio syndrome illustrates:

> "Now that I need to use the manual wheelchair all the time, I cannot get it under the kitchen bench to make a cup of coffee as the drawers and cupboards are in the way. That's really frustrating, because what I should be doing is working on the issue of carbon sequestration in the southern oceans."

This implies that valued outcomes must move beyond fragmented functional and independence measures which attend to capacities such as "mobility" as a discrete function and encompass emerging conceptualisations of life domains [19, 27].

The evidence presented supports the premise that combining interventions into tailored AT solutions is effective as this is in fact how they are used in life. Also, that a lack of joined up service provision exists in Victoria, Australia, along with significant underresourcing of government equipment provision schemes.

This study confirms other recent evidence in identifying that optimal mobility depends upon adequate provision of a range of enablers at both person and environment level [32, 33]. A multilevel or systems approach is required to address these levels [13, 33]. Those practitioners working with people with disabilities to enable participation must also attend to the world in which the person and their mobility device engage. Beyond the garden gate, people operate within broader environments. Facilitators such as continuous paths of travel within the community, accessible public transport networks, welcoming buildings with operable doors and lifts, accessible counters, and educated and friendly staff are essential ingredients for full participation beyond the home.

Who is responsible for the broader community environs? Duty holders in this respect may include local government authorities, government departments dealing with such infrastructure as transport, or individual businesses. While complaints to antidiscrimination bodies such as equal opportunity or human rights commissions can help provide redress for individuals unlawfully denied access to infrastructure or services, proactive measures by these stakeholders are necessary to address the systemic barriers which create inaccessible environments. Rehabilitation practitioners are key stakeholders in the business of enablers for mobility. Occupational therapists, physiotherapists, and other prescribers of AT devices and environmental adaptations to the home rarely advise more widely regarding the built environment. Arguably, practitioners must take on roles beyond individual advocate, towards the more political practice of systemic advocacy [34].

Several other developments may hold answers for improving other facets of inclusive community. The universal design and inclusive design movements [33, 35] offer to both minimize the costs of retrofitting for access through better planning and to destigmatise many enabling elements which can benefit entire communities [36]. From an economic perspective, several authors are beginning to investigate the costs and impacts of nonsocial design [37–39]. This approach potentially allocates costs of access and inclusion out to all community dwellers likely to benefit, so for example parents with prams and retirees share in the benefits of accessible transport and inclusive communities alongside people living with disabilities.

4.1. Limitations of the Study. This study provides a snapshot of enabler-use (broadly defined) and unmet need for a cohort of Victorians with disabilities. It is likely that people with disabilities living outside Victoria or indeed Australia would have similar experiences, although the contextual factors such as government funding or legislative support for community access are likely to differ in other jurisdictions. Efforts were made to ensure the survey tool was universally accessible; however the sample consists largely of adults on substantially low incomes and with low employment rates. Those whose cognition and language skills were insufficient for independent reporting were excluded. A significant issue with the survey design was missing demographic data, and in future studies it would be advisable to place the demographic section at the commencement of the survey, while monitoring impacts on completion particularly for severely impaired participants.

5. Conclusion

Individuals living with impairment face barriers on many levels. In researching community mobility, a valuable perspective is gained through examining barriers and facilitators at both person and environment level. On an individual level, access to tailored enablers is not guaranteed by government equipment schemes despite theoretic commitment to frameworks such as the ICF and the CRPD. From a societal standpoint, barriers remain present within environments and both political and community action be required to transform these environmental barriers into facilitators. If rehabilitation practitioners are committed to optimising community mobility, then the locus of attention must expand to encompass both the individual as well as broader elements of the environment.

Acknowledgment

The data reported in this paper was drawn from *The Equipping Inclusion Studies* which received philanthropic funding from the William Buckland Foundation.

References

[1] B. J. Lutz and B. J. Bowers, "Disability in everyday life," *Qualitative Health Research*, vol. 15, no. 8, pp. 1037–1054, 2005.

[2] *Oxford Dictionary of English*, Oxford University Press, New York, NY, USA, 2nd edition, 2008.

[3] K. L. Rust and R. O. Smith, "Assistive technology in the measurement of rehabilitation and health outcomes: a review and analysis of instruments," *American Journal of Physical Medicine and Rehabilitation*, vol. 84, no. 10, pp. 780–793, 2005.

[4] N. B. Oldridge, "Outcomes measurement: health-related quality of life," *Assistive Technology*, vol. 8, no. 2, pp. 82–93, 1996.

[5] G. Hawthorne, J. Richardson, and R. Osborne, "The Assessment of Quality of Life (AQoL) instrument: a psychometric measure of health-related quality of life," *Quality of Life Research*, vol. 8, no. 3, pp. 209–224, 1999.

[6] M. H. Rioux, "Disability: the place of judgement in a world of fact," *Journal of Intellectual Disability Research*, vol. 41, no. 2, pp. 102–111, 1997.

[7] J. Swain, S. French, C. Barnes, and C. Thomas, Eds., *Disabling Barriers—Enabling Environments*, Sage, London, Uk, 2004.

[8] C. Barnes and G. Mercer, Eds., *Implementing the Social Model of Disability: Theory and Research Leeds*, The Disability Press, 2004.

[9] T. Shakespeare, *Disability Rights and Wrongs*, Routledge, New York, NY, USA, 2006.

[10] T. Shakespeare, "Disability: suffering, social oppression, or complex predicament," in *The Contingent Nature of Life: Bioethics and Limits of Human Existence*, C. Rehmann-Sutter and D. Mieth, Eds., pp. 235–246, Springer, Amsterdam, The Netherlands, 2008.

[11] C. Thomas, *Sociologies of Disability and Illness: Contested Ideas in Disability Studies and Medical Sociology*, Palgrave Macmillan, Basingstoke, UK, 2007.

[12] World Health Organisation, *International Classification of Functioning, Disability and Health*, World Health Organisation, Geneva, Switzerland, 2001.

[13] G. G. Whiteneck, C. L. Harrison-Felix, D. C. Mellick, C. A. Brooks, S. B. Charlifue, and K. A. Gerhart, "Quantifying environmental factors: a measure of physical, attitudinal, service, productivity, and policy barriers," *Archives of Physical Medicine and Rehabilitation*, vol. 85, no. 8, pp. 1324–1335, 2004.

[14] Commonwealth of Australia, *National Disability Strategy 2010–2020*, 2011.

[15] State Government of Victoria, *Victorian State Disability Plan*, Disability Service Division, Victorian Government Department of Human Services, Melbourne, Australia, 2002.

[16] United Nations, *Convention on the Rights of Persons with Disabilities and Optional Protocol*, United Nations, Geneva, Switzerland, 2006.

[17] R. O. Smith, IMPACT 2 MODEL, 2009, http://www.r2d2 .uwm.edu/archive/impact2model.html, 2002.

[18] A. Cook and S. Hussey, Eds., *Assistive Technologies: Principles and Practice*, vol. 3, Mosby Elsevier, St. Louis, Mo, USA, 2008.

[19] N. Layton and E. Wilson, "Re-conceptualizing disability and assistive technology: Australian consumers driving policy change," *Technology and Disability*, vol. 21, no. 4, pp. 135–141, 2010.

[20] Audit Commission, 2002, Fully Equipped: assisting Independence, http://www.audit-commission.gov.uk/reports/ .

[21] A. Molenda, "Equipped for living literature review: identify the monetary benefit to individuals and government of assistive technology," *Journal of Independent Living Centres Australia*, vol. 22, pp. 21–23, 2006.

[22] AAATE, "AAATE position paper: a 2003 view on technology and disability," in *Proceedings of the Association for the Advancement of Assistive Technology in Europe (AAATE '03)*, 2003.

[23] F. Heywood and L. Turner, *Better Outcomes, Lower Costs: Implications for Health and Social Care Budgets of Investment in Housing Adaptations, Improvements and Equipment: a Review of the Evidence*, University of Bristol Office for Disability Issues, Bristol, UK, 2007.

[24] N. Layton, E. Wilson, S. Colgan, M. Moodie, and R. Carter, *The Equipping Inclusion Studies: Assistive Technology Use and Outcomes in Victoria*, Deakin University, Melbourne, Australia, 2010.

[25] A. T. Collaboration, 2009, Assistive Technology-Economics Collaboration, http://www.at.org.au .

[26] AEAA, *Aids and Equipment Action Alliance*, Melbourne, Australia, 2006.

[27] E. Wilson, "Defining and measuring the outcomes of inclusive community for people with disability, their families and the communities with whom they engage," in *From Ideology to Reality: Current Issues in Implementation of Intellectual Disability Policy: Proceedings of the Roundtable on Intellectual Disability Policy*, C. Bigby, C. Fyffe, and J. Mansell, Eds., pp. 24–33, LaTrobe University, Bundoora, Australia, 2006.

[28] D. Gottliebson, N. Layton, and E. Wilson, "Comparative effectiveness report: online survey tools," *Disability and Rehabilitation: Assistive Technology*, vol. 5, no. 6, pp. 401–410, 2010.

[29] ISO 9999, *Assistive Products for Persons with Disability—Classification and Terminology*, ISO, 2007.

[30] G. Hawthorne and R. Osborne, "Population norms and meaningful differences for the Assessment of Quality of Life (AQoL) measure," *Australian and New Zealand Journal of Public Health*, vol. 29, no. 2, pp. 136–142, 2005.

[31] A. Barbara and M. Curtin, "Gatekeepers or advocates? Occupational therapists and equipment funding schemes," *Australian Occupational Therapy Journal*, vol. 55, no. 1, pp. 57–60, 2008.

[32] J. Wee and R. Lysaght, "Factors affecting measures of activities and participation in persons with mobility impairment," *Disability and Rehabilitation*, vol. 31, no. 20, pp. 1633–1642, 2009.

[33] E. Steinfeld and G. S. Danford, *Enabling Environments: Measuring the Impact of Environment on Disability and Rehabilitation*, Kluwer Academic/Plenum, New York, NY, USA, 1999.

[34] F. Kronenberg, S. S. Algado, and N. Pollard, *Occupational Therapy without Borders: Learning from the Spirit of Survivors*, Elsevier Churchill Livingstone, London, UK, 2005.

[35] H. Dong, "Shifting paradigms in universal design," in *Universal Access in Human Computer Interaction: Coping with Diversity*, C. Stephanidis, Ed., pp. 66–74, Springer, Berlin, Germany, 2007.

[36] R. Nissim, *Universal Housing—Universal Benefits: A VCOSS Discussion Paper on Universal Housing Regulation in Victoria*, VCOSS, Melbourne, Australia, 2008.

[37] D. Fouarge, *Costs of Non-Social Policy: Towards an Economic Framework of Quality Social Policies—And the Costs of Not Having Them*, European Commission, 2003.

[38] I. Schraner and N. Bolzan, "Inclusion—what does it cost and how do we measure this?" in *Assistive Technology from Adapted Equipment to Inclusive Environments*, P. L. Emiliani, L. Burzagli, A. Como, F. Gabbanini, and A. Salminen, Eds., pp. 777–782, IOS Press, Amsterdam, The Netherlands, 2009.

[39] D. De Jonge and I. Schraner, "Economics of inclusiveness: can we as a society afford not to provide assistive technology or use universal design?" in *The State of the Science in Universal Design: Emerging Research and Developments*, J. Maisel, Ed., pp. 132–143, Bentham Science, Buffalo, NY, USA, 2010.

9

Does the Motor Level of the Paretic Extremities Affect Balance in Poststroke Subjects?

Kamal Narayan Arya, Shanta Pandian, C. R. Abhilasha, and Ashutosh Verma

Pandit Deendayal Upadhyaya Institute for the Physically Handicapped (University of Delhi),
Ministry of Social Justice and Empowerment, Government of India, 4 VD Marg, New Delhi 110002, India

Correspondence should be addressed to Kamal Narayan Arya; kamalnarya2@gmail.com

Academic Editor: Keh-chung Lin

Background. Poststroke impairment may lead to fall and unsafe functional performance. The underlying mechanism for the balance dysfunction is unclear. *Objective.* To analyze the relation between the motor level of the affected limbs and balance in poststroke subjects. *Method.* A prospective, cross-sectional, and nonexperimental design was conducted in a rehabilitation institute. A convenience sample of 44 patients was assessed for motor level using Brunnstrom recovery stage (BRS) and Fugl-Meyer Assessment: upper (FMA-UE) and lower extremities (FMA-LE). The balance was measured by Berg Balance Scale (BBS), Postural Assessment Scale for Stroke Patients (PASS), and Functional Reach Test (FRT). *Results.* BRS showed moderate correlation with BBS ($\rho = 0.54$ to 0.60; $P < 0.001$), PASS ($r = 0.48$ to 0.64; $P < 0.001$) and FRT ($\rho = 0.48$ to 0.59; $P < 0.001$). FMA-UE also exhibited moderate correlation with BBS ($\rho = 0.59$; $P < 0.001$) and PASS ($\rho = 0.60$; $P < 0.001$). FMA-LE showed fair correlation with BBS ($\rho = 0.50$; $P = 0.001$) and PASS ($\rho = 0.50$; $P = 0.001$). *Conclusion.* Motor control of the affected limbs plays an important role in balance. There is a moderate relation between the motor level of the upper and lower extremities and balance. The findings of the present study may be applied in poststroke rehabilitation.

1. Introduction

Balance is an ability to maintain upright position within the base of support during static and dynamic positions [1]. Balance dysfunction, especially during maintenance of erect upright posture and walking, is a common poststroke consequence. Inability to maintain balance reduces functional performance and increases the fall frequency [2]. The dysfunction leads to various musculoskeletal complications multiplying the rehabilitation challenges [3–7].

In stroke, the exact mechanism underlying balance impairment is ambiguous [8]. The factors such as cognition, perception, and biomechanical alterations were found to be responsible for the impairment [9, 10].

A subject with hemiparesis bears more weight on the nonparetic lower extremity leading to asymmetry and impaired erect posture [11]. The weight-bearing asymmetry is associated with the increased postural sway and poor balance [12, 13]. The inability of the nonaffected lower extremity

to compensate for the paretic limb also contributes to the postural imbalance [11, 14]. In addition, the arm movements have a considerable role in balance control. The movement of upper limbs usually appears prior to and during loss of balance. By reaching and grasping the outside support, the arms provide a protective function during the fall. The upper limb movements also prevent a fall by shifting the centre of gravity opposite to the direction of imbalance [15, 16]. Due to the arm paresis, poststroke subjects exhibit poor protective function to maintain balance [17]. They demonstrate a deficit in anticipatory and reactive postural adjustments [10]. The impairment of affected lower and upper limbs does not permit the subject to recover from perturbations during functional tasks such as walking [11, 18–20].

In stroke, the voluntary limb movements may have a contribution in balance. However, no study has investigated the relation between the voluntary motor control of the limbs and balance impairment. The objective of the present study was to analyze the relation between the motor level of the affected upper and lower extremities and balance in poststroke subject.

2. Methods

2.1. Participants. Forty-four patients (34 men and 10 women) attending the Outpatient Occupational Therapy Department of Pandit Deendayal Upadhyaya Institute for the Physically Handicapped were selected for the study. The study protocol was approved by the ethics committee of the institute. The stroke subjects were briefed about the assessment procedure before they signed the informed consent. The subjects who met the following inclusion criteria were selected for the study: (1) chronic stroke (>6 months of onset), (2) ischemic or hemorrhagic stroke, (3) 35 to 65 years of age [21–23], and (4) Functional Ambulation Classification (FAC) [24] level 2 and above. The subjects were excluded from the study if they exhibited (1) cerebellar lesion, (2) multiple strokes, (3) severe cognitive and perceptual deficit, and (4) any acute medical illness.

This study was a prospective, cross-sectional, and nonexperimental design. The subjects were conveniently selected as per the inclusion criteria. A detailed clinical evaluation was performed and then the standardized assessments were applied. The assessments were carried out by two assessors who had 15 to 20 years of experience in stroke rehabilitation. One of the assessors applied the motor measures for all the subjects, while the other conducted the balance measures for them. Two sessions were allotted for the entire assessments, one for the motor level and the other for the balance assessment. All the assessment procedures were performed as per the standard guidelines of the respective scale.

2.2. Outcome Measures. Motor level was assessed by using Brunnstrom recovery stages (BRS) and Fugl-Meyer Assessment (FMA) for the upper and lower extremities [25, 26]. BRS is classified under six categories (1, flaccidity with no movement, to 6, individual joint movement with little awkwardness) as per the motor recovery process of poststroke hemiparesis. The stages have been separately described for the upper extremity (BRS-UE), hand (BRS-H), and lower extremity (BRS-LE). BRS demonstrated strong responsiveness with the Motricity Index (effect size $d = 0.97$, Wilcoxon $Z = 5.33$, and $P < 0.001$; $d = 0.81$, $Z = 5.09$, and $P < 0.001$) [27]. BRS was found to be highly valid ($r = -0.81$; $P < 0.001$) when compared with neurophysiological measures [28]. However, there is no reporting of its reliability in the literature. FMA, a 3-point ordinal scale, measures the impairment of volitional movement ranging from 0 (items cannot be performed) to two (items can be fully performed). The upper extremity section of this scale (FMA-UE) is divided into two subsections: upper arm (FMA-UA) and wrist hand (FMA-WH). The section comprises nine items (6: upper arm; 3: wrist hand) with a sum score of 66 (36: upper arm; 30: hand). The lower extremity section (FMA-LE) has six items with a maximum score of 34. In both the sections, items are further divided into different subcomponents. FMA demonstrated high reliability ($r = 0.99$) and good validity

($r = 0.63$ to 0.88) [29, 30]. It exhibited good responsiveness for the poststroke motor assessment [31].

The balance of the subjects was assessed by Berg Balance Scale (BBS), Postural Assessment Scale for Stroke Patients (PASS), and Functional Reach Test (FRT). BBS is used to assess static and dynamic balance abilities required for functional tasks. It comprises 14 items, scored on a 5-point ordinal scale (0, poor balance, to 4, good balance) with a maximum score of 56. The items range from unsupported sitting/standing to turn 360°/standing upon one leg. The scale demonstrated excellent interrater as well as test-retest reliability (ICC = 0.91 to 0.99) and internal consistency (Cronbach alpha = 0.92 to 0.98), and its validity ranged from 0.55 to 0.91 (r) [29, 32, 33]. PASS assesses postural control on a 4-point ordinal scale (0, cannot perform, to 3, can perform independently) comprising 12 items (PASS-T), 5 for maintaining (PASS-M) and 7 for changing the posture (PASS-C). It showed excellent interrater agreement (ICC = 0.97) and high internal consistency (Cronbach = 0.93). Further, it showed acceptable validity, ranging from 0.73 to 0.89 (r) [34]. FRT is a quick and performance-based test to assess dynamic postural control during a functional activity. It is measured as a maximal forward-reaching distance beyond the arm's length while maintaining the standing position. The normal range varies from 10.5 to 16.7 inches depending on the age and gender [33]. The reliability of FRT ranges from 0.92 to 0.98 (ICC), while the validity varies from 0.65 to 0.71 (r). In the present study, the measurement was performed on the less-affected upper extremity [29].

2.3. Data Analysis. Data analysis was performed using IBM SPSS, version 21.0. The Spearman test (ρ) was used to find the relation between the measures of motor level and balance. Relation between the individual items of each motor outcome measure with that of the balance measures was analyzed using the same test. The level of relation corresponding to the correlation coefficient was followed as low (<0.5; $P < 0.05$), moderate (0.5 to 0.69; $P < 0.05$), and high (0.7 to 0.89; $P < 0.05$) [35]. Furthermore, subgroup and partial correlation analysis were also conducted. The significance level was set at $P < 0.05$.

3. Results

All the enrolled subjects completed the assessment protocol. The mean age of the participants was 48.82 ± 12.04 years. The average poststroke duration was 19.73 ± 12.21 months. Twenty-six (59%) subjects had right side paresis. Three subjects (7%) exhibited the hand dominance for left side. Table 1 shows the detailed demographic characteristics of the participants. Thirty-two (72.5%) subjects were at stages III to IV of BRS-UE, while 31 (70%) were at stages III to IV of BRS-LE. The mean BBS of the subjects was 42.64 ± 10.35. Table 2 shows the description of the motor level and balance as assessed by the outcome measures.

On analyzing the relation between the measures of motor level and balance, moderate correlation ($\rho = 0.5$ to 0.7) was found between most of the variables. BRS-UE, BRS-H, and

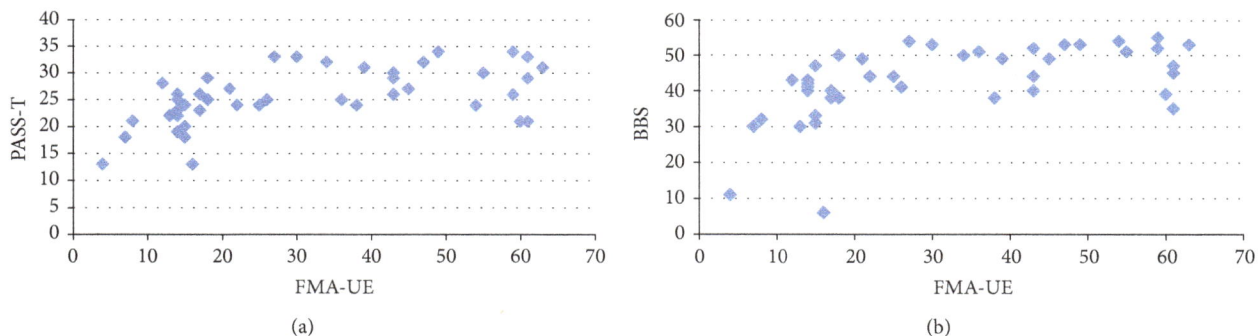

FIGURE 1: (a) Showing the relation between the total score of Fugl-Meyer Assessment: upper extremity (FMA-UE) and Postural Assessment Scale for Stroke (PASS-T). (b) Showing the relation between the total score of Fugl-Meyer Assessment: upper extremity (FMA-UE) and total score of Berg Balance Scale (BBS).

TABLE 1: Demographic characteristics of the participants.

Characteristics	Number (%)/mean ± SD
Number of participants (44)	
Male/female	34 (77%)/10 (23%)
Age (in years)	48.82 ± 12.04
Poststroke duration (in months)	19.73 ± 12.21
Side of involvement (right/left)	26 (59%)/18 (41%)
Handedness (right/left)	41 (93%)/03 (07%)
Type of stroke	
Ischemic/hemorrhagic	28 (64%)/16 (36%)
Area of involvement	
Frontoparietal	12 (27%)
Basal ganglia	04 (09%)
Thalamus	06 (14%)
Internal capsule	02 (4.5%)
Multiple	20 (45.5%)
Risk factor	
Hypertensive	32 (77%)
Hereditary	15 (34%)
Smoking	12 (27%)
Alcoholic	17 (39%)
Diabetic	08 (18%)
Obesity	07 (16%)

SD: standard deviation.

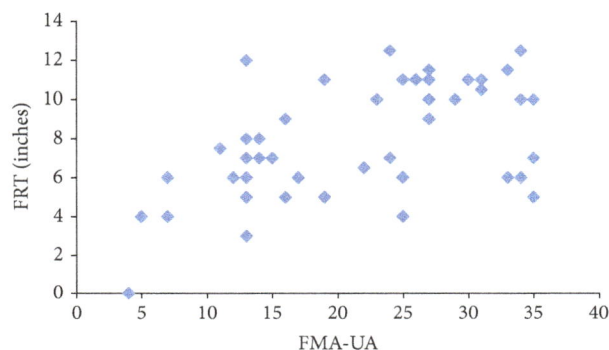

FIGURE 2: Showing the relation between the upper arm subscore of Fugl-Meyer Assessment (FMA-UA) and Functional Reach Test (FRT).

BRS-LE showed moderate correlation with BBS ($\rho = 0.54$ to 0.60; $P < 0.001$), PASS ($\rho = 0.48$ to 0.64; $P \leq 0.001$), and FRT ($\rho = 0.48$ to 0.59; $P \leq 0.001$). FMA-UE, including FMA-UA, also exhibited moderate correlation with BBS ($\rho = 0.59$ to 0.63; $P < 0.001$) and PASS ($\rho = 0.54$ to 0.62; $P < 0.001$). Figures 1(a) and 1(b) show the relation between the FMA-UE and BBS and PASS-T. FMA-UE along with FMA-WH demonstrated low relation with FRT. However, FMA-UA alone was found to be related to FRT ($\rho = 0.50$; $P = 0.002$). Figure 2 showed the relation between FMA-UA and FRT. FMA-LE demonstrated fair correlation with BBS ($\rho = 0.50$; $P = 0.001$) and PASS ($\rho = 0.50$; $P = 0.001$). It showed poor relation with PASS-C while showing no relation with FRT. Table 3 shows the detailed ρ value for all the variables.

Further, on exploring the relation between the individual items of FMA with the same of BBS, FMA-UE items II (flexor synergy), III (extensor synergy), and IV (movement out of synergy) were found to have moderate correlation (0.50 to 0.64; $P = 0.001$ to 0.003) with most of the BBS items (except items 1, 2, 3, 5, and 6). FMA wrist-hand items (VII and VIII) also exhibited moderate relation with BBS items 4, 7, and 9 (0.50 to 0.58 and $P < 0.001$ to 0.002). FMA IX showed moderate relation with BBS items 4 to 12 (ranging from 0.50 to 0.65; $P < 0.001$ to 0.002). FMA-UE items II, III, IV, and IX demonstrated significant correlation with total BBS (0.46 to 0.66; $P < 0.001$ to 0.002). All items of FMA-UE (except I and II) showed good relation with PASS item 3 (standing with support) (0.50 to 0.58; $P < 0.001$). FMA-UE items II to V were found to be significantly related (0.45 to 0.66; $P < 0.001$ to 0.003) with PASS-C items 6 to 10. FMA-UE II to IV also exhibited moderate correlation with total PASS score (0.55 to 0.65; $P < 0.001$). FMA-UE VII, VIII, and IX demonstrated correlation with PASS item 6 (0.45 to 0.53 and $P < 0.001$ to 0.002). FMA-UE VII and IX were found to be related to PASS item 10 (0.45 to 0.47 and $P < 0.001$ to 0.002). Same components of FMA-UE showed good relation with total

TABLE 2: Description of motor recovery and balance measures.

Outcome measures	Stage I	Stage II	Stage III	Stage IV	Stage V	Stage VI
BRS-A	00 (0%)	04 (9%)	20 (45.5%)	12 (27%)	07 (16%)	01 (2%)
BRS-H	00 (0%)	20 (45.5%)	10 (23%)	07 (16%)	06 (13.5%)	01 (2%)
BRS-LE	01 (2%)	02 (4.5%)	12 (27%)	19 (43%)	10 (23%)	00 (0%)
			Mean ± SD			
FMA-UE (*maximum score—66*)			31.98 ± 18.92			
FMA-UA (*maximum score—36*)			21.59 ± 9.23			
FMA-WH (*maximum score—30*)			10.39 ± 9.51			
FMA-LE (*maximum score—34*)			19.64 ± 5.10			
BBS (*maximum score—56*)			42.64 ± 10.35			
PASS-T (*maximum score—36*)			25.75 ± 5.30			
PASS-M (*maximum score—15*)			10.45 ± 2.18			
PASS-C (*maximum score—21*)			15.30 ± 3.46			
FRT (*in inches*)			7.87 ± 2.94			

BRS: Brunnstrom recovery stages, A: arm, H: hand, FMA: Fugl-Meyer Assessment, UE: upper extremity, UA: upper arm, WH: wrist and hand, BBS: Bergs Balance Scale, PASS: Postural Assessment Scale for Stroke Patients, T: total, M: maintenance of posture, C: change in posture, FRT: Functional Reach Test, and SD: standard deviation.

TABLE 3: Relation between the motor recovery and balance measures.

	BBS	PASS-C	PASS-M	PASS-T	FRT
BRS-A	$\rho = 0.60$ ($P < 0.001$)	$\rho = 0.64$ ($P < 0.001$)	$\rho = 0.55$ ($P < 0.001$)	$\rho = 0.63$ ($P < 0.001$)	$\rho = 0.59$ ($P < 0.001$)
BRS-H	$\rho = 0.55$ ($P < 0.001$)	$\rho = 0.50$ ($P = 0.001$)	$\rho = 0.50$ ($P = 0.001$)	$\rho = 0.52$ ($P < 0.001$)	$\rho = 0.55$ ($P < 0.001$)
BRS-LE	$\rho = 0.54$ ($P < 0.001$)	$\rho = 0.51$ ($P < 0.001$)	$\rho = 0.55$ ($P < 0.001$)	$\rho = 0.57$ ($P < 0.001$)	$\rho = 0.48$ ($P = 0.001$)
FMA-UE	$\rho = 0.59$ ($P < 0.001$)	$\rho = 0.56$ ($P < 0.001$)	$\rho = 0.54$ ($P < 0.001$)	$\rho = 0.60$ ($P < 0.001$)	$\rho = 0.38$ ($P = 0.01$)
FMA-UA	$\rho = 0.63$ ($P < 0.001$)	$\rho = 0.59$ ($P < 0.001$)	$\rho = 0.58$ ($P < 0.001$)	$\rho = 0.62$ ($P < 0.001$)	$\rho = 0.50$ ($P = 0.002$)
FMA-WH	$\rho = 0.50$ $P = 0.001$	$\rho = 0.50$ $P = 0.001$	$\rho = 0.43$ $P < 0.003$	$\rho = 0.50$ ($P < 0.001$)	$\rho = 0.30$ $P < 0.04$
FMA-LE	$\rho = 0.50$ ($P = 0.001$)	$\rho = 0.41$ ($P = 0.006$)	$\rho = 0.50$ ($P = 0.001$)	$\rho = 0.50$ ($P = 0.001$)	NS

BRS: Brunnstrom recovery stages, A: arm, H: hand, FMA: Fugl-Meyer Assessment, UA: upper arm, WH: wrist and hand, UE: upper extremity, PASS: Postural Assessment Scale for Stroke Patients, C: change in posture, M: maintenance of posture, FRT: Functional Reach Test, BBS: Berg Balance Scale, ρ: Spearman test, and NS: not significant.

PASS (0.50 to 0.51; $P < 0.001$). FMA-UE items II, III, and IV displayed low relation with FRT (0.45 to 0.48; $P < 0.001$ to 0.002). All other FMA-UE items did not demonstrate any relation with FRT.

BBS and FMA-LE item II (flexor synergy) were found to be related to BBS items 5, 8, 11, 12, and 14 and overall total BBS ($\rho = 0.50$ to 0.60 and $P < 0.001$ for all). FMA-LE item IV showed significant correlation with two items of BBS (8 and 14) and total BBS ($\rho = 0.45$ to 0.47 and $P = 0.001$ to 0.002). Only 2 FMA-LE items (III and IV) were found to be related to PASS items 3, 4, 8, 9, and 10 ($\rho = 0.47$ to 0.58 and $P \leq 0.001$). The items also related to PASS-M ($\rho = 0.49$ to 0.53; $P \leq 0.001$) and total PASS score ($\rho = 0.48$ to 0.52 and $P \leq 0.001$). Figures 3(a) and 3(b) show the relation between the FMA-LE and BBS and PASS-T. None of the items of FMA-LE was found to be related to FRT.

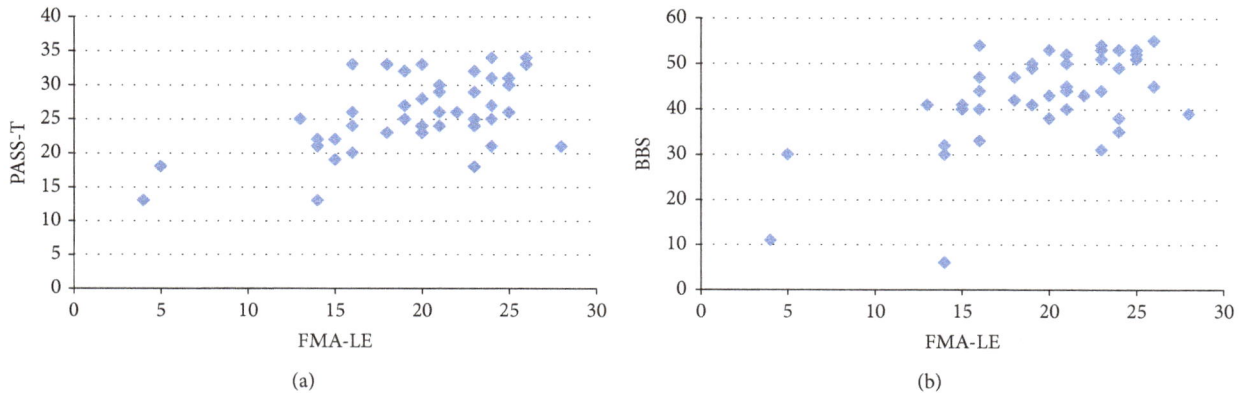

FIGURE 3: (a) Showing the relation between the total score of Fugl-Meyer Assessment: lower extremity (FMA-LE) and Postural Assessment Scale for Stroke (PASS-T). (b) Showing the relation between the total score of Fugl-Meyer Assessment: lower extremity (FMA-LE) and total scores of Berg Balance Scale (BBS).

The scores of balance measures were not found to be significantly different between the subgroups based on the side of involvement (dominant/nondominant side) and gender. Only FRT of male subjects (8.44 ± 2.98 inches) was found to be higher than the female subjects (5.95 ± 1.80 inches) with $P < 0.008$.

Partial correlation analysis was also performed to neutralize the effect of FMA-UE and FMA-LE on one another, when inferring the relation with balance measures. By controlling FMA-LE, no relation was found between FMA-UE and BBS, while, on controlling FMA-UE, FMA-LE demonstrated low significant relation with BBS ($\rho = 0.38$; $P < 0.012$). Both FMA-UE and FMA-LE exhibited no relation with PASS-T when one of the FMA (FMA-LE / FMA-UE) components was controlled.

4. Discussion

Balance is a complex motor behavior and involves multiple sensorimotor, environmental, and functional contexts, required during functional performance [9]. In other words, all factors, such as biomechanical constraint, cognition, perception, somatosensation, and motor control, affect the balance ability. Apart from the paretic lower limb, the upper extremity may also be responsible for poor balance [13, 15].

To date, no study has inferred the relation between the motor level of the limbs and balance in stroke. Most of the studies have been done focusing either on the weight-bearing and functional issues or on the validity aspect of a measure [11, 12, 14, 36, 37]. This study utilized multiple measures for assessing motor level and balance. The three balance measures were used to examine the various simple to complex balance-related tasks. In addition, the relation was investigated between individual movement and balance components. The findings of the present study revealed a positive relation between the motor level of the paretic limbs and balance in stroke subjects.

After stroke, the paretic upper limb is unable to execute voluntary movements, usually needed before and during losing the balance. The findings of the present study indicated that the lower the motor level of the upper limb the poorer the balance. Although the role of arm movement in balance control is evident to the healthy individuals, no study confirms the same in stroke subjects [15, 16].

Due to hemiparesis of the body, the centre of gravity shifts to the stronger side of the body. Weight-bearing asymmetry is the most common reason proposed for balance deficit among stroke survivors [11, 12]. The lower extremity recovery level exhibited moderate relation with BBS and PASS-T. However, FMA-LE assesses only voluntary movements of the lower limb and does not have any weight-bearing item. It may be inferred that the ability to carry out voluntary leg movements is necessary for maintaining balance, for example, the stepping strategy, the ability to take forward or sideward step to prevent falling [33].

Fall is the most common complication in poststroke subjects, and the fear of fall or anticipatory behaviour leads to reduced physical activity [38]. The average BBS of the study participants was 42.6. The scores below 45 were considered as increased risk for falls [39]. However, the relation of BBS scores between fallers and nonfallers is still controversial [20]. In the present study, 18 (41%) subjects reported fear of fall, 14 (32%) had history of occasional fall, and 12 (27%) had the frequent fall prior to the rehabilitation management. All the participants were undergoing conventional rehabilitation for more than 3 months. None of the subjects reported fall after the commencement of the management.

FRT was not found to be related to both FMA-UE and FMA-LE. This could be due to the assessment of FRT using the less-affected upper limb. In comparison to other balance measures, FRT assesses only reaching ability. BBS, apart from reaching, comprises multiple balance-related tasks in static and dynamic positions. PASS exclusively measures stroke-related postural impairment. Although some of the items overlap with that of the BBS, PASS specifically assesses paretic side and bed mobility.

Simultaneous recovery of the affected upper and lower limbs may influence the balance control. In the present study, the effect of motor level of one limb (upper or lower) was controlled while analyzing the relation of recovery with balance. It could be inferred that the balance is not related to either upper or lower limb independently. Rather, balance is an integrated response of the performance of the upper extremities while maintaining upright position by the lower extremities.

A good correlation was found between the recovery of affected limb (upper limb and lower limb independently) and balance. However, the level of relation declined when both the affected limbs were considered as a single unit. Both FMA-UE and FMA-LE exhibited no relation with PASS-T when one of the FMA (FMA-LE/FMA-UE) components was controlled.

FMA-UE components exhibited good relation with the majority of BBS items. The items were either those which required control through protective extension such as stand-to-sit or complex items (9 and beyond) comprising the upper limb control and manipulation. Similarly, FMA-UA components exhibited good relation with most of the PASS-C items, which required the upper extremity control during postural change. Both synergistic and nonsynergistic FMA-LE components demonstrated acceptable association with BBS items such as reaching forward while standing and standing upon one leg.

Different approaches such as task-oriented gait training are used to alleviate balance dysfunction in stroke [40]. Despite evidence, no single approach is considered to be the best to achieve balance in stroke subjects [41]. The arm training improves postural control and independent walking [42, 43]. Exclusive task-oriented arm training in standing may improve postural control (centre of pressure displacement and the anticipatory adjustments) [42, 44]. The role of the limbs in balance control may be utilized in stroke rehabilitation. The present study had few limitations, for instance, variability in age, chronicity, and lesioned area. The number of female participants was considerably low. The trunk impairment may also affect balance. However, the trunk control was not assessed in the study. Further, due to nonavailability of the reliability, only the validity as a psychometric value was considered for BRS.

Advance measures such as kinematic analysis and force place may be used for future studies. Interaction of rehabilitation intervention on recovery and balance may be investigated in the longitudinal studies.

5. Conclusion

Balance, a multifactorial phenomenon, required for safe functional performance, gets impaired in stroke. In the present study, there exists a positive relation between the motor level of the affected upper and lower extremities and balance among poststroke subjects. Voluntary motor control of the paretic limbs may be one of the factors in balance-related functions. The findings may be utilized in planning stroke rehabilitation program.

Conflict of Interests

The authors declare that there is no conflict of interests regarding the publication of this paper.

Acknowledgment

The present study was partially funded by the Pandit Deendayal Upadhyaya Institute for the Physically Handicapped, 4 Vishnu Digamber Marg, New Delhi, India.

References

[1] S. F. Tyson, M. Hanley, J. Chillala, A. Selley, and R. C. Tallis, "Balance disability after stroke," *Physical Therapy*, vol. 86, no. 1, pp. 30–38, 2006.

[2] A. A. Schmid, M. van Puymbroeck, P. A. Altenburger et al., "Balance and balance self-efficacy are associated with activity and participation after stroke: a cross-sectional study in people with chronic stroke," *Archives of Physical Medicine and Rehabilitation*, vol. 93, no. 6, pp. 1101–1107, 2012.

[3] J. E. Harris, J. J. Eng, D. S. Marigold, C. D. Tokuno, and C. L. Louis, "Relationship of balance and mobility to fall incidence in people with chronic stroke," *Physical Therapy*, vol. 85, no. 2, pp. 150–158, 2005.

[4] V. Weerdesteyn, M. de Niet, H. J. R. van Duijnhoven, and A. C. H. Geurts, "Falls in individuals with stroke," *Journal of Rehabilitation Research and Development*, vol. 45, no. 8, pp. 1195–1214, 2008.

[5] M. Rensink, M. Schuurmans, E. Lindeman, and T. B. Hafsteinsdóttir, "Falls: incidence and risk factors after stroke—a systematic literature review," *Tijdschrift voor Gerontologie en Geriatrie*, vol. 40, no. 4, pp. 156–167, 2009.

[6] P. Lisiński, J. Huber, E. Gajewska, and P. Szłapiński, "The body balance training effect on improvement of motor functions in paretic extremities in patients after stroke—a randomized, single blinded trial," *Clinical Neurology and Neurosurgery*, vol. 114, no. 1, pp. 31–36, 2012.

[7] J. Y. Lim, S. H. Jung, W. S. Kim, and N. J. Paik, "Incidence and risk factors of poststroke falls after discharge from inpatient rehabilitation," *PM & R*, vol. 4, no. 12, pp. 945–953, 2012.

[8] M. Mihara, I. Miyai, N. Hattori et al., "Cortical control of postural balance in patients with hemiplegic stroke," *Neuroreport*, vol. 23, no. 5, pp. 314–319, 2012.

[9] C. B. de Oliveira, I. R. T. de Medeiros, N. A. F. Frota, M. E. Greters, and A. B. Conforto, "Balance control in hemiparetic stroke patients: main tools for evaluation," *Journal of Rehabilitation Research and Development*, vol. 45, no. 8, pp. 1215–1226, 2008.

[10] J. Carr and R. Shepherd, *Stroke Rehabilitation: Guidelines for Exercises and Training to Optimize Motor Skill*, Butterworth-Heinemann, London, UK, 1st edition, 2003.

[11] A. Mansfield, G. Mochizuki, E. L. Inness, and W. E. McIlroy, "Clinical correlates of between-limb synchronization of standing balance control and falls during inpatient stroke rehabilitation," *Neurorehabilitation and Neural Repair*, vol. 26, no. 6, pp. 627–635, 2012.

[12] J. F. Kamphuis, D. de Kam, A. C. Geurts, and V. Weerdesteyn, "Is weight-bearing asymmetry associated with postural instability after stroke? A systematic review," *Stroke Research and Treatment*, vol. 2013, Article ID 692137, 13 pages, 2013.

[13] J. Hendrickson, K. K. Patterson, E. L. Inness, W. E. McIlroy, and A. Mansfield, "Relationship between asymmetry of quiet standing balance control and walking post-stroke," *Gait & Posture*, vol. 39, no. 1, pp. 177–181, 2014.

[14] N. Genthon, P. Rougier, A.-S. Gissot, J. Féroger, J. Pélissier, and D. Pérennou, "Contribution of each lower limb to upright standing in stroke patients," *Stroke*, vol. 39, no. 6, pp. 1793–1799, 2008.

[15] M. Shafeie, S. Manifar, M. Milosevic, and K. M. McConville, "Arm movement effect on balance," in *Proceedings of the Annual International Conference of the IEEE Engineering in Medicine and Biology Society (EMBC '12)*, pp. 4549–4552, San Diego, Calif, USA, August-September 2012.

[16] M. Milosevic, K. M. V. McConville, and K. Masani, "Arm movement improves performance in clinical balance and mobility tests," *Gait & Posture*, vol. 33, no. 3, pp. 507–509, 2011.

[17] M. Acar and G. K. Karatas, "The effect of arm sling on balance in patients with hemiplegia," *Gait & Posture*, vol. 32, no. 4, pp. 641–644, 2010.

[18] T. Krasovsky, A. Lamontagne, A. G. Feldman, and M. F. Levin, "Reduced gait stability in high-functioning poststroke individuals," *Journal of Neurophysiology*, vol. 109, no. 1, pp. 77–88, 2013.

[19] M. D. Lewek, C. E. Bradley, C. J. Wutzke, and S. M. Zinder, "The relationship between spatiotemporal gait asymmetry and balance in individuals with chronic stroke," *Journal of Applied Biomechanics*, vol. 30, no. 1, pp. 31–36, 2013.

[20] T. Baetens, A. de Kegel, P. Calders, G. Vanderstraeten, and D. Cambier, "Prediction of falling among stroke patients in rehabilitation," *Journal of Rehabilitation Medicine*, vol. 43, no. 10, pp. 876–883, 2011.

[21] G. F. Fuller, "Falls in the elderly," *The American Family Physician*, vol. 61, no. 7, pp. 2159–2168, 2173–2174, 2000.

[22] D. Griffiths and J. Sturm, "Epidemiology and etiology of young stroke," *Stroke Research and Treatment*, vol. 2011, Article ID 209370, 9 pages, 2011.

[23] B. Ovbiagele and M. N. Nguyen-Huynh, "Stroke epidemiology: advancing our understanding of disease mechanism and therapy," *Neurotherapeutics*, vol. 8, no. 3, pp. 319–329, 2011.

[24] J. Perry, M. Garrett, J. K. Gronley, and S. J. Mulroy, "Classification of walking handicap in the stroke population," *Stroke*, vol. 26, no. 6, pp. 982–989, 1995.

[25] A. R. Fugl-Meyer, L. Jaasko, I. Leyman, S. Olsson, and S. Steglind, "The post stroke hemiplegic patient. I. A method for evaluation of physical performance," *Scandinavian Journal of Rehabilitation Medicine*, vol. 7, no. 1, pp. 13–31, 1975.

[26] K. Sawner and J. LaVigne, *Brunnstrom's Movement Therapy in Hemiplegia: A Neurophysiological Approach*, JB Lippincott, Philadelphia, Pa, USA, 2nd edition, 1992.

[27] I. Safaz, B. Yilmaz, E. Yaşar, and R. Alaca, "Brunnstrom recovery stage and motricity index for the evaluation of upper extremity in stroke: analysis for correlation and responsiveness," *International Journal of Rehabilitation Research*, vol. 32, no. 3, pp. 228–231, 2009.

[28] S. Naghdi, N. N. Ansari, K. Mansouri, and S. Hasson, "A neurophysiological and clinical study of Brunnstrom recovery stages in the upper limb following stroke," *Brain Injury*, vol. 24, no. 11, pp. 1372–1378, 2010.

[29] E. Finch, D. Brooks, P. W. Stratford, and E. N. Mayo, *Physical Rehabilitation Outcome Measures: A Guide to Enhanced Clinical Decision Making*, Canadian Physiotherapy Association, Ontario, Canada, 2nd edition, 2002.

[30] J.-H. Lin, M.-J. Hsu, C.-F. Sheu et al., "Psychometric comparisons of 4 measures for assessing upper-extremity function in people with stroke," *Physical Therapy*, vol. 89, no. 8, pp. 840–850, 2009.

[31] Y.-W. Hsieh, C.-Y. Wu, K.-C. Lin, Y.-F. Chang, C.-L. Chen, and J.-S. Liu, "Responsiveness and validity of three outcome measures of motor function after stroke rehabilitation," *Stroke*, vol. 40, no. 4, pp. 1386–1391, 2009.

[32] L. Blum and N. Korner-Bitensky, "Usefulness of the berg balance scale in stroke rehabilitation: a systematic review," *Physical Therapy*, vol. 88, no. 5, pp. 559–566, 2008.

[33] S. O'Sullivan and T. J. Schmitz, Eds., *Physical Rehabilitation*, F.A. Davis, Philadelphia, Pa, USA, 5th edition, 2007.

[34] C.-H. Wang, I.-P. Hsueh, C.-F. Sheu, and C.-L. Hsieh, "Discriminative, predictive, and evaluative properties of a trunk control measure in patients with stroke," *Physical Therapy*, vol. 85, no. 9, pp. 887–894, 2005.

[35] R. Carter, J. Lubinsky, and E. Domholdt, Eds., *Rehabilitation Research: Principles and Applications*, Elsevier Saunders, St. Louis, Mo, USA, 4th edition, 2011.

[36] M. Likhi, V. V. Jidesh, R. Kanagaraj, and J. K. George, "Does trunk, arm, or leg control correlate best with overall function in stroke subjects?" *Topics in Stroke Rehabilitation*, vol. 20, no. 1, pp. 62–67, 2013.

[37] S. Knorr, B. Brouwer, and S. J. Garland, "Validity of the community balance and mobility scale in community-dwelling persons after stroke," *Archives of Physical Medicine and Rehabilitation*, vol. 91, no. 6, pp. 890–896, 2010.

[38] K. Cho and G. Lee, "Impaired dynamic balance is associated with falling in post-stroke patients," *The Tohoku Journal of Experimental Medicine*, vol. 230, no. 4, pp. 233–239, 2013.

[39] B. L. D. Thorbahn and R. A. Newton, "Use of the berg balance test to predict falls in elderly persons," *Physical Therapy*, vol. 76, no. 6, pp. 576–583, 584–585, 1996.

[40] N. M. Salbach, N. E. Mayo, S. Robichaud-Ekstrand, J. A. Hanley, C. L. Richards, and S. Wood-Dauphinee, "The effect of a task-oriented walking intervention on improving balance self-efficacy poststroke: a randomized, controlled trial," *Journal of the American Geriatrics Society*, vol. 53, no. 4, pp. 576–582, 2005.

[41] A. C. H. Geurts, M. de Haart, I. J. W. van Nes, and J. Duysens, "A review of standing balance recovery from stroke," *Gait & Posture*, vol. 22, no. 3, pp. 267–281, 2005.

[42] M. S. Waller and M. G. Prettyman, "Arm training in standing also improves postural control in participants with chronic stroke," *Gait & Posture*, vol. 36, no. 3, pp. 419–424, 2012.

[43] S. S. Y. Au-Yeung, J. T. W. Ng, and S. K. Lo, "Does balance or motor impairment of limbs discriminate the ambulatory status of stroke survivors?" *The American Journal of Physical Medicine and Rehabilitation*, vol. 82, no. 4, pp. 279–283, 2003.

[44] A. Kubicki, G. Petrement, F. Bonnetblanc, Y. Ballay, and F. Mourey, "Practice-related improvements in postural control during rapid arm movement in older adults: a preliminary study," *Journals of Gerontology A: Biological Sciences and Medical Sciences*, vol. 67, no. 2, pp. 196–203, 2012.

10

Work Status and Return to the Workforce after Coronary Artery Bypass Grafting and/or Heart Valve Surgery: A One-Year-Follow Up Study

Kirsten Fonager,[1,2] Søren Lundbye-Christensen,[1] Jan Jesper Andreasen,[3,4] Mikkel Futtrup,[3] Anette Luther Christensen,[3] Khalil Ahmad,[3] and Martin Agge Nørgaard[3]

[1] *Department of Social Medicine, Center for Cardiovascular Research, Aalborg University Hospital, 9100 Aalborg, Denmark*
[2] *Department of Health Science and Technology, Faculty of Medicine, Aalborg University, 9220 Aalborg, Denmark*
[3] *Department of Cardiothoracic Surgery, Center for Cardiovascular Research, Aalborg University Hospital, 9100 Aalborg, Denmark*
[4] *Department of Clinical Medicine, Aalborg University, 9100 Aalborg, Denmark*

Correspondence should be addressed to Kirsten Fonager; k.fonager@rn.dk

Academic Editor: Jeffrey Jutai

Background. Several characteristics appear to be important for estimating the likelihood of reentering the workforce after surgery. The aim of the present study was to describe work status in a two-year time period around the time of cardiac surgery and estimate the probability of returning to the workforce. *Methods.* We included 681 patients undergoing coronary artery bypass grafting and/or heart valve procedures from 2003 to 2007 in the North Denmark Region. We linked hospital data to data in the DREAM database which holds information of everyone receiving social benefits. *Results.* At the time of surgery 17.3% were allocated disability pension and 2.3% were allocated a permanent part-time benefit. Being unemployed one year before surgery reduced the likelihood of return to the workforce ($RR = 0.74$ (0.60–0.92)) whereas unemployment at the time of surgery had no impact on return to the workforce ($RR = 0.96$ (0.78–1.18)). Sickness absence before surgery reduced the likelihood of return to the workforce. *Conclusion.* This study found the work status before surgery to be associated with the likelihood of return to the workforce within one year after surgery. Before surgery one-fifth of the population either was allocated disability pension or received a permanent part-time benefit.

1. Background

In the early era of cardiac surgery, the main focus was on immediate postoperative survival. The EuroScore (the European System for Cardiac Operative Risk Evaluation) is today probably the most widely implemented scoring system for estimating mortality up to 30 days after surgery [1]; however, with improving results regarding survival, more attention should now be paid to the postoperative quality of life, including the patients' ability to return to the workforce. The ability to return to the workforce must be regarded as a very important part of the postoperative outcome since many patients are still part of the workforce when they undergo cardiac surgery.

Several clinical and sociodemographic factors have been associated with return to the workforce for patients undergoing cardiac surgery, for example, occupation, relief of symptoms, age, and education [2–9]. As expected, the rate of patients returning to work has been found to be lower in patients with comorbidity than in patients with no comorbidity [10] and certain psychological variables have been shown to be important as well [11]. Participation in cardiac rehabilitation programs have been found to be associated with an increasing number of patients returning to work compared with patients not joining such programs [12]. Finally, preoperative work status might also have an impact on the postoperative likelihood of return to work [2, 4–6, 8].

The aim of the present study was to describe work status in a two-year time period around the time of surgery and estimate the probability of returning to the workforce, in Denmark, depending on work status before surgery.

2. Methods

The Danish National Health Service provides tax-funded healthcare and social welfare for all citizens. By use of the unique civil registration number (CPR number) assigned to all Danish citizens, unambiguous linkage between various registers and databases can be performed. This cohort study was conducted within the population of the North Denmark Region (population: 0.6 million) and the study was approved by the Danish Data Protection Agency.

All patients undergoing cardiac surgery in the North Denmark Region are included in the Western Denmark Heart Registry [13]. This registry keeps records of all procedures and operations performed on patients admitted for adult cardiac surgery in the western part of Denmark. Data in this database are registered by the departments at the time of hospitalisation (preoperative data) and by the surgeons, anesthesiologists, and perfusionists (operative data).

The material for this study was consecutive patients receiving first-time coronary artery bypass grafting (CABG) and/or heart valve-procedures. Patients receiving re-do surgery or other concomitant procedures were not included in the study. The patients were operated on during the period from January 1, 2003, to December 31, 2007.

From the Western Denmark Heart Registry we extracted information on all patients aged 62 years or younger at the time of surgery. This age was chosen so the patients had a potential of at least two years of workforce association, after surgery, before ordinary retirement (the retirement age was changed between 65 and 67 years during the observation period). From the database we included information regarding type of operation and the logistic EuroScore I. This score is based on patient-related factors (i.e., neurologic dysfunctional disease, serum creatinine, etc.), heart-related factors (i.e., unstable angina, left ventricular dysfunction, etc.), and operative factors (i.e., other surgeries than isolated CABG, postinfarct septal rupture, etc.) [1].

In Denmark, social security benefits and social services are financed by taxation and all citizens in need are entitled to receive social security benefits and social services—regardless of factors such as their affiliation to the labour market. Short-term sickness benefit (in the study period first two weeks of sick leave) is paid by the employer, and thereafter by the municipality sometimes with a supplement from the employer [13]. Both Self-employed and employees are covered.

Using the unique civil registration number of the patients data were linked to the DREAM database where information on all social benefits is registered on a weekly basis. The DREAM database contains pooled data from all relevant Danish ministries, all Danish municipalities and the national bureau of statistics (Statistics Denmark) since July 1991. This database has been found suitable for public health research [14, 15]. The DREAM database has more than 100 different codes which cover benefits paid to a citizen at any given week. Short-term sick-listing (in the study period less than two weeks) is usually not recorded for working citizens. For the present study we used codes for unemployment (including both benefits for patients with and without private unemployment insurance), sick leave, part-time benefit (flexjob, i.e., job created for persons with a permanent limited working capacity), and disability pension. Patients registered with none of these codes were classified as working. Patients registered with codes, for example, national education grants and early retirement benefits were considered self-supporting and classified in the working group.

Work status was defined by use of DREAM data. We categorized the patients into five groups before and after surgery as follows.

(1) Working.

(2) Unemployed.

(3) On sick leave.

(4) Receiving part-time benefit.

(5) Receiving disability pension.

For each patient we extracted the information from the DREAM database from one year before surgery till one year after.

2.1. Statistical Analysis. The primary endpoint was return to the workforce (defined as being capable to work, that is, working or unemployed 6 months or 12 months after surgery). The objective was to describe the importance of work status (measured by DREAM data) before surgery. Two associations were investigated. Firstly we studied the importance of work status from nine to twelve months before surgery (the main type of benefit in the three months' time period) on return to the workforce. Secondly we studied the influence of work status the week before surgery on return to the workforce.

The relative risks were presented unadjusted and adjusted for EuroScore (included as a continuous variable), type of operation (CABG, valve operation, or both), age (three groups), and gender using a modified Poisson regression model [16].

Statistical tests were two-tailed, and $P < 0.05$ was considered significant. Statistical analyses were performed using Stata version 11.2 (StataCorp. 2009. Stata: Release 11. Statistical Software. College Station, TX: Stata Corp LP, USA).

3. Results

A total of 681 patients operated on during the study period fulfilled the inclusion criteria. Table 1 shows the characteristics of the study population. Most of the patients were men and the age varied between 19 and 62 years. Most of the study population underwent CABG either alone or in combination with valve surgery. One year before surgery 30% of the women and 17% of the men had been allocated either disability pension or permanent part-time benefits and the week before surgery this percentages was 33% and

TABLE 1: Characteristics of patients undergoing coronary artery bypass surgery and/or heart valve surgery in the North Denmark Region, from 2003 to 2007; numbers and percentages.

		Men N = 581 n (%)	Women N = 100 n (%)
Age	Median (range)	56 (19–62)	55.5 (22–62)
Type of operation	CABG*	444 (77)	57 (57)
	Heart valve surgery	107 (19)	32 (32)
	Both	30 (5)	11 (11)
EuroScore**	Median (range)	1.5 (0.9–52.3)	2.4 (1.2–61.9)
Work status 9–12 months before surgery	Working	409 (70)	51 (51)
	Unemployed	46 (8)	11 (11)
	On sick leave	28 (5)	8 (8)
	Receiving part-time permanent benefit***	11 (2)	3 (3)
	Disability pension	87 (15)	27 (27)
Work status the week before surgery	Working	185 (32)	28 (28)
	Unemployed	23 (4)	5 (5)
	On sick leave	272 (47)	34 (34)
	Receiving part-time permanent benefit***	12 (2)	4 (4)
	Disability pension	89 (15)	29 (29)

*CABG: coronary artery bypass grafting. **A scoring system for estimating the 30-day mortality based on patient-related factors, cardiac-related factors, and operation related factors. ***A benefit awarded if the applicant has a permanently reduced ability to work.

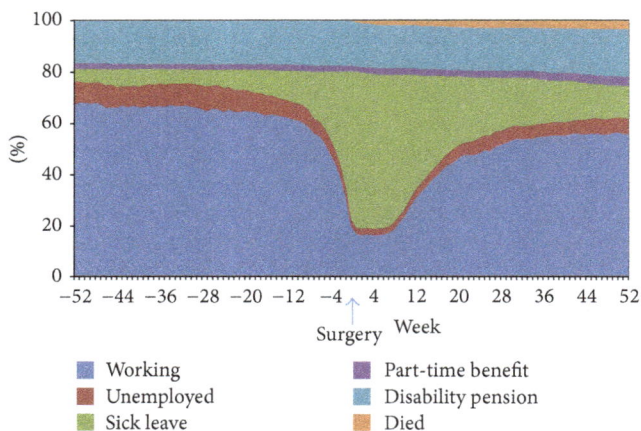

FIGURE 1: Work status for patients undergoing coronary artery bypass surgery and/or heart valve surgery in the North Denmark Region from one year before surgery to one year after.

18%, respectively. In total, 17.3% were allocated disability pension and 2.3% were allocated a permanent part-time benefit before surgery. Overall, less than 5% were on sick leave one year before surgery and one week before surgery this figure increased to 45%.

The percentage of patients on sick leave increased from especially two months before surgery, and at the first weeks after surgery more than 60% of the study population was on sick leave (Figure 1). It is noteworthy that about 16% of the study population did not receive any social benefits around the time of surgery. During the one-year follow-up 22 patients died; nine of them were allocated disability pension or part-time benefits before surgery.

Overall 55% were working or unemployed 6 months after surgery which increased to 62% 12 months after surgery (Table 2). Patients receiving disability pension or part-time benefits before surgery remained on these benefits during the study period.

Being unemployed one year before surgery reduced the likelihood of returning to the workforce ($RR = 0.74$ (0.60–0.92)) whereas unemployment at the time of surgery had no impact in the adjusted model ($RR = 0.96$ (0.78–1.18)) (Table 3). Being on sick leave both one year before and at the time of surgery reduced the likelihood of returning to the workforce but was most pronounced for patients on sick leave one year before surgery ($RR = 0.52$ (0.34–0.78)). 13 out of the 22 patients who died during follow-up did not receive any permanent benefits at the time of surgery. Excluding those who died during the follow-up period from the analyses did not change the relative risks.

4. Discussion

The study showed that one-fifth of the study-group below the age of 63 was allocated either disability pension (17.3%) or a permanent part-time benefit (2.3%) before they underwent CABG and/or valve surgery. Patients being unemployed or on sick leave one year before surgery had a reduced likelihood of returning to the workforce after surgery, whereas unemployment at the time of surgery had no impact. Being on sick leave at the time of surgery had only a minor impact on returning to the workforce one year after the surgery.

TABLE 2: Return to the workforce 6 and 12 months after surgery for patients undergoing CABG and/or heart valve surgery in the North Denmark Region from 2003 to 2007.

		Return to the workforce (working or unemployed)[*]			
		6 months after surgery		12 months after surgery	
		Yes	No	Yes	No
		N (%)	N (%)	N (%)	N(%)
Overall		376 (55)	305 (45)	420 (62)	261 (38)
Work status 9–12 months before surgery	Working	331 (72)	129 (28)	373 (81)	87 (19)
	Unemployed	33 (58)	24 (42)	33 (58)	24 (42)
	On sick leave	12 (33)	24 (67)	14 (39)	22 (61)
	Receiving part-time permanent benefit	0 (0)	14 (100)	0 (0)	14 (100)
	Disability pension	0 (0)	114 (100)	0 (0)	114 (100)
Work status the week before surgery	Working	177 (83)	36 (17)	183 (86)	30 (14)
	Unemployed	23 (82)	5 (18)	21 (75)	7 (25)
	On sick leave	176 (58)	130 (42)	216 (71)	90 (29)
	Receiving part-time permanent benefit	0 (0)	16 (100)	0 (0)	16 (100)
	Disability pension	0 (0)	118 (100)	0 (0)	118 (100)

[*] 22 patients died during the one year follow-up (9 working, 3 unemployed, 1 on sick leave, and 9 receiving part-time benefit or disability pension one year before surgery), included in the No category.

TABLE 3: The chance of having returned to the workforce 12 months after coronary artery bypass surgery and/or heart valve surgery, by work status before surgery.

| | | Return to the workforce (working or unemployed) | | |
		N (%)	RR (95% CI)	RR[*] (95% CI)
Work status 9–12 months before surgery	Working	373 (81)	1	1
	Unemployed	33 (58)	0.71 (0.57–0.89)	0.74 (0.60–0.92)
	On sick leave	14 (39)	0.48 (0.32–0.72)	0.52 (0.34–0.78)
Work status one week before surgery	Working	183 (86)	1	1
	Unemployed	21 (75)	0.87 (0.70–1.09)	0.96 (0.78–1.18)
	On sick leave	216 (71)	0.82 (0.75–0.90)	0.85 (0.78–0.94)

[*] Adjusted for age, gender, type of operation, and EuroScore.

How often the patients return to the workforce after cardiac surgery varies from less than one third to no difference in employment rate one year after surgery compared to before [3–8, 10–12, 17, 18] which might be explained by differences in study populations, time periods, and the socioeconomic support system of the countries. The proportion of patients returning to the workforce in our study was especially high if the patients were working and the lowest for patients at sick leave one year before surgery. The importance of work status before cardiac surgery for returning to the workforce postoperatively has previously been demonstrated [3–6, 8]. One obvious explanation lies in differences in health status between those who work and those who do not, especially looking at patients on sick leave one year before surgery. By including the EuroScore we tried to adjust for the differences in health status among the patients prior to surgery. However, EuroScore is an implemented scoring system for estimating postoperative mortality [1], and the EuroScore alone may not have been able to fully adjust for all comorbidities, for example, diabetes, adiposity, musculoskeletal disorders, and psychiatric diseases which might have an impact on

the patients' ability to reenter the workforce postoperatively. Therefore, there is a risk of residual confounding with respect to comorbidities.

Not only being on sick leave but also being unemployed the year before surgery had a significant negative impact on the chance of returning to the workforce one year after surgery and might indicate that health status alone is not the only factor critical to the patients chance of returning to the workforce. Unemployment has earlier been associated with an increased risk of all-cause mortality but the mechanism is not fully understood [19]. However, a recent study indicated that people with impaired health are forced out of the labor market in times of increasing unemployment rather than pointing towards a negative effect of unemployment on health [20].

The strength of this registry-based study is the uniform data collection at baseline and the complete follow-up which minimizes the risk of selection bias. We had no information regarding the type of work or education which might have had an impact on the patients' chance of returning to the workforce [21]. Furthermore we only had information about the type of benefits the patients received, but not the reason (i.e., the reason for being on sick leave).

The patients were included from 2003 to 2007 and followed the first year after surgery. Since then the number of available jobs in general has been reduced due to the financial crisis. However, focusing on return to the workforce instead of return to work probably made the estimates more robust for the one-year follow-up. Furthermore, the influence of the financial crisis on changes in the social security system would more likely have an impact looking at longer follow-up periods.

It is surprising that 16% of the study population did not receive any social benefit at the time of surgery. This may indicate short-term sick leave for these patients, since only sick leave more than two weeks is registered in the DREAM database. Some of the patients not receiving benefit may reflect that they were economically funded by their spouses. However, this figure is probably low.

In the postoperative period patients may experience fatigue, anxiety, depression, and cognitive dysfunction [22, 23] and these conditions may influence the ability of the patients to return to the workforce. An observational study from Israel indicated more frequent return to the workforce among participants in a cardiac rehabilitation programmes, in a population with a participation rate at 7% [12]. In Denmark complete participation in cardiac rehabilitation has been found even lower for patients with ischaemic heart disease [24]. More knowledge regarding the impact of cardiac rehabilitation on the possibility to return to the workforce is needed among patients who undergo cardiac surgery. Furthermore, the impact of culture and socioeconomic factors present in different countries should be analysed in future studies.

In conclusion, this study found work status before surgery to be important for the likelihood of returning to the workforce after CABG and/or valve surgery. Furthermore, at the time of surgery 17% of patients below the age of 63 were allocated disability pension.

Conflict of Interests

The authors declare that there is no conflict of interests regarding the publication of this paper.

Authors' Contribution

Kirsten Fonager made substantial contributions to the design and to the interpretation of data and drafted the paper. Søren Lundbye-Christensen participated in the design, performed the statistical analysis, and helped to draft the paper. Jan Jesper Andreasen made substantial contributions to the design and to the interpretation of data and helped to draft the paper. Mikkel Futtrup and Khalil Ahmad had participated in acquisition of data. Anette Luther Christensen participated in the design, acquisition of data, and statistical analysis. Martin Agge Nørgaard participated in the design and helped to draft the paper. All authors read and approved the final paper.

References

[1] S. Siregar, R. H. H. Groenwold, F. de Heer, M. L. Bots, Y. van der Graaf, and L. A. van Herwerden, "Performance of the original EuroSCORE," *European Journal of Cardio-thoracic Surgery*, vol. 41, no. 4, pp. 746–754, 2012.

[2] A. Oberman, J. B. Wayne, N. T. Kouchoukos, E. D. Charles, R. O. Russell Jr., and W. J. Rogers, "Employment status after coronary artery bypass surgery," *Circulation*, vol. 65, no. 7, pp. I-115–I-119, 1982.

[3] P. J. Bradshaw, K. Jamrozik, I. S. Gilfillan, and P. L. Thompson, "Return to work after coronary artery bypass surgery in a population of long-term survivors," *Heart Lung and Circulation*, vol. 14, no. 3, pp. 191–196, 2005.

[4] G. Speziale, G. Ruvolo, and B. Marino, "Quality of life following coronary bypass surgery," *Journal of Cardiovascular Surgery*, vol. 37, no. 1, pp. 75–78, 1996.

[5] J. S. Skinner, M. Farrer, C. J. Albers, H. A. W. Neil, and P. C. Adams, "Patient-related outcomes five years after coronary artery bypass graft surgery," *Monthly Journal of the Association of Physicians*, vol. 92, no. 2, pp. 87–96, 1999.

[6] M. A. Hlatky, D. Boothroyd, S. Horine et al., "Employment after coronary angioplasty or coronary bypass surgery in patients employed at the time of revascularization," *Annals of Internal Medicine*, vol. 129, no. 7, pp. 543–547, 1998.

[7] P. Sellier, P. Varaillac, G. Chatellier et al., "Factors influencing return to work at one year after coronary bypass graft surgery: results of the PERISCOP study," *European Journal of Cardiovascular Prevention and Rehabilitation*, vol. 10, no. 6, pp. 469–475, 2003.

[8] V. Hällberg, A. Palomäki, M. Kataja et al., "Working after CABG study group. Return to work after coronary artery bypass surgery. A 10-year follow-up study," *Scand Cardiovasc*, vol. 43, no. 5, pp. 277–284, 2009.

[9] J. Lundbom, H. O. Myhre, B. Ystgaard, K.-D. Bolz, R. Hammervold, and O. W. Levang, "Factors influencing return to work after aortocoronary bypass surgery," *Scandinavian Journal of Thoracic and Cardiovascular Surgery*, vol. 26, no. 3, pp. 187–192, 1992.

[10] S. Davoodi, M. Sheikhvatan, A. Karimi, and M. Sheikhfathollahi, "Determinants of social activity and work status after coronary bypass surgery," *Asian Cardiovascular and Thoracic Annals*, vol. 18, no. 6, pp. 551–556, 2010.

[11] H. Boudrez and G. De Backer, "Recent findings on return to work after an acute myocardial infarction or coronary artery bypass grafting," *Acta Cardiologica*, vol. 55, no. 6, pp. 341–349, 2000.

[12] E. Simchen, I. Naveh, Y. Zitser-Gurevich, D. Brown, and N. Galai, "Is participation in cardiac rehabilitation programs associated with better quality of life and return to work after coronary artery bypass operations? The Israeli CABG study," *Israel Medical Association Journal*, vol. 3, no. 6, pp. 399–403, 2001.

[13] M. Schmidt, M. Maeng, C.-J. Jakobsen et al., "Existing data sources for clinical epidemiology: the western Denmark heart registry," *Clinical Epidemiology*, vol. 2, no. 1, pp. 137–144, 2010.

[14] N. H. Hjollund, F. B. Larsen, and J. H. Andersen, "Register-based follow-up of social benefits and other transfer payments: accuracy and degree of completeness in a Danish interdepartmental administrative database compared with a population-based survey," *Scandinavian Journal of Public Health*, vol. 35, no. 5, pp. 497–502, 2007.

[15] C. M. Stapelfeldt, C. Jensen, N. T. Andersen, N. Fleten, and C. V. Nielsen, "Validation of sick leave measures: Self-reported sick leave and sickness benefit data from a Danish national register compared to multiple workplace-registered sick leave spells in a Danish municipality," *BMC Public Health*, vol. 12, no. 1, article 661, 2012.

[16] G. Zou, "A modified poisson regression approach to prospective studies with binary data," *American Journal of Epidemiology*, vol. 159, no. 7, pp. 702–706, 2004.

[17] S. J. Pocock, R. A. Henderson, P. Seed, T. Treasure, and J. R. Hampton, "Quality of life, employment status, and anginal symptoms after coronary angioplasty or bypass surgery: 3-year follow-up in the randomized intervention treatment of angina (RITA) trial," *Circulation*, vol. 94, no. 2, pp. 135–142, 1996.

[18] B. Geissler and S. Aggestrup, "Qualitative assessment of pain relief and functional improvement after coronary bypass operation," *Ugeskrift for Laeger*, vol. 164, no. 11, pp. 1506–1510, 2002.

[19] D. J. Roelfs, E. Shor, K. W. Davidson, and J. E. Schwartz, "Losing life and livelihood: a systematic review and meta-analysis of unemployment and all-cause mortality," *Social Science and Medicine*, vol. 72, no. 6, pp. 840–854, 2011.

[20] S. Thorlacius and S. Ólafsson, "From unemployment to disability? Relationship between unemployment rate and new disability pensions in Iceland 1992–2007," *European Journal of Public Health*, vol. 22, no. 1, pp. 96–101, 2012.

[21] N. Pinto, P. Shah, B. Haluska, R. Griffin, J. Holliday, and J. Mundy, "Return to work after coronary artery bypass in patients aged under 50 years," *Asian Cardiovascular and Thoracic Annals*, vol. 20, no. 4, pp. 387–391, 2012.

[22] N. Stroobant and G. Vingerhoets, "Depression, anxiety, and neuropsychological performance in coronary artery bypass graft patients: a follow-up study," *Psychosomatics*, vol. 49, no. 4, pp. 326–331, 2008.

[23] J.-H. A. Krannich, P. Weyers, S. Lueger, M. Herzog, T. Bohrer, and O. Elert, "Presence of depression and anxiety before and after coronary artery bypass graft surgery and their relationship to age," *BMC Psychiatry*, vol. 7, article 47, 2007.

[24] M. W. Würgler, L. T. Sonne, J. Kilsmark, H. Voss, and J. Søgaard, "Danish heart patients' participation in and experience with rehabilitation," *Scandinavian Journal of Public Health*, vol. 40, no. 2, pp. 126–132, 2012.

11

Acute Effect of Topical Menthol on Chronic Pain in Slaughterhouse Workers with Carpal Tunnel Syndrome: Triple-Blind, Randomized Placebo-Controlled Trial

Emil Sundstrup,[1,2] Markus D. Jakobsen,[1,2] Mikkel Brandt,[1] Kenneth Jay,[1,2] Juan Carlos Colado,[3] Yuling Wang,[4] and Lars L. Andersen[1]

[1] National Research Centre for the Working Environment, Lersø Parkalle 105, 2100 Copenhagen O, Denmark
[2] Institute for Sports Science and Clinical Biomechanics, University of Southern Denmark, 5230 Odense M, Denmark
[3] Laboratory of Physical Activity and Health, Research Group in Sport and Health, Department of Physical Education and Sports, University of Valencia, 46010 Valencia, Spain
[4] Department of Rehabilitation Medicine, The Sixth Affiliated Hospital of Sun Yat-sen University, No. 26 Yuancun 2nd Cross Road, Guangzhou 510655, China

Correspondence should be addressed to Emil Sundstrup; esu@nrcwe.dk

Academic Editor: Jae-Young Lim

Topical menthol gels are classified "topical analgesics" and are claimed to relieve minor aches and pains of the musculoskeletal system. In this study we investigate the acute effect of topical menthol on carpal tunnel syndrome (CTS). We screened 645 slaughterhouse workers and recruited 10 participants with CTS and chronic pain of the arm/hand who were randomly distributed into two groups to receive topical menthol (Biofreeze) or placebo (gel with a menthol scent) during the working day and 48 hours later the other treatment (crossover design). Participants rated arm/hand pain intensity during the last hour of work (scale 0–10) immediately before 1, 2, and 3 hours after application. Furthermore, global rating of change (GROC) in arm/hand pain was assessed 3 hours after application. Compared with placebo, pain intensity and GROC improved more following application of topical menthol ($P = 0.026$ and $P = 0.044$, resp.). Pain intensity of the arm/hand decreased by −1.2 (CI 95%: −1.7 to −0.6) following topical menthol compared with placebo, corresponding to a moderate effect size of 0.63. In conclusion, topical menthol acutely reduces pain intensity during the working day in slaughterhouse workers with CTS and should be considered as an effective nonsystemic alternative to regular analgesics in the workplace management of chronic and neuropathic pain.

1. Introduction

Carpal tunnel syndrome (CTS) is a neuromuscular condition caused by increased pressure on the median nerve at the level of the wrist and accounts for approximately 90% of all entrapment neuropathies [1, 2]. Commonly reported symptoms of CTS include pain in the wrist and hand [3], paresthesias [4], thenar muscle weakness, and loss of dexterity [4]. Female gender, increasing age, physical illness, repetitive hand use, and occupation are potential risk factors for the development of CTS [1, 5]. However, Falkiner and Myers [6] concluded that except in the case of work that involves very cold temperatures (possibly in conjunction with

load and repetition) such as butchery work is less likely than demographics and disease related variables to cause CTS. In line with this, the prevalence of CTS among Danish slaughterhouse workers was found to be almost 4 times that of reference workers (6.3% versus 1.6%) possibly due to the highly repetitive and forceful work tasks [7].

Conservative treatment is usually offered to individuals with mild to moderate intermittent symptoms of CTS, whereas surgical carpal tunnel release is the preferred treatment of patients with persistent CTS symptoms and those not responding to conservative treatment [2, 4, 8, 9]. Oral medications such as nonsteroidal anti-inflammatory drugs (NSAIDs) and corticosteroids along with corticosteroid injection are offered as a nonsurgical treatment of CTS. These local analgesics have been shown to relieve neuropathic pain by acting as a sodium channel blocker in the affected nerves; however high systemic concentrations of these compounds may increase the likelihood of adverse events [10]. For example, gastrointestinal problems and dyspepsia have been reported following use of NSAIDS [11] and corticosteroid use can lead to adverse osseous and ocular effects [12]. Thus, alternative treatments for temporal pain relieve such as topical analgesics that act at the peripherally located site of injury could provide the symptomatic benefits of oral analgesics on neuropathic pain but without the risk of adverse events [13–15].

Menthol possesses weak analgesic properties when applied to the site of musculoskeletal injury and topical gel containing menthol is thus used as analgesics [16–18]. Topical menthol application produces a cool sensation by activation of the TRPM8 channel also known as the cold and menthol receptor 1, found mainly within thermosensitive neurons [19, 20]. Menthol increases the sensitization of these neurons consequently leading to the perception of coolness, which have an inhibitory effect on nociceptive afferents and on dorsal-horn neurons conducting pain impulses to the thalamus [21]. It is well established that specific sodium channels (Nav 1.8 and Nav 1.9) are greatly involved in pain pathways and tissue specific localization, and the development of type-specific blockers of sodium channels is an important part of the treatment of chronic and neuropathic pain [22, 23]. Hence, Gaudioso et al. [24] found menthol to be a state-selective blocker of Nav 1.8, Nav 1.9, and TTX-sensitive sodium channels in rats and highlighted the role of menthol as topical analgesic compound by its ability to be a sodium channel inactivator.

Johar and coworkers [25] demonstrated that a menthol based topical analgesic was more effective than ice for decreasing DOMS induced symptoms of pain in the elbow flexors and Higashi et al. [15] reported, in a double-blind randomized controlled trial, significant pain relief from muscle strain following 8-hour application of a patch containing methyl salicylate and menthol compared to placebo. Additionally, a randomized controlled study found that topical menthol combined with chiropractic adjustments reduced acute low back pain [26]. Thus, application of topical menthol is used to relieve pain of the musculoskeletal system and is widespread in sport medicine; however, double-blind randomized placebo-controlled trials are lacking and the acute effects of topical menthol application on chronic neuropathic pain remain unclear.

The aim of the study was to evaluate the acute effect of topical menthol and placebo (gel with a menthol scent) on pain in slaughterhouse workers with chronic pain and symptoms of carpal tunnel syndrome.

2. Methods

2.1. Study Design. This triple-blind randomized placebo-controlled crossover trial evaluates the acute effect of topical menthol (Biofreeze) and placebo (gel with a menthol scent) on chronic pain in Danish slaughterhouse workers with symptoms of carpal tunnel syndrome. The study was approved by The Danish National Ethics Committee on Biomedical Research (Ethical Committee of Frederiksberg and Copenhagen; H-3-2010-062) and registered in ClinicalTrails.gov (NCT01716767). The Consolidated Standard of Reporting Trials (CONSORT) checklist was followed to ensure transparent and standardized reporting of the trial. All participants were informed about the purpose and content of the project and gave their written informed consent to participate in the study. All experimental conditions conformed to The Declaration of Helsinki.

2.2. Recruitment and Flow of Participants. Recruitment was established on subjects excluded from participation in another randomized controlled trial [27] due to contraindications of carpal tunnel syndrome. In that study, 19 individuals showed symptoms of carpal tunnel syndrome and were subsequently excluded from an intervention with high-intensity resistance training and were invited to participate in this study. Of the 19 invited individuals, 10 met the inclusion criteria and were willing to participate in the project.

The recruitment was as follows. A screening questionnaire was administered to 645 Danish slaughterhouse workers (aged 18–67 years). In total 595 individuals replied to the questionnaire of which 410 were interested to participate in the research project. The initial inclusion criteria based on the screening questionnaire were (1) currently working at a slaughterhouse for at least 30 hours a week, (2) pain intensity in the shoulder, elbow/forearm, or hand/wrist of 3 or more on a 0–10 VAS scale during the last 3 months, (3) stating at least "some" work disability scoring on a five-point scale: "not at all," "a little," "some," "much," to "very much" when asked the following question: "during the last 3 months, did you have any difficulty performing your work due to pain in the shoulder, arm, or hand," (4) no participation in resistance training during the last year, and (5) no ergonomics instruction during the last year. Of the 410 interested respondents, 145 met the above inclusion criteria and were invited for a clinical examination.

A total of 135 employees presented for the baseline clinical examination. Exclusion criteria were hypertension (Systolic BP > 160, diastolic BP > 100), a medical history of cardiovascular diseases, symptoms of carpal tunnel syndrome, recent traumatic injury of the neck, shoulder, arm, or hand regions, or pregnancy. Furthermore, at the day of the clinical examination participants filled in another questionnaire with the following inclusion criteria: (1) pain intensity in the shoulder, elbow/forearm, or hand/wrist of at least 3 on a 0–10 VAS scale during the last week, (2) pain that lasted more than 3 months, and (3) frequency of pain of at least 3 days per week during the last week.

Based on the clinical examination and associated questionnaire, 69 workers were excluded due to contraindications of which 19 showed symptoms of carpal tunnel syndrome. Symptoms of carpal tunnel syndrome included (1) nocturnal numbness of the hand; (2) paresthesia in the distribution of the median nerve; (3) positive Tinel's sign over the carpal tunnel; (4) positive Phalen's test; (5) decreased sensibility in the distribution of median nerve; (6) decreased strength in

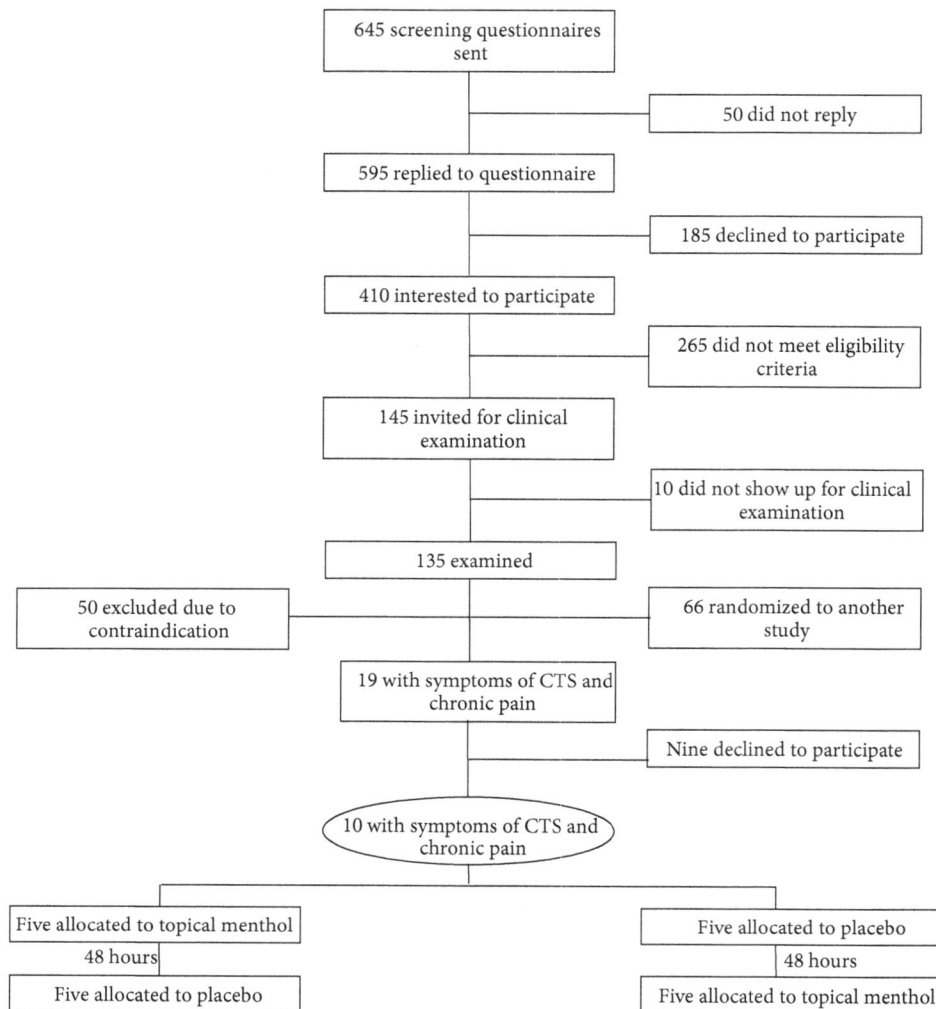

FIGURE 1: Participants flow. CTS denotes carpal tunnel syndrome.

abduction of the thumb; (7) pain intensity of at least 4 in the hand/wrist; and (8) the pain should have lasted at least 3 months. Participants should fulfill all these eight criteria to be defined as having carpal tunnel syndrome. The 19 workers with symptoms of carpal tunnel syndrome were invited to participate in the present study and 10 workers willingly accepted. Figure 1 shows the flow of participants through the study.

2.3. Randomization and Blinding. Using a computer generated random numbers table, participants were randomly distributed into two groups to receive either topical menthol (Biofreeze) or placebo on the first day of testing at a 1:1 menthol/placebo ratio. Interspersed by a minimum of 48 hours, participants received the other treatment (crossover design) on the second day of testing.

Both the active treatment (topical menthol gel) and placebo (gel with a menthol scent) were provided by The Hygenic Corporation (Akron, OH).

Menthol and placebo gels were prepared by technicians from The Hygenic Corporation who also verified proper

labeling of the gel tubes with corresponding allocation code. The menthol and placebo gels were packaged and labeled in the same manner, so that each topical gel tube resembled the other. The menthol and placebo topical gels, which had no other identifiers, were delivered to a blinded study administrator at the National Research Centre for the Working Environment and further delivered by hand to the research assistant who administered the treatment and recorded the allocation on a separate case report form. Following data collection and statistical analyses the allocation code was broken by The Hygenic Corporation and delivered to the researchers at the National Research Centre for the Working Environment.

2.4. Interventions. Participants were invited for two separate days of testing involving topical application of menthol or placebo to the arm, wrist, and hand. On the first day of testing, participants were randomly allocated to receive either topical menthol (Biofreeze) or placebo (gel with a menthol scent) and on the second day of testing, participants received the contrasting treatment, thus acting as their own controls in a crossover design.

The Biofreeze topical gel contained 4% active menthol and the following ingredients: *Aloe barbadensis* leaf extract, *Arnica Montana* flower extract, *Arctium lappa* root extract, *Boswellia carterii* resin extract, *Calendula officinalis* extract, carbomer, *Camellia sinensis* leaf extract, camphor, glycerin, *Ilex paraguariensis* leaf extract, isopropyl alcohol, isopropyl myristate, *Melissa officinalis* leaf extract, silicon dioxide, tocopheryl acetate, triethanolamine, Blue 1, and Yellow 5. The placebo comparator contained no menthol but had a menthol scent, with the following ingredients: *Aloe barbadensis* leaf extract, *Arnica montana* flower extract, *Arctium lappa* root extract, *Boswellia carterii* resin extract, *Calendula officinalis* extract, carbomer, *Camellia sinensis* leaf extract, camphor, fragrance, glycerin, *Ilex paraguariensis* leaf extract, isopropyl alcohol, isopropyl myristate, *Melissa officinalis* leaf extract, silicon dioxide, tocopheryl acetate, triethanolamine, Blue 1, and Yellow 5. The menthol and placebo gels had a similar texture, odor, and color.

Menthol and placebo were applied topically to the hand and wrist by a blinded research assistant at a recommended dosage of 2.5 mL per 500 cm^2 [28]. As the majority of the slaughterhouse workers with CTS also suffered from general elbow and forearm pain, topical menthol and placebo were additionally applied to the forearm. The mode of application involved light strokes with no substantially force, pressure, or rubbing [25]. Topical application was applied to the participants at the end of lunch break during a typical working day at the slaughterhouse, allowing for a 3-hour testing period after lunch. Additionally, all participants were asked about adverse events during every reporting of pain intensity (at 1, 2, and 3 hours following application) by the blinded research assistant.

2.5. Outcome Measures. The primary outcome was the change in arm/hand pain intensity (scale 0–10) during work. The participant rated "pain intensity during the last hour" on the 0–10 modified VAS scale (where 0 indicates "no pain at all" and 10 indicates "worst pain imaginable") immediately before and 1, 2, and 3 hours after application of the gel [29, 30]. The primary outcome is calculated as the change in pain from before to after (average of 1, 2, and 3 hours after) application of the gel. The secondary outcome measure was the global rating of change (GROC), which is a fundamental clinical tool to elucidate whether a patient has improved or worsened and is commonly used among patients with musculoskeletal symptoms, including chronic pain [31, 32]. Thus, the scale is used to asses participants overall evaluation of the topical gel application treatment [33]. Participants rated the change in arm/ hand pain on a scale from −5 (much worsening of pain) to 5 (much improvement of pain) 3 hours after application of the gel.

2.6. Sample Size. Power calculations showed that 10 participants in a paired crossover design were necessary for testing the null hypothesis of equality of treatment at an alpha level of 5%, a statistical power of 80%, a minimal relevant difference in hand/wrist pain intensity of 1.5, and SD of 1.5 on a scale of 0–10.

2.7. Statistical Analysis. Statistical analyses were performed using the SAS statistically software for Windows (SAS Institute, Cary, NC). The primary outcome (change in hand/wrist pain) was analyzed according to intention-to-treat principle using a repeated measures 2 × 2 mixed-factorial design (Proc Mixed), with *time, group,* and *time by group* as independent categorical variables (fixed factors). Subject was entered as a repeated effect. Analyses were adjusted for gender and pain intensity at baseline. The secondary outcome variable (GROC) was analyzed by analysis of variance (ANOVA) and adjusted for gender and pain intensity at baseline. Prior to the ANOVA, a Kolmogorov-Smirnov goodness-of-fit test had shown that the data did not significantly deviate from a normal distribution.

An alpha level of 0.05 was used for statistical significance. The primary outcome variable (change in hand/wrist pain) is reported as between-group least square mean differences and 95% confidence intervals from before to after (average of 1, 2, and 3 hours after) application of the gel. The secondary outcome variable is reported as between-group least square mean differences and 95% confidence intervals. Finally we calculated effect size as Cohen's d [34] based on arm/hand pain intensity (between-group differences divided by the pooled standard deviation).

3. Results

Table 1 shows baseline characteristics of the participants. All participants completed the intervention and none of the participants reported any adverse events to either placebo or menthol topical application.

3.1. Pain and Global Rating of Change. Figure 2 illustrates the change in hand/wrist pain immediately before and 1, 2, and 3 hours after application of Biofreeze and placebo, respectively. A priory hypothesis testing showed a statistically significant *group by time* interaction for pain intensity ($P = 0.026$) from before to after (average of 1, 2, and 3 hours after) topical application. Compared with placebo, hand/wrist pain intensity decreased −1.2 (CI 95%: −1.7 to −0.6) following Biofreeze application. The effect size (Cohen's d) of the change in arm/hand pain was 0.63 and categorized as moderate with topical menthol. Post hoc analyses revealed a significant pain intensity reduction at all timepoints (1, 2, and 3 hours) following menthol application compared to placebo ($P = 0.016$, $P = 0.027$, and $P = 0.009$, resp., Table 2).

Analysis of variance showed a *group* effect for GROC of hand/wrist pain 3 hours following topical application ($P = 0.044$). Compared to placebo, GROC improved to a greater extent with Biofreeze (1.5 point; CI 95%: −2.94 to −0.1, Table 2).

4. Discussion

This triple-blind, randomized placebo-controlled trial found that topical gel containing menthol applied to the hand and arm acutely reduced chronic pain among slaughterhouse workers with carpal tunnel syndrome. The effect persisted all three hours of the experiment.

TABLE 1: Baseline characteristics of the participants. Values are means (SD).

Demographics	
Height, cm	173 (7)
Weight, kg	80 (21)
Body mass index, $kg\,m^{-2}$	26 (5)
Age, year	45 (7)
Number of men/women	8/2
Clinical	
Elbow/forearm pain intensity during the last week (scale 0–10)	6.3 (2.3)
Hand/wrist pain intensity during the last week (scale 0–10)	5.7 (2.8)
Arm/hand pain intensity during the last hour of work (scale 0–10)	4.3 (1.8)
Days with pain during the last week	5.8 (1.9)

TABLE 2: Changes in arm/hand pain intensity and global rating of change (GROC) following menthol and placebo topical application. Differences of each group are shown on the left and post hoc contrasts between the groups on the right. Values are means (95% confidence interval).

	Within-group difference from before to after application		Between-group difference	
	Menthol	Placebo	Menthol versus placebo	P value
Pain at hour 1 (0–10)	−1.3 (−2.2 to −0.4)	−0.1 (−1.0 to 0.8)	−1.2 (−2.1 to −0.2)	0.016
Pain at hour 2 (0–10)	−1.4 (−2.3 to −0.5)	−0.3 (−1.2 to 0.6)	−1.1 (−2.0 to −0.1)	0.027
Pain at hour 3 (0–10)	−1.3 (−2.2 to −0.4)	0.0 (−0.9 to 0.9)	−1.3 (−2.2 to −0.3)	0.009
GROC (−5 to 5)	−1.2 (−2.4 to −0.1)	0.3 (−0.9 to 1.4)	−1.5 (−2.9 to −0.1)	0.044

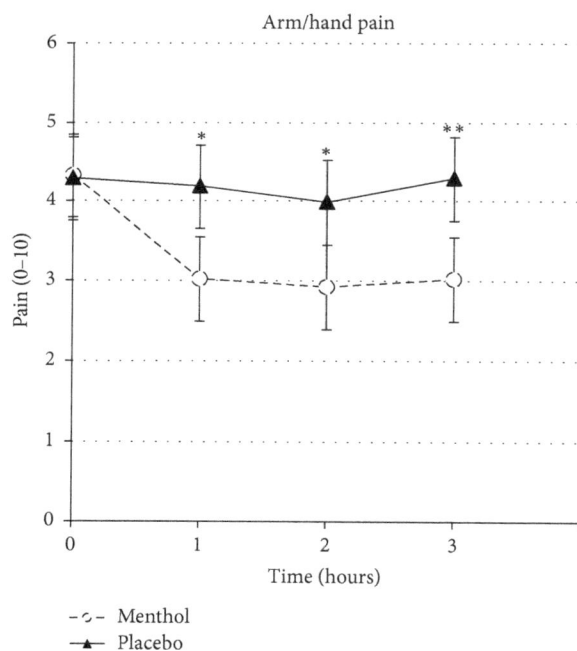

FIGURE 2: Change in arm/hand pain following application of topical menthol (menthol) or topical placebo (placebo) before (time 0) and 1, 2, and 3 hours following application. *, ** denotes significant difference between interventions ($P < 0.05$; $P < 0.01$, resp.).

Topical gel containing menthol led to a 31% (1.3 point on 0–10 VAS) acute reduction in chronic pain associated with carpal tunnel syndrome, and the absolute change in pain symptoms between topical menthol and placebo was 1.2 corresponding to a moderate effect size (Cohen's d ≥ 0.50). In patients with chronic pain a change in pain intensity of 1 on a 0–10 scale is considered a minimal clinical important change [35], and Todd et al. [36] reported the minimum clinically significant change in patients with acute pain measured with a 100 mm scale to be 13 (corresponding to a 1.3 change on a 0–10 scale). Thus, the results of the present study indicate a marginal clinical significant change in chronic pain perception following menthol based application. This is further supported by the observed difference in global rating of change (GROC) in hand/wrist pain in favor of the topical menthol group. Topical menthol application could therefore serve as an alternative to oral analgesics, to produce clinical relevant reductions in chronic pain intensity without resulting in high systemic concentrations of analgesic that may lead to adverse events.

Menthol based topical applications are a widely used analgesic compound acting at the peripherally located site of injury. Zhang et al. [26] reported a significant reduction in acute low back pain following 4 weeks of Biofreeze application combined with chiropractic adjustment compared with chiropractic adjustment alone. However, the study was not blinded, and the acute effects of topical menthol application were not measured. Another study found topically applied menthol to cause higher transepidermal water loss (which is often compromised due to injury) whereas no effect on pain sensation was observed, compared to alcohol [18]. Topical menthol is regularly used in sports medicine, and a topical patch of methyl salicylate—an analgesic—in combination with menthol has been reported to relief pain associated with mild to moderate muscle strain compared to placebo

[15]. However, the direct contribution of menthol on pain is difficult to extract as the patch also contained methyl salicylate.

Menthol applied to the skin increases the sensitization of thermosensitive neurons by activation of the TRPM8 channel consequently leading to the perception of coolness, which has an inhibitory effect on nociceptive afferents and on dorsal-horn neurons conducting pain impulses to the thalamus [21]. It has been reported that the subjective cooling effect following topical menthol application lasts up to 70 min in 12 of 18 subjects, with a mean cooling sensation of 32 min [18]. This knowledge contributed to the study design by Johar et al. [25] who measured DOMS induced pain symptoms and tetanic contraction force 20, 25, and 35 min following application of either menthol gel or ice to the elbow flexors. They demonstrated that the menthol containing gel was more effective than ice for increasing evoked tetanic force; however no significant group by time interaction in pain perception was observed. Our study revealed a decrease in pain intensity 1 hour following menthol application, and this reduction was maintained for both 2 and 3 hours indicating that pain relief lasts longer than the perceived cooling effect. This discrepancy between the sensation of cool and the perception of pain should in a timewise perspective be investigated in future studies.

Workplace risk factors for the development of CTS involve repetitive and forceful hand use, and the prevalence of CTS among Danish slaughterhouse workers was found to be almost 4 times that of reference workers [6, 7]. Workers diagnosed with carpal tunnel syndrome may be treated by surgical procedures, while others will have to rely on conservative treatments. However, physical exercise such as strength training, which has shown to relieve other types of musculoskeletal pain [37, 38] (refs), may be contraindicated in carpal tunnel syndrome. Thus, topical menthol may provide acute pain reduction for this group of workers. For instance, the gel can be applied in the morning and again at lunch to provide pain relief during the entire working day. Nevertheless, it should be remembered that the acute analgesic effect of topical menthol does not treat the underlying cause of carpal tunnel syndrome, and the workloads may need to be adjusted to prevent further aggravation of the symptoms.

4.1. Strengths and Limitations. The randomized, triple-blind placebo-controlled crossover design protects against systematic bias. As we did not measure nerve conduction velocity or ultrasound waves over the carpal tunnel we were not able to conclusively establish the diagnose of carpal tunnel syndrome. However, to be regarded as a worker with symptoms of carpal tunnel syndrome all participants were to experience all of the following symptoms: (1) nocturnal numbness of the hand; (2) paresthesia in the distribution of the median nerve; (3) positive Tinel's sign over the carpal tunnel; (4) positive Phalen's test; (5) decreased sensibility in the distribution of median nerve; (6) decreased strength in abduction of the thumb; (7) pain intensity of at least 4 in the hand/wrist; and (8) pain that lasted at least 3 months. A limitation of the study is that only subjective rating scales are used as outcome variables. However, even without objective measures to support the subjective variables, the triple-blind, placebo-controlled design eliminates the probability of a placebo effect. The exclusion and inclusion criteria used in the present study confine the generalizability of our results to workers with chronic pain and symptoms of carpal tunnel syndrome exposed to highly and repetitive and forceful work. The size of the study allows us to test the effectiveness of topical menthol, but for evaluating adverse events a much larger study is needed. However, topical gels are generally considered safe.

5. Conclusion

Topical menthol application acutely reduces pain intensity among slaughterhouse workers with chronic pain and symptoms of carpal tunnel syndrome compared with placebo. Thus, topical menthol should be considered as an effective nonsystemic alternative to regular analgesics in the workplace management of chronic, localized musculoskeletal, and neuropathic pain.

Conflict of Interests

The authors declare that there is no conflict of interests regarding the publication of this paper.

Acknowledgments

The authors would like to thank Stine Dam Søndergaard for valuable practical help during the data collection. Furthermore, thanks are due to the Hygenic Corporation for supporting this study.

References

[1] S. Aroori and R. A. J. Spence, "Carpal tunnel syndrome," *Ulster Medical Journal*, vol. 77, no. 1, pp. 6–17, 2008.

[2] M. J. Page, D. O'Connor, V. Pitt, and N. Massy-Westropp, "Exercise and mobilisation interventions for carpal tunnel syndrome," *Cochrane Database of Systematic Reviews*, vol. 6, Article ID CD009899, 2012.

[3] D. Rempel, B. Evanoff, P. C. Amadio et al., "Consensus criteria for the classification of carpal tunnel syndrome in epidemiologic studies," *American Journal of Public Health*, vol. 88, no. 10, pp. 1447–1451, 1998.

[4] A. J. Viera, "Management of carpal tunnel syndrome," *American Family Physician*, vol. 68, no. 2, pp. 265–279, 2003.

[5] I. Atroshi, C. Gummesson, R. Johnsson, E. Ornstein, J. Ranstam, and I. Rosén, "Prevalence of carpal tunnel syndrome in a general population," *Journal of the American Medical Association*, vol. 282, no. 2, pp. 153–158, 1999.

[6] S. Falkiner and S. Myers, "When exactly can carpal tunnel syndrome be considered work-related?" *ANZ Journal of Surgery*, vol. 72, no. 3, pp. 204–209, 2002.

[7] P. Frost, J. H. Andersen, and V. K. Nielsen, "Occurrence of carpal tunnel syndrome among slaughterhouse workers," *Scandinavian Journal of Work, Environment and Health*, vol. 24, no. 4, pp. 285–292, 1998.

[8] A. A. M. Gerritsen, H. C. W. de Vet, R. J. P. M. Scholten, F. W. Bertelsmann, M. C. T. F. M. de Krom, and L. M. Bouter, "Splinting vs surgery in the treatment of Carpal tunnel syndrome: a randomized controlled trial," *The Journal of the American Medical Association*, vol. 288, no. 10, pp. 1245–1251, 2002.

[9] J. G. Jarvik, B. A. Comstock, M. Kliot et al., "Surgery versus non-surgical therapy for carpal tunnel syndrome: a randomised parallel-group trial," *The Lancet*, vol. 374, no. 9695, pp. 1074–1081, 2009.

[10] M. S. Wallace, J. B. Dyck, S. S. Rossi, and T. L. Yaksh, "Computer-controlled lidocaine infusion for the evaluation of neuropathic pain after peripheral nerve injury," *Pain*, vol. 66, no. 1, pp. 69–77, 1996.

[11] O. Mathiesen, J. Wetterslev, V. K. Kontinen, H.-C. Pommergaard, L. Nikolajsen, and J. Rosenberg, "Adverse effects of perioperative paracetamol , NSAIDs, glucocorticoids, gabapentinoids and their combinations: a topical review," *Acta Anaesthesiologica Scandinavica*, 2014.

[12] L. Fardet, A. Flahault, A. Kettaneh et al., "Corticosteroid-induced clinical adverse events: frequency, risk factors and patient's opinion," *British Journal of Dermatology*, vol. 157, no. 1, pp. 142–148, 2007.

[13] S. P. Stanos and K. E. Galluzzi, "Topical therapies in the management of chronic pain," *Postgraduate Medicine*, vol. 125, upplement 1, no. 4, pp. 25–33, 2013.

[14] J. Sawynok, "Topical and peripheral ketamine as an analgesic," *Anesthesia & Analgesia*, vol. 119, no. 1, pp. 170–178, 2014.

[15] Y. Higashi, T. Kiuchi, and K. Furuta, "Efficacy and safety profile of a topical methyl salicylate and menthol patch in adult patients with mild to moderate muscle strain: a randomized, double-blind, parallel-group, placebo-controlled, multicenter study," *Clinical Therapeutics*, vol. 32, no. 1, pp. 34–43, 2010.

[16] G. Wasner, D. Naleschinski, A. Binder, J. Schattschneider, E. M. Mclachlan, and R. Baron, "The effect of menthol on cold allodynia in patients with neuropathic pain," *Pain Medicine*, vol. 9, no. 3, pp. 354–358, 2008.

[17] N. Galeotti, L. di Cesare Mannelli, G. Mazzanti, A. Bartolini, and C. Ghelardini, "Menthol: a natural analgesic compound," *Neuroscience Letters*, vol. 322, no. 3, pp. 145–148, 2002.

[18] G. Yosipovitch, C. Szolar, X. Y. Hui, and H. Maibach, "Effect of topically applied menthol on thermal, pain and itch sensations and biophysical properties of the skin," *Archives of Dermatological Research*, vol. 288, no. 5-6, pp. 245–248, 1996.

[19] A. M. Peier, A. Moqrich, A. C. Hergarden et al., "A TRP channel that senses cold stimuli and menthol," *Cell*, vol. 108, no. 5, pp. 705–715, 2002.

[20] J. Vriens, B. Nilius, and R. Vennekens, "Herbal compounds and toxins modulating TRP channels," *Current Neuropharmacology*, vol. 6, no. 1, pp. 79–96, 2008.

[21] C. J. Proudfoot, E. M. Garry, D. F. Cottrell et al., "Analgesia mediated by the TRPM8 cold receptor in chronic neuropathic pain," *Current Biology*, vol. 16, no. 16, pp. 1591–1605, 2006.

[22] R. S. Swanwick, A. Pristerá, and K. Okuse, "The trafficking of $Na_V1.8$," *Neuroscience Letters*, vol. 486, no. 2, pp. 78–83, 2010.

[23] E. V. Bird, C. R. Christmas, A. R. Loescher et al., "Correlation of Nav1.8 and Nav1.9 sodium channel expression with neuropathic pain in human subjects with lingual nerve neuromas," *Molecular Pain*, vol. 9, no. 1, article 52, 2013.

[24] C. Gaudioso, J. Hao, M.-F. Martin-Eauclaire, M. Gabriac, and P. Delmas, "Menthol pain relief through cumulative inactivation of voltage-gated sodium channels," *Pain*, vol. 153, no. 2, pp. 473–484, 2012.

[25] P. Johar, V. Grover, R. Topp, and D. G. Behm, "A comparison of topical menthol to ice on pain, evoked tetanic and voluntary force during delayed onset muscle soreness," *International Journal of Sports Physical Therapy*, vol. 7, no. 3, pp. 314–322, 2012.

[26] J. Zhang, D. Enix, B. Snyder, K. Giggey, and R. Tepe, "Effects of Biofreeze and chiropractic adjustments on acute low back pain: a pilot study," *Journal of Chiropractic Medicine*, vol. 7, no. 2, pp. 59–65, 2008.

[27] E. Sundstrup, M. D. Jakobsen, C. H. Andersen et al., "Effect of two contrasting interventions on upper limb chronic pain and disability: a randomized controlled trial," *Pain Physician*, vol. 17, no. 2, pp. 145–154, 2014.

[28] J. L. Olive, B. Hollis, E. Mattson, and R. Topp, "Vascular conductance is reduced after menthol or cold application," *Clinical Journal of Sport Medicine*, vol. 20, no. 5, pp. 372–376, 2010.

[29] L. L. Andersen, C. A. Saervoll, O. S. Mortensen, O. M. Poulsen, H. Hannerz, and M. K. Zebis, "Effectiveness of small daily amounts of progressive resistance training for frequent neck/shoulder pain: Randomised controlled trial," *Pain*, vol. 152, no. 2, pp. 440–446, 2011.

[30] T. Pincus, M. Bergman, T. Sokka, J. Roth, C. Swearingen, and Y. Yazici, "Visual analog scales in formats other than a 10 centimeter horizontal line to assess pain and other clinical data," *Journal of Rheumatology*, vol. 35, no. 8, pp. 1550–1558, 2008.

[31] S. J. Kamper, C. G. Maher, and G. Mackay, "Global rating of change scales: A review of strengths and weaknesses and considerations for design," *The Journal of Manual & Manipulative Therapy*, vol. 17, no. 3, pp. 163–170, 2009.

[32] R. H. Dworkin, D. C. Turk, J. T. Farrar et al., "Core outcome measures for chronic pain clinical trials: IMMPACT recommendations," *Pain*, vol. 113, no. 1-2, pp. 9–19, 2005.

[33] M. J. Stewart, C. G. Maher, K. M. Refshauge, R. D. Herbert, N. Bogduk, and M. Nicholas, "Randomized controlled trial of exercise for chronic whiplash-associated disorders," *Pain*, vol. 128, no. 1-2, pp. 59–68, 2007.

[34] J. Cohen, *Statistical Poer Analysis for the Behavioral Sciences*, Lawrence Erlbaum Associates, New York, NY, USA, 1988.

[35] R. H. Dworkin, D. C. Turk, M. P. McDermott et al., "Interpreting the clinical importance of group differences in chronic pain clinical trials: IMMPACT recommendations," *Pain*, vol. 146, no. 3, pp. 238–244, 2009.

[36] K. H. Todd, K. G. Funk, J. P. Funk, and R. Bonacci, "Clinical significance of reported changes in pain severity," *Annals of Emergency Medicine*, vol. 27, no. 4, pp. 485–489, 1996.

[37] L. L. Andersen, J. L. Andersen, C. Suetta, M. Kjær, K. Søgaard, and G. Sjøgaard, "Effect of contrasting physical exercise interventions on rapid force capacity of chronically painful muscles," *Journal of Applied Physiology*, vol. 107, no. 5, pp. 1413–1419, 2009.

[38] L. L. Andersen, C. H. Andersen, E. Sundstrup, M. D. Jakobsen, O. S. Mortensen, and M. K. Zebis, "Central adaptation of pain perception in response to rehabilitation of musculoskeletal pain: randomized controlled trial," *Pain Physician*, vol. 15, no. 5, pp. 385–393, 2012.

12

An Individualized and Everyday Life Approach to Cognitive Rehabilitation in Schizophrenia: A Case Illustration

M.-N. Levaux,[1,2] **B. Fonteneau,**[1] **F. Larøi,**[1] **I. Offerlin-Meyer,**[2]
J.-M. Danion,[2] **and M. Van der Linden**[1,3]

[1] *Cognitive Psychopathology Unit, Department of Psychology: Cognition and Behavior, University of Liège, 4000 Liège, Belgium*
[2] *Psychiatry Service I, Inserm 666 Unit, 67091 Strasbourg, France*
[3] *Cognitive Psychopathology and Neuropsychology Unit, University of Geneva, 1211 Geneva, Switzerland*

Correspondence should be addressed to M.-N. Levaux, mnlevaux@ulg.ac.be

Academic Editor: Susan R. McGurk

Objective. The effectiveness of an individualized and everyday approach to cognitive rehabilitation for schizophrenia was examined in a case study. *Method.* After cognitive and functional assessment, concrete objectives were targeted for the person's everyday complaints. Strategies were constructed based on an analysis of the cognitive profile, daily life functioning, and processes involved in activities. They included a memory strategy for reading, a diary to compensate memory difficulties, and working memory exercises to improve immediate processing of information when reading and following conversations. Efficacy was assessed with outcome measures. *Results.* The program had beneficial effects on the person's cognitive and everyday functioning, which persisted at a 3-year follow-up. *Conclusion.* Findings provide suggestive evidence that an individualized and everyday approach may be a useful alternative in order to obtain a meaningfully lasting transfer of training to daily life, compared to the nomothetic ones which dominate the field.

1. Introduction

Cognitive rehabilitation therapy refers to "a behavioral training based intervention that aims to improve cognitive processes ... with the goal of durability and generalization" [1]. Recently, two meta-analyses in schizophrenia [1, 2] revealed that cognitive rehabilitation has a positive, small-moderate effect on overall cognition (resp., 0.41 and 0.45; 0.43 at follow-up [1]), psychosocial functioning (resp., 0.35 and 0.42; 0.37 at follow-up [1]), and symptoms (resp. 0.28 and 0.18; no longer significant at follow-up [1]). Moreover, stronger effects on psychosocial functioning were found when cognitive rehabilitation was provided together with psychiatric rehabilitation [1, 2]. The effect size on functioning was larger in Wykes et al. (.59, [1]) than in McGurk et al. (.47, [2]), while the number of studies both evaluating psychosocial functioning and combining it with cognitive rehabilitation were increased in the recent meta-analysis [1]. The analyses indicated that the studies which did not have a significant impact on functioning were providing cognitive rehabilitation in "stand alone" cognitive programs with no functional interventions [1, 2]. Thus, the combination of cognitive rehabilitation and psychosocial rehabilitation served to significantly enhance the response to cognitive intervention.

Generalization and the ability to produce a meaningfully lasting effect represent two major goals of cognitive rehabilitation. Unfortunately, however, a large number of cognitive rehabilitation studies have overlooked both issues. In terms of the ability to produce a meaningfully lasting effect, Wykes et al. [1] report that only 28% and 30% of studies included in their meta-analysis comprised a follow-up assessment for global cognition and functional outcome, respectively, and only 23% of studies included such an assessment for cognition in McGurk et al. [2]. Moreover, when follow-up periods are included, they are many times limited to only few weeks or months.

The issue of generalization has also been neglected by studies, yet the ultimate goal of remediating cognitive deficits is not simply to improve cognitive test scores but to generalize improvements to durable real-world application [3]. In Wykes et al. [1], only 48% of studies evaluated psychosocial functioning, and, in McGurk et al. [2], this was only 42%.

In our opinion, there are at least two major reasons why cognitive rehabilitation, until now, has had a limited effect on functional outcome. First, specific difficulties in patients' everyday lives have not been given the importance they deserve when designing and proposing cognitive rehabilitation programs, yet it is these difficulties that should be the main focus of interventions. Few current cognitive remediation programs take functioning into account in their design. Persons with specific functional difficulties (rather than cognitive difficulties) are included in two of these programs. Among those, the "Thinking Skills for Work program" by McGurk et al. [4, 5] has worked as the primary outcome and combines cognitive and vocational rehabilitation, which consists of comprehensive assessment of obstacles to employment, identification of cognitive and behavioral strengths and weaknesses, provision of restorative and compensatory cognitive remediation strategies that are individualized, tracking of functioning, and full integration of work services so that employment specialist can help the client adapt compensatory strategies learned in the intervention to the specific work place. The "Attention Training" intervention by Silverstein et al. [6] is another example, which is fully integrated into social skills training with the goal of improving social functioning. Second, previous studies and interventional strategies have not taken into account the vast heterogeneity inherent in schizophrenia. Taking both these issues into account will hopefully render cognitive rehabilitation programs even more effective, especially in terms of improvements in psychosocial functioning.

Thus, in addition to identifying the impaired and preserved cognitive domains in a patient with schizophrenia, it is equally important to define the consequences of the cognitive deficits on daily life activities and to develop ecological rehabilitation strategies (i.e., which can be transferred to real-world situations) based on concrete objectives in daily life. Consequently, the efficacy of a cognitive rehabilitation should be based not only on the results of cognitive measures but also on everyday life measures. Moreover, cognitive rehabilitation programs have generally not focused on the real-world difficulties of persons with schizophrenia, but rather, on patients' cognitive difficulties. This has been based on the supposition that the trained cognitive tasks share some common cognitive processes with daily life activities, such that improvement of performance on a cognitive task will lead to beneficial effects on everyday functioning. However, due to the complex nature of the relations between cognitive and real-life functioning, such an approach might not necessarily lead to a significant improvement in daily life functioning. Therefore, we favor an approach which identifies patients' difficulties on everyday activities and endeavors to understand the nature (cognitive or otherwise) of these difficulties and thus to be able to identify which (cognitive or otherwise) processes to remediate (see [7, 8]).

Secondly, schizophrenia is unmistakably a vastly heterogeneous disorder (e.g., [9, 10]), but this fact has not been taken into account in most cognitive rehabilitation studies, where the same program is administered to all patients. Detailed analyses of the profiles of persons are not carried out, even though people with schizophrenia clearly differ in terms of the degree and type of their cognitive deficits (e.g., [11, 12]), and on a large number of other dimensions including, for example, difficulties in everyday activities, goals, coping capacities, and environmental contexts. The adoption of a single-case methodology is one manner of taking this heterogeneity into account. Indeed, in light of evidence of the heterogeneity of people with neurological lesions, the neuropsychological literature also advocates the use of a single-case methodology in cognitive rehabilitation [13]. In schizophrenia, this approach was primarily used by Velligan and collaborators [14, 15] who developed a Cognitive Adaptation Training (CAT) that utilizes compensatory strategies and supports (such as pill containers with alarms, organization of belongings, and activity checklists) in the home environment and tailored to the specific cognitive impairments of each participant.

In sum, the beneficial effects of cognitive rehabilitation in schizophrenia could be improved by adopting an approach that individualizes treatment and that directly focuses on decreasing the person's everyday difficulties. For this purpose, we concretely propose four steps. (1) The patient's goals and needs are identified, in addition to specific activities that pose problems in everyday life. This information can be assembled using various methods such as open discussions (e.g., with the patient, the patient's caregivers, the clinical team), observations (e.g., of the patient in various contexts or when performing performance-based tasks of everyday activities), or questionnaires of psychosocial functioning. (2) Detailed evaluations are carried out, which include cognitive assessments of both defective and intact processes and the identification of the optimizing factors (i.e., strategies that may improve or facilitate cognitive performance). (3) Based on these cognitive and functional evaluations, reasons are established as to why the patient might have difficulties in the various everyday activities. (4) Ecological rehabilitation strategies, which are combined and chosen according to the rehabilitation objectives, are then proposed to the patient and a "rehabilitation contract" is mutually agreed upon between the patient, and the mental health professional. Such a contract may include information such as what will be remediated and why, how it will be remediated, and the duration and frequency of sessions. In this approach, the patient's needs are directly addressed in a treatment context, thus undoubtedly increasing intrinsic motivation, which is a central issue in treatment programs [3]. What follows is a description of a case study, which will serve as an illustration of this individualized and everyday life approach to cognitive rehabilitation.

2. Case Illustration

D.S. is a 42-year-old woman without a profession and who lives with her husband. She completed one year of superior studies in chemistry when her first psychotic episode appeared at 22 years of age leading to a diagnosis of paranoid schizophrenia according to DSM-IV criteria. She has had approximately 20 hospitalizations; the last one being approximately two years before the rehabilitation program. During acute phases of the disease, D.S. presented delusions, visual and auditory hallucinations, stereotypies, and obsessions. D.S. was clinically stable for at least six months before the rehabilitation apart from occasionally experiencing auditory hallucinations. At the time of the study, her treatment consisted of two atypical antipsychotics (olanzapine: 2×10 mg; quetiapine: 1×200 mg) and one benzodiazepine (lorazepam: 1×2.5 mg), and she was seen by her psychiatrist about twice a month.

2.1. Daily Functioning Complaints.

D.S. expressed a desire to be more autonomous and to not have to rely on her husband all the time. She described a number of difficulties in everyday activities: following and retaining television or radio programs, following and retaining conversations, reading and maintaining text information (e.g., from a book or newspaper), remembering appointments, dates, activities (forcing her to write everything down on sheets of paper in order not to forget). These difficulties had a deleterious impact on her everyday functioning, such as social withdrawal. For instance, D.S. did not dare communicate with others as she feared that she would not be able to follow and understand the discussions. Also, if she constantly asked people to repeat what was said, she feared this will get on peoples' nerves or lead them to suspect that she is insane.

2.2. Pre-Rehabilitation Cognitive Assessment.

An extensive cognitive battery was administered to D.S., which covered various aspects of cognitive functioning (see Table 1). A score indicating a deficit was set at < -1.65 for the z-score and at <10 for the percentile score (in order to be less strict in comparison to a threshold <1.96 and <5; some scores were presented as z-scores and others as percentiles, depending on the given norms for each test). Performance was impaired on working memory tests assessing processing load and updating, while storage was preserved. Analysis of executive functioning revealed deficits related to flexibility and planning, but not inhibition. Performance was impaired on the verbal episodic memory tests, but not on the visual episodic memory test. Performances in divided and sustained attentional functions were all impaired. Processing speed was slow, but not impaired.

3. Treatment Study

3.1. Design.

The rehabilitation consisted of two 90-minute sessions per week (20 in total) and lasted three months. The intervention plan was designed to evaluate the effect of cognitive rehabilitation on functional targets. For this purpose, outcome measures at two different times were used: pre-rehabilitation and post-rehabilitation assessment.

3.2. Targets and Strategies.

Based on an analysis of D.S.'s daily functioning complaints and cognitive assessment, three rehabilitation target objectives were defined to improve her daily life functioning. Rehabilitation strategies were constructed according to processes involved in these target activities, analysis of preserved and impaired processes, and the optimizing factors.

3.2.1. Macrostructure Use.

Based on cognitive assessment, D.S. presented verbal episodic memory deficits, and in particular encoded text information in an unsystematic way. These impairments could explain difficulties she had in reading and remembering the contents of books or newspapers. In order to improve her memory for texts, a structured encoding strategy was proposed to D.S. This involved extracting the main information of a text in an organized manner, by omitting unimportant details and by highlighting significant elements. This strategy could help D.S. both at encoding and consequently at retrieval of a text (i.e., the use of a macrostructure at retrieval could serve as a cue that elicits recall of the text).

3.2.2. Working Memory Training.

D.S. also expressed difficulties in following conversations, and TV or radio programs. These difficulties, in addition to difficulties in maintaining information from texts from books or newspapers, could be related to a reduction of working memory resources observed in D.S. Thus, improving D.S.'s capacity to process immediate information in working memory could favor the extraction of main information and the binding between external information and mental representation in reading or conversational activities. Consequently, working memory training was implemented with several processing load and dual-task monitoring exercises.

3.2.3. Diary Use.

Memory (working and episodic) and planning deficits were observed in D.S., which were implicated in her difficulties to remember and plan everyday activities. Thus, an external aid was proposed to compensate for memory and planning deficits and to decrease the anxiety related to forgetting. A personalized diary was created, which was structured with various headings according to her activities, and was implemented in D.S.'s daily life.

3.3. Tasks and Stimuli

3.3.1. Macrostructure Use.

The macrostructure consisted of six headings: (1) title; (2) spatial context (where?); (3) temporal context (when?); (4) person(s); (5) facts; (6) results and conclusions. Two types of texts that D.S. had particular difficulties with were chosen by her: chapters from a book and newspaper articles. These texts did not differ according to their difficulty, length, and number of essential information contained in the six headings. In total, 17 chapters and 13 articles were used for the rehabilitation sessions (1 chapter and 1 article per session). They were analyzed in order to extract the total number of essential information contained in each of them and in order to construct a scoring grid (according to the six headings).

TABLE 1: Pre-rehabilitation, post-rehabilitation, and follow-up cognitive assessment.

Cognitive tests	Pre-rehabilitation	Post-rehabilitation	Follow-up
Working memory			
Storage			
(i) Digit span (forward) (MEM-III)	−0.7	0.49	−0.7
Processing load			
(i) Digit span (backward) (MEM-III)	−1	0.76	0.17
(ii) Number of trials for digit span (MEM-III)	**−2.33**	0.33	−0.33
(iii) Letter-number sequencing (MEM-III)	−1.33	−0.66	−0.66
Updating			
(i) Working memory (TAP): median RT/SD RT/omission(s)	P84/P50/**P4**	P79/P50/P18	P76/P50/P18
Executive functions			
Inhibition			
(i) Go/no-go (TAP): median RT/SD RT/error(s)	P14/P27/P<46	**P1**/P38/P42	P34/P46/<P42
Flexibility			
(i) Flexibility (TAP): median RT/SD RT/error(s)	−P10/**P7**/P27	**P7/P2**/P82	P12/P16/**P8**
(ii) Verbal fluency: phonological/semantic	−0.33/−1.42	0.18/−2.37	0.16/−0.71
Planning			
(i) Six Elements Test: total score/error(s)	−1.48/−1.5	−2.62/−0.08	0.01/0.32
Episodic Memory			
Explicit verbal episodic memory*			
(i) Logical memory (MEM-III): (I) First recall/total recall/	−1.33/**−1.67**	/	/
learning curve/theme	−1/−1	/	/
(II) Total recall/retention%/theme	**−1.67**/−1/−1	/	/
(ii) California Verbal Learning Test:			
First recall A/fifth recall A/total recall A/	**−1.93**/P5-25/−2	0.2/P50/−0.91	/
Short-term recall A/cued recall A	−1.6/**−1.67**	−0.44/−1.2	/
Delayed recall A/delayed cued recall A	−2/−2.42	−1.62/−1.49	/
Recognition/false recognition	**P5-25/P5-25**	P50/**P5-25**	/
(iii) RL/RI-16: immediate recall/free recall I/cued recall I	/	/	P99/−1.5/P99
Free recall II/cued recall II	/	/	**−1.84**/P25
Free recall III/cued recall III	/	/	−1.57/P99
Delayed free recall/delayed cued recall/recognition (/16)	/	/	**−3.6/P5-25**/16
Explicit visual episodic memory			
(i) Face recognition (MEM-III): part I/part II/retention	0.33/−0.33/−0.67	/	/
Attentional functions			
Divided attention			
(i) Divided attention (TAP): median RT/SD RT/omission(s)	P62/P42/**P4**	P38/P14/P12	P76/P16/<P18
Sustained attention			
(i) Digit continuous ordination: mean efficiency: 0–10 min/	**−2.62**	**−2.76**	**−2.83**
10–20 min/0–20 min	**−2.72/−2.82**	**−2.72/−2.79**	**−3.22/−3.1**
Processing speed			
(i) Digit symbol—coding (WAIS-III)	−1	−0.67	−0.33

*Different episodic memory tests were used at different moments of evaluation (pre-rehabilitation, post-rehabilitation, follow-up) in order to avoid learning effects; numbers in bold indicate a deficit score (<−1.65 for the z-scores, <10 for the percentiles); RT: reaction time; SD: standard deviation; digit span, letter-number sequencing, logical memory (MEM-III; [16]); working memory, go/no-go, flexibility, divided attention (TAP; [17]); digit symbol (WAIS-III; [18]); verbal fluency [19]; Six Elements Test ([20]; French adaptation, [21]); California Verbal Learning Test ([22]; French adaptation, [23]); RL/RI-16 [24]; digit continuous ordination [25].

After reading a text, D.S. was asked to complete the various headings of the macrostructure (for an example from a newspaper article, see Table 3). Then, she was asked to read this macrostructure once or twice. Finally, D.S. had to recall the text without using the macrostructure both immediately after the session and in the next session, in order to check for long-term retention of the information. The task lasted about 45 minutes and was realized in 18 rehabilitation sessions.

3.3.2. Working Memory Training. Several types of working memory exercises (36 in total across 14 sessions) were proposed to D.S. (2 to 4 per session, each exercise lasting about 10 minutes): (1) 10-word reconstruction exercises: a word was orally spelt to D.S. beginning with the last letter and she had to find the correct word; 10-number reconstruction exercises: a series of digits were orally read to D.S. who was then asked to provide the number formed by the digits; the words and numbers were of different lengths (4 to 6 letters; 4 to 5 digits) (1 point for each correct response; maximum score for each task = 15); (2) 3 alphabetical ordination exercises of orally presented words (3 to 4 words) (1 point for each correct response; maximum score = 10); (3) 8 exercises from a Brown-Peterson task: a number of four digits and then three words were read to D.S. who had to repeat the words and then recall the number (1 point for each recalled number; maximum score = 15); (4) 5 exercises from a market task: D.S. received a list containing the price of articles in a market. The name of a person and the purchases (2 to 3 articles) were orally presented to D.S. who had to memorize them and calculate the total price (1 point for each correct response, that is, articles, name of the person, and total price; maximum score = 40 to 50).

3.3.3. Diary Use. The diary consisted of four headings based on D.S.'s daily functioning: "important dates" (e.g., doctor appointments), "outings" (e.g., with friends), "shopping list," and "housework". On one sheet of the diary representing a week, the four headings were positioned on top horizontally and the days of the week were positioned to the left vertically.

During the first session, D.S. was taught how to use the diary correctly. Two main objectives were proposed: (1) to gather all the information to be remembered in one place by respecting the headings and (2) to consult this diary at the same time of the day (i.e., morning, midday, and evening). For the following sessions, D.S. was asked to bring her diary with her in order to examine whether it was used in a regular and correct manner in daily life. If this was not the case, a discussion of how to improve diary use followed (e.g., use all the headings, make changes in her diary according to her timetable). In total, interviews concerning diary use were carried out in 10 sessions and lasted about 10 minutes each.

3.4. Outcome Measures. Outcome measures (administered before and after the rehabilitation program) consisted of assessing macrostructure use, working memory performance, and diary use (parallel versions of macrostructure use and working memory performance were used in order to minimize practice effects). The Subjective Scale to Investigate Cognition in Schizophrenia (SSTICS, [26]) was also administered before and after the rehabilitation program to obtain an index of the person's subjective cognitive complaints for five cognitive domains (memory, attention, executive function, language, and praxis). Finally, a subjective assessment questionnaire for the three rehabilitation objectives was administered at post-rehabilitation.

4. Results

4.1. Pre-Rehabilitation versus Post-Rehabilitation Comparison. The post-rehabilitation results (see Table 1) revealed an improvement (i.e., when a performance previously impaired at pre-rehabilitation is within the norms at post-rehabilitation) in both processing load and the updating component of working memory. There was a decrease in the number of errors for planning abilities. Flexibility remained impaired. Verbal episodic memory showed clear improvement. Divided attention (i.e., number of omissions) improved slightly, but sustained attention remained impaired. Finally, working memory storage improved.

Performance of pre- and post-rehabilitation outcome measures was compared (see Table 2) for macrostructure use, working memory tasks, diary use, and the SSTICS. A statistical analysis using chi-square tests was carried out to compare the scores regarding macrostructure use, working memory tasks, and SSTICS.

4.1.1. Macrostructure Use. The mean immediate recall percentage for chapters and for articles was calculated. Significant improvements were noted for chapters ($\chi^2(1) = 35.17$; $P < .001$) and articles ($\chi^2(1) = 200$; $P < .001$).

4.1.2. Working Memory. Scores on the word reconstruction task and the number reconstruction task improved significantly (resp., $\chi^2(1) = 6.5$; $P = .01$; $\chi^2(1) = 12.53$; $P < .001$). The scores on the Brown-Peterson task did not significantly improve from pre-rehabilitation to post-rehabilitation ($\chi^2(1) = .08$; $P = .78$). Finally, the market task improved significantly ($\chi^2(1) = 56.23$; $P < .001$).

4.1.3. Diary Use. D.S. used the diary and its headings correctly from the first session. After three sessions, D.S. stopped using numerous separate reminders scattered around the house as they were now centralized in her diary, and she consulted it regularly (i.e., morning, midday, and evening).

4.1.4. SSTICS. The total SSTICS score decreased (nonsignificantly) at post-rehabilitation ($\chi^2(1) = 1.79$; $P = .18$). The decrease essentially concerned attentional complaints that showed a significant decrease ($\chi^2(1) = 28.57$; $P < .001$), while memory ($\chi^2(1) = .74$; $P = .39$) and executive complaints ($\chi^2(1) = 1.73$; $P = .19$) did not significantly diminish.

4.1.5. Qualitative Self-Assessment. Based on replies on the subjective questionnaire, D.S. reported that the macrostructure headings helped her "very much" in structuring her thoughts and in concentrating when reading. Moreover, D.S. reported that she spontaneously used the macrostructure procedure. She also mentioned that she found herself talking to people more often and giving responses due to an increased ability to comprehend and follow conversations. When asked whether there was an improvement in attention when watching movies or during conversations, she answered "very much." The use of the diary helped her to plan her week in a more efficient manner (without

TABLE 2: Pre-rehabilitation, post-rehabilitation, and follow-up outcome measures.

Outcome measures	Pre-rehabilitation	Post-rehabilitation	Follow-up
Macrostructure use			
(i) Chapter: mean immediate recall percentage	40	81*a	62*b
(ii) Article: mean immediate recall percentage	0	100*a	71*b
Working memory			
(i) Word reconstruction task: correct response (/16)	6	9*a	8
(ii) Number reconstruction task: correct response (/20)	7	12*a	8
(iii) Brown-Peterson task: correct response (/64)	36	37	48*b
(iv) Market task: correct response (/60)	13	45*a	29*b
SSTICS			
(i) Total score (/84)	59	51	54
(ii) Memory complaints score (/44)	27	24	27
(ii) Attentional complaints score (/20)	20	15*a	13*b
(iv) Executive complaints score (/12)	8	7	9

*a Significant effect for pre-rehabilitation versus post-rehabilitation comparison; *b significant effect for pre-rehabilitation versus follow-up comparison.

TABLE 3: Example of macrostructure training for a newspaper article entitled "Oil, the luxury product."

Title: oil, the luxury product

Spatial context (where?): in the world, and in Belgium

Temporal context (when?): present day

Person(s): OPEP or the Organization of Petroleum Exporting Countries

Facts: the increase of oil price creates an important world problem. This is due to the fact that China buys oil so that there is no competition and, moreover, the capacities of refining are decreasing

Results and conclusions: in Europe, the European Commission is revising its forecasts (less oil production)

forgetting), thus decreasing her anxiety level. She reported being better organized when everything was gathered in one place. Finally, she had the feeling of having made progress and was very satisfied with the rehabilitation.

4.2. Follow-Up. A follow-up assessment took place three years after the end of the cognitive rehabilitation. During this period, D.S. remained clinically stable without any hospitalizations. As previously, she continued to see her psychiatrist twice a month, and her treatment consisted of two atypical antipsychotics (olanzapine: 2×7.5 mg; quetiapine: 2×300 mg) and one benzodiazepine (lorazepam 1×2.5 mg). Moreover, she did not take part in any kind of rehabilitation (cognitive rehabilitation, cognitive-behavioral therapy, etc.) during this follow-up period.

Assessments carried out at the follow-up were the same as those for pre- and post-rehabilitation. The results of the follow-up cognitive assessment (see Table 1) indicated that the post-rehabilitation improvements in both processing load and the updating component of working memory, planning, and divided attention remained stable at follow-up. Flexibility remained impaired. Scores for verbal episodic

memory, which revealed a general improvement after rehabilitation, indicated no change at follow-up. Finally, her performance in sustained attention remained impaired.

Performance on pre-rehabilitation and follow-up baseline measures were compared (see Table 2) for macrostructure use, working memory tasks, and the SSTICS.

4.2.1. Macrostructure Use. The same types of texts (book chapter and newspaper article) as those used for pre- and post-rehabilitation were administered: one chapter from another book of the same author and one new article.

Pre-Rehabilitation versus Follow-Up. Significant improvements on immediate recall scores for the chapters and the articles persisted (for chapters: χ^2 (1) = 9.68; P = .002; for articles: χ^2 (1) = 110.08; $P < .001$).

Qualitative Analysis. D.S.'s recalls (immediate and delayed) were structured according to the various macrostructure headings and respected the chronological order of the events.

4.2.2. Working Memory Training. The same tasks as those carried out at pre- and post-rehabilitation were administered albeit parallel versions (i.e., different materiel) were used in order to minimize test-retest effects.

Pre-Rehabilitation versus Follow-Up. The significant post-rehabilitation improvement disappeared for the word reconstruction task ($\chi^2(1)$ = 2.92; P = .087) and for the number reconstruction task ($\chi^2(1)$ = .53; P = .47). On the contrary, scores on the Brown-Peterson task significantly improved ($\chi^2(1)$ = 7.99; P = .005), and the significant improvement on the market task persisted ($\chi^2(1)$ = 14.86; $P < .001$).

4.2.3. Diary Use. D.S. reported that the regular use of her diary helped her to better memorize her fixed appointments and that she continued to centralize all the important information in one place. Moreover, she has created another diary where she noted (every evening), on the day page, the activities realized during the day in order to have a better awareness of past personal events.

4.2.4. SSTICS

Pre-Rehabilitation versus Follow-Up. The significant decrease after rehabilitation concerning attentional complaints persisted ($\chi^2(1) = 42.42$; $P < .001$). Stable scores were noted on the total score ($\chi^2(1) = .81$; $P = .37$) and specifically for memory complaints (27/44 versus 27/44) and executive complaints ($\chi^2(1) = 1.55$; $P = .21$).

4.2.5. Qualitative Self-Assessment.
The same subjective questionnaire as the one used at post-rehabilitation was administered at follow-up. First, D.S. noted that the use of the macrostructure still helped her "very much" to structure her thoughts when reading. When asked whether there was an improvement in attention when watching movies or during conversations, she answered "moderately," explaining that she followed the news on the TV better but experienced some difficulties in concentrating during longer activities, which could be due to objective deficits in attentional functions. She indicated that the use of the diary had calmed her down because she no longer had to worry about forgetting important events, therefore allowing her to think about other things. She also expressed that she is more autonomous in her daily-life and that she is still very satisfied with the work realized during the cognitive rehabilitation program.

5. Discussion

Despite numerous appeals in the literature for developing other methodological approaches to cognitive rehabilitation research and practice and in light of findings revealing that "stand alone" cognitive rehabilitation programs have not hitherto succeeded in improving patients' everyday functioning in a significant and durable manner, many studies continue to adopt the same approach. Yet, a change is unmistakably needed. In particular, we call for an individualized and everyday life approach to cognitive rehabilitation in schizophrenia in order to attain this goal. In order to do so, a number of issues need to be addressed and carried out in future studies. In particular, specific and crucial difficulties in patients' everyday lives should be the focus of rehabilitation programs. The vast heterogeneity inherent in schizophrenia must also be considered in forthcoming interventions. It has been argued that taking both these issues into account will result in more effective intervention programs in their ability to provide improvements in patients' psychosocial functioning.

The present case study wished to provide an example of how to work within an individual and everyday life approach to cognitive rehabilitation in schizophrenia. In particular, the study showed that it had a beneficial effect on D.S.'s everyday functioning. The efficacy of the rehabilitation program was especially demonstrated based on results from outcome measures. Furthermore, the beneficial effect of

the cognitive rehabilitation program was transferred to the person's daily life, as disclosed in her responses to self-assessment questionnaires and subjective reports. Thus, D.S. became autonomous in the application of strategies learned during the rehabilitation program. Indeed, for instance, she spontaneously used the macrostructure procedure and expressed the fact that this strategy helped her to retain more information when reading texts. D.S. also mentioned that the use of her diary allowed her to plan her week in a more efficient manner without forgetting events and furthermore helped decrease her level of anxiety. D.S. also reported an improvement in attention when watching movies or when following conversations and discussions. This resulted in D.S. talking to people more often, compared to before the cognitive rehabilitation program. Finally, D.S. reported less attentional complaints in her daily life.

The meaningfully lasting beneficial effects were largely evident in that they were still present when pre-rehabilitation and follow-up scores were compared. However, for some of these measures, significant post-rehabilitation improvement disappeared after the 3-year period. These results suggest that the meaningfully lasting effects were less robust for rehabilitation targets that were not directly associated with compensatory interventions that D.S. still used at the follow-up assessment and/or that rehabilitation sessions aimed at refreshing acquisition would have been necessary. Moreover, D.S. had transferred the learned strategies to her daily-life on a long-term basis: she continued to employ her diary in an efficient manner and continued to structure her reading according to the macrostructure headings. Thus, compensatory approaches, which teach a strategy, have showed to produce life-long changes in function as long as the intervention is effective and the person continues to use the compensatory strategy. Additionally, D.S. expressed being more organized and autonomous—two crucial goals of any rehabilitation program.

In sum, the originality and interest of this study was to take into account the various complaints that a person diagnosed with schizophrenia experienced in her daily life and to use these as rehabilitation objectives. Different rehabilitation strategies were implemented for each of the complaints, and they were adapted according to her cognitive profile. These elements undoubtedly contributed to the fact that the cognitive rehabilitation program was well accepted by D.S. Thus, an individualized and everyday life approach appears to be an effective alternative to improving the effects of cognitive rehabilitation on both cognitive and daily life functioning in people with schizophrenia. Furthermore, these benefits were shown to be maintained at long-term follow-up.

Some limitations of the study should be mentioned. Firstly, there are limits related to an ABA design (A: outcome measures; B: intervention), which are less capable of establishing a causal relation. However, a protocol with multiple outcome measures or other designs (e.g., type ABAB) was not possible to implement for practical reasons: such a protocol requires numerous assessments and, consequently, is very tiresome and tedious for the patient and such protocol is difficult to design, especially when ecological measures are involved. Moreover, the quality of the case study would have been improved with the inclusion of measures defining the severity of psychiatric symptoms pre- and post-rehabilitation. This will be taken into account in future cognitive rehabilitation studies.

Finally, it is also important to underline that the other psychological dimensions (such as auditory hallucinations, obsessional symptoms, social anxiety), which had an impact on D.S.'s everyday functioning, would also have been important to take into account in the individualized rehabilitation program in order to further increase its efficacy. Indeed, cognitive functioning is by far not the sole factor involved in functional outcome in schizophrenia. Fett et al. [27], in their meta-analysis examining relations between cognitive functioning (both neurocognitive and social cognitive) and functional outcome in patients with nonaffective psychosis, found that cognitive functioning explains 25% of the variance of functional status of patients with schizophrenia, and thus as much as 75% of the variance in outcome was left unexplained. There are at least two implications related to this finding. First, it is necessary that other factors significantly related to functional outcome be identified. Secondly, intervention programs must integrate strategies that remediate and improve these additional areas. Indeed, as observed in Wykes et al. [1] and McGurk et al. [2], cognitive rehabilitation approaches clearly need to be combined with other forms of intervention in order to maximize their impact on functional outcome. Studies have shown that a number of other factors are also significantly related to functional outcome in patients with schizophrenia. These factors include (but are not limited to) symptomatology (especially negative symptoms; [28]), various psychological processes such as social cognition [29], dysfunctional attitudes [30], metacognitive processes [31], poor insight [32], and finally environmental factors, such as family attitudes [33], negative stereotypes [34], and internalized stigma [35].

Therefore, we advocate an individualized, integrative, and everyday rehabilitation approach, which includes interventional strategies that help improve, in addition to cognitive factors, other factors that also play a significant role in functional outcome in schizophrenia. Further, we propose to carry out multidimensional evaluations, which include not only cognitive and functional assessments, but also comprise a large array of other dimensions. This integrative approach is important to take into account as schizophrenia is a disorder that affects many different areas and levels of functioning. Moreover, these areas are complementary and interdependent. That is, patients will have difficulties in a number of different areas (e.g., cognitive, motivational, affective) at the same time, and one area may have an impact on the other (e.g., motivational problems may negatively affect affective and cognitive functioning).

Conflict of Interests

The authors declared no potential conflict of interests with respect to the research, authorship, and/or publication of this paper.

Acknowledgments

The authors would like to thank *asbl Réflexions* for their help in the realization of the project. This study was supported by a grant from an Interreg IIIB project and a grant from a MiRe-DRESS project.

References

[1] T. Wykes, V. Huddy, C. Cellard, S. R. McGurk, and P. Czobor, "A meta-analysis of cognitive remediation for schizophrenia: methodology and effect sizes," *American Journal of Psychiatry*, vol. 168, no. 5, pp. 472–485, 2011.

[2] S. R. McGurk, E. W. Twamley, D. I. Sitzer, G. J. McHugo, and K. T. Mueser, "A meta-analysis of cognitive remediation in schizophrenia," *American Journal of Psychiatry*, vol. 164, no. 12, pp. 1791–1802, 2007.

[3] A. Medalia and J. Choi, "Cognitive remediation in schizophrenia," *Neuropsychology Review*, vol. 19, no. 3, pp. 353–364, 2009.

[4] S. R. McGurk, K. T. Mueser, and A. Pascaris, "Cognitive training and supported employment for persons with severe mental illness: one-year results from a randomized controlled trial," *Schizophrenia Bulletin*, vol. 31, no. 4, pp. 898–909, 2005.

[5] S. R. McGurk, K. T. Mueser, K. Feldman, R. Wolfe, and A. Pascaris, "Cognitive training for supported employment: 2-3 Year outcomes of a randomized controlled trial," *American Journal of Psychiatry*, vol. 164, no. 3, pp. 437–441, 2007.

[6] S. M. Silverstein, W. D. Spaulding, A. A. Menditto et al., "Attention shaping: a reward-based learning method to enhance skills training outcomes in schizophrenia," *Schizophrenia Bulletin*, vol. 35, no. 1, pp. 222–232, 2009.

[7] M. N. Levaux, J. Vezzaro, F. Larøi, I. Offerlin-Meyer, J. M. Danion, and M. Van der Linden, "Cognitive rehabilitation of the updating sub-component of working memory in schizophrenia: a case study," *Neuropsychological Rehabilitation*, vol. 19, no. 2, pp. 244–273, 2009.

[8] M.-N. Levaux, F. Larøi, I. Offerlin-Meyer, J.-M. Danion, and M. Van der Linden, "The effectiveness of the Attention Training Technique for the reduction of intrusive thoughts in schizophrenia: a case study," *Clinical Case Studies*, vol. 10, no. 6, pp. 464–482, 2009.

[9] B. W. Palmer, R. K. Heaton, J. Kuck et al., "Is it possible to be schizophrenic yet neuropsychologically normal?" *Neuropsychology*, vol. 11, no. 3, pp. 437–446, 1997.

[10] M. T. Tsuang, M. J. Lyons, and S. V. Faraone, "Heterogeneity of schizophrenia. Conceptual models and analytic strategies," *British Journal of Psychiatry*, vol. 156, pp. 17–26, 1990.

[11] B. E. Seaton, G. Goldstein, and D. N. Allen, "Sources of heterogeneity in Schizophrenia: the role of neuropsychological functioning," *Neuropsychology Review*, vol. 11, no. 1, pp. 45–67, 2001.

[12] T. Shallice, P. W. Burgess, and C. D. Frith, "Can the neuropsychological case-study approach be applied to schizophrenia?" *Psychological Medicine*, vol. 21, no. 3, pp. 661–673, 1991.

[13] A. Caramazza and A. Hillis, "For a theory of remediation of cognitive deficits," *Neuropsychological Rehabilitation*, vol. 3, no. 3, pp. 217–234, 1993.

[14] D. I. Velligan and C. C. Bow-Thomas, "Two case studies of cognitive adaptation training for outpatients with schizophrenia," *Psychiatric Services*, vol. 51, no. 1, pp. 25–29, 2000.

[15] D. I. Velligan, C. C. Bow-Thomas, C. Huntzinger et al., "Randomized controlled trial of the use of compensatory strategies to enhance adaptive functioning in outpatients with

schizophrenia," *American Journal of Psychiatry*, vol. 157, no. 8, pp. 1317–1323, 2000.

[16] D. Wechsler, *MEM-III: Manuel de L'échelle Clinique de Mémoire*, Les éditions du Centre de Psychologie, Paris, France, 3rd edition, 2001.

[17] P. Zimmerman and B. Fimm, *Test for Attentional Performance (TAP)*, PsyTest, Herzogenrath, Germany, 1994.

[18] D. Wechsler, *WAIS-III: Echelle D'Intelligence de Wechsler Pour Adultes*, Les éditions du Centre de Psychologie, Paris, France, 3rd edition, 2000.

[19] D. Cardebat, B. Doyon, M. Puel, P. Goulet, and Y. Joanette, "Formal and semantic lexical evocation in normal subjects. Performance and dynamics of production as a function of sex, age and educational level," *Acta Neurologica Belgica*, vol. 90, no. 4, pp. 207–217, 1990.

[20] T. Shallice and P. W. Burgess, "Deficits in strategy application following frontal lobe damage in man," *Brain*, vol. 114, no. 2, pp. 727–741, 1991.

[21] C. Garnier, F. Enot-Joyeux, C. Jokic, F. Le Thiec, B. Desgranges, and F. Eustache, "Une évaluation des fonctions exécutives chez les traumatisés crâniens: L'adaptation du test des six éléments," *Revue de Neuropsychologie*, vol. 8, no. 3, pp. 385–414, 1998.

[22] D. C. Delis, J. Freeland, J. H. Kramer, and E. Kaplan, "Integrating clinical assessment with cognitive neuroscience: construct validation of the California verbal learning test," *Journal of Consulting and Clinical Psychology*, vol. 56, no. 1, pp. 123–130, 1988.

[23] J. Poitrenaud, B. Deweer, M. Kalafat, and M. Van der Linden, *Adaptation en langue française du California Verbal Learning Test*, Les Editions du Centre de Psychologie Appliquée, Paris, France, 2007.

[24] M. Van der Linden, in *L'épreuve de Rappel Libre/Rappel Indicé à 16 Items (RL/RI-16L'évaluation des Troubles de la Mémoire. Présentation de Quatre Tests de Mémoire Episodique (avec leur étalonnage)*, M. Van der Linden, Ed., Solal, Marseille, France, 2004.

[25] A. Rey, F. Marchand, R. Rappaz, M. Richelle, and M. Schaechtlin, "Centration soutenue sur une tâche intellectuelle simple: ordination continue de chiffres," *Archives de Psychologie*, vol. 36, pp. 29–61, 1957.

[26] E. Stip, J. Caron, S. Renaud, T. Pampoulova, and Y. Lecomte, "Exploring cognitive complaints in schizophrenia: the subjective scale to investigate cognition in Schizophrenia," *Comprehensive Psychiatry*, vol. 44, no. 4, pp. 331–340, 2003.

[27] A.-K. J. Fett, W. Viechtbauer, M. D. G. Dominguez, D. L. Penn, J. van Os, and L. Krabbendam, "The relationship between neurocognition and social cognition with functional outcomes in schizophrenia: a meta-analysis," *Neuroscience and Biobehavioral Reviews*, vol. 35, no. 3, pp. 573–588, 2011.

[28] J. Ventura, G. S. Hellemann, A. D. Thames, V. Koellner, and K. H. Nuechterlein, "Symptoms as mediators of the relationship between neurocognition and functional outcome in schizophrenia: a meta-analysis," *Schizophrenia Research*, vol. 113, no. 2-3, pp. 189–199, 2009.

[29] F. Mancuso, W. P. Horan, R. S. Kern, and M. F. Green, "Social cognition in psychosis: multidimensional structure, clinical correlates, and relationship with functional outcome," *Schizophrenia Research*, vol. 125, no. 2-3, pp. 143–151, 2011.

[30] W. P. Horan, Y. Rassovsky, R. S. Kern, J. Lee, J. K. Wynn, and M. F. Green, "Further support for the role of dysfunctional attitudes in models of real-world functioning in schizophrenia," *Journal of Psychiatric Research*, vol. 44, no. 8, pp. 499–505, 2010.

[31] D. Koren, L. J. Seidman, M. Goldsmith, and P. D. Harvey, "Real-world cognitive— and metacognitive—dysfunction in schizophrenia: a new approach for measuring (and remediating) more "right stuff"," *Schizophrenia Bulletin*, vol. 32, no. 2, pp. 310–326, 2006.

[32] P. H. Lysaker, G. J. Bryson, and M. D. Bell, "Insight and work performance in schizophrenia," *Journal of Nervous and Mental Disease*, vol. 190, no. 3, pp. 142–146, 2002.

[33] M. Girón and M. Gómez-Beneyto, "Relationship between family attitudes and social functioning in schizophrenia: a nine-month follow-up prospective study in Spain," *Journal of Nervous and Mental Disease*, vol. 192, no. 6, pp. 414–420, 2004.

[34] J. D. Henry, C. Von Hippel, and L. Shapiro, "Stereotype threat contributes to social difficulties in people with schizophrenia," *British Journal of Clinical Psychology*, vol. 49, no. 1, pp. 31–41, 2010.

[35] P. T. Yanos, P. H. Lysaker, and D. Roe, "Internalized stigma as a barrier to improvement in vocational functioning among people with schizophrenia-spectrum disorders," *Psychiatry Research*, vol. 178, no. 1, pp. 211–213, 2010.

13

Effects of Posteroanterior Thoracic Mobilization on Heart Rate Variability and Pain in Women with Fibromyalgia

**Michel Silva Reis,[1] João Luiz Quagliotti Durigan,[2] Ross Arena,[3]
Bruno Rafael Orsini Rossi,[4] Renata Gonçalves Mendes,[5] and Audrey Borghi-Silva[5]**

[1] *Department of Physical Therapy, School of Medicine, Federal University of Rio de Janeiro, 8° Floor 3 (8E-03),
Prof Rodolpho Paulo Rocco Street, 21941-913 Rio de Janeiro, RJ, Brazil*

[2] *Physical Therapy Division, University of Brasília, QNN 14 Área Especial, Ceilândia Sul, 72220-140 Brasília, DF, Brazil*

[3] *Department of Physical Therapy and Integrative Physiology Laboratory, College of Applied Health Sciences,
University of Illinois, 1919 W. Taylor Street (MC 898), Chicago, IL 60612, USA*

[4] *Healthy-School Unit, Federal University of Sao Carlos, 235 Km. Washington Luis Rodovia, 13565-905 Sao Carlos, SP, Brazil*

[5] *Laboratory of Cardiopulmonary Physiotherapy, Federal University of Sao Carlos, 235 Km. Washington Luis Rodovia,
13565-905 Sao Carlos, SP, Brazil*

Correspondence should be addressed to Michel Silva Reis; msreis@hucff.ufrj.br

Academic Editor: Francois Prince

Fibromyalgia (FM) has been associated with cardiac autonomic abnormalities and pain. Heart rate variability (HRV) is reduced in FM with autonomic tone dominated by sympathetic activity. The purpose of this study was to evaluate the effects of one session of a posteroanterior glide technique on both autonomic modulation and pain in woman with FM. This was a controlled trial with immediate followup; twenty premenopausal women were allocated into 2 groups: (i) women diagnosed with FM ($n = 10$) and (ii) healthy women ($n = 10$). Both groups received one session of Maitland mobilization grade III posteroanterior central pressure glide, at 2 Hz for 60 s at each vertebral segment. Autonomic modulation was assessed by HRV and pain by a numeric pain scale before and after the intervention. For HRV analyses, heart rate and RR intervals were recorded for 10 minutes. FM subjects demonstrated reduced HRV compared to controls. Although the mobilization technique did not significantly reduce pain, it was able to improve HRV quantified by an increase in rMSSD and SD1 indices, reflecting an improved autonomic profile through increased vagal activity. In conclusion, women with FM presented with impaired cardiac autonomic modulation. One session of Maitland spine mobilization was able to acutely improve HRV.

1. Introduction

Fibromyalgia (FM) is a chronic disorder, which is accompanied by myriad of symptoms such as pain, fatigue, depression, insomnia, and reduced cognitive performance [1]. Chronic fatigue and pain syndromes may precipitate increased sympathetic nervous system activity [2–7]. Specific to the current study, although the exact cause of FM is unknown, some studies suggest autonomic imbalance mechanistically contributes to the symptoms [8, 9].

The autonomic imbalance for FM is characterized by sympathetic hyperactivity at rest and an inability to appropriately respond to physiological stressors [4, 5, 9, 10]. Sympathetic hyperactivity may also be responsible for frequent complaints of cold extremities. Interestingly, a correlation between autonomic dysfunction and symptom severity or quality of life has been previously described [11]. Heart rate variability (HRV) has been used to investigate cardiovascular autonomic modulation as a simple, sensitive, and noninvasive tool [12]. Given the link between abnormal ratios of sympathovagal balance in patients with FM, HRV analysis at rest as well as posttherapeutic interventions may prove to be valuable.

Several therapy strategies [13] have been applied to FM patients with the intention of minimizing the cascade of physically debilitating symptoms. Although there is no consensus, it seems that manual techniques improve quality of life and symptomatology [14]. In a recent study, manual therapy was effective in improving pain intensity, widespread pressure pain sensitivity, impact of FM symptoms on a given patient, sleep quality, and depressive symptoms [15]. The Maitland mobilization is a well-established manual technique that has been applied to a number of musculoskeletal disorders [16].

In relation to HRV, Buttagat et al. [17] demonstrated that manual therapy is effective in increasing cardiac parasympathetic activity, reducing sympathetic activity, and reducing pain and stress in patients with back pain associated with myofascial trigger points. Other authors [18] observed that myofascial trigger-point therapy to the head, neck, and shoulder areas is effective in increasing cardiac parasympathetic activity and improving measures of relaxation.

However, there is no evidence that the Maitland mobilization, focused on mobilizing the thoracic spine, improves autonomic function and pain in FM. The aim of this study was to evaluate the effects of a posteroanterior glide mobilization technique on both HRV and pain. We hypothesize that one session of this manual intervention improves both HRV and pain in woman with FM.

2. Methods

2.1. Design and Study Population.
This was a controlled trial with immediate followup enrolling twenty women. Inclusion criteria were as follows: (1) being in the premenopausal phase and (2) no present history of smoking, lung disease, hypertension, diabetes, hypothyroidism, coronary insufficiency, or other relevant clinical conditions known to affect autonomic control of heart rate, including inflammatory and autoimmune disorders. To the FM group ($n = 10$), the patients were diagnosed with FM by clinicians according to the criteria of the American College of Rheumatology [19]; and the control group ($n = 10$) was composed of apparently healthy women without FM. All subjects were submitted to the following: (1) a clinical assessment (current and past clinical history, family background, lifestyle habits, and physical exam) and (2) physiotherapeutic assessment (postural assessment and muscle tests). The volunteers were informed of experimental procedures and signed an informed consent form before taking part in the study, which was approved by the Ethics Committee of the Federal University of Sao Carlos (109/2006).

2.2. Experimental Procedure.
Data collection was carried out in an air-conditioned laboratory with a 22°C to 24°C temperature and a 50 to 60 percent relative humidity between 8 a.m. and 12 p.m. The subjects were familiarized with the experimental environment and research personnel. The volunteers were instructed to avoid caffeinated beverages; not

to perform physical exercise 24 hours prior to evaluation; have a light meal the morning of data collection; and have an adequate period of sleep the night before (at least 8 hours).

A posteroanterior glide mobilization technique was performed as previously described [20]. The women were instructed to remain in the prone position and an experienced physiotherapist administered the Grade III posteroanterior central pressure glide (III-PAC) at 2 Hz for 60 s at each vertebral segment. Specifically, this manual mobilization was applied between T1 and T12 vertebral structures, corresponding to the thoracic sympathetic preganglionic neurons. The intervention was performed in the control group and FM group by the same physiotherapist that was blinded to each subject's group assignment.

2.3. Pain Assessment.
Pain was assessed with the numeric pain scale (NPS), which assesses the pain intensity and degree of relief experienced by the patient following an intervention (score of 0 = no pain; 10 = unbearable pain) [21].

2.4. Heart Rate and RR Interval Data Acquisition.
Heart rate and RR intervals (RRi) were registered beat-to-beat, through a heart rate monitor (Polar S810i) with a 1,000 Hz sampling frequency, fastened by an elastic band to the lower third of the sternum, providing simultaneous transmission to a watch where the data were stored. Afterwards, through a serial port interface and an infrared sensor, data was transported and stored in a personal computer to be analyzed. This assessment was performed at rest in the supine position for 10 min before and after the posteroanterior glide technique. During the data acquisition, the volunteers were instructed to maintain spontaneous breathing to ensure eupneic conditions (the respiratory frequency was monitored). The protocol transition points were also accurately marked to allow for an adequate data analysis.

2.5. Signal Processing and HRV Analysis.
After acquisition, the signals were transferred to the Polar Precision Performance Software and the section of highest stability for RRi, which included a simple line comprised of at least 256 points, was selected by visual inspection according to the criterion set forth by the Task Force of European Society of Cardiology and the North American Society of Pacing and Electrophysiology [12]. The data were entered into the Kubios HRV Analysis software (MATLAB, version 2 beta, Kuopio, Finland).

Heart rate variability was analyzed by mathematical and statistical models in time and frequency domains and by nonlinear models [19]. In the time domain, the mean RRi, which is all the cyclic components responsible for variability during the recording period and is an estimate of overall HRV, and root mean square of the squares of the differences between successive RRi (rMSSD), in ms, representative of parasympathetic activity, were analyzed. The frequency domain analysis utilized the fast Fourier transform (FFT) on the time series. The application of this algorithm permitted the identification of the power spectral density (PSD) as well as its frequency bands: low frequency (LF) and high frequency (HF), both in

TABLE 1: Demographic, anthropometric, clinical, and medication use data in both groups.

	Fibromyalgia ($n = 10$)	Control ($n = 10$)	P
Age, years	52 ± 10	45 ± 9	0.109
Weight, kg	62 ± 9.9	57 ± 6.0	0.321
Height, cm	157 ± 5.0	163 ± 6.0	0.122
Body mass index, kg/m^2	23.1 ± 3.2	22.6 ± 2.5	0.119
Antidepressant use, %	90	0	<0.001
Anxyolitic use, %	70	0	<0.001
Analgesic use, %	60	0	<0.001
Opiate use, %	10	0	<0.001

Data are presented as mean ± SD or %.

normalized units (nu). Two frequency bands that best represent vagal and sympathetic activities of HR control were used in this study. The LF (0.04 to 0.15 Hz) has been attributed to a mixture of sympathetic and parasympathetic modulation, with sympathetic predominance, as well as baroreflex activity. On the other hand, the HF (0.15 to 0.4) has been attributed to parasympathetic activity [12].

For nonlinear analysis, we used Poincaré plot measure indices SD1 and SD2 (the standard derivation of the Poincaré plot perpendicular and along the line of identity, resp.) representative of parasympathetic autonomic activity and total HRV, respectively [22]. Detrended fluctuation analysis (DFA) was also carried out using DFAα1 (short-term correlation properties of RRi) and DFAα2 (long-term correlation properties of RRi) indices. The technique of the analyses, previously developed by Peng et al. [22], quantifies the presence or absence of fractal-like correlation properties in biological times series and has been used to evaluate the risk of mortality in various groups, given it is a predictor of benign and malignant arrhythmias, sudden cardiac death, and total mortality in patients with reduced left ventricle ejection fraction, acute myocardial infarction, and other cardiovascular diseases [22].

2.6. Statistical Analysis. Sample size was determined a priori using G*Power (version 3.1.3; University of Trier, Trier, Germany) with the level of significance set at $P = 0.05$ and power $(1 - \beta) = 0.95$ in order to detect a large effect ($f^2 > 0.47$). We conducted a pilot study with 5 participants to evaluate the effect size for the main dependent variable (rMSSD). Based on these a priori calculations and the pilot study, we set the final sample size at $n = 20$ (10 per group). For continuous data, parametric statistical tests were used given data presented with a normal distribution (Shapiro-Wilk test) and homogenous variances (Levene's test). For demographic and clinical variables, was performed unpaired t test. The two-way analysis of variance (ANOVA) assessed the group effect (control versus FM), mobilization effect, and interaction between them. Then, Bonferroni post-hoc was performed to identify differences. All analyses were carried out in SPSS software Release 10.0.1 (Chicago, IL) and all statistical tests with a $P < 0.05$ were considered significant.

3. Results

Table 1 lists demographic, anthropometric, clinical characteristics and medication use data for the cohort assessed. We did not observe significant differences between age, weight, height, and body mass index. All women with FM were medicated to manage mood, anxiety, and pain (Table 1).

Table 2 lists HRV indices of the FM and control groups at rest and after the posteroanterior glide mobilization. The FM group presented with significantly lower rMSSD ($F = 11.107$; $P = 0.003$), HF (nu) ($F = 2.386$; $P = 0.036$), and SD1 ($F = 10.410$; $P = 0.003$) values compared to control at rest. Complementarily, LF (nu) ($F = 2.836$; $P = 0.016$), DFAα1 ($F = 3.151$; $P = 0.088$), and DFAα2 ($F = 5.476$; $P = 0.026$) were higher in the FM group compared to control. After the manual intervention, rMSSD ($F = 8.344$; $P = 0.035$) and SD1 ($F = 0.076$; $P = 0.003$) indices were significantly higher when compared to baseline only in the FM group. We did not observe significant changes in perceived pain following manual therapy in the FM group. Figure 1 shows the SD1 and SD2 indices of two women: one of them with FM group and the other in the control group.

4. Discussion

To our knowledge, this was the first study to demonstrate the effect of a posteroanterior glide mobilization technique (III-PAC) to the thoracic spine on autonomic modulation in patients with FM.

The main finding of our study was that patients with FM presented important deleterious alterations in HRV at rest suggesting increased sympathetic and decreased parasympathetic activity. Additionally, although manual manipulation did not significantly reduce pain, it was able to significantly improve HRV, as demonstrated by an increase in the rMSSD and SD1 indices (representative of parasympathetic modulation).

Previous studies have shown that FM may be related to changes in autonomic tone, shifting toward an increase in sympathetic activity. Moreover, it has been proposed that dysautonomia is involved in the pathogenesis of FM, which could serve as a mechanism for some of the signs and symptoms associated with this condition [8, 10, 23, 24].

TABLE 2: Pain assessment and linear and nonlinear indices of heart rate variability before and after posteroanterior glide mobilization.

| | Fibromyalgia | | Control | | P values | | |
	Before	After	Before	After	D	M	I
Pain score	6 ± 1	4 ± 1	—	—	—	—	—
HRV indices							
HR, bpm	81 ± 10	77 ± 9	73 ± 9	69 ± 7	ns	ns	ns
iRR, ms	733.5 ± 99.6	749.3 ± 74.6	823.9 ± 99.5	875.6 ± 92.6	ns	<0.05	ns
rMSSD, ms	12.9 ± 6.7	$26.3 \pm 13.6^{\dagger}$	$34.7 \pm 19.0^{\ddagger}$	37.8 ± 18.7	<0.05	<0.05	ns
SDNN, ms	22.9 ± 13.7	26.3 ± 13.6	40.8 ± 20.0	44.5 ± 15.2	ns	ns	ns
LF, nu	68.6 ± 14.5	51.9 ± 16.9	$47.5 \pm 8.3^{\ddagger}$	45.7 ± 13.9	<0.05	ns	ns
HF, nu	31.4 ± 14.5	48.1 ± 16.9	$52.4 \pm 8.3^{\ddagger}$	54.2 ± 13.9	<0.05	ns	ns
LF/HF	3.2 ± 3.0	1.4 ± 1.4	0.5 ± 0.3	0.9 ± 0.6	ns	ns	ns
SD1, ms	9.19 ± 4.7	$11.0 \pm 5.3^{\dagger}$	$24.2 \pm 14.0^{\ddagger}$	26.7 ± 13.2	<0.05	<0.05	ns
SD2, ms	31.0 ± 18.9	35.3 ± 19.1	52.3 ± 26.3	56.9 ± 17.9	ns	ns	ns
DFAα1	1.2 ± 0.1	1.1 ± 0.1	$1.0 \pm 0.1^{\ddagger}$	0.95 ± 0.2	<0.05	ns	<0.05
DFAα2	1.0 ± 0.1	0.9 ± 0.1	$0.71 \pm 0.2^{\ddagger}$	0.93 ± 0.2	<0.05	ns	<0.05

Data are presented as mean ± standard deviation. Two-way ANOVA test with Bonferroni post-hoc test. D: disease effect; M: mobilization effect; I: interaction; ns: nonsignificant. $^{\dagger}P < 0.05$: before versus after posteroanterior glide technique; $^{\ddagger}P < 0.05$: fibromyalgia versus control.

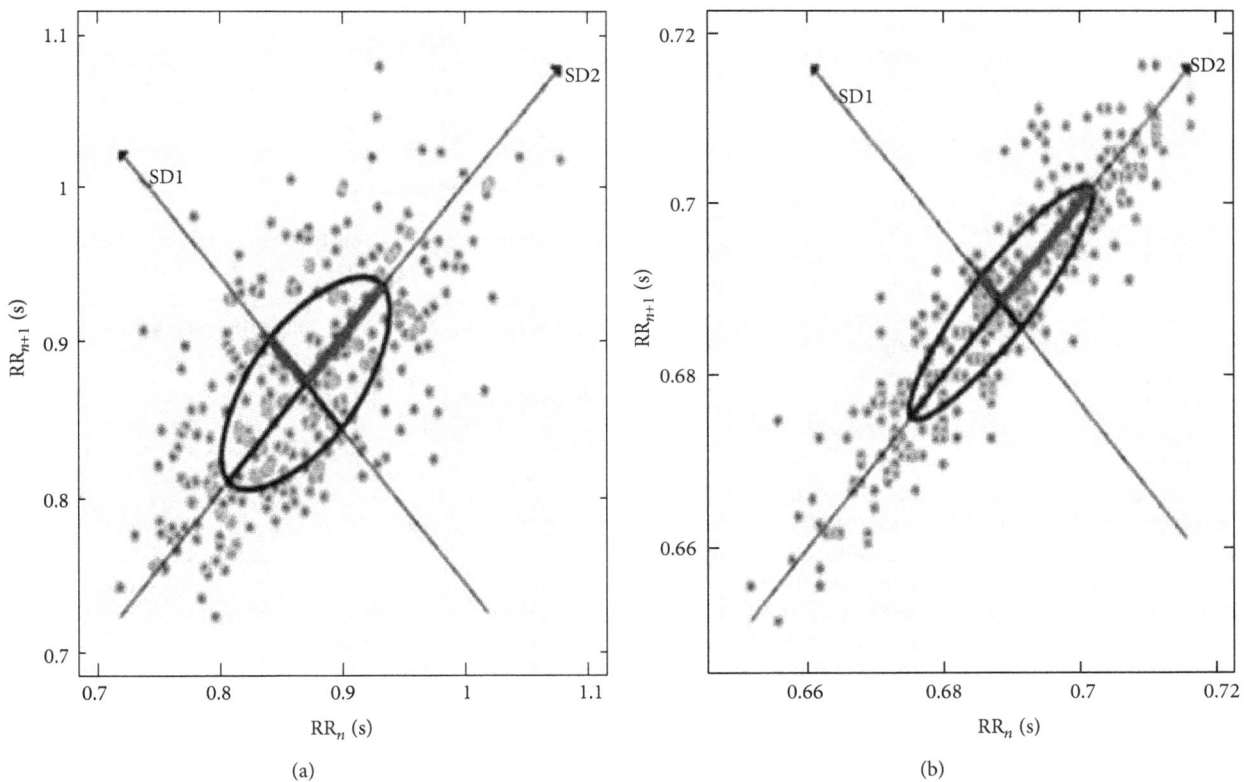

FIGURE 1: Visual differences in Poincare plot of two women at rest after posteroanterior glide technique mobilization. (a) Healthy woman and (b) woman with fibromyalgia.

The present study also demonstrates that patients with FM have increased sympathetic activity and decreased activity in the vagal control of HR, demonstrated by linear and nonlinear HRV indices. This sympathetic excitation could contribute to the diffuse pain and tenderness at specific points experienced by patients with FM.

In this context, several interventions have been proposed to minimize the deleterious signs and symptoms caused by FM. Kingsley et al. [25] assessed the acute effects of strengthening exercises on HRV of FM patients and demonstrated lower sympathetic and higher vagal modulation compared to controls after training. Gamber et al. [26] applied chronic osteopathic manipulation in female patients with FM. These patients received craniosacral manipulation for 23 weeks, one treatment for week, for 15 to 30 minutes per session. The authors emphasized that osteopathic manipulation was able to raise pain thresholds, improve comfort levels, effect components related to chronic illness, and increase perceived functional capacity. Castro-Sánchez et al. [27] demonstrated that massage-myofascial release therapy reduces the sensitivity to pain at tender points in patients with FM, improving their pain perception.

Our findings showed that the employed posteroanterior glide technique did not reduce pain. A previous study demonstrated that manual therapy protocol was effective in improving pain intensity [15]. However, the intervention was applied over 5 sessions and the current study assessed the acute effect of a single session on pain, which could help to explain differences in our findings.

However, the potentially significant impact of our findings is the demonstration that only one session of this manual intervention to the thoracic spine was able to modify HRV in women with FM. Considering that there is a correlation between autonomic dysfunction and symptom severity or quality of life [11], these results may represent clinical benefits to patients who suffer from this condition.

In the current investigation, this mobilization technique was performed to each thoracic spine segment, which has an anatomic relationship with the sympathetic chain ganglia. Some studies have shown that spinal manipulation is able to modulate autonomic nervous activity [28, 29]. Yates et al. [19] examined the effect of chiropractic manipulation to T1–T5 spine segments in patients with arterial hypertension. Immediately after the intervention, they observed a reduction in systolic and diastolic blood pressure and anxiety level. A separate case study showed the effects of 10 sessions of chiropractic manipulation (2 sessions per week) applied throughout the spine (C3 to L5) for 6 weeks. After the first session, there was a reduction in sympathetic activity as measured in the band reflecting parasympathetic tone [30].

Interestingly, it was clearly demonstrated in the current investigation that both SD1 and rMSSD significantly increased after one session of manual mobilization in the FM group, which reflects increased parasympathetic activity (Beckers et al., 2006) [31]. The higher vagal activity is an important finding because it may contribute to improvement in vagal-sympathetic balance. Given these findings, it is plausible to hypothesize that the posteroanterior glide technique utilized in the current study may significantly contribute to reducing the debilitating signs and symptoms of FM, improve quality of life, and reduce cardiovascular risk when applied for more than one session.

It is important to recognize a study limitation regarding the acute effect of manual mobilization on pain and HRV and only assessing the outcomes of a single session in FM subjects. Future studies are needed to evaluate the linkage between this and other manual therapy techniques on pain control and autonomic function in patients with FM over multiple treatment sessions. Follow-up studies are also necessary to confirm the long-term effect of spine manual mobilization in FM in order to elucidate the effects after intervention, that is, to observe whether the short-term effects have an accumulative or permanent influence after repeated application in patients with FM. Lastly, patients with FM oftentimes take medications with potential effects on the autonomic nervous system that were not considered in this study. These aspects deserve to be considered in future research.

5. Conclusion

In conclusion, the current study observed that women with FM present with altered HRV indices reflecting sympathetic hyperactivity at rest. Additionally, after FM subjects underwent one session of a posteroanterior glide mobilization technique to the thoracic spine, we observed a significant increase in rMSSD and SD1 indices, reflecting an improved autonomic profile through increased vagal activity.

Conflict of Interests

The authors declare that there is no conflict of interests regarding the publication of this paper.

Authors' Contribution

Michel Silva Reis and João Luiz Quagliotti Durigan have contributed equally to this paper.

Acknowledgments

The authors thank Conselho Nacional de Desenvolvimento Científico e Tecnológico (CNPq, Brazil) for financial support. M. S. Reis and A. Borghi-Silva are recipients of fellowships from CNPq and FAPESP (2009/01842-0).

References

[1] F. Wolfe, H. A. Smythe, M. B. Yunus et al., "The American College of Rheumatology 1990. Criteria for the classification of fibromyalgia. Report of the Multicenter Criteria Committee," *Arthritis and Rheumatism*, vol. 33, no. 2, pp. 160–172, 1990.

[2] H. Cohen, L. Neumann, M. Shore, M. Amir, Y. Cassuto, and D. Buskila, "Autonomic dysfunction in patients with fibromyalgia: application of power spectral analysis of heart rate variability," *Seminars in Arthritis and Rheumatism*, vol. 29, no. 4, pp. 217–227, 2000.

[3] H. Cohen, L. Neumann, A. Alhosshle, M. Kotler, M. Abu-Shakra, and D. Buskila, "Abnormal sympathovagal balance in men with fibromyalgia," *Journal of Rheumatology*, vol. 28, no. 3, pp. 581–589, 2001.

[4] M. Martínez-Lavín, A. G. Hermosillo, C. Mendoza et al., "Orthostatic sympathetic derangement in subjects with fibromyalgia," *Journal of Rheumatology*, vol. 24, no. 4, pp. 714–718, 1997.

[5] M. Martínez-Lavín and A. G. Hermosillo, "Autonomic nervous system dysfunction may explain the multisystem features of fibromyalgia," *Seminars in Arthritis and Rheumatism*, vol. 29, no. 4, pp. 197–199, 2000.

[6] M. Meeus, D. Goubert, F. de Backer et al., "Heart rate variability in patients with fibromyalgia and patients with chronic fatigue syndrome: a systematic review," *Seminars in Arthritis and Rheumatism*, vol. 43, no. 2, pp. 279–287, 2013.

[7] S. R. Raj, D. Brouillard, C. S. Simpson, W. M. Hopman, and H. Abdollah, "Dysautonomia among patients with fibromyalgia: a noninvasive assessment," *Journal of Rheumatology*, vol. 27, no. 11, pp. 2660–2665, 2000.

[8] M. Fishman, F. J. Jacono, S. Park et al., "A method for analyzing temporal patterns of variability of a time series from Poincaré plots," *Journal of Applied Physiology*, vol. 113, no. 2, pp. 297–306, 2012.

[9] G. A. Reyes del Paso, S. Garrido, Á. Pulgar, and S. Duschek, "Autonomic cardiovascular control and responses to experimental pain stimulation in fibromyalgia syndrome," *Journal of Psychosomatic Research*, vol. 70, no. 2, pp. 125–134, 2011.

[10] R. Staud, "Heart rate variability as a biomarker of fibromyalgia syndrome," *Future Rheumatology*, vol. 3, no. 5, pp. 475–483, 2008.

[11] C. Solano, A. Martinez, L. Becerril et al., "Autonomic dysfunction in fibromyalgia assessed by the composite autonomic symptoms scale (COMPASS)," *Journal of Clinical Rheumatology*, vol. 15, no. 4, pp. 172–176, 2009.

[12] M. Malik, "Heart rate variability: standards of measurement, physiological interpretation, and clinical use," *Circulation*, vol. 93, no. 5, pp. 1043–1065, 1996.

[13] G. Bronfort, M. Haas, R. Evans, B. Leininger, and J. Triano, "Effectiveness of manual therapies: the UK evidence report," *Chiropractic and Osteopathy*, vol. 18, article 3, 2010.

[14] L. Terhorst, M. J. Schneider, K. H. Kim, L. M. Goozdich, and C. S. Stilley, "Complementary and alternative medicine in the treatment of pain in fibromyalgia: a systematic review of randomized controlled trials," *Journal of Manipulative and Physiological Therapeutics*, vol. 34, no. 7, pp. 483–496, 2011.

[15] A. M. Castro-Sánchez, M. E. Aguilar-Ferrándiz, G. A. Matarán-Peñarrocha, M. D. Sánchez-Joya, M. Arroyo-Morales, and C. Fernández-de-Las-Peñas, "Short-term effects of a manual therapy protocol on pain, physical function, quality of sleep, depressive symptoms and pressure sensitivity in women and men with fibromyalgia syndrome: a randomized controlled trial," *The Clinical Journal of Pain*, 2014.

[16] D. A. Hurley, S. M. McDonough, G. D. Baxter, M. Dempster, and A. P. Moore, "A descriptive study of the usage of spinal manipulative therapy techniques within a randomized clinical trial in acute low back pain," *Manual Therapy*, vol. 10, no. 1, pp. 61–67, 2005.

[17] V. Buttagat, W. Eungpinichpong, U. Chatchawan, and S. Kharmwan, "The immediate effects of traditional Thai massage on heart rate variability and stress-related parameters in patients with back pain associated with myofascial trigger points," *Journal of Bodywork and Movement Therapies*, vol. 15, no. 1, pp. 15–23, 2011.

[18] J. P. A. Delaney, K. S. Leong, A. Watkins, and D. Brodie, "The short-term effects of myofascial trigger point massage therapy on cardiac autonomic tone in healthy subjects," *Journal of Advanced Nursing*, vol. 37, no. 4, pp. 364–371, 2002.

[19] R. G. Yates, D. L. Lamping, N. L. Abram, and C. Wright, "Effects of chiropractic treatment on blood pressure and anxiety: a randomized, controlled trial," *Journal of Manipulative and Physiological Therapeutics*, vol. 11, no. 6, pp. 484–488, 1988.

[20] G. D. Maitland, *Vertebral Manipulation*, Butterworth Heinemann, London, UK, 6th edition, 2000.

[21] G. Borg, *Borg's Perceived Exertion and Pain Scales*, Human Kinetics, Champaign, Ill, USA, 1998.

[22] C.-K. Peng, S. Havlin, J. M. Hausdorff, J. E. Mietus, H. E. Stanley, and A. L. Goldberger, "Fractal mechanisms and heart rate dynamics: long-range correlations and their breakdown with disease," *Journal of Electrocardiology*, vol. 28, supplement, pp. 59–64, 1995.

[23] A. M. Castro-Sánchez, G. A. Matarán-Peñarrocha, N. Sánchez-Labraca, J. M. Quesada-Rubio, J. Granero-Molina, and C. Moreno-Lorenzo, "A randomized controlled trial investigating the effects of craniosacral therapy on pain and heart rate variability in fibromyalgia patients," *Clinical Rehabilitation*, vol. 25, no. 1, pp. 25–35, 2011.

[24] S. M. Mostoufi, N. Afari, S. M. Ahumada, V. Reis, and J. L. Wetherell, "Health and distress predictors of heart rate variability in fibromyalgia and other forms of chronic pain," *Journal of Psychosomatic Research*, vol. 72, no. 1, pp. 39–44, 2012.

[25] J. D. Kingsley, L. B. Panton, V. McMillan, and A. Figueroa, "Cardiovascular autonomic modulation after acute resistance exercise in women with fibromyalgia," *Archives of Physical Medicine and Rehabilitation*, vol. 90, no. 9, pp. 1628–1634, 2009.

[26] R. G. Gamber, J. H. Shores, D. P. Russo, C. Jimenez, and B. R. Rubin, "Osteopathic manipulative treatment in conjunction with medication relieves pain associated with fibromyalgia syndrome: results of a randomized clinical pilot project," *Journal of the American Osteopathic Association*, vol. 102, no. 6, pp. 321–325, 2002.

[27] A. M. Castro-Sánchez, G. A. Matarán-Pearrocha, J. Granero-Molina, G. Aguilera-Manrique, J. M. Quesada-Rubio, and C. Moreno-Lorenzo, "Benefits of massage-myofascial release therapy on pain, anxiety, quality of sleep, depression, and quality of life in patients with fibromyalgia," *Evidence-Based Complementary and Alternative Medicine*, vol. 2011, Article ID 561753, 9 pages, 2011.

[28] M. Sterling, G. Jull, and A. Wright, "Cervical mobilisation: concurrent effects on pain, sympathetic nervous system activity and motor activity," *Manual Therapy*, vol. 6, no. 2, pp. 72–81, 2001.

[29] A. Wright, "Hypoalgesia post-manipulative therapy: a review of a potential neurophysiological mechanism," *Manual Therapy*, vol. 1, no. 1, pp. 11–16, 1995.

[30] M. D. Driscoll and M. J. Hall, "Effects of spinal manipulative therapy on autonomic activity and the cardiovascular system: a case study using the electrocardiogram and arterial tonometry," *Journal of Manipulative and Physiological Therapeutics*, vol. 23, no. 8, pp. 545–550, 2000.

[31] F. Beckers, B. Verheyden, and A. E. Aubert, "Aging and nonlinear heart rate control in a healthy population," *The American Journal of Physiology—Heart and Circulatory Physiology*, vol. 290, no. 6, pp. H2560–H2570, 2006.

14

Assessing Function and Endurance in Adults with Spinal and Bulbar Muscular Atrophy: Validity of the Adult Myopathy Assessment Tool

Michael O. Harris-Love,[1,2,3] Lindsay Fernandez-Rhodes,[4,5] Galen Joe,[3] Joseph A. Shrader,[3] Angela Kokkinis,[4] Alison La Pean Kirschner,[4,6] Sungyoung Auh,[7] Cheunju Chen,[4,8] Li Li,[3,9] Ellen Levy,[3] Todd E. Davenport,[10] Nicholas A. Di Prospero,[4] and Kenneth H. Fischbeck[4]

[1] Research Service/Geriatrics and Extended Care, Washington, DC Veterans Affairs Medical Center, 50 Irving Street, NW, Room 11G, Washington, DC 20422, USA

[2] School of Public Health and Health Services, George Washington University, 2033 K Street, NW, Suite 210, Washington, DC 20006, USA

[3] Rehabilitation Medicine Department, Clinical Center, Department of Health and Human Services (DHHS), National Institutes of Health (NIH), 10 Center Drive, Bethesda, MD 20892, USA

[4] National Institute of Neurological Disorders and Stroke (NINDS), Neurogenetics Branch, Department of Health and Human Services (DHHS), National Institutes of Health (NIH), Building 35, Room 2A-1000, 35 Convent Drive, MSC 3705, Bethesda, MD 20892, USA

[5] Department of Epidemiology, University of North Carolina at Chapel Hill Gillings, School of Global Public Health, 170 Rosenau Hall, Campus Box 7400, 135 Dauer Drive, Chapel Hill, NC 27599, USA

[6] Center for Patient Care and Outcomes Research, Medical College of Wisconsin, 8701 Watertown Plank Road, Milwaukee, WI 53226, USA

[7] Clinical Neurosciences Program, NINDS, NIH, 10 Center Drive, Room 5N230, Bethesda, MD 20814, USA

[8] Neurology Department, University of Maryland, 110 South Paca Street, Baltimore, MD 21201, USA

[9] Physical Medicine and Rehabilitation Service, Veterans Affairs Medical Center, 650 East Indian School Road, Phoenix AZ 85012, USA

[10] Department of Physical Therapy, Thomas J. Long School of Pharmacy & Health Sciences, University of the Pacific, 3601 Pacific Avenue, Stockton, CA 95211, USA

Correspondence should be addressed to Michael O. Harris-Love; michael.harris-love@va.gov

Academic Editor: Jeffrey Jutai

Purpose. The adult myopathy assessment tool (AMAT) is a performance-based battery comprised of functional and endurance subscales that can be completed in approximately 30 minutes without the use of specialized equipment. The purpose of this study was to determine the construct validity and internal consistency of the AMAT with a sample of adults with spinal and bulbar muscular atrophy (SBMA). *Methods.* AMAT validity was assessed in 56-male participants with genetically confirmed SBMA (mean age, 53 ± 10 years). The participants completed the AMAT and assessments for disease status, strength, and functional status. *Results.* Lower AMAT scores were associated with longer disease duration ($r = -0.29$; $P < 0.03$) and lower serum androgen levels ($r = 0.49$–0.59; $P < 0.001$). The AMAT was significantly correlated with strength and functional status ($r = 0.82$–0.88; $P < 0.001$). The domains of the AMAT exhibited good internal consistency (Cronbach's $\alpha = 0.77$–0.89; $P < 0.001$). *Conclusions.* The AMAT is a standardized, performance-based tool that may be used to assess functional limitations and muscle endurance. The AMAT has good internal consistency, and the construct validity of the AMAT is supported by its significant associations with hormonal, strength, and functional characteristics of adults with SBMA. This trial is registered with Clinicaltrials.gov identifier NCT00303446.

1. Introduction

The adult myopathy assessment tool is a standardized, observed, physical performance test designed to be administered relatively quickly in clinical and research settings with common clinical equipment and minimal training (see Table 6 for the list of the AMAT tasks and scoring criteria). The AMAT consists of a 13-item battery with an ordinal grading scale for each item and a summated composite functional subscale (range = 0–21), endurance subscale (range = 0–24), and total score (range = 0–45), where lower AMAT subscale scores and total score indicate decreased physical performance. The functional and endurance domains that comprise the AMAT reflect the contribution of impaired muscle force on functional limitations [1–4] and incorporate recent findings that physical performance in people with and without myopathy are also affected by excessive fatigue [5, 6].

The AMAT items include common movements found in other field tests and clinical assessments [7–13], and have been adapted to feature integrated timed and criterion-based scoring within discrete measurement domains (i.e., functional and endurance AMAT subscales). In addition, the functional and endurance AMAT subscales are organized to be congruent with the disability models proposed by both the Institute of Medicine (IOM) [14] and the World Health Organization (WHO) [15]. The functional and endurance subscales were combined for the total AMAT score to imbue the assessment tool with important analytic advantages specifically in assessing patients with myopathy. A strict functional assessment battery based on the attainment of a transfer or mobility task may exhibit a significant ceiling effect (more than 15% of subjects attain the maximum score) if patients have muscle force above what is needed to complete the task for a single repetition. However, impairments in these individuals could be revealed during a more demanding endurance task. In contrast, an endurance battery may display a significant floor effect (more than 15% of subjects attain the minimum score) if patients do not have adequate muscle capacity to meet the criteria for a sustained or repetitive task [16]. Yet, these same individuals may demonstrate the requisite strength to complete a single repetition of a less demanding functional task. Integrating these high and low demand tasks into the AMAT total score diminishes the potential floor and ceiling effects of the assessment tool. Additionally, the AMAT items were sequenced to minimize the effects of fatigue by avoiding consecutive endurance tests of a given agonist muscle group. This assessment was also designed to have clinical utility. Therefore, it may be completed in 25–35 minutes and requires only common equipment such as a stopwatch, adjustable height examination table, standard stairs, and a goniometer. Moreover, the AMAT subscales and total score have been shown to have high interrater and intrarater reliability ($ICC_{2,1}$ = 0.95–0.98, $P < 0.0001$) [17].

A sample of individuals with spinal and bulbar muscular atrophy (SBMA or Kennedy disease), an X-linked degenerative neuromuscular disorder caused by a CAG trinucleotide repeat expansion in the first exon of the androgen receptor gene (AR) [18], participated in this study. Briefly, SBMA is characterized by muscle fasciculations and cramping, bulbar weakness that may result in dysphagia and dysarthria [19, 20], and weakness of the proximal and distal muscles that often leads to impaired mobility and perceptions of excessive fatigue during upright mobility [19]. This sample was initially recruited for a larger clinical trial [21] and was used as a model of neuromuscular disease to help determine selected analytic properties of the AMAT.

There are few standardized scales available for the assessment of impairments and functional limitations due to SBMA [19, 25]. Furthermore, self-report assessment tools may not adequately capture observed functional performance or physical status [26–28]. The purpose of this study was to determine the construct validity of the AMAT for adult participants with SBMA disease. Secondary aims included determining the internal consistency of the AMAT domains and the relationship between functional AMAT subscale items and anatomic regional strength values. Our final aim was to determine if AMAT cut scores can be defined to reflect significant differences in strength, activities of daily living (ADL), timed 2 min walk, or self-reported physical status.

2. Methods

2.1. Participants. Fifty-six subjects (mean age, 53 ± 10 years) were recruited to the National Institutes of Health (NIH) Clinical Research Center in Bethesda, MD, for the purpose of participating in a trial to examine the efficacy and safety of dutasteride in SBMA [21, 29] (The trial is registered with Clinicaltrials.gov identifier NCT00303446); all data were obtained prospectively at the initial screening visit prior to the administration of dutasteride. Patient demographic information has been previously presented [29]. The study was approved by the National Institute of Neurological Disorders and Stroke Institutional Review Board. Signed photograph/recording release forms were obtained from healthy research volunteers in support of this project, and signed informed consent was obtained from study participants in accordance with the Declaration of Helsinki and Federal regulations. Inclusion criteria included: genetically confirmed SBMA, neurological symptoms of SBMA, ability to walk 100 feet with or without the use of an assistive device, male sex, and 18 years of age or older. Exclusion criteria included: female sex, less than 18 years of age, nonambulatory status, and any joint instability or other medical condition deemed by the investigators to pose an undue risk to participants engaging in the performance-based measures associated with the study.

2.2. Genetic Testing and Serum Androgen Profile. Blood samples were obtained after an overnight fast and processed in a CLIA-approved laboratory to assess androgen receptor gene CAG repeat length and serum androgen levels including total testosterone (TT), free testosterone (FT), and dihydrotestosterone (DHT).

2.3. Quantitative Muscle Strength Testing. Isometric maximal voluntary contraction (MVC) testing via quantitative

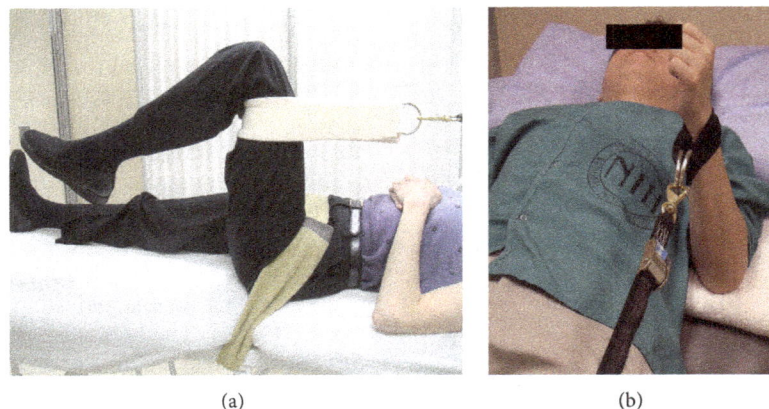

FIGURE 1: Isometric maximal voluntary contraction testing via the quantitative muscle assessment device. (Participant positioning shown for the: (a) hip extensors and (b) elbow flexors.)

muscle assessment (QMA) was used to measure peak force of bilateral muscle groups. The muscle groups and testing positions are listed in Table 7. All QMA tests were performed on a fixed-dynamometer (AEVERL Medical, LLC, P.O. Box 170, Gainesville, GA 30503) using load cells (Interface, 7401 East Butherus Drive, Scottsdale, AZ 85260) with computer-assisted data acquisition. The position of the strap (Figure 1) was adjusted to avoid contact with the participant and maintain a parallel orientation to the force vector. The dynamometer was calibrated per manufacturer guidelines and reset to "zero" prior to each MVC attempt to account for the passive force exerted against the strap. The mean value of the two MVC attempts was used for summation into a composite total score and anatomic region score (i.e., upper extremity and lower extremity).

2.4. Ambulation Status. Ambulation was assessed with the 2-minute walk test [25–30]. The timed 2-minute walk test has high reproducibility [30, 31] based on ICCs of 0.93. We administered 3 trials of the 2-minute walk test [32] as previously described [33], allowing for 2 practice trials before recording distance walked and gait speed. We compared the walk distance with the results of Selman and colleagues [24] to determine the predicted distance for age and gender matched controls.

2.5. Activities of Daily Living and Self-Reported Health Status. ADL assessment was modified [21, 29] from the ADL survey from the Friedreich ataxia rating scale (FARS) [34] by substituting a question about bladder control for one regarding difficulty with handwriting. While this questionnaire is validated for individuals with Friedreich ataxia [35], the ADL items reflect many of the limitations experienced by individuals with SBMA (i.e., walking, falling, swallowing, speech, dressing, personal hygiene, food handling and utensil use, and sitting position quality). The ADL assessment scores were inverted for statistical analysis, producing an ordinal 0–4 item scale (0 = maximum limitation; 4 = unaffected) and a summated composite total score of 36 (range = 0–36) with higher scores indicating increased levels of functioning.

"Walking" and "falling" were individual ADL assessment items selected for additional analyses to better understand their relationship with AMAT performance.

Modules from the Medical Outcomes Study 36-item short form (version 2) questionnaire (SF-36v2) were used to obtain self-reported information on physical functioning and mental status. The SF-36v2 is a 36-item, 4-week recall health-related quality of life assessment that has been used in multiple disorders and can be condensed into 2 summary measures: the physical component summary (PCS) and the mental component summary (MCS) [36, 37]. Using the SAS code provided by QualityMetric Inc., raw scores were converted into normative-based scores with a mean score of 50 (standard deviation, ±10). The scoring algorithms for all SF-36v2 scales and summaries are gender- and age-matched and facilitate simple and valid comparisons between groups [38, 39].

2.6. Administration of the AMAT. A single physician with five years of experience with the AMAT administered the observed, physical performance test to the study participants. The test administrator issued instructions along with task demonstration for each AMAT activity before the participants attempted a given task. In addition, all participants were informed of the criteria to end each task (see Table 6) and the test administrator provided "standby" guarding to ensure participant safety during tasks requiring upright mobility. The participants were allowed a single attempt at completing each AMAT task; however, additional task attempts were allowed in the event of a procedural error during testing. The AMAT was initiated without warm up or preparatory activities and performed a minimum of 4 hours apart from the QMA and 2-minute walk test to avoid the negative impact of fatigue incurred from prior activity.

2.7. Data Analysis. Descriptive statistics were used to depict participant characteristics and all outcome measures. All data are expressed as means and standard deviations except individual AMAT item scores. The ordinal item scores are shown as median values and the interquartile range (IQR).

Additionally, only the data distribution of the MCS and the functional subscale of the AMAT exhibited a significant departure from normality. Therefore, the data associated with these measures were the only variables requiring the use of nonparametric statistics [40]. In this study, the construct validity of the AMAT was based on the strength of its association with outcome measures that influence or reflect functional limitations and submaximal muscle endurance: androgen and genetic markers, muscle strength, timed 2-minute walk, ADL, and self-reported physical status. Construct validity is the extent that inferences may be made from the operational definitions within an assessment tool to the larger theory or concept of interest [40, 41]. Self-reported physical status, via the PCS, was expected to correlate with the AMAT and was used with the other outcome measures to assess construct validity. In contrast, self-reported mental status via the MCS was not expected to correlate with the AMAT and was used to establish divergent validity. Divergent validity of a given assessment tool is supported by a test outcome that lacks a significant association with variables presumed to measure different domains and should be independent of the outcome or construct of interest [41].

Pearson product-moment correlation coefficients (PMCC, r) and Spearman's correlation coefficients (Spearman's rho, ρ) were used to assess the association between variables, and the strength of the association among the variables was based on Munro's criteria [42]. Stepwise multiple linear regression analysis was used to determine the association between variables while accounting for the covariation among disease duration, CAG repeat length, TT, FT, and DHT [43]. All linear regression analyses and correlation coefficients involving QMA strength data included the values scaled to body weight (kg of MVC force/kg of body weight, resulting in a unitless value). This method of scaling strength data facilitated our analysis of the relationship between muscle strength and the functional tasks featured in the AMAT that involve the movement of body weight [44, 45]. QMA values were also expressed as a composite score (total QMA) and anatomic region scores (i.e., upper extremity and lower extremity QMA). Normative-based reference strength values, obtained from the National Isometric Muscle Strength (NIMS) Database Consortium [22] and Andrews and associates [23], were used for comparison with the SBMA group.

Low, moderate, and high levels of physical performance were determined by organizing subgroups of subjects based on cut scores derived from the AMAT total score tertiles. An analysis of variance (ANOVA) was used to discriminate among subjects with higher and lower levels of impairment [43]. The Kruskal Wallis test with Mann Whitney U post hoc tests were used for ADL falling and walking items since they involve ordinal data. Internal consistency of the functional and endurance AMAT subscales was assessed using Cronbach's alpha (α). These AMAT subscales represent related, but heterogeneous, aspects of physical functioning. Therefore internal consistency was evaluated for both AMAT subscales. Internal consistency is based on the pairwise correlations among the items within a subscale used to represent a given construct [40]. An *a priori* decision was made to

consider Cronbach's α values of >0.70 as acceptable internal consistency of an AMAT subscale. In contrast, values exceeding 0.95 were considered indicative of a subscale with excessive item redundancy. Intra-item correlations were also calculated and coefficient values exceeding 0.85 indicated a redundant subscale item. The alpha level (two-tailed) was set at 0.05, and the statistical analyses were performed using SAS 9.1.3 (SAS Institute, Inc., Cary, NC), SUDAAN 9.0 for Windows (Research Triangle Institute Inc., Cary, NC), and SPSS statistical software version 10.0 for Windows (SPSS Inc., Street 233 S. Wacker Drive, Chicago, IL 60606).

3. Results

3.1. Participant Demographics and Disease Characteristics. The mean age of study sample at the time of trial participation was 53 (±10) years with a mean *AR* gene repeat length of 47 CAGs (range = 41–53). Detailed patient demographic information and serum androgen levels have been previously presented [29].

The participants with SBMA had diminished strength levels in comparison to the normative data. The MVC forces represented by the scaled total QMA score, scaled upper extremity (UE) QMA score, and scaled lower extremity (LE) QMA score were 42% to 65% of the reference values (Table 1). The mean distance travelled during the timed 2-minute walk was 109 ± 50 m for the participants corresponding to a mean velocity of 0.9 m/s (Table 1). Twenty-two of the 56 participants (39%) opted to use assistive devices (e.g., canes, walkers, or ankle-foot orthoses). These participants attained a mean distance of 66 ± 23 m with a mean speed of 0.55 m/s, whereas the individuals who did not use assistive devices achieved a mean distance of 136 ± 44 m (n = 34) with a mean speed of 1.13 m/s.

The ADL assessment score indicated that the participants experienced difficulties with physical functioning; the mean ADL assessment score was 25.9 ± 5.0 (range 15.0–35.3), representing 72% of the maximum attainable score. This is in agreement with the self-reported physical status in which the subjects had a mean PCS score of 34.3 ± 11.0 (16.0–57.8) which is 68% of the national age-matched normative data for men (35–74 years of age). In contrast, the self-reported mental status was noted by MCS mean scores of 52.2±11.6 (14.2–67.2) which is 102% of normative values [38, 39].

3.2. The AMAT Subscale Scores and Total Score. Observed physical functioning, as measured with the AMAT, also revealed impaired performance of the participants. The mean total AMAT score was 29.2 ± 10.3 (i.e., 65% of the maximum AMAT total score) and no significant floor or ceiling effects were found in the AMAT total scores [16]. Of the 56 subjects, no one attained the low score of 0, and 2 participants achieved the maximum score of 45. In addition, slightly greater deficits were noted in the endurance AMAT subscale (60% of the maximum score) in comparison to the functional AMAT subscale (70% of the maximum score; Table 1). A range of performance ability was observed in both the functional and endurance AMAT subscales. Median item scores ranged from 1.0 to 3.0 for functional AMAT subscale items

TABLE 1: Physical performance assessments in patients with SBMA.

	SBMA mean ± SD (range)	Percentage of reference values[†]
Quantitative muscle assessment (kg)		
Upper extremity composite	66 ± 25 (18–140)	42%
Lower extremity composite	98 ± 41 (28–231)	65%
Total force	164 ± 63 (63–372)	55%
Adult Myopathy Assessment Tool		
Endurance score (range = 0–24, 24 = max score)	14.5 ± 5.3 (4–24)	60%
Functional score (range = 0–21, 21 = max score)	14.7 ± 5.4 (2–21)	70%
Total score (range = 0–45, 45 = max score)	29.2 ± 10.3 (9–45)	65%
Timed 2-minute walk (m)		
Distance walked	109 ± 50 (15–208)	51%

[†]Normative QMA values obtained from published reference values [22, 23]; AMAT results expressed as a percentage of the maximum attainable score; timed 2 minute walk results compared with published age and gender matched normal reference values [24].
Abbreviations: SBMA: spinal bulbar muscular atrophy; kg: kilograms; m: meters.

TABLE 2: AMAT item scores for patients with SBMA.

	Median score	IQR
Functional AMAT subscale items (range = 0–3)		
Supine to prone	3.0	2.0–3.0
Modified push-up	3.0	2.0–3.0
Sit-up	1.0	0.0–2.0
Supine to sit	3.0	2.0–3.0
Arm raise	3.0	2.0–3.0
Sit to stand	2.0	1.0–3.0
Step-up	2.0	1.0–3.0
Endurance AMAT subscale items (range = 0–4)		
Sustained head elevation	3.0	2.0–4.0
Repeated modified push-ups	1.0	0.0–2.0
Sustained arm raise	3.0	1.3–4.0
Sustained hip flexion	4.0	2.0–4.0
Sustained knee extension	4.0	4.0–4.0
Repeated heel raises	0.0	0.0–1.0

Abbreviations: SBMA: spinal bulbar muscular atrophy; IQR: interquartile range; AMAT: Adult Myopathy Assessment Tool.

(item scale = 0–3) with the sit-up, sit to stand, and step-up tasks being the most difficult to perform. Median item scores varied across the full range of 0 to 4 for endurance AMAT subscale items (item scale = 0–4), with the repeated heel raises and repeated modified push-ups scoring the lowest (Table 2).

3.3. Outcome Variables Associated with the AMAT Total Score. The serum androgen levels had a moderate degree of association with the AMAT (r = 0.49–0.62; P < 0.001). The AMAT was significantly associated with CAG repeat length (t = −3.95; P < 0.001) when the multiple linear regression model corrected for age at evaluation and total testosterone as covariates. There was a stronger relationship between the AMAT and outcome measures related to physical performance. The total QMA score, timed 2-minute walk distance, and ADL assessment score all showed a high degree of association with the AMAT (r = 0.82–0.91; P < 0.0001). The self-reported physical status, as estimated by the PCS score, also correlated well with AMAT (r = 0.62; P < 0.0001) and, as hypothesized, the self-reported mental status via the

MCS did not (r = 0.13; P = 0.355). Correlations between the AMAT total score and the outcome variables are summarized in Table 3.

3.4. Internal Consistency of the AMAT Subscales. The internal consistency of both AMAT subscales was acceptable based on the criteria established by Munro [42]. However, the internal consistency of the AMAT domains was stronger in the functional AMAT subscale (Cronbach's α = 0.89) than in the endurance AMAT subscale (Cronbach's α = 0.77). Intra-item associations of the AMAT subscales did not suggest item redundancy, as none of the correlation coefficients exceeded 0.85. The inter-item Spearman's ρ ranged from 0.39 to 0.74 for the functional AMAT subscale and 0.11 to 0.73 for the endurance AMAT subscale.

3.5. Strength-Function Relationships. Association between the functional AMAT subscale items and the QMA values was used to characterize strength-function relationships (Table 4). The total QMA, UE QMA, and LE QMA scores

TABLE 3: Pearson's correlation coefficients of the AMAT total score and SBMA outcome measures and phenotypic variables.

	AMAT Total Score	P value
Scaled total QMA	0.91	<0.0001
Timed 2-minute walk	0.85	<0.0001
ADL assessment	0.82	<0.0001
Physical component summary[§]	0.82	<0.0001
Total testosterone	0.62	<0.0001
Dihydrotestosterone	0.51	<0.0001
Free testosterone	0.49	0.0002
Age	−0.40	0.002
Disease duration[†]	−0.29	0.03
Mental component summary[§]	0.13	0.355

[§]Self-report of physical and mental status obtained from the physical component summary and mental component summary of the Medical Outcomes Study 36-item short form, version 2.
[†]Disease duration is defined as time from genetic diagnosis to study initial evaluation.
Abbreviations: SBMA: spinal bulbar muscular atrophy; AMAT: Adult Myopathy Assessment Tool; QMA: Quantitative Muscle Assessment; ADL: activities of daily living.

TABLE 4: Spearman's correlation coefficients of the scaled QMA strength values and AMAT Functional subscale items.

	Supine to prone	Push-up	Sit-up	Supine to sit	Arm raise	Sit to stand	Step-up
UE QMA	0.379	0.616	0.623	0.570	0.588	0.614	0.637
LE QMA	0.524	0.559	0.756	0.724	0.471	0.764	0.813
TOTAL QMA	0.487	0.628	0.745	0.687	0.553	0.739	0.777

Note: all P values are <0.001, except UE QMA and supine to prone, P = 0.004; all QMA values are scaled to body weight.
Abbreviations: UE: upper extremity; LE: lower extremity; AMAT: Adult Myopathy Assessment Tool; QMA: quantitative muscle assessment.

were significantly correlated with all of the functional tasks. The anatomic region QMA scores were more strongly associated with the functional tasks than the total QMA score, with the exception of the modified push-up. The UE QMA score had the highest degree of association with arm raise (ρ = 0.59; $P < 0.001$). In comparison, the LE QMA score had the highest degree of association with the supine to prone, sit-up, supine to sit, sit to stand, and the step-up tasks (ρ = 0.72–0.81; $P < 0.001$).

3.6. AMAT Cut Scores. Total AMAT score tertiles led to cut scores that separate the sample into low ≤ 24, moderate 25–34, and high ≥ 35 functioning groups. Significant differences were found among all 3 groups for the total QMA, timed 2-minute walk, total ADL, ADL falling, and ADL walking assessment scores ($P < 0.001$ for all main effects). Post hoc differences for ADL falling and walking were significant among all three groups; $P < 0.001$ in all comparisons except between the moderate and high functioning groups (P = 0.023). The low and high AMAT cut score groups showed significant differences in FT ($P < 0.001$), TT ($P < 0.001$), and DHT ($P = 0.012$), but not CAG repeat length ($P = 0.41$). In addition, the low and high and moderate and high AMAT cut score groups had significantly different physical status self-report scores ($P < 0.001$). All comparisons of the AMAT cut scores and outcome values in the functional domain are summarized in Table 5.

4. Discussion

4.1. Construct Validity of the AMAT. The findings of this investigation support the construct validity and internal consistency of the AMAT in participants with SBMA disease. Dependent measures obtained to characterize disease status and validate the AMAT included serum androgen levels, AR gene CAG trinucleotide repeat length, QMA scores, timed 2-minute walk, ADL assessment, and self-reported physical and mental status. Androgen levels are linked to the maintenance of muscle mass and strength [46], which in turn, leads to improved physical functioning [3, 47]. The relationship between the higher androgen levels and better functional performance was reflected in the significant correlation between the AMAT score and TT, FT, and DHT in the participants. We found a significant relationship between AR gene CAG trinucleotide repeat length and the AMAT total score, when accounting for the covariation of age at evaluation and TT. This finding supports other reports that CAG repeat length affects phenotypic measures of disease status [29, 48]. Additionally, previous work from our group [21] showed that there was an inverse correlation between CAG repeat length and QMA values scaled to body weight ($P = 0.04$).

The participants had significant impairment based on strength levels and walking distances that were approximately half of the normal adult reference values [24]. Also, the ADL assessment scores of the participants (25.9 ± 5.0; maximum attainable score = 36) were diminished, but similar to

TABLE 5: AMAT cut scores. Use of AMAT cut scores to discriminate among low, moderate, and high levels of performance across several ICF domains of function.

AMAT			QMA	2MWT (m)	PCS	ADL
Functional level	Score	N		Mean (SD)		
1-low	0–24	19	2.48 (±0.70)	58.7 (±24.0)	27.3 (±7.3)	21.0 (±3.0)
2-moderate	25–34	18	3.27 (±0.77)	103.1 (±27.7)	31.5 (±8.3)	26.0 (±3.1)
3-high	35–45	19	5.48 (±1.26)	163.7 (±24.3)	43.9 (±9.81)	30.7 (±3.4)
ANOVA				F value (all P values, <0.001)		
			52.9	60.1	18.3	44.7
Tukey's HSD				P values		
1-2			0.02	0.003	0.341	<0.001
2-3			<0.001	<0.001	<0.001	<0.001
1–3			<0.001	<0.001	<0.001	<0.001

Note: Cut scores are based on the tertiles of the AMAT total score. QMA values have been scaled to body weight.
Abbreviations: AMAT: Adult Myopathy Assessment Tool; ICF: International Classification of Functioning; QMA: quantitative muscle assessment; 2MWT: timed 2 minute walk; (m) meters; PCS: Physical Component Summary (obtained from the Medical Outcomes Study 36-Item Short Form, Version 2); ADL: activities of daily living; (SD) standard deviation; ANOVA: analysis of variance; Tukey's HSD: Tukey's Honestly Significant Difference.

the clinical measures reported in other studies [49, 50]. The mean AMAT total score of 29.2 (±10.3; maximum attainable score = 45) reflects the decreased physical performance of the participants and is consistent with the findings regarding impaired muscle strength, ADL assessment, and self-reported physical status.

4.2. AMAT Subscale and Item Assessment. The AMAT subscales and items vary in their level of difficulty. Task difficulty is based on the proportion of body weight being moved and the distance traversed. However, task performance may be influenced by patterns of muscle weakness in people with neuromuscular disease. Based on the median item scores, supine to prone, modified push-up, supine to sit, and arm raise were the least demanding tasks of the functional AMAT subscale, while the sit-up, sit to stand, and step-up tasks posed the largest challenge to the participants. Sit to stand and ascending a step were expected to be challenging tasks due to the requirement to move one's total body weight and the reports of difficulty with these tasks in other cohorts. However, the data suggesting that the sit-up was the most difficult task was unexpected and has not been previously described in SBMA. Trunk weakness is a notable finding that has been observed in myopathies such as polymyositis and dermatomyositis [51]. Muscle groups of the extremities are typically more readily tested with dynamometry than trunk muscles, so the trunk musculature is typically omitted from objective strength assessment studies. Nevertheless, the observed difficulty with the sit-up task suggests that the trunk muscles may merit standardized objective strength assessment.

Sustained knee extension and hip flexion were the least difficult tasks of the endurance AMAT subscale, but even these tasks detected impairments in our sample (13 and 25 participants, resp., failed to reach the maximum score). Repeated heel raises and modified push-ups were clearly the most difficult tasks of the endurance AMAT subscale. The repeated heel raise task performance revealed the extent of distal weakness in the participants. The ankle plantar flexors can generate a large magnitude of force based on the lever

type of the ankle joint and the muscle architecture of the gastrocnemius [52]. Despite these physiologic advantages, 39/56 subjects (70%) were unable to perform a single limb heel raise. The diminished performance of the participants for the repeated push-up task was of interest given the high scores attained on the single repetition version of this task in the functional AMAT subscale. The decreased performance of the repeated version of the push-up item may indicate sufficient strength to complete the task, but inadequate muscle endurance capacity to sustain task performance. Indeed, investigators have cited the need for endurance tests in addition to single repetition functional tasks alone to capture this important aspect of physical performance in persons with myopathy [6]. Repeated movements such as heel raises may be noted by performance deficiencies due to diminished strength and anaerobic capacity at ancillary muscle groups that contribute to stability during tasks with substantial multijoint involvement [53]. Additionally, SBMA is notable for being a lower motor neuron disease with significant muscle tissue abnormalities. Signs of significant muscle fiber damage such as elevated levels of serum creatine kinase often precede stereotypic SBMA clinical symptoms [54]. Also, muscle tissue in those with SBMA is distinguished by aberrant features such as fiber type grouping and centrally located nuclei which reflect characteristics of both neurogenic and myogenic pathology [55]. These morphological and histological abnormalities would contribute to the physical deficits observed in our sample during AMAT testing.

4.3. Characterizing the Strength-Function Relationship Based on AMAT Performance. Construct validity of the AMAT was also supported by the observed strength-function relationships. For example, the UE and LE QMA scores were more strongly associated with the functional AMAT subscale items than the total QMA score. Specificity of the composite regional strength scores moderately improved the observed strength-function relationships for nearly every task. Interestingly, LE QMA was strongly correlated with the sit-up task. However, a stronger correlation may have been attained with

TABLE 6: The adult myopathy assessment tool (AMAT).

	Item instructions and descriptions	Scoring
1	†**Head elevation endurance**: "Raise your head off of the table." Patient in supine; patient flexes head and neck forward and attempts to maintain self-selected position; test ends when occiput touches table.	0 <5 seconds or unable 1 5–30 seconds 2 31–60 seconds 3 61–90 seconds 4 >90 seconds
2	**Supine to prone**: "Roll onto your stomach without stopping and place your arms at your side." Patient begins in supine with arms at side; test ends when patient is prone with arms at side.	0 >10 seconds to attempt transfer or unable 1 completion in >6 seconds <10 seconds or rolls without freeing dependent arm 2 completion in >3 seconds ≤6 seconds 3 completion in ≤3 seconds
3	**Modified push-up**: "Perform a push-up, ending with your elbows as straight as possible; your knees will touch the table during the movement." Patient begins with hands facing forward on table with arm in 0 degrees abduction.	0 unable to do 1 partial elbow extension; sternum in partial contact with table 2 partial elbow extension; sternum NOT in contact with table 3 full elbow extension achieved

Table 6: Continued.

	Item instructions and descriptions	Scoring
4	†**Repeated modified push-up:** "Perform as many push-ups as you can, ending with arms straight, in 2 minutes; your upper chest should touch the table with each repetition." Patient begins with hands on table and shoulders in 0 degrees abduction; self-selected pace; test ends if cueing for faulty technique occurs on 2 consecutive attempts; faulty attempts are not counted.	**0** unable to do **1** 1–10 repetitions **2** 11–20 repetitions **3** 21–30 repetitions **4** 31–40 repetitions
5	**Sit-up:** "Perform a sit-up." Patient begins from supine position with knees fully extended and with hands on thighs or across abdomen; tester applies counter balance at distal lower extremities for grades 0–2.	**0** unable to do **1** scapulae and T7 vertebra not in contact with table (rectus phase) with counter balance **2** L1 vertebra not in contact with table: completion of full sit-up (hip flexor phase) with counter balance **3** completion of full sit-up without counter balance
6	**Supine to sit:** "Move to a sitting position at the edge of the table as quickly as you can." Patient begins from supine position, legs straight, and arms at side. Test ends when feet touch the floor and torso is vertical.	**0** ≥12 seconds to attempt transfer or unable **1** completion in >7 and <12 seconds **2** completion in >4 and ≤7 seconds **3** completion in ≤4 seconds

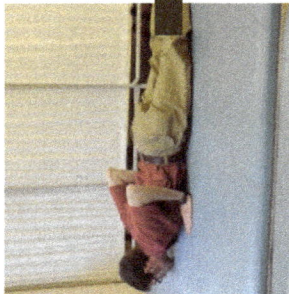

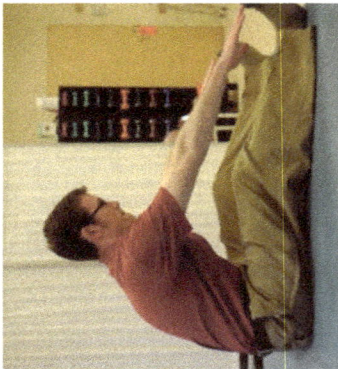

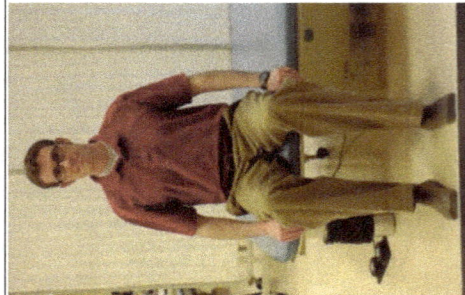

TABLE 6: Continued.

	Item instructions and descriptions	Scoring
7	**Arm raise:** "Raise both hands as high as you can above your head with the elbows straight." Complete within available PROM; apply grade to weakest upper extremity if asymmetry is present.	**0** unable to raise arms to level of acromioclavicular joint **1** hands raised between acromioclavicular joint and top of head **2** hands raised above top of head without full elbow extension **3** hands raised above top of head with full elbow extension
8	† **Arm raise endurance:** "Raise both hands forward (shoulder flexion) to eye level with elbows straight." Trunk upright without hyperextension and both feet flat on floor; end test if shoulder flexion drops below 90 degrees; apply grade to weakest upper extremity if asymmetry is present.	**0** unable to do or <5 seconds **1** 5–30 seconds **2** 31–60 seconds **3** 61–90 seconds **4** >90 seconds
9	**Sit to stand:** "Stand up with as little arm support as possible." Patient seated on exam table with edge bisecting thigh length, trunk erect, lower legs vertical, and knees at 90 degrees measured via goniometer; contact between posterior aspect of the legs and the table is not allowed.	**0** unable to do **1** completes transfer with two or more extremities in contact with the exam table or thigh **2** completes transfer with one extremity in contact with the exam table or thigh **3** completes transfer without contact of any extremity with the exam table or thigh

TABLE 6: Continued.

	Item instructions and descriptions		Scoring

10	†**Hip flexion endurance:** "Raise and hold your knee in the air on your dominant side." Seated with hips and knees at ninety degrees; no shoes; nondominant foot on floor; trunk upright with edge of table bisecting thigh length; upper extremity support on table allowed; knee height is based on the mid-PROM; test ends when foot contacts the floor.	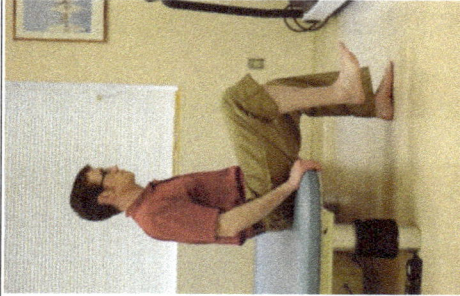	0 unable to do or <5 seconds 1 5–30 seconds 2 31–60 seconds 3 61–90 seconds 4 >90 seconds
11	†**Knee extension endurance:** "Hold your knee as straight as possible on your dominant side." No shoes; nondominant foot on floor; trunk upright with thigh fully supported on table; test ends when the foot contacts the floor; full available PROM.	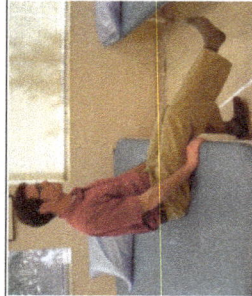	0 unable to do or <5 seconds 1 5–30 seconds 2 31–60 seconds 3 61–90 seconds 4 >90 seconds
12	†**Repeated heel rise:** "While standing on your dominant leg only, raise your heel off of the ground." No shoes; self-selected pace; test ends when 5th metatarsal base or midfoot does not fully rise from the floor; test ends if cueing for faulty technique occurs on 2 consecutive attempts; faulty attempts are not counted; knees remain as straight as possible with no additional flexion during attempts; minimal external support may be provided by a wall; 2 min or 30 repetition limit.	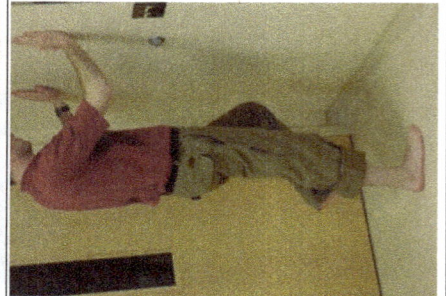	0 unable to do 1 1–7 repetitions 2 8–15 repetitions 3 16–23 repetitions 4 24–30 repetitions

TABLE 6: Continued.

Item instructions and descriptions		Scoring
13	**Step-up:** "Place your dominant leg onto the 7-inch step, step forward with as little arm support as possible, and bring the opposite foot onto the step." Stable upper extremity support should be available for both arms.	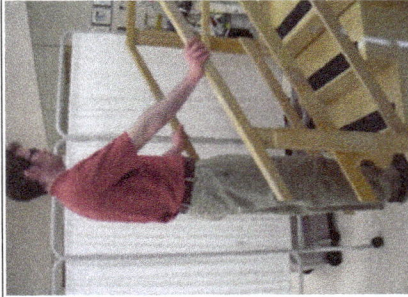 **0** unable to do **1** uses two upper extremities **2** uses one upper extremity **3** completes without upper extremity use

[†] Denotes AMAT endurance subscale items.

General instructions: all AMAT items should be performed in order 1 through 13 with at least one-minute rest period after each item. Rest periods exceeding one minute are dictated by the transition time required to set up proceeding AMAT tasks. Test ending criteria should be provided prior to each task attempt. Standby assistance is required for all items requiring upright mobility. Duration for all timed tasks should be recorded. *Required items:* stopwatch, examination table, goniometer or inclinometer, and stairs with a handrail.

Scoring: Each AMAT item is scored immediately after the task attempt is completed. The AMAT functional subscale (range = 0–21), AMAT endurance subscale (range = 0–24), and AMAT total score (range = 0–45) are calculated after test administration.

Interpretation: AMAT functional level (categorical ranks are based on the AMAT total score)

1-low 0–24

2-moderate 25–34

3-high 35–45

PROM: passive range of motion.

TABLE 7: Quantitative assessment of peak muscle force. The tested muscle groups, subject testing position, and orientation of the dynamometer strap are listed for the quantitative assessment of maximum isometric force$^€$ using a fixed dynamometry load cell$^£$.

Muscle group	Patient position	Strap position
Upper extremity		
Lateral pinch	Seated; elbow at 90°; midrange supination/pronation	None; pinch dynamometer
Hand grip	Seated; elbow at 90°; midrange supination/pronation	None; hand grip dynamometer
Wrist flexors	Seated; elbow at 90°; midrange supination/pronation	Ventral metacarpals with second stabilizing strap at dorsal proximal wrist
Elbow flexors	Supine; elbow at 90°; midrange supination/pronation	Radial distal forearm proximal to wrist
Elbow extensors	Supine; elbow at 90°; midrange supination/pronation	Ulnar distal forearm proximal to wrist
Shoulder abductors	Supine; shoulder and elbow at 90°	Lateral distal arm proximal to elbow
Lower extremity		
Ankle dorsiflexors	Supine; ankle at 90°	Around dorsal metatarsals
Knee extensors	Seated; hip and knee at 90°	Around ankle and proximal to malleolus
Hip flexors	Supine; hip and knee at 90°	Anterior distal femur and proximal to patella
Hip extensors	Supine; hip and knee at 90°	Posterior distal femur
Hip abductors	Seated; hip and knee at 90°	Lateral distal femur

$^€$AEVERL Medical, LLC P.O. Box 170 Gainesville, GA 30503.
$^£$Interface, 7401 East Butherus Drive, Scottsdale, AZ 85260.

a specific measure of trunk strength, which was not included in this study. In addition, it is unclear why the total QMA score was more strongly correlated to the modified push-up task than was the UE QMA score. The muscle groups included in the composite UE QMA score did not include the horizontal adductors of the humerus, and the addition of this group may have improved this relationship. Our results also confirm the findings from other investigators regarding the positive relationship between task difficulty and strength [56]. Among the most difficult AMAT functional tasks were sit to stand and step-up (median score = 2.0). The highest strength-function correlations we observed involved tasks with a clear LE-bias ranging from 0.76 to 0.81. In contrast, the correlations for the UE-biased tasks ranged from 0.59 to 0.62. The large magnitude of association between muscle strength and LE-biased tasks observed in this study is similar to the findings of other studies of participants with neuromuscular disease [57].

4.4. *Internal Consistency of the AMAT.* While both AMAT subscales demonstrated good internal consistency, the functional subscale outperformed the endurance subscale. Frank muscle weakness can confound attempts to measure muscle endurance. Repeated or sustained tasks are designed to measure muscle endurance, but they also demand the requisite strength to attain the testing position. The distal weakness exhibited by the participants rendered the repeated heel raise test, an endurance AMAT subscale item, a *de facto* functional test contingent on strength. Therefore, severe neuromuscular disease that yields specific muscle groups with frank weakness would cause a series of muscle endurance tests to be divergent in their results, thus lowering the intercorrelation of the test items.

4.5. *Utility of the AMAT: Cut Scores and Functional Performance Categories.* The ability to derive meaning from the scores of a given outcome measure is a key arbiter of

assessment tool utility. The determination of AMAT cut scores revealed significant categorical differences in physical performance. These observed differences included strength, walking, total ADL, ADL falling, and self-reported physical status. Participants categorized as having a "high" level of functional performance were at least twice as strong as those categorized as having a "low" level of functional performance. Similarly, walking distance was nearly three times farther in participants demonstrating a higher level of functional performance in comparison to people in the lowest functional category. This sharp contrast in physical functioning suggests that the AMAT cut scores may reveal clinically meaningful differences among the categorical groups. Clinicians may find that AMAT cut scores augment their ability to determine when additional rehabilitative interventions or more detailed assessments are indicated for patients with declining physical status. Moreover, AMAT cut scores may be used by researchers as part of the inclusion or exclusion criteria of a therapeutic trial, to aid group assignment based on the severity of physical impairment or provide a criterion for clinically meaningful improvement or worsening when participant AMAT scores shift in categorical rank. Despite the clear functional distinctions observed in the categorical grouping of our sample, additional study will be needed to better understand how the AMAT cut scores identified in this study apply to other samples and patient populations. Myopathy is a broad category of pathology that encompasses multiple neuromuscular disorders and myogenic diseases. Therefore, the AMAT was not created for the express purpose of assessing individuals with SBMA. Our preliminary data from previous and ongoing clinical studies suggest that the AMAT is a robust measure of physical performance in people with inclusion body myositis and that clinicians exhibit a high degree of reliability scoring AMAT performances by individuals with idiopathic inflammatory myopathies [17].

This performance-based test is intended for use by rehabilitation practitioners such as physicians, therapists, and nurses and may be conducted in physical therapy clinics, outpatient medical facilities, and rehabilitation units within a hospital setting. The emerging analytic properties of the AMAT, including the ability to monitor patient status over time and observe meaningful shifts in the AMAT functional level (i.e., low, moderate, and high), are valuable features of a test designed to characterize the physical performance of people with chronic degenerative conditions. Our findings in support of the construct validity and internal consistency of the AMAT complement our previous observations regarding the ability of the AMAT to assess disease progression. Fernández-Rhodes et al. [29] examined the efficacy and safety of dutasteride in characterizing disease progression over a 24-month period in the placebo-control SBMA group with a variety of secondary measures of impairment level and physical status. Motor unit number estimation, median compound muscle action potentials, and total QMA score detected an annual rate of decline from 1.6% to 2.3%. In contrast, the AMAT and the PCS score showed an annual decline of 4.5% and 5.2%, respectively. However, of these two measures, the AMAT was better at detecting a decline in physical status ($z = 0.68$, $P = 0.004$ versus $z = 0.43$, $P = 0.054$). Therefore, the AMAT may have utility in future clinical trials based on its favorable "signal-to-noise" ratio.

5. Limitations

Although the findings support the construct validity and internal consistency of the AMAT, this study had limitations. Our outcome measures did not include a direct measure of muscle endurance. While the capacity of muscles to exert sustained or repeated submaximal forces is consistent with the requirements of ADL performance and mobility, validation of the endurance AMAT subscale would have been improved by comparisons with an impairment-level measure of anaerobic endurance. The AMAT and other physical performance tests have important advantages over questionnaires regarding physical functioning. Nonetheless, questionnaires such as the ALSFRS-r incorporate important questions regarding bulbar muscle function and various nonmusculoskeletal features of ALS and SBMA that are not included in the AMAT. While the purpose and validity of the AMAT benefits from the integrity of its domains, other tests or questionnaires are required to address the consequences of neuromuscular disease that go beyond physical performance and mobility. Additionally, the cut scores used to categorize participants into AMAT functional levels in this study yielded statistically significant distinctions among the 3 subgroups. However, cut scores based on percentiles are dependent on the distribution of scores within a given sample. An alternative approach would be to use criterion-based cut scores derived from established markers of disablement. A successful implementation of this approach to cut scores and functional categories will require a larger sample size to allow for a sufficient allocation of people in each subgroup and ensure valid statistical comparisons. Finally, other analytic qualities, such as responsiveness, the minimal clinical important difference score, criterion validity of the endurance subscale, and discriminative validity using

normative reference data, need to be explored to fully understand the clinical and research utility of the AMAT.

6. Conclusions

The AMAT is a standardized, performance-based tool that assesses functional limitations and muscle endurance in adults with myopathy. Our findings suggest that the AMAT has excellent construct validity and good internal consistency for adults with SBMA based on its significant associations with strength, objective and subjective physical performance measures, and self-reported physical status. The utility of the AMAT is further supported through the use of cut scores to characterize physical status based on low, moderate, or high levels of performance. These findings support the use of the AMAT as both a clinical assessment tool and outcome measure in future clinical trials of SBMA and merits further study in other adult-onset neuromuscular disease populations.

Conflict of Interests

The authors declare that they have no conflict of interests.

Acknowledgments

The authors wish to thank the Intramural Research Program of the National Institutes of Health (NIH), National Institute of Neurological Disorders and Stroke (NINDS), and Rehabilitation Medicine Department (RMD) of the NIH Clinical Center for supporting this work. Please note that the opinions and information contained in this paper are those of the authors and do not necessarily reflect those of the Department of Veterans Affairs, National Institutes of Health, or the United States Public Health Service. Nicholas A. Di Prospero is currently an employee of Johnson and Johnson, LLC.

References

[1] M. Mänty, C. F. de Leon, T. Rantanen et al., "Mobility-related fatigue, walking speed, and muscle strength in older people," *The Journals of Gerontology A, Biological Sciences and Medical Sciences*, vol. 67, no. 5, pp. 523–529, 2012.

[2] T. Rantanen, J. M. Guralnik, S. Leveille et al., "Racial differences in muscle strength in disabled older women," *Journals of Gerontology A, Biological Sciences and Medical Sciences*, vol. 53, no. 5, pp. B355–B361, 1998.

[3] T. Rantanen, "Muscle strength, disability and mortality," *Scandinavian Journal of Medicine and Science in Sports*, vol. 13, no. 1, pp. 3–8, 2003.

[4] L. P. Lowes, L. Alfano, L. Viollet et al., "Knee extensor strength exhibits potential to predict function in sporadic inclusion-body myositis," *Muscle and Nerve*, vol. 45, no. 2, pp. 163–168, 2012.

[5] B. H. Jacobson, D. Smith, J. Fronterhouse, C. Kline, and A. Boolani, "Assessment of the benefit of powered exercises for muscular endurance and functional capacity in elderly

participants," *Journal of Physical Activity & Health*, vol. 9, no. 7, pp. 1030–1035, 2012.

[6] M. O. Harris-Love, "Physical activity and disablement in the idiopathic inflammatory myopathies," *Current Opinion in Rheumatology*, vol. 15, no. 6, pp. 679–690, 2003.

[7] A. M. Huber, J. E. Hicks, P. A. Lachenbruch et al., "Validation of the childhood health assessment questionnaire in the juvenile idiopathic myopathies," *Journal of Rheumatology*, vol. 28, no. 5, pp. 1106–1111, 2001.

[8] U. Svantesson, U. Österberg, R. Thomeé, and G. Grimby, "Muscle fatigue in a standing heel-rise test," *Scandinavian Journal of Rehabilitation Medicine*, vol. 30, no. 2, pp. 67–72, 1998.

[9] R. T. Moxley III, "Evaluation of neuromuscular function in inflammatory myopathy," *Rheumatic Disease Clinics of North America*, vol. 20, no. 4, pp. 827–843, 1994.

[10] A. Josefson, E. Romanus, and J. Carlsson, "A functional index in myositis," *Journal of Rheumatology*, vol. 23, no. 8, pp. 1380–1384, 1996.

[11] J. M. Guralnik, "Assessment of physical performance and disability in older persons," *Muscle and Nerve*, vol. 20, no. 5, pp. S14–S16, 1997.

[12] M. H. Brooke, G. M. Fenichel, R. C. Griggs et al., "Clinical investigation in Duchenne dystrophy: II. Determination of the "power" of therapeutic trials based on the natural history," *Muscle and Nerve*, vol. 6, no. 2, pp. 91–103, 1983.

[13] C. M. McDonald, R. T. Abresch, G. T. Carter et al., "Profiles of neuromuscular diseases. Duchenne muscular dystrophy," *American Journal of Physical Medicine & Rehabilitation*, vol. 74, no. 5, supplement, pp. S70–S92, 1995.

[14] E. N. Brandt and A. M. Pope, *Enabling America: Assessing the Role of Rehabilitation Science and Engineering*, National Academy Press, Washington, DC, USA, 1997.

[15] World Health Organization, *International Classification of Functioning, Disability and Health (ICF)*, Geneva, Switzerland, 2001.

[16] C. A. McHorney and A. R. Tarlov, "Individual-patient monitoring in clinical practice: are available health status surveys adequate?" *Quality of Life Research*, vol. 4, no. 4, pp. 293–307, 1995.

[17] M. O. Harris-Love, G. Joe, and D. E. Koziol, "Performance-based assessment of functional limitation and muscle endurance: reliability of the Adult Myositis Assessment Tool," *Journal of Neurologic Physical Therapy*, vol. 28, no. 4, pp. 179–180, 2004.

[18] A. R. La Spada, E. M. Wilson, D. B. Lubahn, A. E. Harding, and K. H. Fischbeck, "Androgen receptor gene mutations in X-linked spinal and bulbar muscular atrophy," *Nature*, vol. 352, no. 6330, pp. 77–79, 1991.

[19] N. Chahin, C. Klein, J. Mandrekar, and E. Sorenson, "Natural history of spinal-bulbar muscular atrophy," *Neurology*, vol. 70, no. 21, pp. 1967–1971, 2008.

[20] M. A. Ferrante and A. J. Wilbourn, "The characteristic electrodiagnostic features of Kennedy's disease," *Muscle Nerve*, vol. 20, no. 3, pp. 323–329, 1997.

[21] L. E. Rhodes, B. K. Freeman, S. Auh et al., "Clinical features of spinal and bulbar muscular atrophy," *Brain*, vol. 132, no. 12, pp. 3242–3251, 2009.

[22] The National Isometric Muscle Strength (NIMS) Database Consortium, "Muscular weakness assessment: use of normal isometric strength data," *Archives of Physical Medicine and Rehabilitation*, vol. 77, no. 12, pp. 1251–1255, 1996.

[23] A. W. Andrews, M. W. Thomas, and R. W. Bohannon, "Normative values for isometric muscle force measurements obtained with hand-held dynamometers," *Physical Therapy*, vol. 76, no. 3, pp. 248–259, 1996.

[24] J. P. R. Selman, A. A. de Camargo, J. Santos, F. C. Lanza, and S. Dal Corso, "Reference equation for the two-minute walk test in adults and the elderly," *Respiratory Care*, vol. 59, no. 4, pp. 525–530, 2014.

[25] H. Banno, M. Katsurio, K. Suzuki et al., "Phase 2 trial of leuprorelin in patients with spinal and bulbar muscular atrophy," *Annals of Neurology*, vol. 65, no. 2, pp. 140–150, 2009.

[26] Y. Goverover, A. R. O'Brien, N. B. Moore, and J. DeLuca, "Actual reality: a new approach to functional assessment in persons with multiple sclerosis," *Archives of Physical Medicine and Rehabilitation*, vol. 91, no. 2, pp. 252–260, 2010.

[27] R. J. Shephard, "Limits to the measurement of habitual physical activity by questionnaires," *British Journal of Sports Medicine*, vol. 37, no. 3, pp. 197–206, 2003.

[28] S. F. E. van Weely, J. C. van Denderen, M. P. M. Steultjens et al., "Moving instead of asking? Performance-based tests and BASFI-questionnaire measure different aspects of physical function in ankylosing spondylitis," *Arthritis Research and Therapy*, vol. 14, no. 2, article R52, 2012.

[29] L. E. Fernández-Rhodes, A. D. Kokkinis, M. J. White et al., "Efficacy and safety of dutasteride in patients with spinal and bulbar muscular atrophy: a randomised placebo-controlled trial," *The Lancet Neurology*, vol. 10, no. 2, pp. 140–147, 2011.

[30] P. Rossier and D. T. Wade, "Validity and reliability comparison of 4 mobility measures in patients presenting with neurologic impairment," *Archives of Physical Medicine and Rehabilitation*, vol. 82, no. 1, pp. 9–13, 2001.

[31] J. M. Stolwijk-Swüste, A. Beelen, G. J. Lankhorst et al., "SF36 physical functioning scale and 2-minute walk test advocated as core qualifiers to evaluate physical functioning in patients with late-onset sequelae of poliomyelitis," *Journal of Rehabilitation Medicine*, vol. 40, no. 5, pp. 387–394, 2008.

[32] K. E. Light, A. L. Bebrman, M. Thigpen, and W. J. Triggs, "The 2-minute walk test: a tool for evaluating walking endurance in clients with Parkinson's disease," *Journal of Neurologic Physical Therapy*, vol. 21, no. 4, pp. 136–139, 1997.

[33] R. J. Butland, J. Pang, E. R. Gross, A. A. Woodcock, and D. M. Geddes, "Two-, six-, and 12-minute walking tests in respiratory disease," *British Medical Journal*, vol. 284, no. 6329, pp. 1607–1608, 1982.

[34] S. H. Subramony, W. May, D. Lynch et al., "Measuring Friedreich ataxia: Interrater reliability of a neurologic rating scale," *Neurology*, vol. 64, no. 7, pp. 1261–1262, 2005.

[35] D. R. Lynch, J. M. Farmer, A. Y. Tsou et al., "Measuring Friedreich ataxia: complementary features of examination and performance measures," *Neurology*, vol. 66, no. 11, pp. 1711–1716, 2006.

[36] A. Riazi, J. C. Hobart, D. L. Lamping et al., "Using the SF-36 measure to compare the health impact of multiple sclerosis and Parkinson's disease with normal population health profiles," *Journal of Neurology Neurosurgery and Psychiatry*, vol. 74, no. 6, pp. 710–714, 2003.

[37] D. Finas, M. Bals-Pratsch, J. Sandmann et al., "Quality of life in elderly men with androgen deficiency," *Andrologia*, vol. 38, no. 2, pp. 48–53, 2006.

[38] J. E. Ware, M. Kosinski, J. B. Bjorner, D. M. Turner-Bowker, B. Gandek, and M. E. Maruish, *User's Manual for the SF-36v2 Health Survey*, QualtiyMetric, Lincoln, Mass, USA, 2nd edition, 2007.

[39] J. E. Ware, M. Kosinski, and J. E. Dewey, *How to Score Version Two of the SF-36—Health Survey*, QualityMetric, Lincoln, Mass, USA, 2000.

[40] L. G. Portney and M. P. Watkins, *Foundations of Clinical Research: Applications to Practice*, Pearson/Prentice Hall, Upper Saddle River, NJ, USA, 2009.

[41] S. L. Foster and J. D. Cone, "Validity issues in clinical assessment," *Psychological Assessment*, vol. 7, no. 3, pp. 248–260, 1995.

[42] B. H. Munro, *Statistical Methods for Health Care Research*, Lippincott Williams & Wilkins, Philadelphia, Pa, USA, 4th edition, 2001.

[43] A. Field, *Discovering Statistics Using SPSS*, Sage, Los Angeles, Calif, USA, 2009.

[44] S. Jaric, "Role of body size in the relation between muscle strength and movement performance," *Exercise and Sport Sciences Reviews*, vol. 31, no. 1, pp. 8–12, 2003.

[45] S. Jaric, "Muscle strength testing: use of normalisation for body size," *Sports Medicine*, vol. 32, no. 10, pp. 615–631, 2002.

[46] M. Brown, "Skeletal muscle and bone: effect of sex steroids and aging," *American Journal of Physiology—Advances in Physiology Education*, vol. 32, no. 2, pp. 120–126, 2008.

[47] T. Rantanen, J. M. Guralnik, G. Izmirlian et al., "Association of muscle strength with maximum walking speed in disabled older women," *American Journal of Physical Medicine and Rehabilitation*, vol. 77, no. 4, pp. 299–305, 1998.

[48] M. Doyu, G. Sobue, E. Mukai et al., "Severity of X-linked recessive bulbospinal neuronopathy correlates with size of the tandem CAG repeat in androgen receptor gene," *Annals of Neurology*, vol. 32, no. 5, pp. 707–710, 1992.

[49] A. R. La Spada, D. B. Roling, A. E. Harding et al., "Meiotic stability and genotype—phenotype correlation of the trinucleotide repeat in X-linked spinal and bulbar muscular atrophy," *Nature Genetics*, vol. 2, no. 4, pp. 301–304, 1992.

[50] N. Atsuta, H. Watanabe, M. Ito et al., "Natural history of spinal and bulbar muscular atrophy (SBMA): a study of 223 Japanese patients," *Brain*, vol. 129, no. 6, pp. 1446–1455, 2006.

[51] H. Alexanderson, L. Broman, A. Tollbäck, A. Josefson, I. E. Lundberg, and C. H. Stenström, "Functional Index-2: validity and reliability of a disease-specific measure of impairment in patients with polymyositis and dermatomyositis," *Arthritis Care and Research*, vol. 55, no. 1, pp. 114–122, 2006.

[52] R. L. Lieber, *Skeletal Muscle Structure, Function, and Plasticity: the Physiological Basis of Rehabilitation*, Lippincott Williams & Wilkins, Baltimore, Md, USA, 2010.

[53] M. O. Harris-Love, J. A. Shrader, T. E. Davenport et al., "Are repeated single-limb heel raises and manual muscle testing associated with peak plantar-flexor force in people with inclusion body myositis?" *Physical Therapy*, vol. 94, no. 4, pp. 543–552, 2014.

[54] J. G. Boyer, A. Ferrier, and R. Kothary, "More than a bystander: the contributions of intrinsic skeletal muscle defects in motor neuron diseases," *Frontiers in Physiology*, 2013.

[55] N. Chahin and E. J. Sorenson, "Serum creatine kinase levels in spinobulbar muscular atrophy and amyotrophic lateral sclerosis," *Muscle and Nerve*, vol. 40, no. 1, pp. 126–129, 2009.

[56] G. J. Salem, M.-Y. Wang, J. T. Young, M. Marion, and G. A. Greendale, "Knee strength and lower- and higher-intensity functional performance in older adults," *Medicine and Science in Sports and Exercise*, vol. 32, no. 10, pp. 1679–1684, 2000.

[57] L. Merlini, E. Bertini, C. Minetti et al., "Motor function-muscle strength relationship in spinal muscular atrophy," *Muscle and Nerve*, vol. 29, no. 4, pp. 548–552, 2004.

15

Obstacles to Obtaining Optimal Physiotherapy Services in a Rural Community in Southeastern Nigeria

Chinonso Igwesi-Chidobe

Department of Medical Rehabilitation, Faculty of Health Sciences and Technology, College of Medicine, University of Nigeria, Enugu Campus, 400006 Enugu, Nigeria

Correspondence should be addressed to Chinonso Igwesi-Chidobe, noamyks@yahoo.com

Academic Editor: Luc Vanhees

Background. Many people continue to live with physical disabilities across the globe, especially in rural Africa despite expertise of Physiotherapists and available evidence of effectiveness of Physiotherapy. *Objective.* To determine the obstacles to obtaining Optimal Physiotherapy services in a rural community in Southeastern Nigeria. *Methods.* Population-based cross-sectional study of individuals and health facilities in a rural community in Southeastern Nigeria. *Results.* The obstacles to obtaining optimal physiotherapy services in this community were unavailability of physiotherapy services, poor knowledge of health workers and community dwellers of the roles and scope of physiotherapy, poor health care seeking behavior of community dwellers, patronage of traditional health workers, and poor referral practices by health workers. *Conclusion.* Rural health workers in Nkanu West Local Government and other rural communities in Nigeria and Africa should be educated on the roles and scope of physiotherapy. There is a need for raising awareness of the management options for movement/functional problems for rural indigenous communities in Nigeria in particular and Africa in general. Physiotherapists should be made aware of the growing need for physiotherapy in rural areas of Nigeria and Africa largely comprising of the elderly.

1. Introduction

Concomitant with the aging of our population is a significant rise in the prevalence of chronic diseases. This in turn has increased the need for physical therapists and physical therapy services by all health agencies. The unprecedented need for services may outstrip the capabilities of the existing medical facilities. There is also an increasing need for out-of-hospital treatment programs with a concurrent shortage of competent physical therapists to staff them [1].

Despite the expertise in therapeutic exercises and the available evidence of effectiveness, many people continue to live with physical disabilities across the globe, especially in Africa [2–4]. Access to rehabilitation for people with disability is inadequate, more so in rural communities, with the attendant economic and social implications if the status quo is maintained [2–4]. Webster et al. in 2008 stated that despite physiotherapy being regarded positively by all referral groups of patients, there is still a distinct lack of knowledge about the profession by the general public, which affects self-referral [4]. Different referral practices exist among doctors based on the different views held by these doctors as to the conditions considered amenable to physiotherapy or their therapeutic intentions when prescribing physiotherapy with or without other medications as discussed by Akpala et al. [5]. They stated that other factors that might influence referral patterns could be the age, sex of individual doctors, medical school attended, and previous experience of hospital or other rehabilitation services, and particularly of physical therapy [5]. There is also a problem in the employment of evidence-based practice by many physical therapists. Jette et al. noted that physical therapists had a need to increase the use of evidence in their daily practice [6]. The low concept of public-health-oriented physical therapy can be seen among several physical therapists. Raman and Levi in USA stated that many conceptualized disability as individual limitations within specific contexts and infrequently conceptualized disability as a societal phenomenon affecting persons across

TABLE 1

Ward	Population	Private health facility	Primary health centers	Secondary health facility	Tertiary health facility	Traditional health facility	Total health facilities
Agbani (studied)	20,612	5	3: Ogbeke, Ojiagu and Mgbogodo Health Center	1: Agbani General Hospital	none	1	10
Akegbe Ugwu 1	8,756	1	1: Akegbugwu Health Center	None	None	None	2
Akegbe Ugwu 2 (studied)	8,349	1	1: Our Lady Health of the Sick Health Center	None	None	None	2
Amodu (studied)	9,902	None	1: Amodu Health Center	None	None	1	2
Amurri (studied)	19,385	None	2: Amurri Health Centers 1&2	None	None	1	3
Ndiuno Uwani (studied)	8,632	1	1: Ndiuno Uwani Health Center	None	None	None	2
Obe (studied)	9,635	None	1: Obe Health Center	None	None	None	1
Obinagu Uwani (studied)	12,656	1	1: Obinagu Uwani Health Center	None	None	None	2
Obuno	9,856	None	1: Obuno Health Center	None	None	None	1
Obuoffia	10,141	1	2: Obuoffia and Amangwu Health Centers	None	None	None	3
Ogonogo-ejindiagu	18,306	1	1: Ogonogo-ejindiagu health Center	None	None	None	2
Ogonogo-ejindiuno (studied)	10,848	None	1: Ogonogo-ejindiuno health Center	None	None	None	1
Ozalla	9,311	None	2: Ozalla and Model health Centers	None	1: University of Nigeria Teaching Hospital	None	3
Umueze (studied)	4,108	None	1: Umueze health Center	None	None	None	1
Total	160,497	11	19	1	1	3	35

most settings and circumstances. They believed that a concept of disability that is more inclusive of broad, as well as specific contexts of disability may lead to improved physical therapy management for individuals with a wide range of performance capacities [3].

According to the chartered society of physiotherapy in 2010, physiotherapy workforce has a key role to play in the public health agenda through its contribution to the prevention of disease, promotion of good health, particularly through physical activity and improvement in the general quality of life [7]. Studies indicate the need to address these shortcomings in physiotherapy especially in the Nigerian environment [8–13].

Despite there being a large literature supporting the importance of physiotherapy for optimal public health of every nation's citizenry, there remains a need for a more public health-oriented evidence-based physical therapy practice [14–25]. This should be improved as well as improving other challenges of the profession like improper referral practices, suboptimal treatment choices like the use of oral NSAIDs in place of Physiotherapy, decreased awareness of others of the role and scope of the profession, poor team approach in patient management, patronage of traditional healers, and so many others [26–39].

Significance of Work. Majority of the populace in Nigeria reside in rural areas without any access to rehabilitation services. Furthermore these groups are often poor and marginalized with the highest level of disability and functional dependence, therefore with the highest need for rehabilitation. Unfortunately rehabilitation services are in the urban areas in Nigeria.

2. Materials and Method

2.1. Background of Study Area. Nkanu West Local Government is one of the 17 Local Government Areas (L.G.As) in Enugu State with a population of about 160,497. Enugu State is one of the five states that constitute South Eastern Nigeria with a population of 3, 257, 298 constituting 2.33% of Nigeria's total population of 140, 003, 542 people at the 2006 census. Majority of Nigeria's elderly reside in the rural areas where they engage majorly in subsistence agriculture [40].

The headquarters of Nkanu West are based at Agbani. The L.G.A has an area of 225 km^2 with 14 wards. Nkanu West Local Government is bounded on the north by Enugu South Local Government Area, on the east by Nkanu East L.G.A., on the south by Awgu Local Government Area, and on the west by Udi Local Government. The health facilities in the 14 wards in Nkanu West Local Government include those listed on Table 1.

Therefore, there was a total of 11 private health facilities, 19 primary health centers, 1 secondary health facility,

1 tertiary health facility, and 3 traditional health facilities in the entire L.G.A but the 9 wards randomly studied from the L.G.A had a total of 24 health facilities comprising 8 private health facilities, 12 primary health centers, 1 secondary health facility, 3 traditional health facilities and had no tertiary health facility.

There are about 120 registered physiotherapists in Enugu state out of the total 2,560 registered in Nigeria.

2.2. Design of Study.
Population-based cross-sectional study design.

2.3. Sampling Plan.
Study population:

(i) household members in the communities of the study area,

(ii) directors/Managers of health facilities in the communities.

2.4. Survey Instruments

(i) Interview of heads of households employing interviewer-administered questionnaire to assess the people's knowledge and utilization of physiotherapy services.

(ii) Interview of the directors/managers of the 24 health facilities in the 9 chosen wards using interviewer-administered questionnaire to assess their need and knowledge of Physiotherapy: their perceived need for physiotherapy services and Physiotherapy services offered in their institution. There was also observation to assess the available manpower, equipment, and treatment protocol for physiotherapy services in each health institution by the researcher.

Three copies of these questionnaires were then sent to three experts in questionnaires design to determine their content validity. Corrections based on their input were reflected on the questionnaire before their final versions were produced. Before administration, the questionnaire, which was written in English language, was pretested by a few Physiotherapists in communities outside the study area in order to eliminate ambiguities and ensure comprehension by all respondents.

2.5. Sample Size Estimation, Sampling, and Data Collection

2.5.1. Households.
There is no reasonable estimate of the proportion of people having or lacking knowledge of physiotherapy in any community in Nigeria, hence 50% was used (0.50). Since Nkanu West Local Government has a finite population of about 160,497 people in an area of 225 km^2, sample size formula for proportions with population greater than 10,000 was used

$$n = \frac{z^2 pq}{d^2}, \quad (1)$$

where: n = the desired sample size (when population is greater than 10,000), z = the standard normal deviate, set at 1.96 corresponding to 95% confidence level, p = the proportion of persons requiring physiotherapy services, because it is not available from literature, 50% will be used (0.50), q = 1.0-p, d = error tolerated, set at 0.05 [14], $n = (1.96^2 \times 0.5 \times 0.5)/(0.05)^2 = 384$ participants.

Since the questionnaires were interviewer administered, nonresponse was not anticipated hence minimum sample size was 384 participants but a total of 408 participants were studied.

Study participants in the communities were selected using a 3-stage cluster sampling method. The nine selected wards were composed of 115 villages and 12 of these villages were selected randomly. Approximately each village was located 1 km or less from the health facilities. All consenting members of alternate households in each selected village were enrolled for the study. A total of 34 participants (heads of households) were enrolled in each village making a total of 408 participants but data for 400 participants were finally analyzed.

2.5.2. Health Facilities.
Cluster sampling method was used to select health facilities. Nine wards out of the fourteen wards that make up Nkanu West Local Government Area were chosen randomly. All the health facilities in the 9 wards comprising 8 private health facilities, 12 primary health centers, 1 secondary health facility, and 3 traditional health facilities were studied making a total of 24 health facilities. The director or manager of the health facility and the most senior health worker were interviewed in each selected health facility.

2.6. Method of Data Collection.
Interviewer-administered questionnaires were used to obtain information from the heads of households. A household is skipped if on the second visit, the head of household is not found.

Questionnaires were administered to the director or manager or the most senior staff in charge of physiotherapy services in the health facility on the day of visit. Observation and inspection of available manpower, equipment, and treatment protocols for physiotherapy services at each of the health facility was also carried out. These were carried out by the researcher assisted by eleven paid physiotherapists. There was no Physiotherapy service or Physiotherapist found in all.

2.7. Method of Data Analysis.
Data was organized bearing in mind the objectives of the study. Tables and figures were used to highlight relationship between variables. Data analysis was done using SPSS 19.0 computer software. Descriptive statistics (frequency, percentage) were utilized. Confidence limit was set at 95%.

2.8. Ethical Considerations.
Ethical approval for the study was obtained from the research ethics committee of the University of Nigeria Teaching Hospital Enugu, Nigeria. Permission to carry out the study was obtained from the "Igwes" (Community heads) of the study areas, while verbal

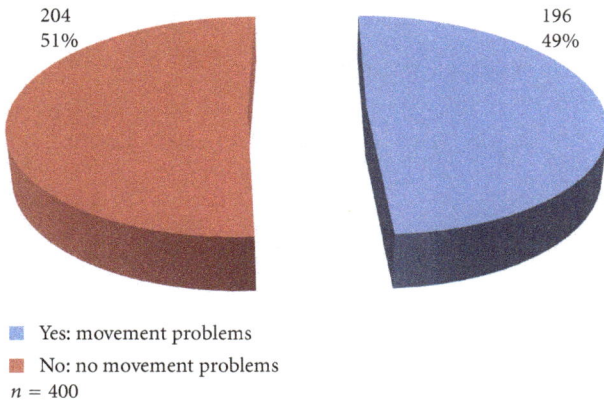

Figure 1: Prevalence of movement/functional problems in households.

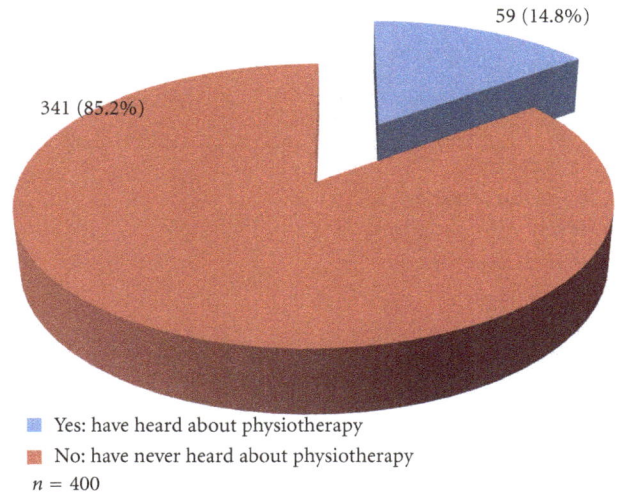

Figure 2: Knowledge of physiotherapy by respondents in the communities.

consent was obtained from the heads of the households in the communities of the study area.

3. Results

No Physiotherapy service or Physiotherapist was found in all the health facilities and communities.

Results showed that nearly half of all the participants interviewed 196 (49.0%) complained of having some movement/functional problems (Figure 1).

The majority of respondents with movement/functional problems were having spinal problems 75 (18.8%), followed by those having multiple joint problems 51 (12.8%) and lower limb joint problem 43 (10.8%). The least problem was upper limb joint problem 8 (2.0%).

A fifth 79 (19.8%) of the respondents were experiencing these problems occasionally, while 60 (15.0%) were having these problems all the time (Table 2).

The majority (55, 28.1%) of these respondents visited chemist for treatment of their movement/functional problems followed by those who used home remedy 33 (16.8%). Only few visited a tertiary or general hospital 12 (6.1%) each, while 39 (19.9%) sought no therapy for the problem (Table 2).

Of those who sought help for movement/functional problems, a majority of 115 (73.3%) either received drugs, traction, and/or Plaster of Paris (POP) as treatment. Only one person (0.6%) had physiotherapy included in the treatment regimen.

The major reasons for choice of health facility include cheap 66 (33.7%), accessibility 44 (22.4%), and expert care 26 (13.3%) (Table 3).

On the whole, 53 (27.0%) visited a traditional health facility of which the majority 29 (54.7%) received topical herbs as treatment followed by 14 (26.4%) who received traditional bone setting (Table 4).

A majority (341, 85.2%) of the respondents have never heard about physiotherapy (Figure 2).

Results show that none of the respondents acknowledged having any physiotherapy outfit nearby (Figure 3).

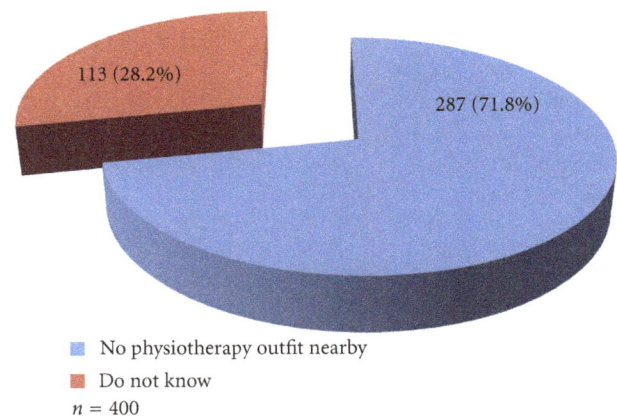

Figure 3: Availability of physiotherapy facilities within the community.

All the health facilities neither have nor offer physiotherapy services.

Many health workers 10 (41.7%) reported having no qualified personnel for physiotherapy services as their reason for lacking physiotherapy services, while an equal number 10 (41.7%) felt physiotherapy services were not needed in their health facility (Table 5).

Results show that many of the health workers 11 (45.8%) had never heard about physiotherapy (Figure 4).

4. Discussion

It was discovered that the majority of the respondents having movement/functional problems visited "chemist," sought no help or used home remedy for their movement/functional problems with majority being treated with drugs, traction and, or Plaster of Paris (POP). Only few visited tertiary health facility, out of which only one person was referred

TABLE 2: Household respondent's movement/functional problems and frequency of occurrence.

Movement/functional problems	Frequency of occurrence			Total no (%)
	All the time	Most times	Occasionally	
	no	no	no	
Spinal problems	14	23	38	75 (18.8)
Multiple joint problems	14	17	20	51 (12.8)
Lower limb joint problem	16	12	15	43 (10.8)
Upper limb joint problem	5	1	2	8 (2.0)
Limb weakness	11	4	4	19 (4.8)
None	—	—	—	204 (51.0)
Total no (%)	60 (15.0)	57 (14.3)	79 (19.8)	400 (100.0)

$n = 400$.

TABLE 3: Management of movement/functional problems at household level.

	Number of respondents	Percentage (%)
First health care provider		
Tertiary hospital	12	6.1
General hospital	12	6.1
Private hospital/clinic	16	8.2
Health center	10	5.1
Chemist	55	28.1
Traditional health facility	18	9.2
Prayer house	1	0.5
Home remedy	33	16.8
No action	39	19.9
Total	196	100.0
Initial treatment received		
Drugs, traction, and/or pop	115	73.3
Herbs and/or traditional bone setting	22	14.0
Hot water and balm	11	7.0
Referral to secondary or tertiary health facility	3	1.9
Massage	2	1.3
Surgery	2	1.3
Prayers	1	0.6
Physiotherapy and others	1	0.6
None	39	19.9
Total	196	100.0
Reasons for choice of facility		
Cheap	66	33.7
Accessibility	44	22.4
Expert care	41	20.9
Referral	26	13.3
Afraid of therapy	19	9.7
Total	196	100.0

$n = 196$.

for physiotherapy. This highlights the poor knowledge and referral status for physiotherapy. Their main reasons for choice of health facility were affordability, accessibility, and expert care. This finding is similar to the findings of Vindigni et al. [15] that the main barriers to managing musculoskeletal conditions for rural Aboriginal communities were that majority of the respondents that reported musculoskeletal conditions did not receive treatment or management because they had learned to live with the problem, were unaware of what might help, or found private therapies too expensive [15]. A similar result was given by Akinpelu et al. in 2010, which showed that very few participants with functional

TABLE 4: Use of traditional health facility for functional problems by households.

	Number of respondents	Percentage (%)
Visit to traditional health facility		
Yes	53	27.0
No	143	73.0
Total	196	100.0
Traditional treatment received		
Topical herbs	29	54.7
Traditional bone setting	14	26.4
Nothing	6	11.3
Oral herbs	2	3.8
Massage	2	3.8
Did not seek traditional treatment	143	73.0
Total	196	100.0

$n = 196$.

TABLE 5: Reasons for lack of physiotherapy services in the 24 health facilities in the study area.

	Number of respondents	Percentage (%)
Why is there no physiotherapy services in your facility		
Lack of trained personnel	10	41.7
Not necessary	10	41.7
Lack resources for equipments	2	8.3
Lack space for such services	2	8.3
Total	24	100.0

$n = 24$.

problems as a result of musculoskeletal pain in rural communities sought hospital treatment while majority used self-prescribed drugs for pain alleviation [16].

Over four-fifths of the respondents in the households had never heard about physiotherapy, and there was no physiotherapy outfit in the community. This result agrees with several other studies supporting that rural communities lack knowledge of physiotherapy and lack physiotherapy services [1, 5, 9, 17–25].

A significant number of the respondents eventually visited traditional health facility for their movement/functional problems with majority either receiving topical herbs or traditional bone setting as treatment. The health workers in the study area were mainly primary health care workers though a significant number were Traditional Birth Attendants and traditional healers. Several studies support that traditional health workers significantly contribute to the number of medical complications presenting to hospitals especially in developing nations [26–30].

More than half of the health workers encountered movement/functional problems in their facility, which is mainly treated using oral NSAIDs and herbs/traditional bone setting. Very few are referred to tertiary health facility.

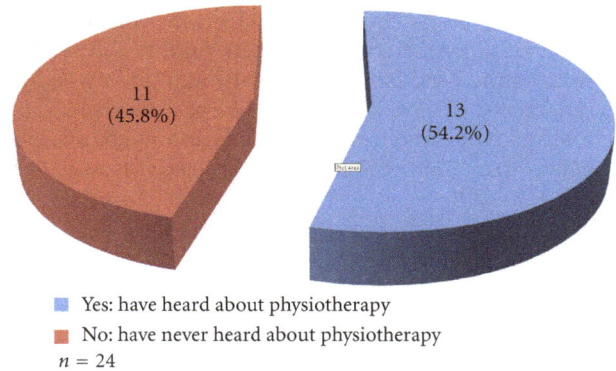

Yes: have heard about physiotherapy
No: have never heard about physiotherapy
$n = 24$

FIGURE 4: Knowledge of physiotherapy by health workers.

Many health workers reported having no qualified personnel for physiotherapy and physiotherapy not necessary as their reasons for lacking physiotherapy services in their health facility. Additionally, nearly half (45.8%) reported having no knowledge of physiotherapy. This shows that though there was a high burden of movement/functional deficits especially involving the spine, multiple joints, and muscles in the communities, many people may not be appropriately referred for physiotherapy. Many of the health workers feel they had no need for physiotherapy probably because they did not know the role and scope of physiotherapy and think their treatment options involving mainly the use of oral NSAIDs are optimal. Studies, however, have shown that oral NSAIDs produce short-term relief and are associated with increased risk of gastrointestinal haemorrhage especially when taken for prolonged periods of time [31–36]. Physiotherapy, on the other hand, has been shown to be better in the long term with effects that can be sustained. However, physiotherapy when combined with short-term topical NSAIDs produces the best results [31–36]. This is because the pain relieving effects of the NSAIDs allowed for better exercise tolerance.

The obstacles to receiving optimal physiotherapy in this community were that the people have poor health care seeking behavior. They made their health care choices based on affordability, accessibility, and "expert care" (Table 3). They may have also felt that the movement and functional loss was inevitable, hence some did not seek help nor do anything for their movement/functional loss. Majority of them have no knowledge of physiotherapy, hence may not have the choice of self-referral for Physiotherapy. There were also no physiotherapy services available neither in the communities nor in the health facilities to address the movement and functional problems. Also quite a number of the health workers completely had no knowledge of physiotherapy therefore may not refer patients appropriately. A significant number of the health workers felt they had no need for physiotherapy in their health facilities most probably because they did not know the role and scope of physiotherapy and because few people were presenting to the health facilities with movement/functional problems, a typical "ice-berg" phenomenon.

These obstacles are, however, different for developed countries like Australia, Canada, United Kingdom, and United States of America, where their rural health workers appreciated the need for physiotherapy and understood the role and scope of physiotherapy. The rural residents knew the role and scope of physiotherapy hence could be available for self-referral if optimal physiotherapy services were to be provided [37–39].

5. Conclusion

The obstacles to obtaining optimal physiotherapy services in this community were unavailability of physiotherapy services, poor knowledge of health workers 11 (45.8%) and the community dwellers 341 (85.2%) of the roles and scope of physiotherapy, poor health care seeking behavior of the community dwellers 50 (25.5%), patronage of traditional health workers 53 (27.0%), and poor referral practices by the health workers 1 (0.6%).

Recommendations

Rural Health workers in Nkanu West Local Government and by extension other rural communities in Nigeria should be educated on the roles and scope of physiotherapy. There is a need for raising awareness of the management options for movement/functional problems for rural indigenous communities in Nkanu West Local Government in particular and Nigeria in general. They should be educated on their need for physiotherapy services. Physiotherapists should be made aware of the growing need for physiotherapy in rural areas of Nigeria largely comprising of the elderly according to World Bank's report of 1994 [40].

Author's Contributions

Igwesi-Chidobe CN was the project leader, performed most of the experiments, data analysis and written manuscript.

References

[1] J. B. Allis, "Orienting the physical therapist to public health practice," *Public Health Reports*, vol. 80, no. 11, pp. 975–980, 1965.

[2] B. L. Snow, E. Shamus, and C. Hill, "Physical therapy as primary health care: public perceptions," *Journal of Allied Health*, vol. 30, no. 1, pp. 35–38, 2001.

[3] S. Raman and S. J. Levi, "Concepts of disablement in documents guiding physical therapy practice," *Disability and Rehabilitation*, vol. 24, no. 15, pp. 790–797, 2002.

[4] V. S. Webster, L. K. Holdsworth, A. K. McFadyen, and H. Little, "Self-referral, access and physiotherapy: patients' knowledge and attitudes-results of a national trial," *Physiotherapy*, vol. 94, no. 2, pp. 141–149, 2008.

[5] C. O. Akpala, A. P. Curran, and J. Simpson, "Physiotherapy in general practice: patterns of utilisation," *Public Health*, vol. 102, no. 3, pp. 263–268, 1988.

[6] D. U. Jette, K. Bacon, C. Batty et al., "Evidence-based practice: beliefs, attitudes, knowledge, and behaviors of physical therapists," *Physical Therapy*, vol. 83, no. 9, pp. 786–805, 2003.

[7] Chartered Society of Physiotherapy. Charting thefuture of Physiotherapy, http://www.csp.org.uk/uploads/documents/csp_charting_the future.pdf, 2008.

[8] S. R. A. Akinbo, D. O. Odebiyi, T. E. Okunola, and O. T. Aderoba, "Evidence-based practice: knowledge, attitudes and beliefs of physiotherapists in Nigeria," in *Nigeria Society of Physiotherapy (NSP) Conference*, 2008.

[9] L. O. Ganiyu, "Physiotherapy in primary health care: are we ready?" *Journal of the Nigeria Society of Physiotherapy*, 2008.

[10] A. L. Oyeyemi and A. Y. Oyeyemi, "Professional Outlook and clinical practice pattern of physiotherapy in Nigeria," in *Nigeria Society of Physiotherapy (NSP) Conference*, 2008.

[11] B. Birabi, A. Okunuga, and U. C. Okafor, "Survey of knowledge and the use of stroke assessment scales by physiotherapists in selected Nigeria health institutions," in *Nigeria Society of Physiotherapy (NSP) Conference*, 2008.

[12] B. Birabi, "Physical fitness, a must have for the urban dweller," in *Nigeria Society of Physiotherapy (NSP) Conference*, 2008.

[13] A. L. Oyeyemi and B. O. A. Adegoke, "Neighbourhood environment as determinants of physical activity and health promotion," in *Nigeria Society of Physiotherapy(NSP) Conference*, 2008.

[14] M. O. Araoye, "Sample size determination," in *Research Methodology with Statistics for Health and Social Sciences*, M. O. Araoye, Ed., pp. 115–122, Nathadox, Ilorin, Nigeria, 2004.

[15] D. Vindigni, D. Griffen, J. Perkins, C. Dacosta, and L. Parkinson, "Prevalence of musculoskeletal conditions, associated pain and disability and the barriers to managing these conditions in a rural, Australian Aboriginal community," *Rural Remote Health*, vol. 4, no. 3, article 230, 2004.

[16] A. O. Akinpelu, A. C. Odole, and A. S. Odejide, "Prevalence and pattern of musculoskeletal pain in a rural community in Southwestern Nigeria," *Internet Journal of Epidemiology*, vol. 8, no. 2, 2010.

[17] R. Blau, S. Bolus, T. Carolan et al., "The experience of providing physical therapy in a changing health care environment," *Physical Therapy*, vol. 82, no. 7, pp. 648–657, 2002.

[18] C. Kigin, "A systems view of physical therapy care: shifting to a new paradigm for the profession," *Physical Therapy*, vol. 89, no. 11, pp. 1117–1119, 2009.

[19] V. A. Obajuluwa, O. K. Abereoje, and M. O. B. Olaogun, "First-contact physiotherapy practice in Nigeria," *Physiotherapy Theory and Practice*, vol. 6, no. 2, pp. 85–89, 1990.

[20] M. Hurley, K. Dziedzic, L. Bearne, J. Sim, and T. Bury, The clinical and cost effectiveness of physiotherapy in the management of older people with common rheumatological conditions. The chartered Society of Physiotherapy, 2002, http://www.csp.org.uk/.

[21] S. Ambwani, "Pain management in the elderly," *Journal of the Indian Academy of Geriatrics*, vol. 5, no. 4, pp. 191–196, 2009.

[22] CSP, *Inquiry into Out-of-Hours Care Provision in Rural Areas*, CSP, Newcastle, UK, 2007.

[23] O. Abereoje, "An evaluation of the effectiveness of itinerant and community physiotherapy schemes in meeting the primary health care needs in Oyo State, Nigeria," *Physiotherapy Practice*, vol. 4, no. 4, pp. 194–200, 1988.

[24] T. Miller Mifflin and M. Bzdell, "Development of a physiotherapy prioritization tool in the Baffin Region of Nunavut: a remote, under-serviced area in the Canadian Arctic," *Rural and Remote Health*, vol. 10, no. 2, article 1466, 2010.

[25] M. Ellangovin, "Innovations in community physiotherapy," *The Journal of Field Actions*, vol. 2, 2009.

[26] B. U. Ngohi, U. Aliyu, U. N. Jibril, A. Lawal, and M. B. Ngohi, "Causes of bone injuries and patronage of traditional

bone setters in Maiduguri, Nigeria," *Sierra Leone Journal of Biomedical Research*, vol. 1, no. 1, pp. 50–54, 2009.

[27] J. D. Ogunlusi, I. C. Okem, and L. M. Oginni, "Why patients patronize traditional bone setters," *Internet Journal of Orthopaedic Surgery*, vol. 4, no. 2, pp. 1–7, 2007.

[28] A. M. Udosen, O. O. Otei, and O. Onuba, "Role of traditional bonesSetters in Africa: experience in Calabar, Nigeria," *Annals of African Medicine*, vol. 5, no. 4, pp. 170–173, 2006.

[29] T. O. Alonge, A. E. Dongo, T. E. Nottidge, A. B. Omololu, and S. O. Ogunlade, "Traditional bonesetters in South Western Nigeria—friends or foes?" *West African Journal of Medicine*, vol. 23, no. 1, pp. 81–84, 2004.

[30] B. A. Solagberu, "Long bone fractures treated by traditional bonesetters: a study of patients' behaviour," *Tropical Doctor*, vol. 35, no. 2, pp. 106–108, 2005.

[31] H. Ulusoy, N. Sarica, S. Arslan, C. Olcay, and U. Erkorkmaz, "The efficacy of supervised physiotherapy for the treatment of adhesive capsulitis," *Bratislava Medical Journal*, vol. 112, no. 4, pp. 204–207, 2011.

[32] W. J. J. Assendelft, E. M. Hay, R. Adshead, and L. M. Bouter, "Corticosteroid injections for lateral epicondylitis: a systematic overview," *British Journal of General Practice*, vol. 46, no. 405, pp. 209–216, 1996.

[33] L. Bisset, A. Paungmali, B. Vicenzino, and E. Beller, "A systematic review and meta-analysis of clinical trials on physical interventions for lateral epicondylalgia," *British Journal of Sports Medicine*, vol. 39, no. 7, pp. 411–422, 2005.

[34] R. P. Calfee, A. Patel, M. F. DaSilva, and E. Akelman, "Management of lateral epicondylitis: current concepts," *Journal of the American Academy of Orthopaedic Surgeons*, vol. 16, no. 1, pp. 19–29, 2008.

[35] E. Ernst, *Desktop Guide to Complementary and Alternative Medicine*, Mosby, London, UK, 2001.

[36] J. J. Wilson and T. M. Best, "Common overuse tendon problems: a review and recommendations for treatment," *American Family Physician*, vol. 72, no. 5, pp. 811–818, 2005.

[37] P. A. Margolis, C. M. Lannon, R. Stevens et al., "Linking clinical and public health approaches to improve access to health care for socially disadvantaged mothers and children: a feasibility study," *Archives of Pediatrics and Adolescent Medicine*, vol. 150, no. 8, pp. 815–821, 1996.

[38] S. Ueki, T. Kasai, J. Takato et al., "Production of a fall prevention exercise programme considering suggestions from community-dwelling elderly," *Nippon Koshu Eisei Zasshi*, vol. 53, no. 2, pp. 112–121, 2006.

[39] R. L. Craik, "A responsibility to put 'health policy in perspective,'" *Physical Therapy*, vol. 89, no. 11, pp. 1114–1115, 2009.

[40] World Bank, *The World Bank Activities and Position on Ageing*, Oxford University Press, New York, NY, USA, 1994.

16

Allocation of Attentional Resources toward a Secondary Cognitive Task Leads to Compromised Ankle Proprioceptive Performance in Healthy Young Adults

Kazuhiro Yasuda,[1] Yuki Sato,[1] Naoyuki Iimura,[2] and Hiroyasu Iwata[2]

[1] *Global Robot Academia Laboratory, Green Computing Systems Research Organization, Waseda University, 27 Waseda-cho, Shinjuku-ku, Tokyo 162-0042, Japan*
[2] *Graduate School of Creative Science and Engineering, Waseda University, 3-4-1 Okubo, Shinjuku-ku, Tokyo 169-8555, Japan*

Correspondence should be addressed to Hiroyasu Iwata; jubi@waseda.jp

Academic Editor: K. S. Sunnerhagen

The objective of the present study was to determine whether increased attentional demands influence the assessment of ankle joint proprioceptive ability in young adults. We used a dual-task condition, in which participants performed an ankle ipsilateral position-matching task with and without a secondary serial auditory subtraction task during target angle encoding. Two experiments were performed with two different cohorts: one in which the auditory subtraction task was easy (experiment 1a) and one in which it was difficult (experiment 1b). The results showed that, compared with the single-task condition, participants had higher absolute error under dual-task conditions in experiment 1b. The reduction in position-matching accuracy with an attentionally demanding cognitive task suggests that allocation of attentional resources toward a difficult second task can lead to compromised ankle proprioceptive performance. Therefore, these findings indicate that the difficulty level of the cognitive task might be the possible critical factor that decreased accuracy of position-matching task. We conclude that increased attentional demand with difficult cognitive task does influence the assessment of ankle joint proprioceptive ability in young adults when measured using an ankle ipsilateral position-matching task.

1. Introduction

Ankle proprioception is critical to maintaining balance during functional activities such as standing and walking [1, 2]. Although there is general consensus on the role of visual, vestibular, and proprioceptive senses in the maintenance of upright posture [3, 4], studies have indicated that the somatosensory system is an important contributor to the feedback for postural control [5]. Previous studies have also suggested that decreased in proprioception in the lower limbs contributes significantly to instability and falls [5, 6].

In rehabilitation, proprioception should be evaluated because of its significance in motor control. Although several methods are available, the joint position-matching task is one of the most reliable tools for the assessment of proprioceptive acuity in the clinic and the laboratory [7–10]. In this test, a participant is asked to reposition a reference joint angle without observing the positioning and repositioning of the joint. Specifically, in ipsilateral position-matching tasks, where the same limb is used for reference and position matching, it is necessary to use memory in order to remember the target position [7]. Hence it is likely that some portion of any position-matching error reflects cognitive capacity.

A recent study by Goble et al. [11] reported that older adults with low working memory were prone to compromised proprioceptive encoding during an ipsilateral elbow position-matching task when a secondary cognitive task was executed concurrently. In the study, older adults with high working memory ability and those with low working memory ability, along with healthy younger adults, performed an ipsilateral elbow position-matching task with and without a secondary task (i.e., counting by 3 s) during target position encoding. The older adults with low working memory ability made significantly more elbow-repositioning errors when a secondary task was performed during target encoding, compared with both younger and older adults who had high working memory ability. The interesting conclusion of their report was that the allocation of attentional resources toward a task led to compromised sensorimotor performance because of a limitation in the resources available for concurrently coping with both tasks [11].

The current study was designed to extend previous findings and to determine whether attentional load influences ankle joint proprioceptive ability in young adults when an ipsilateral position-matching condition is adopted. We selected the ankle joints as the target joints because of the importance of ankle joints for locomotor and postural control. Previous work has shown differences during dual-task performance that included proprioception-dependent tasks, such as standing and walking [12]. In the present study, participants were instructed to perform two concurrent tasks. The primary task was an ipsilateral ankle joint position-matching task, and it was performed with or without a secondary cognitive task—a computerized auditory serial subtraction task [13]. In order to clarify the influence of the difficulty of the secondary task, we performed two experiments: one with an easy secondary task (experiment 1a) and the other with a difficult secondary task (experiment 1b). We hypothesized that increasing the difficulty of the cognitive task would result in decreased accuracy in the ankle position-matching task.

We also examined whether accurate position matching was enhanced when a position was encoded by active movement rather than passive movement. Several studies have demonstrated that participants make smaller errors when a target position is established through their own active movement than when the same target position is determined passively by the experimenter [14, 15]. The effect is thought to be the consequence of two movement-related features: an efferent copy of the motor command [16, 17] and the afferent proprioceptive information within the gamma motor system [18]. On the basis of these studies, we hypothesized that the ability to reproduce ankle position accurately is enhanced when position is encoded by active movement, compared with when it is encoded by passive movement.

2. Materials and Methods

2.1. Participants

2.1.1. Experiment 1a (Easy Cognitive Task). Sixteen young adults participated in this study. The study cohort included 8 males and 8 females, aged 25.4 ± 5.6 years, with an average body weight of 54.29 ± 5.28 kg and an average height of 162±7.32 cm. The inclusion criteria were that the participants had no neurological, muscular, or hearing disorders that could influence voluntary movement and auditory sense. Participants provided written informed consent prior to participation. Waseda University's ethics committee for human

research approved the procedures employed in the study. The tenets of the Declaration of Helsinki were followed.

2.1.2. Experiment 1b (Difficult Cognitive Task). A separate cohort of 16 young adults participated in experiment 1b. This cohort consisted of 8 males and 8 females, aged 26.2 ± 3.6 years, with an average body weight of 56.34 ± 6.34 kg and an average height of 161 ± 8.11 cm. The inclusion criteria were identical to those used in experiment 1a. Each participant gave written informed consent prior to participation.

2.2. Apparatus. We used a custom-made rotating paddle that included a rotary angle encoder (E6A2-CW3C, OMRON, Japan) to measure the joint angle and a motor (USR60-E3N, Shinsei Corporation, Japan) to move the rotating paddle. A custom-made hand switch was used to determine the target joint angle. Custom software (Visual Studio 2010, Microsoft, USA) was used to control the rotating paddle and perform real-time sampling of the joint angle. This software was also used to manipulate a computerized version of the auditory cognitive task. Headphones (HP-RX700, Victor, Japan) were used for listening during the cognitive task.

2.3. Tasks and Procedure

2.3.1. Ipsilateral Ankle Position-Matching Task. Blindfolded participants were seated with their dominant foot (right for all participants) secured with straps onto rotating paddles (Figure 1). In the target-encoding phase, the participants plantarflexed the ankle joint to 20° or 25° from the 0° (neutral) position using either active movement or operation of the rotating paddle (passive movement). This target position was maintained for 12 s, allowing the participants to encode it into their memories. After the target-encoding phase, the ankle was returned to the start position, and then the paddle automatically moved the ankle toward the target angle. The participants were asked to press a hand switch when they felt that their ankle had reached the target angular position. Participants performed the position-matching task 9 times, and the target joint angle was randomly assigned.

2.3.2. Cognitive Task (Computerized Version of the Auditory Serial Subtraction Task). The cognitive task was a computerized version of the auditory serial subtraction task (ASST), in which participants were instructed to continuously subtract a selected number from a randomly selected two-digit number [13, 19]. Participants performed the subtraction task during the 12 s position-encoding phase. The initial number and the pitch of ASST were produced through the headphones, while participants had to provide an answer for ASST verbally. ASST was selected because (a) processing of the task was based on mental arithmetic and (b) it allowed the investigation of different levels of cognitive difficulty and manipulation of the pitch with a programming algorithm.

In experiment 1a, the participants were asked to continuously subtract 3 from the randomly selected two-digit number for 3 s during the 12 s position-encoding phase (i.e., 4 subtraction tasks during 12 s). In experiment 1b, the

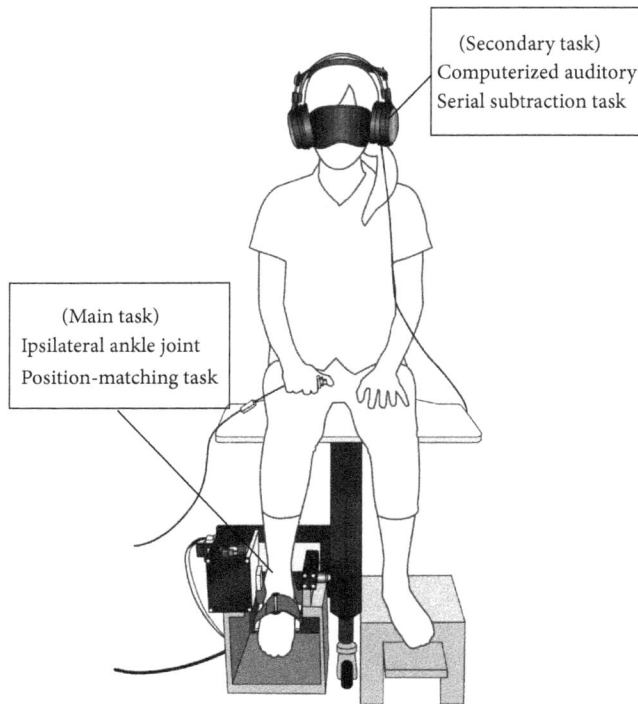

FIGURE 1: Experimental setup.

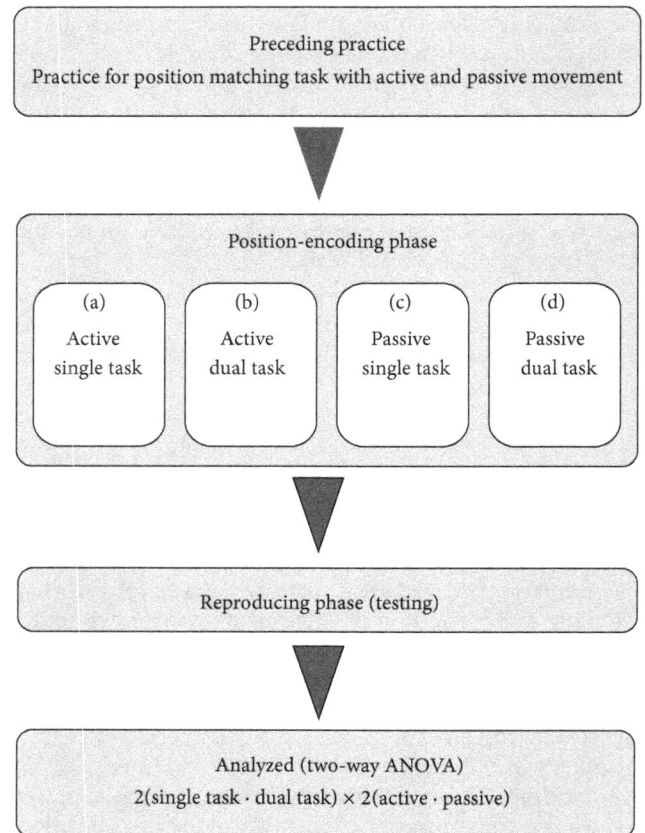

FIGURE 2: Experimental procedure flow diagram.

participants were instructed to continuously subtract 7 from a randomly selected two-digit number for 1 s during the 12 s position-encoding phase (i.e., 12 subtraction tasks during 12 s).

2.3.3. Procedure. The entire procedure (Figure 2) was carried out in an experiment room. At the beginning of the experiment, the participants practiced an ipsilateral position-matching task, in which they tried as accurately as possible to detect a predefined target angle. Two minutes after the end of the initial practice session, the participants moved on to the experimental session. Participants were subjected to 2 (single task, dual task) × 2 (active, passive) experimental conditions for the ankle position-matching task. The conditions were defined as follows: (a) AS, active × single task; (b) AD, active × dual task; (c) PS, passive × single task; (d) PD, passive × dual task. The order of these conditions was counterbalanced among the participants.

2.4. Outcome Measurements

2.4.1. Position-Matching Errors. Three common error scores were used to measure movement accuracy [18]: AE, absolute error; CE, constant error; VE, variable error. AE is the measurement of the magnitude of the error regardless of the direction. CE is the measurement of response bias in relation to a target. VE measures the consistency of the movement.

Each mean AE of joint reproduction was calculated using the following formula:

$$AE = \frac{\sum |X - C|}{K}. \tag{1}$$

In this formula, AE represents the sum of the error for each trial divided by the number of trials in the block. The variable X represents the raw score, C represents the criterion score desired, and K represents the number of trials. The sign of the value of X is to be ignored when calculating AE.

CE was calculated using the following formula:

$$CE = \frac{\sum (X - C)}{K}. \tag{2}$$

This formula is similar to AE except that the relative sign of each score is considered. VE was calculated using the following formula:

$$VE = \sqrt{\frac{\sum (X - C)^2}{K} - (CE)^2}. \tag{3}$$

In this formula, VE is calculated by taking the square root of the sum of the squared difference between each individual error score and the CE score for that block divided by the number of trials in the block.

TABLE 1: Average joint position-matching errors in experiment 1a (mean ± standard deviation).

	Active/single	Active/dual	Passive/single	Passive/dual
AE	1.73 ± 0.52	1.44 ± 0.46	1.54 ± 0.72	1.63 ± 0.61
CE	0.67 ± 1.16	−0.14 ± 1.09	−0.81 ± 1.06	−0.87 ± 1.12
VE	1.68 ± 0.75	1.49 ± 0.48	1.45 ± 0.47	1.38 ± 0.53

AE: absolute error (degrees); CE: constant error (degrees); VE: variable error (degrees).

2.4.2. Percentage of Correct Answers to the Cognitive Task.
Each time a participant gave an answer during the subtraction task, it was determined to be correct or incorrect. These data were used to calculate the percentage of correct answers.

2.5. Statistical Analysis.
For AE, CE, and VE, a separate statistical analysis was performed. A two-way (attention, movement patterns) analysis of variance (ANOVA) with repeated measures on both factors was performed on each dependent variable. A P value of <0.05 was considered statistically significant. A post hoc comparison using Bonferroni's multiple comparison was performed to determine which comparisons were different.

3. Results

3.1. Experiment 1a

3.1.1. Position-Matching Errors.
The means and standard deviations in the position-matching errors AE, CE, and VE are shown in Table 1. For CE, a two-way ANOVA showed that the main effect, the movement pattern, was significant ($F(1, 60) = 16.14$, $P < 0.01$) (Table 2, Figure 3), which indicated that participants made smaller errors when matching a reference position that was established through passive movement rather than active movement. No other main effects or interactions were significant for any of the measurements.

3.1.2. Percentage of Correct Answers to the Cognitive Task.
The average percentage of correct answers to the cognitive task in the AD condition was 98.4% ± 3.35% and was 97.9% ± 4.68% in the PD condition.

3.2. Experiment 1b (Difficult Cognitive Task)

3.2.1. Position-Matching Errors.
The means and standard deviations of each position-matching error are shown in Table 3. For AE, a 2-way ANOVA showed that the main effect, attention, was significant [$F(1, 60) = 6.80$, $P < 0.05$] (Table 4, Figure 4), which indicated that participants made significantly greater errors in the dual-task conditions than in the single-task conditions. No other main effects or interactions were significant for any of the measurements.

3.2.2. Percentage of Correct Answers to the Cognitive Task.
The average percentage of correct answers to the cognitive task in

TABLE 2: Two-way ANOVA results of the joint position-matching error parameters in experiment 1a. P values derived from ANOVA for the main effects of attention and movement. Interaction between attention and movement.

Joint position-matching errors ($n = 16$)		
	F	P
AE		
Attention (A)	0.43	0.51
Movement (B)	0.00	0.97
A × B	1.73	0.19
CE		
Attention (A)	2.53	0.11
Movement (B)	16.14	0.00**
A × B	1.80	0.18
VE		
Attention (A)	0.82	0.37
Movement (B)	1.38	0.24
A × B	0.19	0.65

AE: absolute error; CE: constant error; VE: variable error. $^{**}P < 0.01$.

the AD condition was 56.1% ± 18.19%; in the PD condition, it was 57.9% ± 18.76%.

4. Discussion

In this study, young adults performed an ipsilateral ankle position-matching task in single- and dual-task conditions. The goal of these experiments was to extend previous findings and to determine whether attentional load influences ankle joint proprioceptive ability in young adults when an ipsilateral position-matching paradigm is adopted. The results showed that participants made significantly more ankle position-matching errors under difficult dual-task conditions than under single-task conditions. These findings support previous findings that allocation of attentional resources toward a secondary task can lead to compromised sensorimotor performance, because of a limitation in the available resources for dealing with two tasks concurrently. Furthermore, we found that the difficulty level of the cognitive task might be the possible critical factor that decreased the accuracy of the position-matching task under dual-task conditions.

To our knowledge, this is the first study to demonstrate that increased attentional demands influence the acuity of the ipsilateral ankle position-matching task in young adults. This result suggests that allocation of limited attentional resources during dual-task conditions interferes with the encoding of ankle position. The reduction in ipsilateral ankle position-matching accuracy seen under the difficult dual-task condition suggests that encoding proprioceptive target information shares a common neural substrate with the ability to allocate memory to encode and perform an arithmetic task. Previous research has shown that older adults with low working memory ability made significantly more elbow-repositioning errors when secondary tasks were present during target

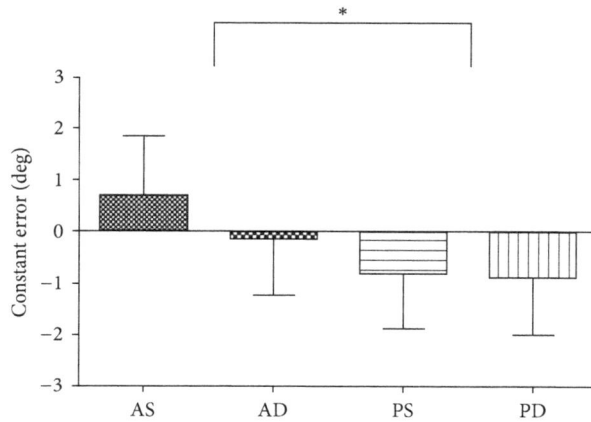

FIGURE 3: Mean ± SD constant errors for each condition in experiment 1a. AS: active/single task, AD: active/dual task, PS: passive/single task, PD: passive/dual task.

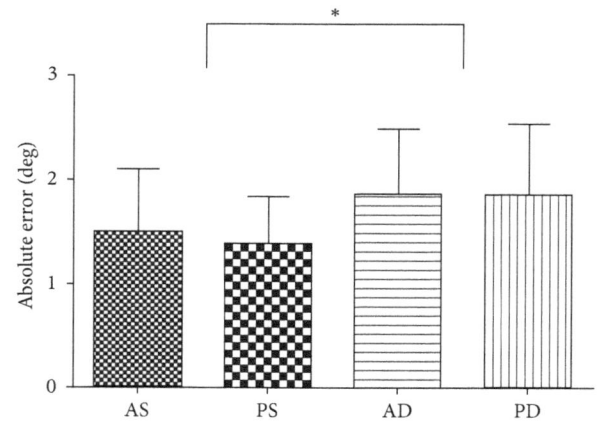

FIGURE 4: Mean ± SD absolute errors for each condition in experiment 1b AS: active/single task, PS: passive/single task, AD: active/dual task, PD: passive/dual task.

TABLE 3: Average joint position-matching errors in experiment 1b (mean ± standard deviation).

	Active/single	Active/dual	Passive/single	Passive/dual
AE	1.56 ± 0.59	1.88 ± 0.65	1.43 ± 0.46	1.90 ± 0.66
CE	−0.15 ± 0.78	−0.19 ± 1.53	−0.37 ± 0.86	−0.33 ± 1.39
VE	1.72 ± 0.54	1.91 ± 0.61	1.44 ± 0.37	1.70 ± 0.43

AE: absolute error (degrees); CE: constant error (degrees); VE: variable error (degrees).

TABLE 4: Two-way ANOVA results of the joint position-matching error parameters in experiment 1b. P values derived from ANOVA for the main effects of attention and movement. Interaction between attention and movement.

Joint position-matching errors ($n = 16$)		
	F	P
AE		
Attention (A)	6.80	0.01 *
Movement (B)	0.14	0.71
A × B	0.27	0.60
CE		
Attention (A)	0.00	1.00
Movement (B)	0.38	0.53
A × B	0.02	0.89
VE		
Attention (A)	3.27	0.07
Movement (B)	3.99	0.05
A × B	0.10	0.75

AE: absolute error; CE: constant error; VE: variable error. * $P < 0.05$.

encoding than both younger and older adults with high working memory ability [11]. In the present study, we selected the ankle joints as the target joints, and in order to clarify the effects of the difficulty of the secondary task, we performed two experiments with two different cohorts: one in which the auditory subtraction task was easy (experiment 1a) and one in which it was difficult (experiment 1b). Our results allow for a streamlined interpretation of the finding that the difficulty of the cognitive task influenced performance in the ipsilateral ankle position-matching task, implying that there is a role for attentional resource in the assessment of ankle proprioception with an ipsilateral position-matching task.

In the present study, although position-matching accuracy (i.e., AE) was not enhanced by active movement during the position-encoding phase of experiment 1a, the results in CE showed that the participants produced undershoot when matching a target position established through passive movement than when matching the same target position encoded actively. This result indicates that the participants tended to underestimate the target position when it was encoded using the passive movement of a rotatory paddle. Some previous studies have demonstrated that CE is not dependent on the mode of target presentation [20, 21], whereas other studies have demonstrated that passive target presentation results in overshooting [22, 23]. These inconsistent findings suggest that the undershooting of passively generated target positions is task dependent. Furthermore, as this tendency was not

replicated in experiment 1b, further studies are necessary to clarify the exact nature of this effect.

Given that most proprioceptive assessments conducted in clinical environments use position-matching tasks administered by therapists, clinicians should note that some portion of the position-matching error reflects cognitive or memory capacity, rather than proprioception itself, when ipsilateral position matching is used in individuals who are prone to having memory issues, such as older people or stroke patients. Furthermore, a previous study has reported differences in dual-task performance that included proprioception-dependent tasks, such as standing and walking [12]. For instance, Harley et al. reported that increased attentional demands during an obstacle-crossing task led to a decrease in obstacle clearance or increased variability in older adults [24]. They predict that, as attention demands increased further, older individuals would show greater reductions in obstacle-crossing performance. When clinical training contains the memory of a movement (i.e., ascending the stairs or stepping over obstacles), cognitive aspects should be taken into account during the assessment of training performance.

There is a methodological issue that limits the conclusions to be drawn from this study. Because the experiments were conducted with relatively young participants, other cohorts where these results could potentially be more relevant (i.e., stroke patients or elderly people) should be included in future studies to exclude the potential for bias occurring in this group of participants. Another limitation of the study is that different cohorts were chosen for the easy (1a) and difficult (1b) tasks in the present study. The reason for the choice of two different cohorts was to avoid a learning effect (i.e., by allowing the participants to become familiar with the dual task procedure). In our pilot study, it became apparent that if someone experiences a difficult cognitive task, they would be able to perform an easier cognitive task without requiring a cognitive load. Thus, we conducted this research with two different cohorts. However, there might be a risk that the difference found was a group effect, rather than an effect of the cognitive task complexity. This is an important issue that warrants additional research (e.g., comparing randomised easy and difficult tasks within the same cohort). In future work, it would also be of interest to address this possibility using a more extensive battery of cognitive tests and to compare the results to standardized norms. Our results raise the question whether other cognitive factors might also influence performance on tests of ankle proprioceptive performance.

5. Conclusion

The present study showed that performing a secondary cognitive task resulted in decreased ipsilateral ankle position-matching performance relative to single-task conditions in young healthy participants. This tendency was observed only for the cohort that performed a difficult cognitive task. Therefore, the difficulty level of the cognitive task might be the possible critical factor that decreased accuracy in the position-matching task under dual-task conditions. These results indicate that allocation of attentional resources toward a difficult cognitive task can lead to compromised sensorimotor performance, because of a limitation in resources available for concurrently coping with both tasks. Further studies that include a larger sample and greater diversity of individuals are necessary to validate our conclusions and findings in a clinical setting.

Conflict of Interests

There is no conflict of interests to declare.

Acknowledgment

This study was supported by the Japanese Society for the Promotion of Science (JSPS) under the Founding Program for Next Generation World-Leading Researchers (NEXT Program).

References

[1] J. H. Pasma, T. A. Boonstra, S. F. Campfens, A. C. Schouten, and H. van der Kooij, "Sensory reweighting of proprioceptive information of the left and right leg during human balance control," *Journal of Neurophysiology*, vol. 108, no. 4, pp. 1138–1148, 2012.

[2] J. Duysens, V. P. Beerepoot, P. H. Veltink, V. Weerdesteyn, and B. C. M. Smits-Engelsman, "Proprioceptive perturbations of stability during gait," *Neurophysiologie Clinique*, vol. 38, no. 6, pp. 399–410, 2008.

[3] J. Jeka, K. S. Oie, and T. Kiemel, "Multisensory information for human postural control: integrating touch and vision," *Experimental Brain Research*, vol. 134, no. 1, pp. 107–125, 2000.

[4] H. van der Kooij, R. Jacobs, B. Koopman, and H. Grootenboer, "A multisensory integration model of human stance control," *Biological Cybernetics*, vol. 80, no. 5, pp. 299–308, 1999.

[5] R. W. M. van Deursen and G. G. Simoneau, "Foot and ankle sensory neuropathy, proprioception, and postural stability," *Journal of Orthopaedic and Sports Physical Therapy*, vol. 29, no. 12, pp. 718–726, 1999.

[6] F. B. Horak, L. M. Nashner, and H. C. Diener, "Postural strategies associated with somatosensory and vestibular loss," *Experimental Brain Research*, vol. 82, no. 1, pp. 167–177, 1990.

[7] D. J. Goble, "Proprioceptive acuity assessment via joint position matching: from basic science to general practice," *Physical Therapy*, vol. 90, no. 8, pp. 1176–1184, 2010.

[8] D. E. Adamo, B. J. Martin, and S. H. Brown, "Age-related differences in upper limb proprioceptive acuity," *Perceptual and Motor Skills*, vol. 104, no. 3, part 2, pp. 1297–1309, 2007.

[9] W. G. Darling, "Perception of forearm angles in 3-dimensional space," *Experimental Brain Research*, vol. 87, no. 2, pp. 445–456, 1991.

[10] O. Bock, "Joint position sense in simulated changed-gravity environments," *Aviation Space and Environmental Medicine*, vol. 65, no. 7, pp. 621–626, 1994.

[11] D. J. Goble, M. A. Mousigian, and S. H. Brown, "Compromised encoding of proprioceptively determined joint angles in older adults: the role of working memory and attentional load," *Experimental Brain Research*, vol. 216, no. 1, pp. 35–40, 2012.

[12] M. Woollacott and A. Shumway-Cook, "Attention and the control of posture and gait: a review of an emerging area of research," *Gait and Posture*, vol. 16, no. 1, pp. 1–14, 2002.

[13] P. A. Pope and R. C. Miall, "Task-specific facilitation of cognition by cathodal transcranial direct current stimulation of the cerebellum," *Brain Stimulation*, vol. 5, no. 2, pp. 84–94, 2012.

[14] G. E. Stelmach, J. A. Kelso, and S. A. Wallace, "Preselection in short-term motor memory," *Journal of Experimental Psychology*, vol. 1, no. 6, pp. 745–755, 1975.

[15] Y. Laufer, S. Hocherman, and R. Dickstein, "Accuracy of reproducing hand position when using active compared with passive movement," *Physiotherapy Research International*, vol. 6, no. 2, pp. 65–75, 2001.

[16] M. Kawato and D. Wolpert, "Internal models for motor control," *Novartis Foundation Symposium*, vol. 218, pp. 291–307, 1998.

[17] D. M. Wolpert and Z. Ghahramani, "Computational principles of movement neuroscience," *Nature Neuroscience*, vol. 3, pp. 1212–1217, 2000.

[18] R. Granit, "Constant errors in the execution and appreciation of movement," *Brain*, vol. 95, no. 4, pp. 451–460, 1972.

[19] D. M. A. Gronwall, "Paced auditory serial addition task: a measure of recovery from concussion," *Perceptual and Motor Skills*, vol. 44, no. 2, pp. 367–373, 1977.

[20] S. V. Adamovich, M. B. Berkinblit, O. Fookson, and H. Poizner, "Pointing in 3D space to remembered targets. I. Kinesthetic versus visual target presentation," *Journal of Neurophysiology*, vol. 79, no. 6, pp. 2833–2846, 1998.

[21] S. V. Adamovich, M. B. Berkinblit, O. Fookson, and H. Poizner, "Pointing in 3D space to remembered targets. II: effects of movement speed toward kinesthetically defined targets," *Experimental Brain Research*, vol. 125, no. 2, pp. 200–210, 1999.

[22] R. G. Marteniuk, "Retention characteristics of motor short-term memory cues," *Journal of Motor Behavior*, vol. 5, no. 4, pp. 249–259, 1973.

[23] E. A. Roy and C. MacKenzie, "Handedness effects in kinesthetic spatial location judgements," *Cortex*, vol. 14, no. 2, pp. 250–258, 1978.

[24] C. Harley, R. M. Wilkie, and J. P. Wann, "Stepping over obstacles: attention demands and aging," *Gait and Posture*, vol. 29, no. 3, pp. 428–432, 2009.

17

Game Analysis, Validation, and Potential Application of EyeToy Play and Play 2 to Upper-Extremity Rehabilitation

Yu-ping Chen,[1,2] **Michelle Caldwell,**[1] **Erica Dickerhoof,**[1] **Anastasia Hall,**[1] **Bryan Odakura,**[1] **Kimberly Morelli,**[1] **and Hsin-Chen Fanchiang**[2]

[1]*Department of Physical Therapy, Georgia State University, P.O. Box 4019, Atlanta, GA 30302-4019, USA*
[2]*Center for Pediatric Locomotion Sciences, Georgia State University, Atlanta, GA 30302-3975, USA*

Correspondence should be addressed to Yu-ping Chen; ypchen@gsu.edu

Academic Editor: Nicola Smania

Objective. To describe and analyze the potential use of games in the commercially available EyeToy Play and EyeToy Play 2 on required/targeted training skills and feedback provided for clinical application. *Methods.* A summary table including all games was created. Two movement experts naïve to the software validated required/targeted training skills and feedback for 10 randomly selected games. Ten healthy school-aged children played to further validate the required/targeted training skills. *Results.* All but two (muscular and cardiovascular endurance) had excellent agreement in required/targeted training skills, and there was 100% agreement on feedback. Children's performance in required/targeted training skills (number of unilateral reaches and bilateral reaches, speed, muscular endurance, and cardiovascular endurance) significantly differed between games ($P < .05$). *Conclusion.* EyeToy Play games could be used to train children's arm function. However, a careful evaluation of the games is needed since performance might not be consistent between players and therapists' interpretation.

1. Introduction

Recently, virtual reality (VR) has been explored as a training device for improving arm function in adults following stroke [1–5] and for children with cerebral palsy (CP) [6–8]. VR is a computer technology that creates an artificial but highly realistic graphical context and populates it with dynamic objects that allow users to interact with that context [9–12]. The process enables the creation of an exercise environment in which participants, either patients with stroke or children with CP, can practice their arm movements intensively and receive visual and auditory feedback. There are several inexpensive, commercial VR gaming systems available now (e.g., PlayStation 2 with EyeToy Camera, Nintendo Wii systems, and Microsoft Kinect system), which increase the accessibility of utilizing VR systems for rehabilitation purposes like training arm function. Consequently, researchers have begun to investigate the effects of these commercially available games on the improvement of arm function in patients with stroke or children with CP [1, 2, 5–8]. The research has shown

the potential for using the games to improve some aspects of arm function.

There are challenges in applying commercially available VR systems that were designed for recreation to do rehabilitation [13]. Deutsch et al. [13] noted that some interfaces might require adaptation (e.g., the Wii remote controller requires good hand control) and the level of difficulty of the games might not be suitable for some players, especially those with impaired arm function. Moreover, the skills required to play games might vary, which makes game selection difficult.

Deutsch et al. [13] created a detailed "game analysis table" to describe the games listed in Wii Sports and Wii Fit (Nintendo of America, Inc., Redmond, Washington), including game-related features (description, scoring, and progression), equipment used, length of game, feedback provided (knowledge of results or knowledge of performance), and impairments that can potentially benefit from the training (balance, coordination, endurance, strength, and upper-extremity control). They validated their game analyses by rating the agreement of two experienced physical therapists who were naïve to the games on feedback and impairment type. The researchers reported 100% agreement between raters on ratings for impairment type and between 50% to 100% agreement on feedback provided.

In this study, we analyzed and validated games in the SONY PlayStation 2 EyeToy Play and EyeToy Play 2 (Sony Computer Entertainment American LLC, San Meteo, CA). EyeToy Play was selected because this system uses a USB camera as the method to capture players' motions, so that the players can see themselves as they are immersed in the virtual world. This software has been used in several studies to train arm movements in patients with stroke or children with CP and has been found effective [1, 2, 5–8]. Moreover, at $150 for a new system, the selected unit is at the low end of the price range for commercially available video consoles. It thus has the greatest potential to be widely used in clinics and in children's homes. The purpose of this paper is to (1) provide a detailed summary table describing all the games in EyeToy Play and EyeToy Play 2 and (2) analyze and validate the specific games in EyeToy Play and EyeToy Play 2 for their potential to train for upper-extremity function in children. Finally, specific recommendations for upper-extremity function in children are also discussed.

2. Materials and Methods

This study included two phases: Phase I—creating a game summary table and Phase II—validating the items in the summary table using two movement experts (Phase II-1) and 10 typically developing children (Phase II-2).

2.1. Phase I: Game Analysis and Game Summary Table Creation. The first author (YC), who was experienced in using EyeToy Play and EyeToy Play 2 games to train children with cerebral palsy, created the items needed for inclusion in the game analysis table. These items were similar to Deutsch et al. [13] and included game features (e.g., goal of the game as listed by the software brochure, object to interact with), required/targeted training skills (e.g., unilateral reaching, bilateral reaching), feedback provided (e.g., knowledge of results), and special notes/comments (e.g., "game rules are unclear"). All items in the required/targeted training skills and feedback categories were defined based on motor learning and rehabilitation references (see Table 1 for definitions) [14–18]. Next, the first author and five physical therapy students played all the games as many times as needed to become conversant with them (range 5–8 times) and worked together to summarize each game in EyeToy Play and EyeToy Play 2 using the items listed earlier to describe the game, required/targeted training skills, feedback provided, and special comments. Table 2 provides an example of the "Beat Freak" game from EyeToy Play.

2.2. Phase II: Validation Process of Game Summary Table

2.2.1. Validation by Movement Experts. To determine agreement on the required/targeted training skills and feedback sections of the game summary table, a physical therapist

rater (KM) with more than 10 years of clinical experience in physical therapy and a movement scientist (HF) with a background in motor learning, biomechanics, and motion analysis evaluated 10 games randomly. The games were selected by putting all the relevant names from the game list into a bag and then randomly picking 10, similar to the method used by Deutsch et al. [13]. Six games from the EyeToy Play (Beat Freak, Kung Fu, Rocket Rumble, Slap Stream, Soccer Craze, and Wishi Washi) and four games from the EyeToy Play 2 (Bubble Pop, Goal Attack, Table Tennis, and Kung 2) were selected.

The two raters were naïve EyeToy players and seldom played video games. A short instruction session was conducted to go over the definitions of each item in the required/targeted training skills and feedback sections. The raters took turns playing and observing each other playing the game, and they were allowed as much time as they wanted for this phase. They then made ratings independently of each other after playing the game. Ratings were based on each rater's own playing experience as well as their observations of the other person. All items were rated either a "yes" or a "no." The raters also commented on whether to recommend the game as part of a therapeutic program for children who need to train their upper-extremity function. Percentage of agreement between the raters was then calculated. After the rating process was completed, a discussion session was held between the two raters and the first author in order to arrive at consensus on any inconsistent ratings. Changes were made in the game summary table if the consensus was different from the summary table (2 games on muscular endurance and 2 games on cardiovascular endurance were changed after discussion).

2.2.2. Validation by Testing Healthy Typically Developing Children. We further validated the required/targeted training skills section in our game summary table by having healthy, typically developing children play EyeToy Play and EyeToy Play 2 games. In this paper, we presented only unilateral reaching, bilateral reaching, speed, muscular endurance, and cardiovascular endurance as these items did not reach 100% agreement during the validation process by two movement experts (see Section 3 for details). We intentionally used children with typical development in this validation process because we needed to establish our reasonable expectations for children's regular performance in the commercial games before using a group of children with clinical diagnosis.

Participants. Ten children aged 6 to 12 years participated in this validation process (mean age: 8.20 ± 1.69 years old, 6 females 4 males). All participants were recruited from flyers or by word of mouth and were reported by their parents to be free of any neurological or orthopedic diseases and to have typical physical and cognitive development. Parents or legal guardians of the children signed an informed consent form prior to testing, and oral assents were obtained from the children.

Apparatus. The game console used was PlayStation 2 with EyeToy camera. The image was projected to a large screen

TABLE 1: Definitions of required/targeted training skills and feedback provided.

	Conceptual definition used in Phases I and II-1 validation by two movement experts	Operational definition used in Phase II-2 validation by testing healthy children
Required/targeted training skills		
Unilateral reaching	Movements of the upper extremities that use 1 hand or arm.	Number of upper-extremity movements using 1 hand between 30 seconds after play started and 1 minute and 30 seconds.
Bilateral reaching	Movements of the upper extremities that use 2 hands or arms. Bilateral reaching can be symmetrical (both arms perform the same joint motions) or alternative (e.g., one arm is extending while the other is flexing).	Number of upper-extremity movements using both hands between 30 seconds after play started and 1 minute and 30 seconds.
Speed	The game requires the player to reach faster, since faster is better.	Number of arm movements per minute
Cognition	This game requires some cognitive abilities. For example, someone with intellectual disabilities may not understand the game rules and may not be able to play the game.	†
Accuracy	The game requires some precision.	†
Muscular endurance	The ability of muscle to sustain forces repeatedly or to generate forces over a period of time. Muscular endurance refers to the body's ability to continue using muscular strength and endure repeated contractions for an extended period of time. Usually, if the game requires the player to constantly repeat the same arm movements over time, it requires muscular endurance.	Total number of arm movements performed in the 3-minute interval
Cardiovascular endurance	The ability of the body to sustain prolonged rhythmical exercise and perform work and participate in an activity over time. Cardiovascular endurance is the power, strength, or ability of the heart to supply enough oxygen to muscles during a physical activity for a prolonged period of time. It essentially indicates how strong one's heart is and can potentially add years to one's life. This can be measured by heart rate change.	Four heart rate related indicators: maximal heart rate change, maximal heart rate, average heart rate, and percentage of heart rate reserve = (maximal heart rate during the game—resting heart rate)/[(208—age $*$ 0.7) —resting heart rate]
Eye-hand coordination	The coordinated control of eye movement with hand movement. The ability to guide the movements of the hand with the eyes.	†
Strength	Muscle force exerted by a group of muscles to overcome a resistance in a specific set of circumstances.	†
Feedback provided		
Knowledge of results	Information about the outcome of the action Individual action: information about the outcome of each action (e.g., a banging sound after hitting an object). Whole game: information about the outcome after playing the whole game (e.g., the total score of the game, number of opponents being hit)	†
Knowledge of performance	Information about the pattern of action, for example, the player can see his/her movement while performing the task.	†

†: reach 100% agreement during the validation process by two movement experts in Phase II-1. It did not include Phase II-2 validation.

on the wall (size: 264 cm × 220 cm) to create better visibility for the children to interact with the virtual objects in the game. Nine games from the Validation Phase 1 were tested with these children, including Beat Freak, Bubble Pop, Goal Attack, Kung Fu, Rocket Rumble, Slap Stream, Soccer Craze, Table Tennis, and Wishi Washi. One game (Kung 2) from the previous list was not used because (1) this game was very similar to the original Kung Fu, which might have left the children feeling bored and uninterested, and (2) the agreement on this game between the two movement experts was already excellent. The order of games to be played was randomized (using a table of random numbers) by a student who was not aware of the study purpose and naïve to these games.

Participants' heart rate was measured using a Puma Children's Heart Rate monitoring system. A digital camera

TABLE 2: Example of a complete game analysis table, using "Beat Freak" from EyeToy Play.

	Beat freak
(I) Game features	
Goal of the game	Follow the CDs to hit the speakers to play the music.
Context	Reach to strike the speakers in the four corners of the screen just as the CD reaches them. There are a few cartoon characters at the bottom of the screen dancing and cheering for the player; however, they may impede the player's view of their movements when hitting the speakers at the two lower corners.
Objects to interact with	CDs
Object location	From the center to one of the 4 speakers located in the 4 corners.
Appearance of the object	About 1.3-1.4 seconds
Total duration of the game	3 minutes
Number of objects to interact with at once	1–4
Disturbing effects	None
Avoiding objects/effects	None
Speed of object appearance	10 CDs/the first 20 seconds
Method to advance to different levels within the same game	None
Method to end the game	Time is up or miss 3 CDs
(II) Required skills	
Unilateral reaching	Yes
Bilateral reaching	Yes (for both symmetrical or asymmetrical)
Speed	Yes
Cognition	Yes
Accuracy	Yes
Muscular endurance	Yes
Cardiovascular endurance	No
Eye-hand coordination	Yes
Strength	Yes
(III) Feedback provided	
Knowledge of results: individual action	Yes: auditory (when hitting the speaker) and visual (speaker lights up)
Knowledge of results: whole game	Yes: score
Knowledge of performance	Yes: the player can see his/her movement
(IV) Special notes	Increase in speed and randomness throughout the game

(Apple, iPhone 5, at 30 Hz) was placed about 15 degrees from the child's midline in front of the child to record the whole play sessions.

Procedures. All the testing took place in a university classroom. After assent and consent were obtained from children and their parent or legal guardians, participants placed the heart rate monitor strap around their chest and were asked to sit quietly for 5 minutes in order to measure their resting heart rate. Then the participants played nine EyeToy games in random order. One researcher was seated behind the participant to obtain the heart rate measurement from the heart rate monitor. For each game, the participant practiced the game for about 30 seconds before the recording started. The participant was instructed to play the game for 3 minutes, and heart rate was recorded at initiation and at 1-minute intervals. Rarely, if the game was accidentally interrupted before 3 minutes, a researcher reactivated the game immediately.

Participants took a 5-minute break after finishing each game and listened to the researcher explaining the rules for the next game. This break allowed participants' heart rate to return to its regular level. The parent was present throughout the testing period.

Data Reduction. Video data were exported to a computer and coded by the first author using Windows Movie Maker. The number of unilateral reaches, bilateral reaches, and total reaches was coded from the video using slow-motion and a frame-by-frame mode. Unilateral reaches were defined as the unilateral extension of one arm towards the location of a virtual object [19]. While one arm was moving, the other arm was held still, regardless of position (e.g., held at shoulder height or at the side of the body). Bilateral reaches were defined as simultaneous performance of both arm movements. To constitute a bilateral reach, the two arms did not need to move in the same direction, but both arms had to be moving. Our definitions were consistent with those of Deutsch et al. [13] and Corbetta and Thelen [20]. Unilateral and bilateral reaches were coded starting around 30 seconds after play started and coding continued for 1 minute. We did not code the complete trial or use the complete dataset to avoid the possible influence of fatigue on reaching frequency and also to avoid having a familiarization period, even though the participants had practiced before data collection. Since children could have a different number of reaches in the period of data collection, we converted the number of unilateral and bilateral reaches into percentages to normalize individual differences. The number of reaches per minute was used to represent speed. Reaches per minute were derived by combining the number of unilateral reaches and bilateral reaches within the coded minute. The higher number of reaches per minute is produced, the faster movement is required (i.e., faster speed).

We used the total number of reaches in the 3-minute interval as an indicator of muscular endurance since the more the reaches done by players, the greater the chance that the players would experience fatigue of the arm. If their muscular endurance was not good, they might do fewer reaches during the 3-minute session.

We also determined whether playing the games required cardiovascular endurance by measuring players' heart rate at initiation and at 1-minute intervals. Four different heart-rate related variables were computed to represent the potential usefulness of each game for training cardiovascular endurance: maximal heart rate change, maximal heart rate, average heart rate, and percentage of heart rate reserve ([maximal heart rate during the game − resting heart rate]/[(208 − age ∗ 0.7) − resting heart rate]) [21–23].

Analysis. For this observational study, we used descriptive statistics to report reaches and heart rate change in each game. The percentages of unilateral and bilateral reaches with each game, the number of reaches per minute, total number of reaches, and maximal heart rate change, maximal heart rate, average heart rate, and percentage of heart rate reserve with each game were compared between games using repeated analysis of variance (ANOVA), with games as the repeated factor. A preplanned paired t test was used to determine where the differences were once the repeated ANOVA reached significance. All the analyses were conducted using SPSS 18.0.

3. Results

3.1. Game Summary Table. The completed game summary table for the EyeToy Play and EyeToy Play 2 games is in Table 3, which includes game related features, required/targeted training skills, feedback provided, and recommendations. A summary of the number of games in EyeToy Play and EyeToy Play 2 that could potentially train the required/targeted skills is given in Table 4.

There are 12 games each in the EyeToy Play and EyeToy Play 2 software. Our analyses showed that 11 games in EyeToy Play and 10 games in EyeToy Play 2 enabled players to practice unilateral reaching; all the games in EyeToy

Play and 8 games in Play 2 enabled practice of bilateral reaching. Most of the games targeted speed, accuracy, eye-hand coordination, and strength. Muscular endurance was targeted in 9 games each in EyeToy Play and EyeToy Play 2. Only 3 games in EyeToy Play and 1 game in EyeToy Play 2 targeted cardiovascular endurance, but this finding might be due to the difficulty in monitoring a player's heart rate without the proper apparatus (i.e., a heart rate monitor). All the games provided "Knowledge of Results" (KR) feedback, and all games but one provided "Knowledge of Performance" (KP) feedback.

Seven games from EyeToy Play and 9 games from EyeToy Play 2 are recommended to children who need to train upper-extremity function (see Table 3). Games were not recommended for children for the following reasons: four games (Plate Spinner, Mirror Game, UFO Juggler, and Monkey Bar) were not recommended because of difficult or confusing game rules, one game (Ghost Eliminator) was not recommended because of the scary scene, one game (Air Guitar) had no real reaching movements, and one game (Home Run) has a small and blurred display of the player on the screen. Among the recommended games, all but one (Goal Attack) can be used to train unilateral reaching, and all but two (Table Tennis and Secret Agent) can be used to train bilateral reaching. All of the recommended games target speed and strength and can provide KR and KP feedback. Four games in EyeToy Play and 8 games in EyeToy Play 2 require some cognition involvement; five games in EyeToy Play and all games in EyeToy Play 2 target accuracy during play.

3.2. Validation of Game Summary Table—by Two Independent Raters. Agreement between the two experts on items in the required/targeted training skills section ranged between 70% and 100%; agreement on items in the feedback category was 100%. The lowest agreement scores were on endurance-related items (70% and 80% for muscular and cardiovascular endurance, resp.). Agreement between raters on each game ranged between 83% and 100%, with the lowest agreement on Soccer Craze (83%). Percent agreement between the raters is shown in Table 5.

3.3. Validation of Game Summary Table—by Testing 10 Children

Unilateral and Bilateral Reaching. All these games produced both unilateral and bilateral reaches. However, there were statistically significant differences between games ($F(8, 32) = 4.565$, $P = .001$). Children who played Slap Stream used mainly unilateral reaching, rather than bilateral reaching. Kung Fu, Rocket Rumble, Beat Freak, Table Tennis, Bubble Pop, and Soccer Craze also elicited more unilateral than bilateral reaching (see Table 6). Children used equal amount of unilateral and bilateral reaching when they played Wishi Washi, and they mainly used bilateral reaching when playing Goal Attack. These differences were statistically significant ($P < .05$).

TABLE 3: Game analysis table for the games in EyeToy Play and EyeToy Play 2.

EyeToy Play

Game	Goal	Context	Unilateral	Bilateral	Speed	Cognition	Accuracy	Muscular endurance	CV endurance	Eye-hand coordination	Strength	KR individual	KR-whole game	KP	Recommendation
Beat Freak	Follow the CDs to hit the speakers to play the music.	Reach to strike the speakers in the four corners of the screen just as the CD reaches them.	Y	Y	Y	Y	Y	Y	N	Y	Y	Auditory and visual	Score	Player's mvts	Y
Slap Stream	Hit the mice, but not the bunny girls.	Four clouds located at 4 corners with mouse or bunny appearing randomly.	Y	Y	Y	Y	Y	Y	N	Y	Y	Auditory and visual	Score	Player's mvts	Y
Wishi Washi	Clean as many windows as possible before the time runs out.	A window with soap all over needs to be cleaned using any upper-extremity movements. When soap is cleaned, the player will be seen.	Y	Y	Y	N	N	Y	Y	N	Y	Visual	Number of windows	Trajectory of hand mvts	Y
Kung Foo	Knock off the creatures and break the boards during bonus game.	Two towers located at the sides with creatures coming out from upper or lower windows or from the ground.	Y	Y	Y	N	Y	Y	N	Y	Y	Auditory and visual	Score	Player's mvts	Y
Soccer Craze	Keep the soccer ball(s) from hitting the ground as well as trying to hit the "bad guys" in the windows.	Two buildings located at each side with "bad guys" randomly appearing from one of the windows to interrupt hitting the soccer ball. The soccer ball is falling from the sky and the player needs to keep it up.	Y	Y	Y	Y	Y	Y	N	Y	Y	Visual	Score	Player's mvts	Y
Rocket Rumble	Catch the rocket to create a firework show.	Rockets appear from the bottom of the screen. The player needs to touch the rockets with the same color and then push handle at either side to create a firework show.	Y	Y	Y	Y	Y	Y	N	Y	Y	Auditory and visual	Score	Player's mvts	Y

TABLE 3: Continued.

Game	Goal	Context	Unilateral	Bilateral	Speed	Cognition	Accuracy	Muscular endurance	CV endurance	Eye-hand coordination	Strength	KR individual	KR-whole game	KP	Recommendation
Boxing Chump	Try to knock out the opponent in the boxing match.	Player must sit at an angle to the screen and use as many arm movements as possible to knock out the opponent and avoid being hit.	Y	Y	Y	N	N	Y	Y	Y	Y	Auditory	Score and energy bar	Player's mvts	Y
Plate Spinner	Spin the plates and try to keep the monkeys from knocking the plates over.	Four plate spinners located at each side with two higher and two lower. The player needs to constantly move the spinners to prevent the plates from falling.	N	Y	Y	Y	N	Y	Y	Y	Y	Visual	Score	Player's mvts	N
Mirror Game	Hit the green balls but avoid the red ones.	Four balls located at 4 corners of the screen. The player needs to hit the green balls but not the red ones. The screen will flip right/left and upside down (mirrored images) to make this game very difficult	Y	Y	Y	Y	Y	N	N	Y	Y	Auditory and visual	Score	Player's mvts	N
Ghost Eliminator	Wave the player's hand over the ghosts and bats to make them disappear.	Ghosts and bats appear from different locations of the screen. The scene displays a cemetery and a dark castle at night, which may be scary to kids.	Y	Y	Y	N	Y	N	N	Y	Y	Visual	Score	Player's mvts	N
Disco Stars	Imitate the dance moves of the disco girl on stage.	A disco star dances on the stage, and the player needs to copy her moves and rhythm. The star will point to 1 or 2 of the 5 lights on the top of the screen and the player needs to imitate the moves and tempo.	Y	N	N	Y	Y	N	N	Y	Y	Visual (written comment)	Score	Player's mvts	N
UFO Juggler	Spin the UFOs so they can elevate and fly off to safety.	UFOs randomly appear from the bottom of the screen. The player needs to constantly wave to keep spinning the UFOs, but too much spinning will also cause UFOs to blow up.	Y*	Y*	N	Y	Y	Y	N	Y	Y	Visual	Score	Player's mvts	N

TABLE 3: Continued.

Game	Goal	Context	Unilateral	Bilateral	Speed	Cognition	Accuracy	Muscular endurance	CV endurance	Eye-hand coordination	Strength	KR individual	KR-whole game	KP	Recommendation
		EyeToy Play 2													
Bubble Pop	Reach with one or both arms to pop all the blue bubbles and avoid popping the red bubbles before the time runs out.	The locations and proportions of the blue and red bubbles vary at different levels. The more advanced the level is, the harder it is to pop all the blue bubbles as they may require very precise aiming movements.	Y	Y	Y	Y	Y	Y	N	Y	Y	Auditory and visual	Score	Player's mvts	Y
Goal Attack	Use both arms to block the soccer ball to the side or above the player's head.	The player needs to successfully block the soccer ball from entering the net during practice trial (a ball machine) or from the opponent team member.	Y	Y	Y	Y	Y	N	N	Y	Y	Auditory and visual	Score	Player's mvts	Y
Table Tennis	Use the player's hands as paddles to hit the ping-pong balls.	Different opponents to compete and bonus round (e.g., to break the glass bottles, to squeeze tankers, etc.)	Y	N	Y	Y	Y	Y	N	Y	Y	Visual	Score	Player's mvts	Y
Kung 2	Punch all small ninjas appearing from different parts of the screen.	Small ninjas may appear from any location of the screen. The player needs to hit the ninjas and ninjas' weapons to avoid losing "lives."	Y	Y	Y	Y	Y	Y	N	Y	Y	Auditory and visual	Score and energy bar	Player's mvts	Y
DIY	Successfully complete common household tasks and chores.	Eight household tasks randomly appear: grab saw, leaky pipes, stack bricks, wood chipper, demolish wall, tiles, and cutting logs, and hammer the nails.	Y†	Y†	Y	Y	Y	Y	N	Y	Y	Auditory and visual	Score	Player's mvts	Y
Air Guitar	The player pretends to play a guitar, constantly strumming and cued to "grasp" the cord on the neck of the guitar at regular intervals.	A guitar appears on the screen and the player pretends to play. A cue is offered and the player needs to "catch" the falling "cues" and then strum the guitar in order to play music.	N	N	N	N	N	N	N	N	N	Auditory and visual	Score and music	Only player's fingers appear on screen. No KP	N

TABLE 3: Continued.

Game	Goal	Context	Unilateral	Bilateral	Speed	Cognition	Accuracy	Muscular endurance	CV endurance	Eye-hand coordination	Strength	KR individual	KR-whole game	KP	Recommendation
Secret Agent	Reach in all directions to capture the assigned objects that are falling from the top of the screen or present at any locations of the screen.	Different scenarios with different assignments: (1) prison cell—grab 6 hacksaws to avoid the cameras or be perfectly still to avoid detection; (2) rooftop—collect 8 ropes to avoid the search light or be perfectly still to avoid detection; (3) courtyard—steal 8 keys and avoid the search light.	Y	N	Y	Y	Y	Y	N	Y	Y	Visual	Score and words ("mission complete")	Player's mvts	Y
Drumming	Strike certain drums as the game cues them to	Six drums on the lower half of the screen: 3 at each side. A red note cue flies from the center to the drum and the player needs to strike the drum accordingly.	Y	Y	Y	Y	Y	Y	N	Y	Y	Auditory and visual	Score and music	Player's mvts	Y
Home Run	To hit the baseball to make it a home run. An indicator shows in front of the player to help the player determine the timing to hit the ball.	The player would be positioned as a hitter to hit the baseball. There are crowds cheering, and there is a virtual pitcher that throws the baseball. The virtual distance the ball flies will be displayed like a real baseball game.	Y	Y	Y	Y	Y	Y	N	Y	Y	Auditory and visual	Score	Player's mvts	Y/N
Mr. Chef	The player makes burgers, milkshakes, and other food.	The player needs to follow the order to grasp the ingredients to make the order within a desired time limit, or to follow the instructions to make the food (e.g., to shake the shaker).	Y	Y	Y	Y	Y	Y	N	Y	Y	Visual	Score	Player's mvts	Y
Knock out	To hit the opponent	Similar to Box Chump in EyeToy Play. The player needs to hit the matched opponent at different angles.	Y	Y	Y	N	Y	Y	Y	Y	Y	Auditory	Score and energy	Player's mvts	Y‡
Monkey Bars	Quite difficult to figure out how to play this game.	A tall building with lots of windows. A monkey needs to climb up and down the building using the 4 corner bottoms but not sure how to activate and move the monkey.	Y	?	Y	Y	Y	?	?	Y	Y	Visual	Score	Unclear	N

Abbreviations: CV: cardiovascular; KR: knowledge of results; KP: knowledge of performance; Y: yes; N: no; mvts: movements; Y*: For UFO juggler, it is more a waving motion than an arm reaching movement. †For DIY game, it depends on the tasks to involve unilateral and/or bilateral reaching; Y‡: although this game can train the child's arm movements, be mindful of violence of this game.

TABLE 4: Summary of number of games that could potentially train the required/targeted skills in EyeToy Play and EyeToy Play 2.

	EyeToy Play	EyeToy Play 2
Unilateral reaching	11 (91.67%)	10 (83.33%)
Bilateral reaching	12 (100%)	8 (66.67%)
Speed	10 (83.33%)	11 (91.67%)
Cognition	8 (66.67%)	10 (83.33%)
Accuracy	9 (75.00%)	11 (91.67%)
Muscular endurance	9 (75.00%)	9 (75.00%)
Cardiovascular endurance	3 (25.00%)	1 (8.33%)
Eye-hand coordination	11 (91.67%)	11 (91.67%)
Strength	12 (100.00%)	11 (91.67%)
Knowledge of results: individual action	12 (100.00%)	12 (100.00%)
Knowledge of results: Whole game	12 (100.00%)	12 (100.00%)
Knowledge of performance	12 (100.00%)	11 (91.67%)
Recommendation	7 (58.33%)	9 (75.00%)

TABLE 5: Percent agreement between two independent raters by game and by item.

By game	Agreement	By item	Agreement
Beat Freak	100.00%	Unilateral reaching	100.00%
Kung Fu	92.31%	Bilateral reaching	90.00%
Rocket Rumble	100.00%	Speed	90.00%
Slap Stream	100.00%	Cognition	100.00%
Soccer Craze	84.62%	Accuracy	100.00%
Wishi Washi	92.31%	Muscular endurance	70.00%
Bubble Pop	92.31%	Cardiovascular endurance	80.00%
Goal Attack	92.31%	Eye-hand coordination	100.00%
Kung 2	100.00%	Strength	100.00%
Table Tennis	92.31%	Feedback provided	100.00%
		Knowledge of results: Individual action	100.00%
		Knowledge of results: Whole game	100.00%
		Knowledge of performance	100.00%
		Recommendation	90.00%

Speed. Number of arm movements ranged from 15.17 to 79.10 per minutes and differed statistically different between games ($F(8, 32) = 3.416$, $P = .006$). Children did more movements per minute when playing WishiWashi and Rocket Rumble and fewer when playing Goal Attack.

Muscular Endurance. Muscular endurance was operationalized as the total number of reaching movements in the 3-minute playing interval. Wishi Washi produced the greatest number of reaches, followed by Bubble Pop, Rocket Rumble, Kung Fu, Soccer Craze, and Beat Freak. Goal Attack produced the smallest number of reaches. Table Tennis and Slap Stream also tended to produce fewer reaches than other games. The difference between games for number of reaches was statistically significant ($F(8, 64) = 3.55$, $P = .002$).

Cardiovascular Endurance. Cardiovascular endurance was operationalized using maximal heart rate change, maximal heart rate, average heart rate, and percentage of heart rate reserve as indicators. All of these variables indicated similar trends: Soccer Craze, Kung Fu, and Wishi Washi elicited the largest maximal heart rate change, maximal heart rate, average heart rate, and percentage of heart rate reserve, followed by Beat Freak, Rocket Rumble, and Table Tennis. Slap Stream, Goal Attack, and Bubble Pop had the smallest heart rate change, maximal heart rate, average heart rate, and percentage of heart rate reserve.

4. Discussion

The primary goals of this study were to provide summary of the games in EyeToy Play and EyeToy Play 2 and to validate the game table for future use by clinicians. Seven games from the EyeToy Play and 9 games from the EyeToy Play2 are recommended for children who need to train upper-extremity function. Almost all of the 16 games can be used to train unilateral and bilateral reaching movements and provide proper feedback. Some games, however, require more cognitive involvement than others, and some games can be specifically used to train for accuracy or for speed of reaching movements. The detailed game analysis table can also help clinicians select the games they recommend to their clients for use in training reaching movements.

Agreement by movement experts on the required/targeted training skills rating ranged from 70% to 100%. As expected, the two items with the lowest agreement were related to endurance (muscular endurance and cardiovascular endurance). Muscular endurance was defined as "the ability of muscle to sustain forces repeatedly or to generate forces over a period of time," but even though we suggested the use of total arm movements during the 3-minute period, this was hard to operationalize because the strategies used to play the games varied slightly between players. For example, when playing the game of Soccer Craze, the two movement experts (i.e., the two raters) in our study used different strategies to complete the game: Rater 1 used quick and short arm movements to keep the soccer ball in the air, while Rater 2 used a different strategy, moving the arm slowly but more precisely. Both strategies worked since both raters were able to play the game for at least 3 minutes. Cardiovascular endurance was also difficult to rate since it is difficult to be measured directly. The rest of the required/targeted training skills were highly consistent between the two raters, showing excellent validity of the game analysis table.

TABLE 6: Quantitative validation of the game analysis table using 10 children with typical development.

Game	Unilateral reaching[*]	Bilateral reaching[*]	Speed[*] (# arm mvts/min)	Number of total arm mvts[*]	Maximal heart rate change[*]	Maximal heart rate[*]	Average heart rate[*]	Percentage of heart rate reserve[*]
Beat Freak	75.04% (12.42%)	24.96% (12.42%)	51.00 (11.32)	187.88 (97.96)	23.60 (18.33)	132.70 (13.14)	122.40 (12.69)	36.10% (14.51%)
Kung Fu	84.76% (12.75%)	15.24% (12.75%)	49.22 (13.84)	166.89 (82.44)	35.10 (17.52)	147.20 (17.62)	130.13 (16.21)	44.63% (17.87%)
Rocket Rumble	81.42% (23.46%)	18.58% (23.46%)	62.78 (36.21)	253.33 (234.52)	23.00 (18.97)	140.90 (25.43)	128.55 (16.75)	41.24% (19.30%)
Slap Stream	98.78% (2.74%)	1.22% (2.74%)	41.11 (13.73)	125.44 (54.02)	16.30 (9.55)	128.60 (10.52)	120.47 (13.58)	33.18% (10.72%)
Soccer Craze	65.80% (36.88%)	34.20% (36.88%)	35.90 (13.63)	159.89 (64.76)	38.60 (21.14)	154.70 (24.82)	137.78 (17.89)	53.18% (20.47%)
Wishi Washi	54.67% (42.15%)	45.33% (42.15%)	79.10 (32.78)	456.78 (415.93)	33.50 (17.83)	145.60 (17.65)	131.43 (17.23)	46.74% (18.40%)
Bubble Pop	75.52% (12.56%)	24.48% (12.56%)	40.14 (21.42)	335.22 (421.66)	19.10 (7.52)	131.60 (15.79)	121.30 (14.44)	33.84% (11.46%)
Goal Attack	21.00% (22.26%)	79.00% (22.26%)	15.17 (5.85)	67.33 (38.68)	16.00 (9.80)	129.20 (12.02)	121.15 (12.52)	33.30% (11.46%)
Table Tennis	76.59% (34.19%)	23.41% (34.19%)	33.56 (15.37)	125.56 (68.38)	25.20 (16.61)	133.40 (16.22)	121.65 (12.58)	35.17% (16.82%)

[*]$P < .05$: a statistical significance was found between games; the value in parentheses is the standard deviation; mvts: movements.

Unlike the rating scheme for feedback (KR or KP) developed by Deutsch et al. [13], the two raters agreed 100% on whether the individual games they rated could provide KR and/or KP. One possible explanation would be that we used a dichotomous variable (yes/no) to rate feedback, rather than a Likert scale, which narrowed the range of responses and thus increased the likelihood of agreement. Another possible explanation is that the EyeToy games had a USB camera to capture the player's movements on screen, providing one-to-one corresponding movements, which made the rating of feedback for KP very easy since the player could see his/her movement on the screen.

Our study further validated those games which did not have a perfect agreement by 10 healthy, typically developing children playing the games. We videotaped the children playing the games in a random order and used a heart rate monitor to measure their heart rates. We coded their reaches and counted their total reaching movements during the 3-minute game. Interestingly, although all 9 games elicited unilateral and bilateral reaching, some games produced more unilateral reaches than others (e.g., Slap Stream) and some games elicited more bilateral reaches than others (e.g., Goal Attack). The number of arm movements per minute was used to represent the speed in the required/targeted training skills. Wishi Washi and Rocket Rumble were the two games required fast speed, whereas Goal Attack did not. We used the count of total arm movements during the entire 3-minute session to represent muscular endurance and four heart rate related measures to represent cardiovascular endurance. Wishi Washi, Bubble Pop, and Rocket Rumble produced more arm movements than the other games, indicating that these games might be used for training more muscular endurance if players can finish the game. Interestingly, all 4

heart rate related measures indicated similar trends among the 9 games: Soccer Craze, Kung Fu, and Wishi Washi increased heart rate more than Slap Stream, Goal Attack, and Bubble Pop.

Generally, the ratings between the movement experts and children's performance were quite consistent in unilateral reaching, bilateral reaching, speed, and muscular endurance. Only one game (Goal Attack) differed between the experts and children's performance in speed, which was operationally defined as number of arm movements per minute. The experts rated all games as requiring/targeting speed; however, the children's performance showed that Goal Attack generated just 15 arm movements per minute (in other words, it was relatively slow). Using the standard reported by Lythgo et al. [24, 25], a typical school-aged child doing a daily activity like walking can generate about 30 arm movements per minute, yet Goal Attack produced a slower frequency of arm movements, which was different from the experts' rating. Unilateral reaching, bilateral reaching, and muscular endurance were consistent between the experts' ratings and the children's performance.

Cardiovascular endurance was the item showing the most inconsistency between the experts' rating and children's performance. In the expert's rating, only Wishi Washi required/targeted cardiovascular endurance. However, from the children's performance, all games on average reached at least 33% of their heart rate reserve. It is worth noting that 4 games (Kung Fu, Rocket Rumble, Soccer Craze, and Wishi Washi) exceeded 40% of heart rate reserve, which is the recommendation of the American College of Sport Medicine for aerobic training [18]. This suggests that these games would have the potential to train children's cardiovascular endurance. This inconsistency when rating cardiovascular endurance suggests that therapists might be based on their own experience and expertise to make the exercise prescription to children which may not be accurate because children's movement strategies may differ from adults. If this is true, then therapists would need to observe the children in action in order to make correct recommendations.

There are some limitations in this study. The sample size used in this study was only 10, though the children performed quite consistently among themselves. Future studies should include a larger sample and should also include children with need to train arm function (e.g., cerebral palsy) since their responses may not be the same as those of children with typical development. In addition, the heart rate monitor used in the current study could not store heart rate data; therefore, the actual amount by which heart rate exceeded the training zone (40% of heart rate reserve) could not be calculated. Future studies should include a more sensitive heart rate monitor to examine the effect of VR games on cardiovascular endurance. Also, our definition of "speed" was based on number of arm movements per minute which might not be the best definition, as we did not directly measure the speed of the arm movements. A sensitive motion analysis system and eye tracker may be needed to examine the speed and accuracy of participants' movements and even eye-hand coordination.

5. Conclusion

Our study provides a detailed summary table for the games in Sony PlayStation 2 EyeToy Play and EyeToy Play2. Moreover, although these games are not designed specifically for children who need to train their arm function, our research shows that some of the games studied could be useful therapeutic tools to improve their reaching abilities. For example, if the goal is to target unilateral reaching, Slap Stream might be a good game to train for that. If the goal is to train muscular endurance, Wishi Washi, Bubble Pop, and Rocket Rumble might be the best choices. If cardiovascular endurance is the training goal, Soccer Craze, Kung Fu, and Wishi Washi might be the best games. The advancement of new technology has promise to move treatment forward at a low cost; however, a careful evaluation of the games is needed since performance might not be consistent between players and therapists' interpretation.

Conflict of Interests

The authors declare that there is no conflict of interests regarding the publication of this paper.

Acknowledgments

The authors acknowledge and thank Dr. Shih-Yu Lee for her comments on an earlier draft of this paper. Danielle August, PT, DPT, Sarah Harper, PT, DPT, Krista Penninger, PT, DPT, Lauren Perry, PT, DPT, and LaToyia Williams, PT, DPT, contributed to earlier versions of Table 3. This study was supported in part by a GSU internal grant awarded to the first author. The authors alone are responsible for the content and writing of this paper.

References

[1] S. Flynn, P. Palma, and A. Bender, "Feasibility of using the Sony PlayStation 2 gaming platform for an individual poststroke: a case report," *Journal of Neurologic Physical Therapy*, vol. 31, no. 4, pp. 180–189, 2007.

[2] A. Neil, S. Ens, R. Pelletier, T. Jarus, and D. Rand, "Sony PlayStation EyeToy elicits higher levels of movement than the Nintendo Wii: implications for stroke rehabilitation," *European Journal of Physical and Rehabilitation Medicine*, vol. 49, no. 1, pp. 13–21, 2013.

[3] D. M. Peters, A. K. McPherson, B. Fletcher, B. A. McClenaghan, and S. L. Fritz, "Counting repetitions: an observational study of video game play in people with chronic poststroke hemiparesis," *The Journal of Neurologic Physical Therapy*, vol. 37, no. 3, pp. 105–111, 2013.

[4] D. Rand, R. Kizony, and P. T. L. Weiss, "The sony playstation II eye toy: low-cost virtual reality for use in rehabilitation," *Journal of Neurologic Physical Therapy*, vol. 32, no. 4, pp. 155–163, 2008.

[5] G. Yavuzer, A. Senel, M. B. Atay, and H. J. Stam, "'Playstation eyetoy games' improve upper extremity-related motor functioning in subacute stroke: a randomized controlled clinical trial," *European Journal of Physical and Rehabilitation Medicine*, vol. 44, no. 3, pp. 237–244, 2008.

[6] Y.-P. Chen, L.-J. Kang, T.-Y. Chuang et al., "Use of virtual reality to improve upper-extremity control in children with cerebral palsy: a single-subject design," *Physical Therapy*, vol. 87, no. 11, pp. 1441–1457, 2007.

[7] Y.-P. Chen, S.-Y. Lee, and A. M. Howard, "Effect of virtual reality on upper extremity function in children with cerebral palsy: a meta-analysis," *Pediatric Physical Therapy*, vol. 26, no. 3, pp. 289–300, 2014.

[8] M. J. A. Jannink, G. J. van der Wilden, D. W. Navis, G. Visser, J. Gussinklo, and M. Ijzerman, "A low-cost video game applied for training of upper extremity function in children with cerebral palsy: a pilot study," *Cyberpsychology & Behavior*, vol. 11, no. 1, pp. 27–32, 2008.

[9] T. D. Parsons, A. A. Rizzo, S. Rogers, and P. York, "Virtual reality in paediatric rehabilitation: a review," *Developmental Neurorehabilitation*, vol. 12, no. 4, pp. 224–238, 2009.

[10] L. Snider, A. Majnemer, and V. Darsaklis, "Virtual reality as a therapeutic modality for children with cerebral palsy," *Developmental Neurorehabilitation*, vol. 13, no. 2, pp. 120–128, 2010.

[11] P. L. Weiss, D. Rand, N. Katz, and R. Kizony, "Video capture virtual reality as a flexible and effective rehabilitation tool," *Journal of NeuroEngineering and Rehabilitation*, vol. 1, article 12, 2004.

[12] P. N. Wilson, N. Foreman, and D. Stanton, "Virtual reality, disability and rehabilitation," *Disability and Rehabilitation*, vol. 19, no. 6, pp. 213–220, 1997.

[13] J. E. Deutsch, A. Brettler, C. Smith et al., "Nintendo Wii sports and Wii fit game analysis, validation, and application to stroke rehabilitation," *Topics in Stroke Rehabilitation*, vol. 18, no. 6, pp. 701–719, 2011.

[14] R. A. Magill, *Motor Learning and Control: Concepts and Applications*, McGraw-Hill Companies, New York, NY, USA, 9th edition, 2010.

[15] A. Shumway-Cook and M. Woollacott, *Motor Control: Translating Research into Clinical Practice*, Lippincott Williams & Wilkins, Baltimore, Md, USA, 4th edition, 2011.

[16] R. A. Schmidt and T. D. Lee, *Motor Control and Learning: A Behavioral Emphasis*, Human Kinetics, Champaign, Ill, USA, 5th edition, 2011.

[17] APTA, Ed., *Guide to Physical Therapist Practice*, American Physical Therapy Association, Alexandria, Va, USA, 2nd edition, 2003.

[18] ACSM, Ed., *ACSM's Guidelines for Exercise Testing and Prescription*, Lippincott Williams & Wilkins, Philadelplhia, Pa, USA, 9th edition, 2013.

[19] L. Fetters and J. Todd, "Quantitative assessment of infant reaching movements," *Journal of Motor Behavior*, vol. 19, no. 2, pp. 147–166, 1987.

[20] D. Corbetta and E. Thelen, "The developmental origins of bimanual coordination: a dynamic perspective," *Journal of Experimental Psychology: Human Perception and Performance*, vol. 22, no. 2, pp. 502–522, 1996.

[21] F. A. Machado and B. S. Denadai, "Validity of maximum heart rate prediction equations for children and adolescents," *Arquivos Brasileiros de Cardiologia*, vol. 97, no. 2, pp. 136–140, 2011.

[22] A. D. Mahon, A. D. Marjerrison, J. D. Lee, M. E. Woodruff, and L. E. Hanna, "Evaluating the prediction of maximal heart rate in children and adolescents," *Research Quarterly for Exercise and Sport*, vol. 81, no. 4, pp. 466–471, 2010.

[23] M. Robert, L. Ballaz, R. Hart, and M. Lemay, "Exercise intensity levels in children with cerebral palsy while playing with an active video game console," *Physical Therapy*, vol. 93, no. 8, pp. 1084–1091, 2013.

[24] N. Lythgo, C. Wilson, and M. Galea, "Basic gait and symmetry measures for primary school-aged children and young adults whilst walking barefoot and with shoes," *Gait & Posture*, vol. 30, no. 4, pp. 502–506, 2009.

[25] N. Lythgo, C. Wilson, and M. Galea, "Basic gait and symmetry measures for primary school-aged children and young adults. II: walking at slow, free and fast speed," *Gait & Posture*, vol. 33, no. 1, pp. 29–35, 2011.

18

The Effects of Two Different Ankle-Foot Orthoses on Gait of Patients with Acute Hemiparetic Cerebrovascular Accident

Noel Rao,[1] Jason Wening,[2] Daniel Hasso,[2] Gnanapradeep Gnanapragasam,[1] Priyan Perera,[1] Padma Srigiriraju,[1] and Alexander S. Aruin[1,3]

[1] Marianjoy Rehabilitation Hospital, 26W171 Roosevelt Road, Wheaton, IL 60187, USA
[2] Scheck & Siress, 1551 Bond Street, Naperville, IL 60563, USA
[3] Department of Physical Therapy (MC 898), University of Illinois at Chicago, 1919 West Taylor Street, Chicago, IL 60612, USA

Correspondence should be addressed to Alexander S. Aruin; aaruin@uic.edu

Academic Editor: Jeffrey Jutai

Objective. To compare the effects of two types of ankle-foot orthoses on gait of patients with cerebrovascular accident (CVA) and to evaluate their preference in using each AFO type. *Design*. Thirty individuals with acute hemiparetic CVA were tested without an AFO, with an off-the-shelf carbon AFO (C-AFO), and with a custom plastic AFO (P-AFO) in random order at the time of initial orthotic fitting. Gait velocity, cadence, stride length, and step length were collected using an electronic walkway and the subjects were surveyed about their perceptions of each device. *Results*. Subjects walked significantly faster, with a higher cadence, longer stride, and step lengths, when using either the P-AFO or the C-AFO as compared to no AFO ($P < 0.05$). No significant difference was observed between gait parameters of the two AFOs. However, the subjects demonstrated a statistically significant preference of using P-AFO in relation to their balance, confidence, and sense of safety during ambulation ($P < 0.05$). Moreover, if they had a choice, $50.87 \pm 14.7\%$ of the participants preferred the P-AFO and $23.56 \pm 9.70\%$ preferred the C-AFO. *Conclusions*. AFO use significantly improved gait in patients with acute CVA. The majority of users preferred the P-AFO over the Cf-AFO especially when asked about balance and sense of safety.

1. Introduction

Cerebrovascular accident (CVA) is the leading cause of serious, long-term disability among adults. Each year in the United States approximately 795,000 people sustain a new or recurrent CVA [1] and nearly half survive with some level of neurological impairment and disability [2]. CVA often results in dysfunction of one side of the body (hemiparesis) leading to gait impairment and increased probability for falls [3, 4].

Restoration of ambulation and ability to move around in the community is considered a high priority for individuals after CVA [5]. An ankle-foot orthosis is commonly prescribed to assist a patient with hemiparetic CVA to return to ambulation. AFOs can prevent foot drop, control the ankle in the coronal and sagittal planes during standing and walking, and improve the stability of the knee joint during ambulation [6]. Several studies have concluded that plastic AFOs (P-AFOs)

have a positive influence on the walking velocity and other gait parameters of individuals with hemiparetic CVA [7–11]. Recently carbon AFOs (C-AFOs) have been introduced to the marketplace by several manufacturers. The manufacturers of the C-AFOs claim that these devices are appropriate for hemiparetic patients who meet criteria that include minimal equinus contracture of the ankle, minimal coronal plane deformity of the ankle, minimal fluctuating edema, and no or low spasticity. However, the literature on the use of carbon AFOs to improve ambulation of individuals with CVA is insufficient. Moreover, to the best of our knowledge, no information exists on the patients' preference in using carbon AFOs.

There is also a body of literature on the importance of using a custom-made plastic AFO [12, 13]. Thus, it was reported that when a patient with posterior tibial tendon dysfunction was provided with an off-the-shelf ankle-foot orthosis (AFO), a custom solid AFO, and a custom articulated AFO, she selected a custom articulated AFO [14]. However, it is not known whether the patients with CVA would prefer using the prefabricated carbon AFOs when they have a choice to select the type of AFO. Given that the cost of orthoses varies considerably and that choosing an effective orthosis that is affordable to the patient is largely a trial-and-error process [14], it is important to obtain information on the patients' preference when prescribing an AFO.

It was reported that 35.3% of the study subjects who used an AFO indicated that they walked more confidently [15] and that patients reported a 70% increase in self-confidence [13] while using an AFO. These reports suggest a feeling of confidence may be more important to persons with hemiparesis than speed and distance; however, little information exists on the subjective preference in selecting the type of AFO by individuals with stroke.

While the literature provides important information on the beneficial effect of the AFOs, there is a need for more data describing the impact of AFOs on gait of subjects in the acute phase of rehabilitation after CVA. Moreover, there is not enough data on the use of the prefabricated carbon AFOs in gait of individuals with acute stroke. Thus, the aims of the study were (1) to investigate the effect of walking using the prefabricated carbon AFO in comparison with the custom polymer AFO and no AFO and (2) to obtain data on the users' preference in using either the prefabricated carbon AFO or the custom plastic AFO.

We hypothesized that individuals with acute CVA will improve their gait while provided with an AFO and that the improvement will be similar whether they use the prefabricated carbon AFO or the custom plastic AFO. We also hypothesized that when the subjects have a choice, they will prefer using the custom-made plastic AFO.

2. Methods

2.1. Subjects. Subjects in the acute phase of rehabilitation after hemiparetic CVA were referred by a physician during their visit to the orthotic clinic of a free-standing rehabilitation hospital. The inclusion criteria were as follows: CVA less than 12 weeks after onset, Ashworth scale score of less than 2, ability to walk 10 m without an AFO, but with an appropriate assistive device (cane or walker), a need for a custom polymer AFO for ambulation (based on evaluation by the clinic team), and ability to follow instructions. The exclusion criteria were as follows: histories of other significant neurologic or orthopedic disorders, significant coronal plane deformity or plantar flexion contracture, and minimal fluctuating edema. All subjects signed an informed consent approved by the Marianjoy Rehabilitation Hospital Institutional Review Board.

Thirty individuals who satisfied inclusion/exclusion criteria were selected to participate in the study. There were 15 males and 15 females with an average age of 60.4 ± 11.3 years; 16 of the subjects presented with right and 14 with left hemiparesis. The study participants received a full clinical evaluation and assessment. Based on this assessment the clinic team determined the type of a plastic AFO (flexible, semirigid, or rigid) that was most appropriate for each subject. Subjects were molded for the appropriate AFO [16] and measured for an Ossur AFO dynamic carbon off-the-shelf AFO. Thus, based on clinical evaluation, a subject prescribed, for example, with a semirigid AFO was provided with a semirigid plastic AFO or a semirigid carbon off-the-shelf AFO. Individuals who required a different type of AFO, such as a metal AFO, were excluded from the study. Plastic AFOs were custom modified and fabricated from 3/16″ polypropylene and included a proximal calf strap and distal ankle wrap around strap. During the course of the study subjects were provided with minimal information about the design and construction of the different AFOs. Instead, the AFOs were described as AFO A and AFO B for the subjects to prevent their impression of the device from being influenced by words such as "custom" or "carbon" (Figure 1). Subjects were tested at 21 ± 8 days after CVA. While all of the subjects were actively receiving physical and occupational therapy as prescribed by the treating physician, none of them had experience with an AFO prior to the day of fitting and testing. Subjects received clinically appropriate AFO: three subjects received a flexible AFO, twenty received a semirigid AFO, and seven subjects were provided with rigid AFOs.

2.2. Experimental Setup and Procedure. During the tests, the subjects were randomly provided with an off-the-shelf carbon AFO (C-AFO) and a custom plastic AFO (P-AFO). Testing included assessment of gait while walking using different AFOs and walking with no AFO (while each subject used the same own shoes during all the tests) and participation in a survey about the subject's perceptions of each AFO.

Temporal and spatial gait parameters were collected using a GAITRite electronic walkway (CIR Systems Inc., Havertown, PA). This device has been validated to study gait of individuals with stroke [17]. The *L*-test was used to further assess the subjects' functional walking ability. The *L*-test is a variant of the Timed Up and Go (TUG) test that uses an L shaped path instead of a straight line path [18]. Two walks were performed using the GAITRite and the *L*-test for each condition: no AFO, C-AFO, and P-AFO. Prior to the tests, the subjects were allowed for a brief adaptation with the AFOs. The order of the test conditions was randomized across the subjects. Subjects used an appropriate assistive device such as a cane or walker as needed; each subject used the same assistive device during all the tests involving ambulation. Subjects were allowed close supervision by a physical therapist but no direct contact. A minimum of five-minute rest between test conditions was provided to minimize the effect of fatigue.

All the study participants completed the Subject Perception of Functional Benefit Survey about their impression of the device that was just used (with assigned values of 0 being the most positive response and 4 the most negative). This survey was conducted after the use of each AFO type. In addition, at the end of the study, subjects completed the Subject AFO Preference Survey to determine if subjects had a preference for the polymer AFO, carbon fiber AFO, both AFOs, or neither AFO (with assigned values of 0 being

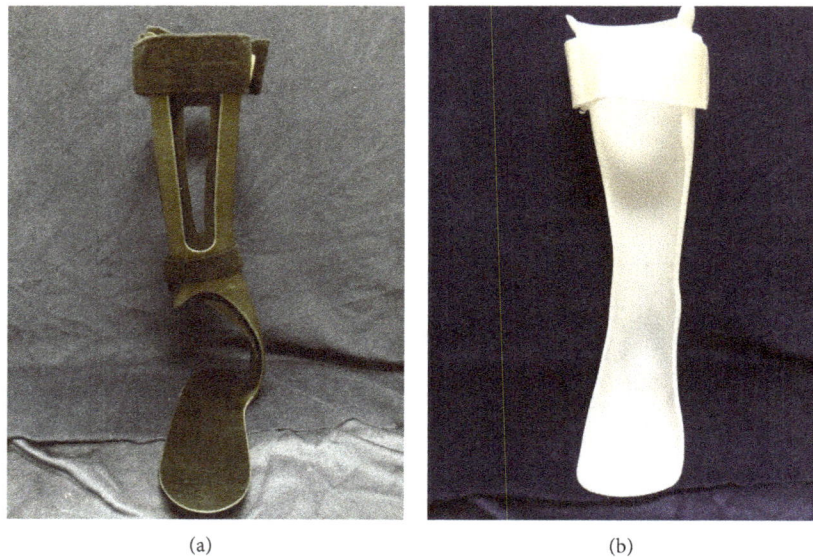

(a)   (b)

FIGURE 1: Off-the-shelf carbon AFO (a) and custom plastic AFO (b) used in the study.

the most positive response and 3 the most negative). These surveys are slightly modified versions of the survey described in the literature [18].

2.3. Data Processing and Analysis. Walking data was processed within the GAITRite software and velocity, cadence, and stride and step length were obtained as outcome measures. All the data were subjected to Shapiro-Wilk test for normality. One-way repeated measures ANOVA was performed with factor AFO (3 levels: no AFO, C-AFO, and P-AFO) separately for velocity, cadence, and stride length. Split-plot ANOVA was performed with factors AFO (3 levels: no AFO, C-AFO, and P-AFO) and side (involved and uninvolved) to analyze the differences in step length. Pairwise comparisons were used for further analyses of significant effects. Mann-Whitney test comparing survey responses for the polymer AFO and the carbon AFO was performed to test for statistical difference in subject perceptions of the functional benefit of the two different devices. For all tests, statistical significance was set at $P < 0.05$. Statistical analysis was performed in SPSS 17 for Windows 7 (SPSS Inc., Chicago, USA).

3. Results

3.1. Gait Velocity. With no AFO, the patients' gait velocity was 30.50 ± 13.58 cm/sec. When they were provided with the off-the-shelf carbon AFO (C-AFO), gait velocity increased to 36.38 ± 16.06 cm/sec. When a custom plastic AFO was used their gait velocity increased further reaching 39.21 ± 18.09 cm/sec. The difference in gait velocity was statistically significant ($F_{2,58} = 20.86$, $P < 0.0001$). Further analysis revealed statistically significant difference between no AFO condition and C-AFO and P-AFO ($P = 0.001$ and $P < 0.0001$, resp.). While the subjects were able to walk faster while being

provided with P-AFO as compared to C-AFO, the difference was not statistically significant ($P = 0.11$) (Figure 2).

3.2. Cadence. While walking without AFO, the subjects' cadence was 54.93 ± 13.95 steps/min. Cadence increased while using the AFOs. Thus, it reached 60.20 ± 14.72 and 62.76 ± 15.81 steps per minute when the subjects were provided with C-AFO and P-AFO, respectively. The difference between conditions was statistically significant ($F_{2,58} = 21.90$, $P < 0.0001$). Pairwise comparison revealed that no AFO condition was statistically significant compared to C-AFO and P-AFO conditions ($P = 0.001$, $P < 0.0001$, resp.). However the difference between C-AFO and P-AFO was not significant ($P = 0.099$) (Figure 2).

3.3. Stride Length. Patients walking without AFOs showed stride length of 64.98 ± 16.86 cm. When they were provided with the off-the-shelf carbon AFO (C-AFO), stride length increased to 70.35 ± 18.83 cm. When a custom polymer AFO was used, the stride length increased further reaching 72.35 ± 20.11 cm. The difference in stride length was statistically significant ($F_{2,58} = 10.23$, $P < 0.0001$). Further analysis revealed statistically significant difference between no AFO condition and C-AFO and P-AFO ($P = 0.006$ and $P < 0.01$, resp.). The difference in stride length between walking while being provided with P-AFO and C-AFO was not statistically significant ($P = 0.79$).

3.4. Step Length. Step length in conditions with no AFO was 36.99 ± 8.65 cm and 27.63 ± 14.01 cm for the involved and uninvolved lower extremities, respectively. When the off-the-shelf carbon AFO (C-AFO) was provided, step length increased to 39.66 ± 9.97 cm and 31.00 ± 11.66 cm on the involved and uninvolved side, respectively. Using the custom P-AFO resulted in the increase of the step length on the

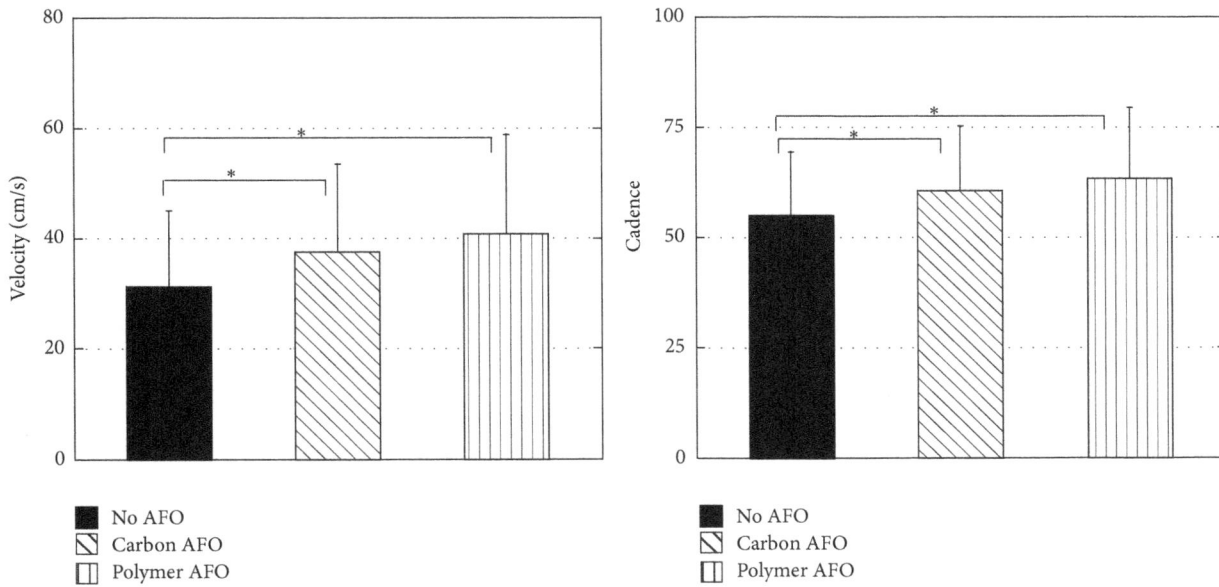

FIGURE 2: Gait velocity and cadence measured while walking without an AFO and with a carbon AFO or plastic AFO. ∗ shows statistical significance ($P < 0.001$).

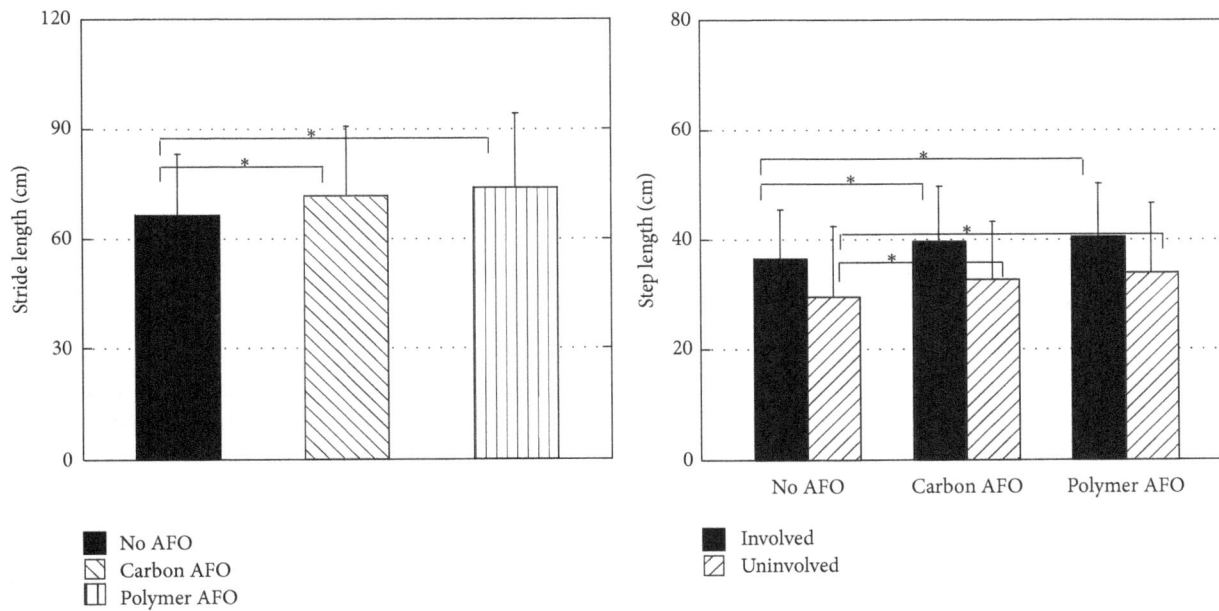

FIGURE 3: Stride length and step length recorded during walking without an AFO and with a carbon AFO or plastic AFO. ∗ shows statistical significance ($P < 0.001$).

involved side to 40.21 ± 9.69 and on the uninvolved side to 31.92 ± 14.09. The difference in step length while provided with AFOs was statistically significant ($F_{2,116} = 12.97$, $P < 0.0001$). The interaction between the AFOs and the involved or uninvolved side was however not statistically significant ($F_{2,116} = 0.24$, $P = 0.79$). Further pairwise comparison of the use of AFOs revealed statistically significant difference between no AFO condition and C-AFO and P-AFO ($P = 0.001$ and $P < 0.0001$, resp.). The difference in step length

between walking while being provided with P-AFO and C-AFO was not statistically significant ($P = 0.99$) (Figure 3).

3.5. L-Test. While walking without AFO, the time needed to cross 10 m distance by the subjects was 1.45 ± 0.71 min. This time decreased to 1.25 ± 0.79 min and to 1.33 ± 0.66 min when the subjects were provided with C-AFO and P-AFO, respectively (L-test data was collected for 26 subjects). The difference between conditions, however, was not statistically

TABLE 1: Subjects perception of Functional Benefit Survey.

	With the AFO I just used…			Response			Significance
(1)	Lifting my toes is…	Much easier	A little easier	No different	A little harder	Much harder	$P = 0.053$
(2)	Swinging my leg forward is…	Much easier	A little easier	No different	A little harder	Much harder	**P = 0.023**
(3)	Taking weight through my foot is…	Much easier	A little easier	No different	A little harder	Much harder	$P = 0.105$
(4)	My walking speed…	Much faster	A little faster	Not changed	A little slower	Much slower	$P = 0.051$
(5)	My balance is…	Much better	A little better	No different	A little worse	Much worse	**P = 0.006**
(6)	My confidence is…	Much higher	A little higher	Not changed	A little less	Much less	**P = 0.014**
(7)	My sense of safety is…	Much higher	A little higher	Not changed	A little less	Much less	**P = 0.005**
(8)	Walking is…	Much easier	A little easier	No different	A little harder	Much harder	**P = 0.009**

TABLE 2: Subjects perceptions regarding the AFO type, $N = 29$.

		Plastic AFO	Carbon AFO	Both	None
(1)	Lifting my toes is easier with…	8 (27%)	5 (17%)	14 (48%)	1 (3%)
(2)	Swinging my leg forward is easier with	17 (58.6%)	8 (27%)	4 (13.8%)	0 (0%)
(3)	Taking weight through my foot is easier with…	16 (55%)	8 (27%)	5 (17%)	0 (0%)
(4)	I walk faster with…	18 (62%)	5 (17%)	6 (21%)	0 (0%)
(5)	My balance is better with…	18 (62%)	5 (17%)	6 (21%)	0 (0%)
(6)	My sense of safety is higher with…	17 (58.6%)	2 (7%)	10 (34%)	0 (0%)
(7)	I like the fit and comfort of…	15 (52%)	11 (38%)	2 (7%)	1 (3%)
(8)	I like the appearance of…	17 (58.6%)	9 (31%)	3 (10%)	0 (0%)
(9)	I would rather use…to assist my walking	7 (24%)	9 (31%)	6 (21%)	7 (24%)

significant ($F_{2,52} = 6.35$, $P = 0.14$). Pairwise comparison revealed that no AFO condition was statistically significant compared to C-AFO ($P = 0.004$). At the same time, the difference between no AFO and P-AFO and between C-AFO and P-AFO was not statistically significant ($P = 0.1417$, $P = 0.46$, resp.).

3.6. Users' Perceptions regarding the AFO Type. The analysis of the outcome of the Perception of Functional Benefit Survey about the device that was just used revealed that in general the study participants preferred P-AFO when compared to the C-AFO (data for 29 subjects). Thus, the users demonstrated statistically significant preference of using P-AFO while answering question 2 ($U = 280.5$, $P = 0.023$), question 5 ($U = 252$, $P = 0.006$), question 6 ($U = 271$, $P = 0.014$), question 7 ($U = 250$, $P = 0.005$), and question 8 ($U = 262.5$, $P = 0.009$). Moreover, the differences between the two types of AFO were just under the level of statistical significance for question 1 ($U = 301$, $P = 0.053$) and question 4 ($U = 301.5$, $P = 0.051$) (Table 1).

The analysis of the outcome of the Subject AFO Preference Survey revealed that the study participants preferred the P-AFO to the C-AFO (Table 2). This was especially true when they were asked about balance and sense of safety during ambulation. On average, $50.87 \pm 14.7\%$ of the study participants preferred P-AFO and $23.56 \pm 9.70\%$ of the subjects preferred C-AFO. It is also important to mention that $18.1 \pm 8.3\%$ preferred using both types of AFOs and only

$3.1 \pm 7.90\%$ of the study participants preferred not using either type of AFO.

4. Discussion

It is documented in the prior literature that individuals after CVA walk slower than healthy individuals [19]. It was also reported that the ability of individuals with stroke to ambulate is improved as a result of wearing an ankle-foot orthosis [20]. Moreover, there is a plethora of evidence on the beneficial effect of AFOs in improving of functional mobility and quality of gait as well as decreasing the likelihood of falls in individuals suffering from a CVA [21, 22]. Thus, individuals with CVA provided with an AFO improved gait parameters such as cadence, stride length, and gait velocity [18, 23, 24]. Moreover, improvement in gait velocity that is believed to reflect progress in mobility, is often used as a measure of recovery after a CVA [20, 25, 26], and is considered an important goal of rehabilitation.

At the same time, the literature on the use of different types of AFOs (especially recently introduced carbon AFOs) to improve ambulation of individuals with CVA is limited. As such, the goals of the study were to investigate the effect of walking using the prefabricated carbon AFO in comparison with the custom polymer AFO and no AFO and to investigate the users' preference in using either the prefabricated carbon AFO or the custom plastic AFO.

The results of the current study demonstrated that individuals with acute CVA increased their gait velocity when using either C-AFO or P-AFO, and, as a result, the gap between "normal" and "hemiparetic" gait velocity decreased. These results are in line with the literature reporting a positive effect of AFOs on gait velocity of individuals with hemiparesis [9, 19, 27]. Similarly, improvements in cadence were associated with the use of an AFO; without an AFO patients walked with lower cadence as compared to healthy individuals. A similar positive effect of AFOs on cadence of individuals with hemiparesis was described in the literature [27, 28]. Since cadence is the number of steps taken in a certain time, the observed increase in the velocity of gait could be due to changes in the number of steps per minute. Nevertheless, the impact of AFOs on cadence remains inconclusive as some studies report an improvement in this variable with the AFO use and others report no significant improvement [22]. Thus, there is a need for more studies focused on the investigation of the role of different types of AFOs on gait velocity and cadence. An increase in the average stride and step length with either type of AFO was evident in the current study and has been also reported in the past literature [27, 28].

While in general there is a consensus in the literature that gait velocity is a powerful indicator of function and prognosis after CVA [26] there is an opinion that gait velocity itself may not be wholly representative of functional mobility and meaningful improvement in performance [29]. To address this possible concern, we added the L-test assessment (that includes rising from a chair, two 90-degree turns in opposite directions, a 180-degree turn, and returning to a seated position) as the task that is indicative of the types of movements that are required in household ambulation. The outcome of the L-test revealed that patients while using AFOs of either type showed better performance compared to walking with no AFO. Moreover, clinically the patients showed improvement as the time needed for the completion of the test was shorter when they were provided with either type of AFO.

The study participants were positive about the use of AFOs as the majority found it comfortable and felt it improved their walking, particularly the functional aspects such as safety and confidence. This finding is in line with the literature reporting that 96% of users felt they walked better with the AFO and found it comfortable [18]. Moreover, the majority of the subjects gave a preference to the custom-made plastic AFOs: the subjects perception was about 2 : 1 in favor of the custom-made plastic AFO. This could be because each plastic AFO was specifically molded and fitted for each subject. Nevertheless, further study is needed to examine the longer-term effects and the cost-effectiveness of prescribing a custom-made or off-the-shelf AFO for people with CVA.

5. Conclusion

Both types of AFO significantly improved gait velocity, cadence, step length, and stride length in patients with acute CVA. The majority of users preferred the custom-made plastic AFO over the prefabricated carbon AFO. This outcome should be taken into consideration while prescribing AFOs. Further study is needed to examine the longer-term effects

and the cost-effectiveness of prescribing different types of AFO for people with CVA.

Conflict of Interests

The authors declare that there is no conflict of interests regarding the publication of this paper.

References

[1] V. L. Roger, A. S. Go, D. M. Lloyd-Jones et al., "Heart disease and stroke statistics—2011 update: a report from the American Heart Association," *Circulation*, vol. 123, no. 4, pp. e18–e209, 2011.

[2] M. Kelly-Hayes, J. T. Robertson, J. P. Broderick et al., "The American heart association stroke outcome classification," *Stroke*, vol. 29, no. 6, pp. 1274–1280, 1998.

[3] C. Detrembleur, F. Dierick, G. Stoquart, F. Chantraine, and T. Lejeune, "Energy cost, mechanical work, and efficiency of hemiparetic walking," *Gait & Posture*, vol. 18, no. 2, pp. 47–55, 2003.

[4] N. Wada, M. Sohmiya, T. Shimizu, K. Okamoto, and K. Shirakura, "Clinical analysis of risk factors for falls in home-living stroke patients using functional evaluation tools," *Archives of Physical Medicine and Rehabilitation*, vol. 88, no. 12, pp. 1601–1605, 2007.

[5] S. E. Lord, K. McPherson, H. K. McNaughton, L. Rochester, and M. Weatherall, "Community ambulation after stroke: how important and obtainable is it and what measures appear predictive?" *Archives of Physical Medicine and Rehabilitation*, vol. 85, no. 2, pp. 234–239, 2004.

[6] J. F. Lehmann, S. M. Condon, R. Price, and B. J. deLateur, "Gait abnormalities in hemiplegia: their correction by ankle-foot orthoses," *Archives of Physical Medicine and Rehabilitation*, vol. 68, no. 11, pp. 763–771, 1987.

[7] H. Beckerman, J. Becher, G. J. Lankhorst, and A. L. M. Verbeek, "Walking ability of stroke patients: efficacy of tibial nerve blocking and a polypropylene ankle-foot orthosis," *Archives of Physical Medicine and Rehabilitation*, vol. 77, no. 11, pp. 1144–1151, 1996.

[8] D. C. M. de Wit, J. H. Buurke, J. M. M. Nijlant, M. J. IJzerman, and H. J. Hermens, "The effect of an ankle-foot orthosis on walking ability in chronic stroke patients: a randomized controlled trial," *Clinical Rehabilitation*, vol. 18, no. 5, pp. 550–557, 2004.

[9] M. Franceschini, M. Massucci, L. Ferrari, M. Agosti, and C. Paroli, "Effects of an ankle-foot orthosis on spatiotemporal parameters and energy cost of hemiparetic gait," *Clinical Rehabilitation*, vol. 17, no. 4, pp. 368–372, 2003.

[10] N. Rao, G. Chaudhuri, D. Hasso et al., "Gait assessment during the initial fitting of an ankle foot orthosis in individuals with stroke," *Disability and Rehabilitation: Assistive Technology*, vol. 3, no. 4, pp. 201–207, 2008.

[11] S. Roehrig and D. A. Yates, "Case report: effects of a new orthosis and physical therapy on gait in a subject with longstanding hemiplegia," *Journal of Geriatric Physical Therapy*, vol. 31, no. 1, pp. 38–46, 2008.

[12] H. B. Kitaoka, X. M. Crevoisier, K. Harbst, D. Hansen, B. Kotajarvi, and K. Kaufman, "The effect of custom-made braces for the ankle and hindfoot on ankle and foot kinematics and

ground reaction forces," *Archives of Physical Medicine and Rehabilitation*, vol. 87, no. 1, pp. 130–135, 2006.

[13] A. Slijper, A. Danielsson, and C. Willen, "Ambulatory function and perception of confidence in persons with stroke with a custom-made hinged versus a standard ankle foot orthosis," *Rehabilitation Research and Practice*, vol. 2012, Article ID 206495, 6 pages, 2012.

[14] C. Neville and J. Houck, "Choosing among 3 ankle-foot orthoses for a patient with stage II posterior tibial tendon dysfunction," *Journal of Orthopaedic & Sports Physical Therapy*, vol. 39, no. 11, pp. 816–824, 2009.

[15] A. Doğan, M. Mengüllüoğlu, and N. Özgirgin, "Evaluation of the effect of ankle-foot orthosis use on balance and mobility in hemiparetic stroke patients," *Disability and Rehabilitation*, vol. 33, no. 15-16, pp. 1433–1439, 2011.

[16] Standards, "AFO Modification/Fabrication/Standards," 2012, http://www.aopsolutions.com/forms/afo_modification_form.pdf.

[17] S. S. Kuys, S. G. Brauer, and L. Ada, "Test-retest reliability of the GAITRite system in people with stroke undergoing rehabilitation," *Disability and Rehabilitation*, vol. 33, no. 19-20, pp. 1848–1853, 2011.

[18] S. F. Tyson and H. A. Thornton, "The effect of a hinged ankle foot orthosis on hemiplegic gait: objective measures and users' opinions," *Clinical Rehabilitation*, vol. 15, no. 1, pp. 53–58, 2001.

[19] H. S. Jorgensen, H. Nakayama, H. O. Raaschou, J. Vive-Larsen, M. Stoier, and T. S. Olsen, "Outcome and time course of recovery in stroke, part II: time course of recovery: the Copenhagen Stroke Study," *Archives of Physical Medicine and Rehabilitation*, vol. 76, no. 5, pp. 406–412, 1995.

[20] R.-Y. Wang, P.-Y. Lin, C.-C. Lee, and Y.-R. Yang, "Gait and balance performance improvements attributable to ankle-foot orthosis in subjects with hemiparesis," *The American Journal of Physical Medicine and Rehabilitation*, vol. 86, no. 7, pp. 556–562, 2007.

[21] E. Cakar, O. Durmus, L. Tekin, U. Dincer, and M. Z. Kiralp, "The ankle-foot orthosis improves balance and reduces fall risk of chronic spastic hemiparetic patients," *European Journal of Physical and Rehabilitation Medicine*, vol. 46, no. 3, pp. 363–368, 2010.

[22] L. A. Ferreira, H. P. Neto, L. A. Grecco et al., "Effect of ankle-foot orthosis on gait velocity and cadence of stroke patients: a systematic review," *Journal of Physical Therapy Science*, vol. 25, no. 11, pp. 1503–1508, 2013.

[23] H. Gök, A. Küçükdeveci, H. Altinkaynak, G. Yavuzer, and S. Ergin, "Effects of ankle-foot orthoses on hemiparetic gait," *Clinical Rehabilitation*, vol. 17, no. 2, pp. 137–139, 2003.

[24] H. Abe, A. Michimata, K. Sugawara, N. Sugaya, and S.-I. Izumi, "Improving gait stability in stroke hemiplegic patients with a plastic ankle-foot orthosis," *Tohoku Journal of Experimental Medicine*, vol. 218, no. 3, pp. 193–199, 2009.

[25] J. Perry, M. Garrett, J. K. Gronley, and S. J. Mulroy, "Classification of walking handicap in the stroke population," *Stroke*, vol. 26, no. 6, pp. 982–989, 1995.

[26] A. Schmid, P. W. Duncan, S. Studenski et al., "Improvements in speed-based gait classifications are meaningful," *Stroke*, vol. 38, no. 7, pp. 2096–2100, 2007.

[27] Å. Bartonek, M. Eriksson, and E. M. Gutierrez-Farewik, "A new carbon fibre spring orthosis for children with plantarflexor weakness," *Gait and Posture*, vol. 25, no. 4, pp. 652–656, 2007.

[28] C. Bleyenheuft, G. Caty, T. Lejeune, and C. Detrembleur, "Assessment of the Chignon dynamic ankle-foot orthosis using instrumented gait analysis in hemiparetic adults," *Annales de Réadaptation et de Médecine Physique*, vol. 51, no. 3, pp. 154–160, 2008.

[29] S. E. Lord and L. Rochester, "Measurement of community ambulation after stroke: current status and future developments," *Stroke*, vol. 36, no. 7, pp. 1457–1461, 2005.

19

Two Different Protocols for Knee Joint Motion Analyses in the Stance Phase of Gait: Correlation of the Rigid Marker Set and the Point Cluster Technique

Takashi Fukaya,[1] Hirotaka Mutsuzaki,[2] Hirofumi Ida,[3] and Yasuyoshi Wadano[2]

[1] Department of Physical Therapy, Faculty of Health Sciences, Tsukuba International University, 6-8-33 Manabe, Ibaraki, Tsuchiura 300-0051, Japan
[2] Department of Orthopedic Surgery, Ibaraki Prefectural University of Health Sciences, 4669-2 Ami, Ibaraki, Ami-machi 300-0394, Japan
[3] Department of Human System Science, Tokyo Institute of Technology, 2-12-1 Oh-okayama, Meguro, Tokyo 152-8550, Japan

Correspondence should be addressed to Takashi Fukaya, t-fukaya@tius-hs.jp

Academic Editor: Arie Rimmerman

Objective. There are no reports comparing the protocols provided by rigid marker set (RMS) and point cluster technique (PCT), which are similar in terms of estimating anatomical landmarks based on markers attached to a segment. The purpose of this study was to clarify the correlation of the two different protocols, which are protocols for knee motion in gait, and identify whether measurement errors arose at particular periods during the stance phase. *Methods.* The study subjects were 10 healthy adults. All estimated anatomical landmarks were which their positions, calculated by each protocol of the PCT and RMS, were compared using Pearson's product correlation coefficients. To examine the reliability of the angle changes of the knee joint measured by RMS and the PCT, the coefficient of multiple correlations (CMCs) was used. *Results.* Although the estimates of the anatomical landmarks showed high correlations of >0.90 ($P < 0.01$) for the Y- and Z-coordinates, the correlations were low for the X-coordinates at all anatomical landmarks. The CMC was 0.94 for flexion/extension, 0.74 for abduction/adduction, and 0.71 for external/internal rotation. *Conclusion.* Flexion/extension and abduction/adduction of the knee by two different protocols had comparatively little error and good reliability after 30% of the stance phase.

1. Introduction

Gait analysis with motion analysis based on a camera system has been widely applied both clinically and in research. It is used to assess changes over time in patients and to evaluate differences in their gait patterns compared with those of normal subjects. Gait analysis for patients with problems such as osteoarthritis and ligament injury of the knee has been previously reported [1–3]. However, measurement errors are caused by the method used to attach the reflective markers to the body in gait analysis with motion analysis, and these errors influence the reliability of the results. In previous studies, sufficiently reliable results were not obtained for movement of either the frontal or horizontal plane, although the reliability was comparatively high for movement of the sagittal plane of the knee joint [4, 5].

A set of at least three noncollinear reflective markers on each segment is required to define a rigid body in three-dimensional space. While measurement of marker sets mounted on bone pins [6] is comparatively accurate, the procedure is invasive and difficult to use. Although the reflective markers are attached directly to the skin in skin-mounted marker sets [7], soft tissue artifacts are increased by muscle contraction and the impact of the initial contact during the stance phase, leading to the development of measurement errors when the joint angle and joint moment are calculated.

The rigid marker set (RMS), a method to estimate the positions of anatomical landmarks in motion by calibrating anatomical landmarks from the three markers mounted on rigid plates in the standing position, has been previously reported [8–10]. The method using markers mounted on rigid plates is possible to prevent the independent movement of each marker compared with the method using skin-mounted marker sets.

The point cluster technique (PCT) reported by Andriacchi et al. [11], which is a calculation method that reduces the measurement error caused by artifacts of each skin marker, was used clinically as a noninvasive method [12, 13]. The PCT involves attachment of multiple reflective markers (usually about 5–20) on the thigh and shank together with anatomical landmarks. In this technique, the three-dimensional movement of the knee joint is calculated from the estimated positions of the femur and tibia bones in vivo, where a principal axis transformation for the segment marker clusters is used to define the local reference system for this estimation. Andriacchi et al. [11] computationally simulated that the PCT could reduce the influence of skin movement artifacts. They also demonstrated that the obtained data were comparable to the relative movement of the thigh and shank bones during walking reported in a previous study [6]. However, it is also considered that the PCT is insufficient to catch the three-dimensional motion of the knee joint during measurements [14]. Both RMS and the PCT were devised as protocols to reduce measurement errors caused by skin movement artifacts. Although these protocols are similar in terms of estimating anatomical landmarks based on markers attached to a segment to describe the three-dimensional motion of the knee joint, there are no previous reports of studies comparing the protocols provided by RMS and the PCT. Evaluation of the results obtained by these two protocols and examination of the estimates of the anatomical landmarks will reveal the influences on the results of both protocols and identify the periods of the stance phase in which errors occur.

The purpose of this study was to clarify the correlation of the two different protocols, RMS and the PCT. For this purpose, we examined changes in the estimates of anatomical landmarks and knee joint angles obtained by RMS and the PCT as protocols for knee joint motion in gait analyses and identified whether measurement errors arose at particular periods during the stance phase.

2. Methods

2.1. Subjects.

The study subjects were 10 healthy adults (7 males and 3 females; mean age ± SD, 29.2 ± 5.0 years; mean height ± SD, 1.70 ± 0.12 m; mean mass ± SD, 67.4 ± 9.5 kg; mean BMI ± SD, 23.3 ± 2.4 kg/m^2) who had neither orthopedic disease of the lower limbs, including ligament injury or bone/spinal fracture, nor neurological impairment and had no limitations in their activities of daily life. All subjects provided written informed consent prior to any assessment. Ethical approval for this study was obtained from the Ibaraki Prefectural University of Health Sciences Ethics Committee.

2.2. Procedure.

A three-dimensional motion analysis system (Vicon, Oxford, UK) and a floor-mounted force plate

(Kistler Instruments, Winterthur, Switzerland), each with a sampling rate of 200 Hz, were used in this study. The subjects walked barefoot along a 10 m walkway at their self-selected habitual speeds and were directed to step on a force plate with the right lower limb. Five trials were performed, with sufficient rest between the trials. Reflective markers of 9.5 mm diameter were attached with double-sided tape to each subject's pelvis and anatomical landmarks on the right thigh, shank, and foot segments. After identification by palpation, markers were directly placed over the following anatomical landmarks: bilateral anterior and posterior superior iliac spines, unilateral greater trochanter, lateral and medial femoral epicondyles, lateral and medial tibial condyles, lateral and medial malleoli, calcaneus, and top of the foot at the base of the second metatarsal. Moreover, RMS with three attached reflective markers was placed on the lateral side of the thigh and shank (Figure 1). In addition, 10 markers on the thigh and 6 markers on the shank were attached to calculate the movement of the knee joint by the PCT (Figure 1). After attachment of the markers, decisions were made regarding the relative positions of the anatomical landmarks to the two rigid plates for the RMS and PCT markers based on a single static calibration to estimate the anatomical landmarks of the thigh and shank from the RMS and the PCT markers. The PCT algorithm described by Ida et al. [15] was showed as following. From a rest trial (e.g., quiet standing), a principal axis transformation determines the local reference system that is fixed to the marker cluster. The positions of anatomical landmarks are described on the local reference system by marker cluster. For a dynamic trial, the positions of the anatomical landmarks are extrapolated on the basis of the marker cluster motions during the trial, where the local reference system is calculated for each frame from the marker cluster data. Using the extrapolated anatomical landmark data, the positions of femur and tibia bones are estimated. The estimations of the anatomical landmarks by RMS were calculated with numerical software (Vicon, Bodybuilder) using three markers on each rigid plate.

2.3. Data Analysis.

Foot strike and toe-off were determined using the force plate data, and the corresponding frame number was identified in the kinematics data. The kinematics data were normalized to the 100% stance phase (foot strike to toe-off = 100%) using spline interpolation. To calculate the kinematics data, the local coordinate systems of the thigh and shank were defined in the three-dimensional position by the anatomical landmarks of the thigh and shank estimated from RMS and the PCT. The knee joint angles during the stance phase were calculated using the joint coordinate system (JCS) approach described by Grood and Suntay [16]. The global coordinate system was defined as follows: the x-axis was lateral, y-axis was anterior, and z-axis was vertical (Figure 1(b)). The coordinate systems for the thigh (T) and shank (S) were defined as follows:

T_x: vector directed laterally from the medial to lateral femoral epicondyle,

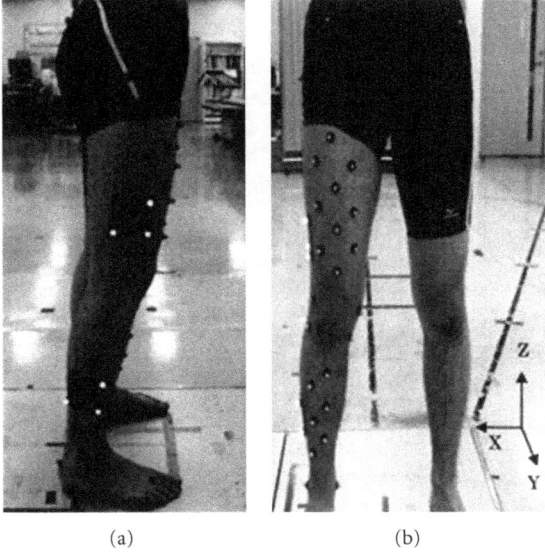

(a)   (b)

FIGURE 1: The rigid marker set (black squares with three reflective markers appearing white attached to the thigh and shank) and the point cluster technique (10 markers on the front of the thigh and 6 markers on the front of the shank). Image (a) shows RMS on the lateral side, and image (b) shows the PCT on the front side. The global coordinate system is shown in (b).

T_y: cross product of a vector directed anteriorly from the knee joint center (midpoint between the medial and lateral femoral epicondyles) to the greater trochanter and T_x,

T_z: cross-product of vectors T_x and T_y,

S_x: cross-product of vectors S_y and S_z,

S_y: cross-product of S_z and a vector directed anteriorly from the medial to lateral tibial condyle,

S_z: vector directed from the ankle joint center (midpoint between the lateral and medial malleoli) to the midpoint between the medial and lateral tibial condyles.

To calculate knee joint angles, two axes of the JCS were embedded in the two segments whose relative motion was to be described. The two vectors were the T_x vector of the thigh coordinate system and the S_z vector of the shank coordinate system. The third axis was called the floating axis and was the common perpendicular to both T_x and S_z. Flexion-extension occurred about the T_x axis. The flexion-extension angle, α, was obtained by the angle between T_y and the floating axis, and flexion was positive when extension was negative. External-internal rotation occurred about the S_z axis. The external-internal angle, γ, was obtained by the angle between S_y and the floating axis, and external was positive when internal was negative. Abduction-adduction occurred about the floating axis. The abduction-adduction angle, β, was obtained by the value in which $\pi/2$ was pulled from δ and was defined by the angle between T_x and the S_z axis. Abduction was positive when adduction was negative.

TABLE 1: Pearson's product moment correlation coefficients of landmarks estimated by RMS and the PCT.

	X	Y	Z
Great trochanter	0.92*	0.99*	0.95*
Lateral epicondyle	0.86*	0.99*	0.99*
Medial epicondyle	0.85*	0.99*	0.96*
Lateral condyle	0.87*	0.99*	0.99*
Medial condyle	0.75*	0.99*	0.93*
Lateral malleolus	0.87*	0.99*	0.99*
Medial malleolus	0.90*	0.99*	0.99*

*Significant difference was $P < 0.01$ for all landmarks.

2.4. Statistical Analysis. The comparison between RMS and the PCT was examined using Pearson's product moment correlation coefficient for each estimation of the anatomical landmarks in the stance phase. In addition, the coefficient of multiple correlations (CMCs) was used to examine the difference in the angle changes of the knee joint motion in the stance phase provided by RMS and the PCT and was calculated using a method described by Kadaba et al. [17].

3. Results

The correlation coefficients for the estimations by RMS and the PCT for the anatomical landmarks in the stance phase are shown in Table 1. The Y- and Z-coordinates showed very high correlations of ≥ 0.90 ($P < 0.01$) for all anatomical landmarks. The X-coordinates showed slightly lower positive correlations than the Y- and Z-coordinates. The X-coordinates of the medial condyle had a particularly low value of 0.75 ($P < 0.01$).

The time-dependent changes in the knee joint angles in the stance phase are shown in Figure 2. The data represent the means $\pm$ SD for all subjects for the two measurement methods during the stance phase. In these results, the CMC values for the angle changes of the knee joint during the stance phase calculated by RMS and the PCT were 0.94 for flexion/extension, 0.74 for abduction/adduction, and 0.71 for external/internal rotation. As shown in Figure 2, the differences were approximately 4° at 28% of the stance phase in flexion/extension, approximately 1.6° at 5% of the stance phase for abduction/adduction, and approximately 9.8° at the initial contact of the stance phase for external/internal rotation. These results indicate that the differences in the knee joint angles measured by RMS and the PCT were the largest. In terms of external-internal rotation, the error gradually decreased from initial contact to approximately 70% of the stance phase, but after 70%, the error tended to increase again.

4. Discussion

This study examined the estimates of anatomical landmarks and the differences in the knee joint motion obtained using RMS and the PCT in the stance phase. The estimates of the anatomical landmarks showed very high positive correlations

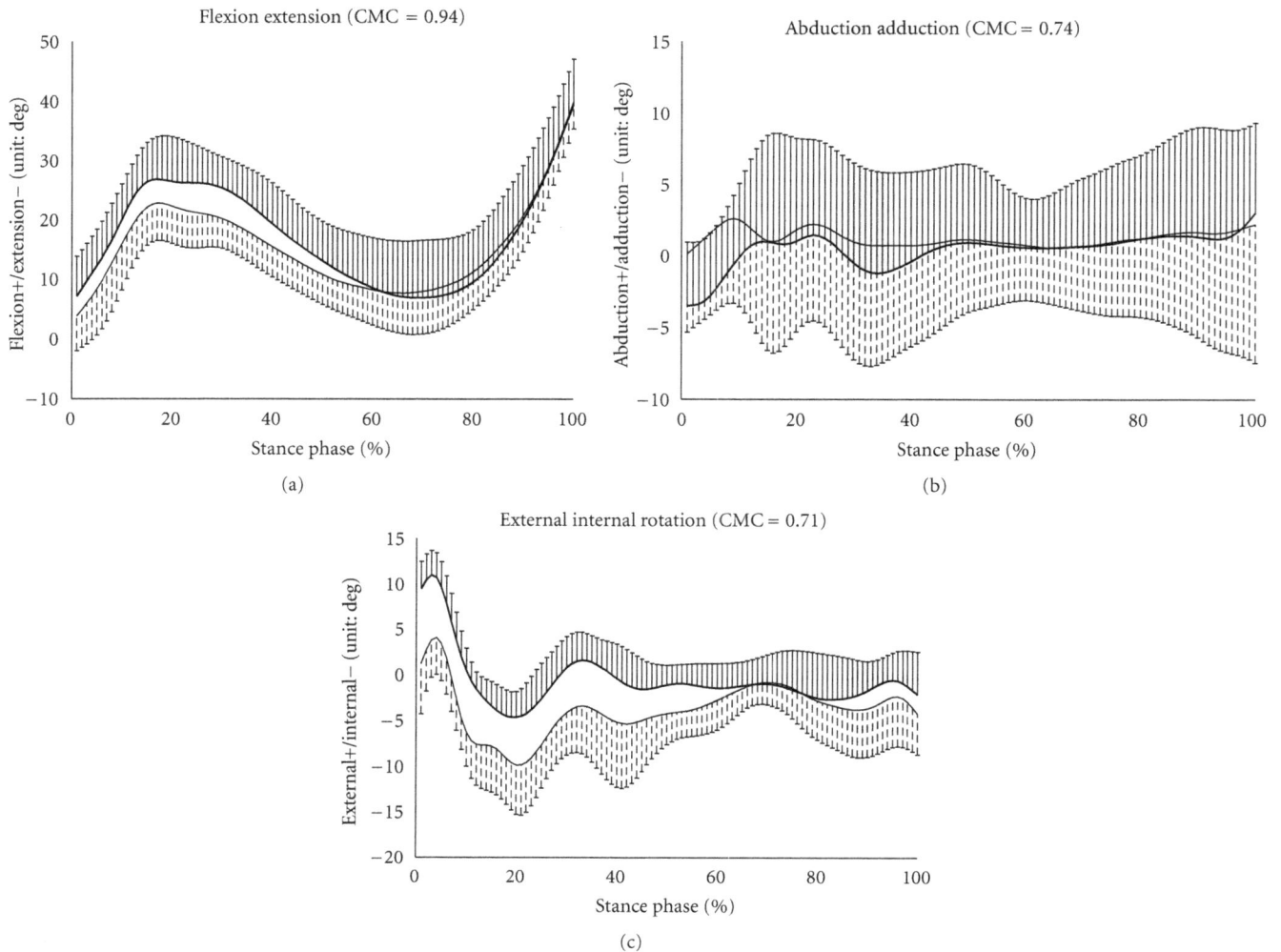

FIGURE 2: Angle changes of the knee joint motion measured by RMS (thin lines) and the PCT (thick lines). The vertical bars show the SD. Image (a) shows flexion/extension, image (b) shows abduction/adduction, and image (c) shows external/internal rotation. The CMC value is shown in each figure.

for the Y- and Z-coordinates, while the X-coordinates showed slightly lower positive correlations than the Y- and Z-coordinates. The X-coordinates of the medial condyle had a particularly low value of 0.75. Because we defined the knee joint center as the link of each middle point of the lateral and medial epicondyles and the long axis of the tibia as the link of each middle point of the lateral and medial malleoli and the middle points of the lateral and medial condyles in this study, the errors in the X-coordinates of each anatomical landmark affected the degree of leaning of the long axis of the thigh and shank. This provides the possibility of increasing the error in the angle calculation and is thought to be a factor in why the CMC values for abduction/adduction and external/internal rotation were low compared with the value for flexion/extension.

Based on the data shown in Figure 2, the error grew to 30% from the initial contact in the stance phase between RMS and the PCT. In addition, in terms of rotational motion of the knee joint, the error grew to be large after 70% of the

stance phase. The tibialis anterior muscle acts as a brake for plantar flexion of the ankle during the early stance phase. The array of markers used in the PCT is assumed to be affected by the skin deformation caused by contraction of the tibial anterior muscle in the PCT to position the front of the shank. On the other hand, RMS attaches to the outside surface of the shank and is estimated to be affected by contraction of the long peroneus muscle rather than of the tibialis anterior muscle. Because the long peroneus muscle was required for the large contraction during the late stance phase [18], it was suggested that the large contraction of the long peroneus muscle affected the error of rotational motion of the late stance phase.

It was thought that errors might be produced in the anatomical landmark estimates by the X-coordinates of the anatomical landmarks estimated from the markers of the shank because the muscles related to the marker attachment position are different. These values may affect the results for abduction/adduction and external/internal rotation. In the early stance phase, the ground reaction force and muscle activity around the thigh become active, and it is thought that large deformation of the skin around the knee is caused by muscle contraction around the thigh. The lateral and medial epicondyles were expected to be particularly affected by muscle contraction around the thigh, and Ishii et al. [19] reported that the medial epicondyle had the largest error compared with the error between the skin marker sets and the PCT. In this study, the lateral and medial epicondyles showed high correlations of >0.90. However, the correlations of the X-coordinates were lower than those of the Y- and Z-coordinates, and this was considered to have an impact on the calculations of the knee angle. In particular, error tended to grow large about the rotational motion of the knee joint during the early and late stance phases; it was supposed that errors of X-coordinates of the thigh and shank were strongly affected when the rotational motion of the knee joint grew to be large.

A limitation of this research is that neither RMS nor the PCT follows the motion of a true bone; therefore, true values cannot be calculated. Although the error by skin movement artifacts remains a problem that cannot be avoided in gait analyses using skin-mounted markers, it is suggested that these analyses may obtain comparatively reliable results by using protocols that estimate anatomical landmarks. In the PCT using many reflective markers, it is difficult to attach markers on a few parts because of the influence of muscle contraction. However, for RMS, it is thought that the measurement results can be brought closer to more exact values by setting three markers on parts with as little influence of muscle contraction as possible. In this study, the correlations between protocols of RMS and the PCT were lower for the X-coordinates at all anatomical landmarks than for the Y- and Z-coordinates. In particular, it was difficult to obtain an adequately reliable measurement of the rotational motion of the knee joint, and the errors of X-coordinates of each anatomical landmark around the knee joint were a large factor for the rotational motion of the knee joint. However, it is suggested that flexion/extension and abduction/adduction of RMS and the PCT had comparatively little error and good reliability after 30% of the stance phase in this study.

5. Conclusions

Flexion/extension and abduction/adduction of the knee by two different protocols had comparatively little error and good reliability after 30% of the stance phase.

Conflict of Interests

The author declared no conflict of interests.

References

[1] N. Foroughi, R. Smith, and B. Vanwanseele, "The association of external knee adduction moment with biomechanical variables in osteoarthritis: a systematic review," *Knee*, vol. 16, no. 5, pp. 303–309, 2009.

[2] C. O. Kean, T. B. Birmingham, J. S. Garland et al., "Moments and muscle activity after high tibial osteotomy and anterior cruciate ligament reconstruction," *Medicine and Science in Sports and Exercise*, vol. 41, no. 3, pp. 612–619, 2009.

[3] J. A. Zeni and J. S. Higginson, "Differences in gait parameters between healthy subjects and persons with moderate and severe knee osteoarthritis: a result of altered walking speed?" *Clinical Biomechanics*, vol. 24, no. 4, pp. 372–378, 2009.

[4] J. Fuller, L. J. Liu, M. C. Murphy, and R. W. Mann, "A comparison of lower-extremity skeletal kinematics measured using skin-and pin-mounted markers," *Human Movement Science*, vol. 16, no. 2-3, pp. 219–242, 1997.

[5] C. Reinschmidt, A. J. Van Den Bogert, A. Lundberg et al., "Tibiofemoral and tibiocalcaneal motion during walking: external versus Skeletal markers," *Gait and Posture*, vol. 6, no. 2, pp. 98–109, 1997.

[6] M. A. Lafortune, P. R. Cavanagh, H. J. Sommer, and A. Kalenak, "Three-dimensional kinematics of the human knee during walking," *Journal of Biomechanics*, vol. 25, no. 4, pp. 347–357, 1992.

[7] M. H. Schwartz, J. P. Trost, and R. A. Wervey, "Measurement and management of errors in quantitative gait data," *Gait and Posture*, vol. 20, no. 2, pp. 196–203, 2004.

[8] A. Cappello, A. Cappozzo, P. F. La Palombara, L. Lucchetti, and A. Leardini, "Multiple anatomical landmark calibration for optimal bone pose estimation," *Human Movement Science*, vol. 16, no. 2-3, pp. 259–274, 1997.

[9] A. Cappozzo, F. Catani, U. Della Croce, and A. Leardini, "Position and orientation in space of bones during movement: anatomical frame definition and determination," *Clinical Biomechanics*, vol. 10, no. 4, pp. 171–178, 1995.

[10] M. Donati, V. Camomilla, G. Vannozzi, and A. Cappozzo, "Enhanced anatomical calibration in human movement analysis," *Gait and Posture*, vol. 26, no. 2, pp. 179–185, 2007.

[11] T. P. Andriacchi, E. J. Alexander, M. K. Toney, C. Dyrby, and J. Sum, "A point cluster method for in vivo motion analysis: applied to a study of knee kinematics," *Journal of Biomechanical Engineering*, vol. 120, no. 6, pp. 743–749, 1998.

[12] Y. Nagano, H. Ida, M. Akai, and T. Fukubayashi, "Biomechanical characteristics of the knee joint in female athletes during tasks associated with anterior cruciate ligament injury," *Knee*, vol. 16, no. 2, pp. 153–158, 2009.

[13] G. Misonoo, A. Kanamori, H. Ida, S. Miyakawa, and N. Ochiai, "Evaluation of tibial rotational stability of single-bundle vs. anatomical double-bundle anterior cruciate ligament reconstruction during a high-demand activity—a quasi-randomized trial," *Knee*, vol. 19, pp. 87–93, 2011.

[14] A. Cereatti, U. Della Croce, and A. Cappozzo, "Reconstruction of skeletal movement using skin markers: comparative assessment of bone pose estimators," *Journal of NeuroEngineering and Rehabilitation*, vol. 3, article 7, 2006.

[15] H. Ida, Y. Nagano, T. Fukubayashi, and M. Akai, "Measurement of in vivo motion of the knee: assessment and application of the point cluster technique," in *Proceedings of the SICE Annual Conference*, pp. 1255–1258, August 2005.

[16] E. S. Grood and W. J. Suntay, "A joint coordinate system for the clinical description of three-dimensional motions: application to the knee," *Journal of Biomechanical Engineering*, vol. 105, no. 2, pp. 136–144, 1983.

[17] M. P. Kadaba, H. K. Ramakrishnan, M. E. Wootten, J. Gainey, G. Gorton, and G. V. B. Cochran, "Repeatability of kinematic, kinetic, and electromyographic data in normal adult gait," *Journal of Orthopaedic Research*, vol. 7, no. 6, pp. 849–860, 1989.

[18] J. Perry, *Gait Analysis: Normal and Pathological Function*, SLACK Incorporated, Thorofare, NJ, USA, 1992.

[19] H. Ishii, Y. Nagano, H. Ida, T. Fukubayashi, and T. Maruyama, "Knee kinematics and kinetics during shuttle run cutting: comparison of the assessments performed with and without the point cluster technique," *Journal of Biomechanics*, vol. 44, no. 10, pp. 1999–2003, 2011.

20

Evaluation of Strength and Irradiated Movement Pattern Resulting from Trunk Motions of the Proprioceptive Neuromuscular Facilitation

Luciana Bahia Gontijo,[1] Polianna Delfino Pereira,[2] Camila Danielle Cunha Neves,[3] Ana Paula Santos,[1] Dionis de Castro Dutra Machado,[4] and Victor Hugo do Vale Bastos[4, 5]

[1] Physical Therapy Department, Federal University of the Valleys of Jequitinhonha and Mucuri, 39100-000 Diamantina, MG, Brazil
[2] Department of Neuroscience and Behavioral Sciences, School of Medicine of Ribeirão Preto, University of São Paulo, 14049-900 Ribeirão Preto, SP, Brazil
[3] Multicenter Post Graduation Program in Physiological Sciences, Federal University of the Valleys of Jequitinhonha and Mucuri, 39100-000 Diamantina, MG, Brazil
[4] Physical Therapy Department, Brain Mapping Lab & Functionality, Federal University of Piauí, 64202-020 Parnaíba, PI, Brazil
[5] CNPq, 71605-001 Brasília, DF, Brazil

Correspondence should be addressed to Dionis de Castro Dutra Machado, dionis@ufpi.edu.br

Academic Editor: Luc Vanhees

Introduction. The proprioceptive neuromuscular facilitation (PNF) is a physiotherapeutic concept based on muscle and joint proprioceptive stimulation. Among its principles, the irradiation is the reaction of the distinct regional muscle contractions to the position of the application of the motions. *Objective.* To investigate the presence of irradiated dorsiflexion and plantar flexion and the existing strength generated by them during application of PNF trunk motions. *Methods.* The study was conducted with 30 sedentary and female volunteers, the PNF motions of trunk flexion, and extension with the foot (right and left) positioned in a developed equipment coupled to the load cell, which measured the strength irradiated in Newton. *Results.* Most of the volunteers irradiated dorsal flexion in the performance of the flexion and plantar flexion during the extension motion, both presenting an average force of 8.942 N and 10.193 N, respectively. *Conclusion.* The distal irradiation in lower limbs became evident, reinforcing the therapeutic actions to the PNF indirect muscular activation.

1. Introduction

Proprioceptive neuromuscular facilitation (PNF) is a concept of treatment [1] in which the basic philosophy considers that every human, including those with disabilities, has an untapped existing potential [2]. PNF is a method used in clinical practice [3] in order to improve development of neuromuscular system by stimulation of muscle and joint proprioceptors [4]. Some concepts characterize the philosophy under the technique: integrated approach (i.e., treatment is directed toward the human as a whole and not only as a body segment), based on an untapped existing potential (mobilizing reserves patients), positive approach (reinforcing patient's ability on a physical and psychological

level) whose goal is reaching the level of function from this patient through the International Classification of Functioning (ICF) model.

Among the PNF's principles, irradiation is a useful aspect for patients with muscle weakness in areas that cannot be directly worked (strengthened) [5]. This principle is based on fact that stimulation of strong and preserved muscle groups produces strong activation of injured and weak muscles, facilitating muscle contraction [6]. So, these weak muscles can develop an increase in the duration and/or intensity by the spread of the response to stimulation or by the synergistic muscle inhibition [7]. Some studies have investigated the presence of irradiation [3, 7–9], but type of muscle (agonist or antagonist) which receives irradiation is not consistent in the literature. According to Sherrigton [7], irradiation only innervates agonist muscles, but Hellebrandt et al. [8] found in their studies that during wrist exercises, the most significant effects were seen in contralateral limb muscles [9]. In order to determine quantitatively and accurately the existence of muscle strength, accurate equipment must be used.

To evaluate force exerted on limb by virtue of irradiation, it is possible to use load cell equipment as force measurement transducer due to its lower cost and greater portability in addition to being one of the most used instruments for measuring force [10–14]. The operating principle of load cells is based on variations in the ohmic resistance of a sensor named as extensometer or strain gauge, when submitted to a deformation. Specialized tools for verifying irradiation to the lower limbs have not been found on the market and in the literature; therefore a specific apparatus was developed for this purpose.

PNF is one of the main concepts of rehabilitation treatment for patients with neurological injuries, being used for several years and spread by known authors such as Kabat, Susan, who defend its efficiency. The trunk is the central region for motor control of lower and upper limbs and can irradiate to them. When an injury of nervous system occurs, as a stroke, this motor control can be disturbed and does not allow effective movements at limbs [1, 2]. However, researches are still scarce nowadays, especially regarding the neurophysiological basis of the irradiation principle. Further studies are necessary to form a more concrete and detailed definition, which can trigger improvements in physical conditions and life quality for the patient, avoiding its erroneous applications. In this sense, the study objective was to evaluate strength, using load cell, and motion pattern (dorsiflexion or plantar flexion) triggered by irradiation resulting from PNF motions of trunk flexion and extension.

2. Methodology

2.1. Subjects. Sample of this cross-sectional study consisted of 30 female volunteers aged 18–30, university students, sedentary, who performed less than 20 minutes of physical activity in less than 3 days in a week, in the last six months [15]. The selection for only female volunteers occurred due to the fact that the researcher was a woman, which would prevent performance of the maximum strengthening from male volunteers since they possibly have higher force range. Smokers, male gender, subjects with presence of any cardiac, pulmonary, musculoskeletal, or neurological diseases, with functional limitation to perform resistance exercises or those having baseline blood pressure above 140/90 mmHg, were excluded. This study covers standards required for researches involving human subjects contained in Declaration of Helsinki and was approved by the Ethics Committee in Research of UFVJM under protocol 132/10, also in accordance with the Resolution CNS 196/96.

All volunteers were evaluated about body mass index according to the criteria of the National Health and Nutrition Examination Survey, proposed in United States and to blood pressure, using the same aneroid and stethoscope

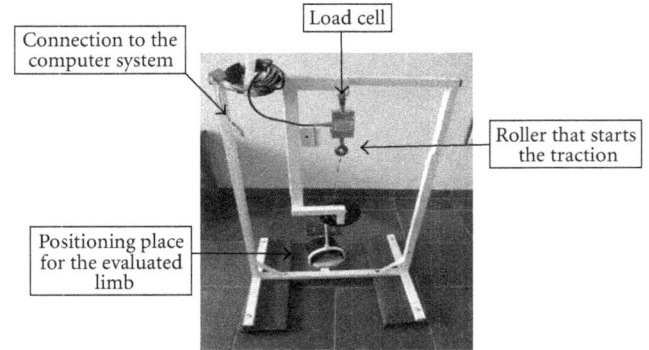

FIGURE 1: Measuring instrument, coupled to the load cell, used to measure the irradiation and the force generated by the PNF motions.

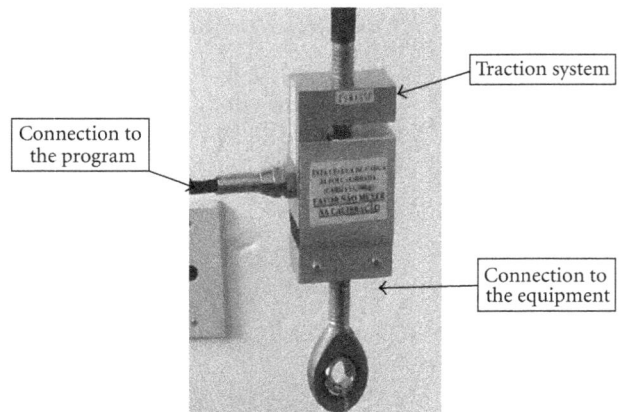

FIGURE 2: Load cell.

sphygmomanometer type, and answered the item related to the lower limb of the Oldfield Handedness Inventory [16]. Subjects were not familiar with the PNF concept to prevent possible bias. Volunteers were instructed not to drink alcohol 24 hours before evaluation, not to ingest caffeine (chocolate, chocolate drinks, coffees, teas, soft drinks, and the like) on the day of evaluation, to have a good sleep on previous night, and not practice any physical activity 24 hours before evaluation. All subjects eligible participated in the study; no desistance occurred.

2.2. Measurement. The instrument used to measure plantar flexion and dorsiflexion pattern (Figure 1) and the force generated by irradiation was developed by researchers with the help of a designers and its efficiency was tested. The device enables foot positioning and starts the rolling to right (indicating dorsiflexion) or to left (indicating plantar flexion) pulling the load cell coupled to the system, generating its deformation and the measurement in a computerized system. The load cell used was from Miotec-Biomedical Equipment 250 kg (Figure 2).

The data was collected in one single moment, according to volunteers availability, at morning or at afternoon. A familiarity with the motions was performed 48 hours before

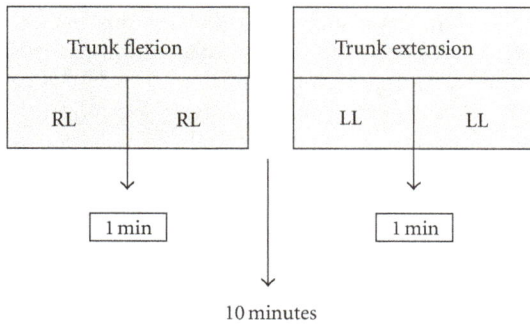

FIGURE 3: Performed motion sequence. RL: right limb; LL: left limb.

the study, but it did not involve any learning due to the given interval. Each volunteer seated at the same wooden chair with a backrest and without armrests, with the foot on the system, the knee flexion at 60° degrees on a foam wedge. Trunk flexion and extension motions were performed using the resistance PNF motion, evaluating both positioning feet, the left and the right one on the system at each motion. The motion of each foot was held in two trials, with one minute rest between them, considering the highest value and standard developed by this value. Between trunk flexion and extension motions, a ten-minute break was given in order to avoid fatigue and the decrease of the maximum developed force (Figure 3).

2.3. Motions. The task was explained to each subject and started with the examiner's command "go." This command is an auditory stimulus and works like a positive reinforcement. The command was repeated some times during the task execution according basic to principles of PNF's concept (positive approach). The motions followed the concepts established by PNF's philosophy [1], in which a continuous manual resistance was applied through lumbrical contact, and an encouragement of voice command was given. Then, the volunteers performed motions of trunk flexion and extension, using their maximum strength. The quantification of maximum strength developed by volunteers was made by overcoming theraband elastic resistance, in which the intensity of force was represented by the following: entire elastic in purple, in gray, and in orange, folded elastic in purple, in gray, and in orange.

Trunk flexion motion was performed with therapist in front of the volunteer, with the elbows extended and one leg in front of the other, with the knees in semiflexion, resting both hands on anterosuperior surface of the volunteer trunk, with lumbrical grip at anterior shoulder region. The volunteer was sitting on a wooden chair, and the limb was evaluated positioned on equipment with knee flexion of 60°. The movement started from neutral position of trunk (upright position) followed by trunk flexion until it reaches 45° against a manual resistance from the therapist (Figure 4).

Extension motion was performed with therapist behind the volunteer, extended elbows and one leg in front of the other, with the knees in semiflexion, resting with lumbrical grip at posterior shoulder region. The volunteer was sitting

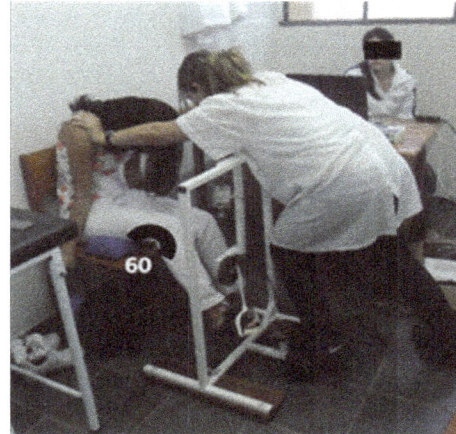

FIGURE 4: Trunk flexion motion.

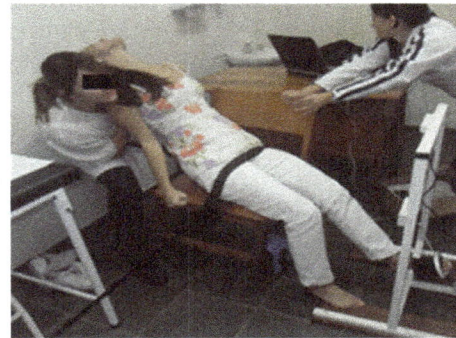

FIGURE 5: Trunk extension motion.

on a chair and involved with a Velcro strip to prevent sliding on the seat during the motion. The movement started from neutral position of trunk and performed an extension until it reaches 45° against the manual resistance from the therapist, so that the volunteer could perform her maximum strength. The remaining positions were the same as the flexion motion (Figure 5).

To perform statistical analysis the Statistical Package for the Social Sciences (SPSS) was used. The Shapiro-Wilk test verified the nonnormality from the data of the strength generated in each shift (morning and afternoon) and limb (right and left), so the comparison of the averages was performed using nonparametric Mann-Whitney test. Normality was found for data of motion (extension and flexion), so the independent *t*-test was performed to compare the averages. Values less than 0.05 were considered as statistically significant, according to the Fisher criteria.

3. Results

The sample was composed of 30 subjects with mean age of 22.57 years old, weight of 57.42 kg, height of 164.23 cm, and BMI equivalent to 21.30 (Table 1).

The execution of trunk flexion motion caused irradiation to dorsal flexion at 96.7% of subjects when right foot was placed on equipment and at 100% when the left foot

TABLE 1: Sample description.

	Age	Weight	Height	BMI
Average	22.57	57.42	164.23	21.30
Standard deviation	1.695	7.238	5.52	2.38
Maximum	27	73	178.00	27.62
Minimum	20	43	154.00	17.33

was positionated. During extension motion, plantar flexion irradiation was generated at 100% of subjects in both of the positioned feet. The dorsiflexion developed an average force of 2.60N on the right limb and 2.84N on the left limb, and the triggered plantar flexion generated an average force of 7.52N on the right limb and of 7.24N on the left one.

From the total sample, 14 volunteers participated at morning and 16 at afternoon. Table 2 shows the mean strength that was triggered by each motion pattern (flexion or extension trunk) with both feet positioning. Comparing this data, higher mean strength generated by volunteers that performed the motion of the right limb at morning was considered significant. It presented $P = 0.013$ in the plantar flexion of the right foot triggered by trunk extension, and $P = 0.029$ on the right foot dorsiflexion triggered by trunk flexion.

Stronger subjects used therabands of higher resistance and so, more force was irradiated. However, the results from these force descriptions will not be presented in this study due to the large number of variables already available, which need the development of new future researches. The laterality questionnaire obtained dominance of the right lower limb in 100% of the volunteers.

The independent t-test was used to compare the total force developed by the flexion and extension motions regardless of the positioned foot. At trunk flexion mean was 2.72N (± 2.40), and at trunk extension it was 7.38N (± 5.61). Significant values were found in relation to a greater force generated by the extension ($P = 0.000$).

4. Discussion

This study aimed to investigate the pattern (dorsiflexion or plantar flexion) and the amount of irradiated strength resulting from the resistance imposed on trunk flexion and extension movement of PNF. The sample was composed of female subjects in which smallest amount of lean mass observed [17] may have reduced the average of the irradiated force. Further studies with male volunteers should be conducted to investigate this hypothesis. This study presents initial data as the first surveys from future researches that are intended to be carried out by the researchers.

Trunk flexion motion significantly irradiated dorsal flexion movement for both right and left ankle. Possibly a need of approximation from the origin and the insertion of the rectus femoris favored the great length tension required in sufficient pelvic stabilization for trunk flexion in its maximum efficiency [18], considering, during the

data collection, an associated ipsilateral hip flexion with dorsiflexion was observed. So, the contraction of hip flexors could lead to shortening of deep lateral myofascial causing ankle dorsiflexion [19]. This fact resembles the primitive patterns of sensory inputs during walking in basic patterns, specifically the swing phase [20]. Therefore, the irradiated movement may be associated to the triggering stimulus of nervous system, which presents among its circuits predetermined sequential activation of muscle contractions to the achievement of efficient walking and lower energy expenditure [21].

It is noteworthy that the present study used a simple technique of trunk flexion and extension to observe irradiation to the lower limbs; another possibility consists in using trunk rotation to cause irradiation to them. In physical therapy practice, irradiation can be used in cases where paresis is noted; that is, stroke or spinal cord injury and other conditions present with weakness by immobility. However, integrity of trunk movements is necessary. If trunk does not have sufficient strength or have an instability, it must be worked on previously to acquire strength and stability sufficient to generate irradiation to the lower limbs.

During trunk extension motion, the movement performed by the ankle was the plantar flexion, on both limbs that were analyzed. A similar pattern triggered by the primitive patterns of walking (pulse phase) was present [21], but initial position of the volunteer (hip and knee flexion) led to changes in patterns considered normal. This event is held by the human body as adapters to atypical stimulus [22, 23]. In this way, trunk extension performed by the erector spinae triggered a hip extension and plantar flexion. However, instead of having knee flexion there was a trend to extension, favoring the biomechanical advantage of rectus femoris contraction as soon as it approximated its insertions, so that it could eccentrically stabilize the pelvis [18]. Since the developed standard was significant in the study, the trunk motions may be directed to the "indirect" strengthening, in which it starts the trunk flexion training to strengthen the dorsal flexors and the plantar flexors with trunk extension.

The origination of higher force ranges in the right limb to perform the task may be related to high incidence of volunteers right-handedness, observed by Oldfield inventory. Studies believe that dominant lower limb has a higher efficiency of force generation [24, 25] since the asymmetric functions are specified in the mobility to perform unipodal tasks due to more complex neuromuscular demands [26]. This event has been explained by neurodevelopmental theory which believes that the influence of asymmetry of ear and labyrinth development, in third trimester of pregnancy, is related to higher efficiency of ipsilateral hemisphere for providing early experience [27]. Another aspect is the fact that social culture tends to create demand for tasks with right limb, favoring its postural control and, consequently, a more efficient contraction [26]. Strength generation itself, as demonstrated numerically in joules, proves the existence of distal strength in irradiation. Therefore, the studied motions can be applied to perform muscle contraction without direct contact to the activated muscle.

TABLE 2: Strength generated in each shift.

Motion pattern	Shift	Mean strength	Standard deviation
Flexion—right foot	Morning	3.67	0.77
Flexion—right foot	Afternoon	1.67	0.36
Flexion—left foot	Morning	3.77	0.74
Flexion—left foot	Afternoon	2.03	0.44
Extension—right foot	Morning	9.71	1.48
Extension—right foot	Afternoon	5.60	1.41
Extension—left foot	Morning	9.02	1.44
Extension—left foot	Afternoon	5.69	1.26

One of the hypotheses to explain better results at morning is that the circadian rhythm might have been influenced because the best development of skeletal muscles occurs as a metabolic consequence of human, which in most cases are more activated by specific hypothalamic hormones [28]. The hormonal peaks vary during the 24 hours of the day for mammals, according to the energy required from the species [29], increasing metabolism in skeletal muscle, which can help effectiveness of its contraction. According to Atkinson [30] this condition is more constant at morning, which may have influenced higher levels of strength during this period, as well as it is possible that the volunteers who performed the motions at afternoon had done more activities during the day, compared to the ones from the morning shift, leading to a greater cumulative muscle fatigue. In accordance with these results, training aiming to achieve higher thresholds of strength will have a greater efficiency at morning. In this study the maneuvers application at afternoon was necessary due to samples availability and was not a study limitation. Another hypothesis that can be explored is examiner's fatigue at afternoon, but on research design was programmed the routine data collection considering examiner rested to apply the correct technique, and it was followed.

The plantar flexion produced a higher average of force range as a consequent movement from trunk extension motion. Newton's Law of Universal Gravitation may have influenced the result of the unleashed force [31, 32], since the volunteer had the sum of the gravity and muscle strengths in the plantar flexion of the determined position. Different from dorsiflexion, that had the force of gravity as a negative element. Another determining factor may have been the combination of gravity to muscle aspect with higher numbers of muscle fibers and muscle favorable biomechanics (by semiflexion of the knee from the initial position of the test), leading to an intrinsic advantage of the physiological mechanisms of mentioned muscle [18, 33]. In order to develop the equipment, some items were established as essential in its design. The possibility of dorsal or plantar flexion execution was one of these items, since it was necessary to have them primarily investigated because of its nondetermination in the literature. However, its application had the influence of gravitational force as a consequence, which can be disregarded by mathematical calculations in future analyses.

5. Conclusion

The results show that trunk flexion and extension motions generate an irradiated movement in dorsiflexion and plantar flexion, respectively. Considerable strength values were measured as a result of the indirect muscle activation of the muscle groups responsible for such action, both in healthy and sedentary women. Therefore, PNF concept enables the performance of muscle activation of dorsal and plantar flexors which cannot be worked directly as in poststroke hemiparetic members.

References

[1] S. Susan, A. D. Beckers, and M. Buck, in *FNP in Practice: An Illustrated Guide*, M. V. Heidelberg, Ed., pp. 80–89, Springer, Berlin, Germany, 2003.

[2] J. W. Youdas, D. B. Arend, J. M. Exstrom, T. J. Helmus, J. D. Rozeboom, and J. H. Hollman, "Comparison of muscle activation levels during arm abduction in the plane of the scapula vs.proprioceptive neuromuscular facilitation upper extremity patterns," *The Journal of Strength & Conditioning Research*, vol. 26, no. 4, pp. 1058–1065, 2012.

[3] P. C. Meningroni, C. S. Nakada, L. Hata, A. C. Fuzaro, W. M. Júnior, and J. E. Araujo, "Contralateral force irradiation for the activation of tibialis anterior muscle in carriers of Charcot-Marie-Tooth disease: effect of PNF intervention program," *Revista Brasileira de Fisioterapia*, vol. 13, no. 5, pp. 438–443, 2009.

[4] K. N. Sharma, *Handbook of Proprioceptive Neuromuscular Facilitation: Basic Concepts and Techniques*, Lambert, Saarbrücken, Germany, 2012.

[5] P. M. S. Pink, "Contralateral effects of upper extremity proprioceptive neuromuscular facilitation patterns," *Physical Therapy*, vol. 61, no. 8, pp. 1158–1162, 1981.

[6] N. Kofotolis, I. S. Vrabas, E. Vamvakoudis, A. Papanikolaou, and K. Mandroukas, "Proprioceptive neuromuscular facilitation training induced alterations in muscle fibre type and cross sectional area," *British journal of sports medicine*, vol. 39, no. 3, p. e11, 2005.

[7] C. Sherrington, *The Integrative Action of the Nervous System*, Yale University Press, New Haven, UK, 1947.

[8] F. A. Hellebrandt, S. J. Houtz, M. J. Partridge, and C. E. Walters, "Tonic neck reflexes in exercise of stress in man," *American Journal of Physical Medicine and Rehabilitation*, vol. 35, pp. 144–159, 1956.

[9] F. A. Hellebrandt and J. C. Waterland, "Indirect learning. The influence of unimanual exercise on related muscle groups of the same and the opposite side," *American Journal of Physical Medicine*, vol. 41, pp. 45–55, 1962.

[10] J. Loss et al., "Recommended method for correlating muscle strength and electromyography," *Movement*, vol. 8, no. 1, pp. 33–40, 1998.

[11] L. Schettino et al., "Comparative study on the strength and autonomy of sedentary versus active elderly women," *Revista Terapia Manual*, vol. 5, no. 20, pp. 131–135, 2007.

[12] M. Papoti et al., "Standardization of a specific protocol for determining the anaerobic conditioning in swimmers using load cells," *Revista Portuguesa de Ciências do Desporto*, vol. 3, no. 3, pp. 36–42, 2003.

[13] M. Gonçalves and F. S. S. Barbosa, "Analysis of strength and resistance parameters of the lumbar spinae erector muscles during isometric exercise at different effort levels," *Revista Brasileira de Medicina do Esporte*, vol. 11, no. 2, pp. 109–114, 2005.

[14] J. M. Miller, J. A. A. Miller, D. Perruchini, and J. O. L. DeLancey, "Test-retest reliability of an instrumented speculum for measuring vaginal closure force," *Neurourology and Urodynamics*, vol. 26, no. 6, pp. 858–863, 2007.

[15] J. M. Jakicic, B. H. Marcus, K. I. Gallagher, M. Napolitano, and W. Lang, "Effect of exercise duration and intensity on weight loss in overweight, sedentary women: a randomized trial," *Journal of the American Medical Association*, vol. 290, no. 10, pp. 1323–1330, 2003.

[16] L. J. Elias, M. P. Bryden, and M. B. Bulman-Fleming, "Footedness is a better predictor than is handedness of emotional lateralization," *Neuropsychologia*, vol. 36, no. 1, pp. 37–43, 1998.

[17] Y. Okamoto, A. Kunimatsu, T. Kono, Y. Kujiraoka, J. Sonobe, and M. Minami, "Gender differences in MR muscle tractography," *Magnetic Resonance in Medical Sciences*, vol. 9, no. 3, pp. 111–118, 2010.

[18] A. D. Neumann, *Kinesiology of the Musculoskeletal System*, Elsevie, Rio de Janeiro, Brazil, 2011.

[19] T. Myers, *Anatomy Trains*, Elsevier, Rio de Janeiro, Brazil, 2010.

[20] A. Frigon and J. P. Gossard, "Evidence for specialized rhythm-generating mechanisms in the adult mammalian spinal cord," *Journal of Neuroscience*, vol. 30, no. 20, pp. 7061–7071, 2010.

[21] Y. P. Ivanenko, R. E. Poppele, and F. Lacquaniti, "Five basic muscle activation patterns account for muscle activity during human locomotion," *Journal of Physiology*, vol. 556, no. 1, pp. 267–282, 2004.

[22] G. Cappellini, Y. P. Ivanenko, N. Dominici, R. E. Poppele, and F. Lacquaniti, "Motor patterns during walking on a slippery walkway," *Journal of Neurophysiology*, vol. 103, no. 2, pp. 746–760, 2010.

[23] R. Cham and M. S. Redfern, "Changes in gait when anticipating slippery floors," *Gait and Posture*, vol. 15, no. 2, pp. 159–171, 2002.

[24] L. J. Elias, M. P. Bryden, and M. B. Bulman-Fleming, "Footedness is a better predictor than is handedness of emotional lateralization," *Neuropsychologia*, vol. 36, no. 1, pp. 37–43, 1998.

[25] B. D. McLean and M. D. Tumilty, "Left-right asymmetry in two types of soccer kick," *British Journal of Sports Medicine*, vol. 27, no. 4, pp. 260–262, 1993.

[26] C. Gabbard and S. Hart, "A Question of foot dominance," *Journal of General Psychology*, vol. 123, no. 4, pp. 289–296, 1996.

[27] F. H. Previc, "A general theory concerning the prenatal origins of cerebral lateralization in humans," *Psychological Review*, vol. 98, no. 3, pp. 299–334, 1991.

[28] X. Zhang, T. J. Dube, and K. A. Esser, "Working around the clock: circadian rhythms and skeletal muscle," *Journal of Applied Physiology*, vol. 107, no. 5, pp. 1647–1654, 2009.

[29] R. R. Almon, E. Yang, W. Lai et al., "Relationships between circadian rhythms and modulation of gene expression by glucocorticoids in skeletal muscle," *American Journal of Physiology—Regulatory Integrative and Comparative Physiology*, vol. 295, no. 4, pp. R1031–R1047, 2008.

[30] G. Atkinson, H. Jones, and P. N. Ainslie, "Circadian variation in the circulatory responses to exercise: relevance to the morning peaks in strokes and cardiac events," *European Journal of Applied Physiology*, vol. 108, no. 1, pp. 15–29, 2010.

[31] V. M. Zatsiorsky, F. Gao, and M. L. Latash, "Motor control goes beyond physics: differential effects of gravity and inertia on finger forces during manipulation of hand-held objects," *Experimental Brain Research*, vol. 162, no. 3, pp. 300–308, 2005.

[32] V. Baltzopoulos and D. A. Brodie, "Isokinetic dynamometry. Applications and limitations," *Sports Medicine*, vol. 8, no. 2, pp. 101–116, 1989.

[33] H. Degens, R. M. Erskine, and C. I. Morse, "Disproportionate changes in skeletal muscle strength and size with resistance training and ageing," *Journal of Musculoskeletal Neuronal Interactions*, vol. 9, no. 3, pp. 123–129, 2009.

21

Functional Stretching Exercise Submitted for Spastic Diplegic Children: A Randomized Control Study

Mohamed Ali Elshafey,[1] **Adel Abd-Elaziem,**[2] **and Rana Elmarzouki Gouda**[3]

[1] *Department of Physical Therapy for Growth and Developmental Disorder in Children and Its Surgery, Faculty of Physical Therapy, Cairo University, Egypt*
[2] *Faculty of Medicine, Zagazig University, Egypt*
[3] *Physical Therapy Department, General Hospital of Mit Ghamr, Egypt*

Correspondence should be addressed to Mohamed Ali Elshafey; elrahmapt@gmail.com

Academic Editor: Nicola Smania

Objective. Studying the effect of the functional stretching exercise in diplegic children. *Design.* Children were randomly assigned into two matched groups. *Setting.* Outpatient Clinic of the Faculty of Physical Therapy, Cairo University. *Participants.* Thirty ambulant spastic diplegic children, ranging in age from five to eight years, participated in this study. *Interventions.* The control group received physical therapy program with traditional passive stretching exercises. The study group received physical therapy program with functional stretching exercises. The treatment was performed for two hours per session, three times weekly for three successive months. *Main Outcome Measure(s).* H\M ratio, popliteal angle, and gait parameters were evaluated for both groups before and after treatment. *Results.* There was significant improvement in all the measuring variables for both groups in favor of study group. H\M ratio was reduced, popliteal angle was increased, and gait was improved. *Conclusion(s).* Functional stretching exercises were effectively used in rehabilitation of spastic diplegic children; it reduced H\M ratio, increased popliteal angle, and improved gait.

1. Background

Spastic children are the commonest type of cerebral palsy (CP) [1] characterized by increased resistance to passive movement due to spasticity [2]. The loss of supraspinal control over reflex arc causes spasticity [3] depending on location and severity of lesion [4, 5]. Spasticity leads to muscle contractures and bone deformities as a result of secondary structure changes of the muscles fibers [6, 7]. These changes in fiber bundles and fewer sarcomeres [8, 9] cause a decreased range of motion (ROM) [10]. Spastic diplegic children had hip flexors, hamstrings, psoas, and calf muscles tightness, leading to flexed posture [11–13].

Stretching exercises were developed to manage spasticity, including passive and active stretching, positioning, and isotonic and isokinetic stretching. The effect of stretching depends on tension applied to the soft tissue, duration, repetition in session, and daily frequency [14, 15]. Static stretching splint reduced spasticity and improved motor function [16, 17]. Stretching prevented adhesion of the joint capsule [18]. Stretching followed by passive exercise reduced hyperactive stretch reflexes [19, 20]. Slowly sustained stretch managed painful contractures [21, 22]. Prolonged muscle stretch reduced motor neuron excitability [23]. Stretching exercises increased Achilles tendon cross-sectional area, decreased gastrocnemius and soleus muscle fascicular stiffness [24], and improved walking and crouch posture [25].

On the other hand, some researches stated that stretching did not improve joint mobility in people with contractures if performed for less than seven months [26]. Prolonged muscle stretch did not efficiently treat or prevent contracture [27] and failed to provide proper treatment for spasticity [28].

A systematic review of stretching exercises for CP children reported limited evidence that manual stretching increased ROM, reduced spasticity, and improved walking because of methodological issues, small sample sizes, small number of studies, and little attention in the evaluation of active stretching in children with CP [29]. There is no

TABLE 1: Description of block randomization.

Severity according to gross motor function classification system	Treatment	
	Control	Study
Grade I	8	8
Grade II	8	8

evidence that stretching improved ROM during walking or other functional activities [30]. A systematic review of physical therapy treatment for CP demonstrated that stretching exercise for CP is limited because the mechanism and etiology of muscle contractures are not clear and clinical research evaluating the effectiveness of stretching techniques is inconclusive and cannot guide therapists' clinical decision making [31].

2. Subjects, Materials, and Methods

2.1. Study Design. This study was a randomized controlled trial. The study was performed over one year during the period from January 2013 to January 2014.

2.2. Subjects. Thirty-two ambulant spastic diplegic CP children were selected from the Outpatient Clinic of the Faculty of Physical Therapy, Cairo University. Their range of age was 5–8 years old. The experiments divided subjects into blocks according to severity of mild and moderate. Then, within each block subjects are randomly assigned to control and study groups to ensure that each treatment condition has proportion equal to control and study group. The randomized block removes dividing of the children groups as source of variability and as confounding variable (Table 1).

All children were ambulant with crouch gait pattern and had grades I and II according to gross motor function classification system and spasticity of grade 1 or grade 1^+ according to modified Ashworth scale. All children can follow orders and have neither auditory nor visual disorders. Children were excluded if they had hip dislocation, fixed contractures or deformity, surgical intervention as surgical release, rhizotomy and tenotomy, Botulinum toxin injections, baclofen pump, osteoporosis, heart diseases, uncontrolled convulsions, and leg length discrepancy.

2.3. Materials. EMG Neuropac S1, Model DI 90B, SN 00030, made in Japan, Motion analysis system, Hocoma 00034, made in USA, and universal goniometry were used.

2.4. Methods. Each group was evaluated before and after three months of treatment by the Hoffmann reflex of soleus muscle. The soleus H-reflex is obtained by anodal stimulation of the posterior tibial nerve at the popliteal fossa. Small intensities of stimulation preferentially activate Ia fibers that excite alpha-motor neurons, thus giving rise to reflex response in the soleus H-wave that was recorded by EMG and then stimulation with higher intensities to activate axons of alpha-motor neurons and M-response was recorded. The popliteal angle was measured by the universal geometry, with the child placed in supine position and hip flexed to right angle.

The stationary arm of the goniometer was placed parallel to the longitudinal axis of the femur, in line bisecting greater trochanter and the movable arm parallel to the longitudinal axis of fibula, in line bisecting lateral malleolus and the axis of the goniometer was placed over the lateral epicondyle of the femur, while the other leg in neutral extension. Stride length, stride speed, and stance phase percentages were evaluated in both groups before and after treatment by 3D motion analysis system.

3. Treatment Methods

The control group received the selected physical therapy program; the program included function training, balance exercise, trunk control, and passive stretching exercises for the hip flexors, hip adductors, hamstring, and calf muscle; stretching was applied for 30 sec with 30 sec rest 3–5 times for each muscle group within pain limit followed by strengthening exercise for weak muscles which was performed in three groups; each group contained ten repetitions for each weak muscle group.

The study group received the same selected physical therapy program also; however, stretching exercise and function training were performed together. The functional stretching exercises were performed by training the child to maintain walk standing and stride standing positions with gradual increase of distance between lower limbs with extended knees to stretch lower limb muscle, and the child was trained to stoop and recover from these positions. The child was trained to walk with full extended knees and hips in slight abduction with correction of lower limb rotation. Strengthening of abdominal and back muscles was performed with hip joint abductions and knee joint extension. The program was performed gradually according to child tolerance within pain limit also and rest given when required (Figure 1).

3.1. Functional Stretching Exercise Program. The child was trained to be maintained standing in walk stand position and gradually increase distance between both legs to stretch lower extremities muscles with RT leg forward then with LT leg forward.

The child was trained to be maintained standing in stride standing position and gradually increase distance between legs to stretch tight hip adductors muscles of both sides.

The child was trained to stand on RT leg in complete extension while holding the other leg in abduction to stretch hip adductor of the raised leg and then reverse the leg position.

The child was trained to walk while manually holding knee joint in full extension and hip joint in slight abduction to stretch all lower limb muscles with correction of lower extremities rotation.

Stoop and recovery were performed from walk and stride stand position and gradually increased distance between both legs according to the child tolerance.

Strengthening of lower back extensor and hip extensors was performed prone on wedge and both legs abducted and knees extended; also strengthening of abdominal muscles

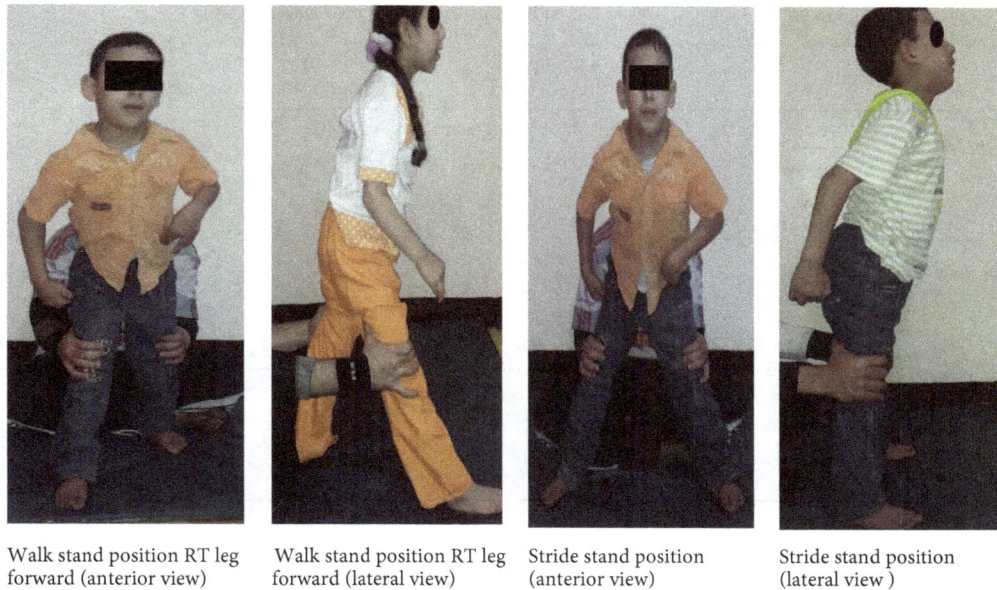

Walk stand position RT leg forward (anterior view)

Walk stand position RT leg forward (lateral view)

Stride stand position (anterior view)

Stride stand position (lateral view)

FIGURE 1: Illustration of walk stand and stride stand positions.

TABLE 2: Pretreatment comparison between right and left sides in each group.

Variables	Control group			Study group		
	RT $\overline{X} \pm$ SD	LT $\overline{X} \pm$ SD	P value	RT $\overline{X} \pm$ SD	LT $\overline{X} \pm$ SD	P value
H\M ratio	0.75 ± 0.09	0.77 ± 0.07	0.348*	0.76 ± 0.07	0.75 ± 0.01	0.792*
Popliteal angle	77.2 ± 5.58	76.93 ± 5.63	0.77*	7.6 ± 7.32	76.3 ± 7.56	0.313*
Stride length	79.46 ± 7.8	81.13 ± 5.82	0.16*	75.46 ± 19.5	80.53 ± 6.0	0.269*
Stride speed	0.56 ± 0.09	0.59 ± 0.6	0.234*	0.6 ± 0.11	0.59 ± 0.085	0.539*
Stance phase %	72.86 ± 3.7	71.66 ± 3.19	0.212*	71.33 ± 4.16	70.6 ± 4	0.469*

$\overline{X} \pm$ SD: mean ± standard deviation; P: level of significant; *nonsignificant.

was performed supine on mat with legs abducted and knees extended.

Balance exercise was performed also from walk stand and stride stand positions.

Both groups wear ankle foot orthosis during day time and knee ankle foot orthosis at bed time. Both groups received the treatment program for two hours three times weekly for three successive months.

3.2. Data Analysis. The statistical analyses were performed with the aid of the statistical package of social sciences (SPSS) version 20. Descriptive statistics (mean and standard deviation) were computed for all data. The paired t-test was applied for comparison within the group and the independent t-test was applied to compare between both groups before and after treatment. Cronbach's alpha applied for measuring internal consistency, the statistical power, and minimal clinical difference depending on the Anchor method were calculated.

4. Result

There was no significant difference between both groups in age ($P > 0.05$); the mean age was 6.23 ± 0.942 and 6.06 ± 0.951 for control and study group, respectively. There was

TABLE 3: The internal consistency of the different measured variables.

Variable	Cronbach's alpha
H\M ratio	0.97*
Stride length	0.96*
Stride speed	0.96*
Stance phase	0.95*
Popliteal angle	0.94*

*Excellent validity.

also no significant difference between both groups in gender, spasticity, and gross motor function classification system level distributed between both groups; the Chi-squared value was 0.67, 0.8, and 0.7, respectively ($P > 0.05$).

Comparison between right and left leg in both groups revealed that there was no significant difference between both sides ($P > 0.05$) as illustrated in Table 2. The internal consistency was expressed as excellent validity according to the values of Cronbach's alpha for the different measured variables according to Table 3.

Comparison between pre- and posttreatment for both groups revealed that there was significant improvement in

TABLE 4: Comparison between both groups in all measured variable.

Variable	Time	Control group $\overline{X} \pm$ SD	Study group $\overline{X} \pm$ SD	P value	Standard error
H\M ratio	Before	0.75 ± 0.09	0.76 ± 0.07	0.66**	0.28
	After	0.55 ± 0.04	0.39 ± 00.7	0.001*	0.27
	P value	0.001*	0.001*		
	Standard error	0.192	0.14		
Popliteal angle	Before	77.2 ± 5.58	77.6 ± 7.32	0.868**	1.53
	After	85 ± 5.71	91.8 ± 5.7	0.003*	1.36
	P value	0.001*	0.001*		
	Standard error	0.3	0.63		
Stride length	Before	79.46 ± 7.8	75.46 ± 19.5	0.468**	1.77
	After	87.4 ± 7.45	94.46 ± 3.87	0.003*	1.61
	P value	0.001*	0.001*		
	Standard error	0.3	0.98		
Stride speed	Before	0.56 ± 0.09	0.6 ± 0.11	0.325**	0.03
	After	0.836 ± 0.89	0.94 ± 0.038	0.001*	0.01
	P value	0.001*	0.001*		
	Standard error	0.27	0.26		
Stance phase %	Before	72.86 ± 3.7	71.33 ± 4.16	0.296**	1.45
	After	67.5 ± 3.79	63.73 ± 1.48	0.001*	1.14
	P value	0.001*	0.001*		
	Standard error	1.54	1.19		

$\overline{X} \pm$ SD: mean ± standard deviation; P: level of significant; *significant; **nonsignificant.

both groups after treatment in all measured variables ($P <$ 0.05) as illustrated in Table 4 and Figures 2, 3, 4, 5, and 6. The posttreatment comparison revealed that there was significant improvement in favor of the study group ($P < 0.05$) as illustrated in Table 4.

The statistical power values showed greater effect for both groups in favor of the study group. The minimal clinical difference was ≤ 0.5 SD representing a moderate effect size and this is corresponding to the minimal important difference (Table 5).

5. Discussion

Spastic diplegic CP children suffered from muscular tightness and loss of flexibility, leading to mechanical problems, loss of range of motion, and limited executive function abilities. Stretching exercise was applied to increase soft tissue flexibility in CP children; some researchers reported that regular stretching does not produce clinical changes in joint mobility, spasticity, and function activities [32].

The functional stretching exercises were designed to treat soft tissue flexibility problems during function training; stretching is applied in unique way depending on the concepts of overcorrection of deformities and prolonged stretching to utilize the inhibitory effect of stretching in improving function training during physical therapy treatment in order to optimize motor performance. Different techniques were used for spasticity evaluation but we used H-reflex because it is standardized procedure and had greater evidence of validity [33]. The popliteal angle was measured because it

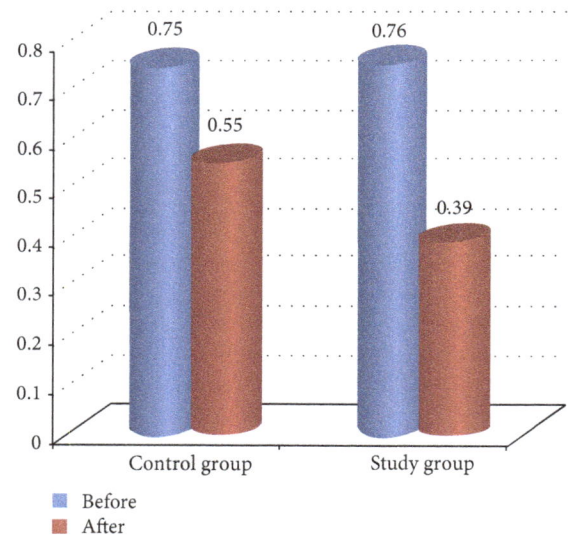

FIGURE 2: Comparison between pre- and posttreatment in H\M ratio for both groups.

is a strong clinical indicator for hamstring muscle tightness and needed for surgical intervention. Stride length, stride speed, and stance phase percentages were measured by 3D gait analysis as indicator of program effect on gait parameters.

The result of the study demonstrated that there was no significant difference between and within the groups before treatment and the internal consistency expressed excellent

TABLE 5: Statistical power and minimal clinical difference for both groups.

Variables	Statistical power (%)		Minimal clinical difference	
	Control group	Study group	Control group	Study group
H\M ratio	83*	98*	0.02	0.015
Popliteal angle	80*	86.9*	2.5	2.7
Stride length	83*	94*	3.2	1.8
Stride speed	80*	86*	0.04	0.012
Stance phase	87*	93*	1.5	0.5

*Statistical power ≥ 80% has large effect.

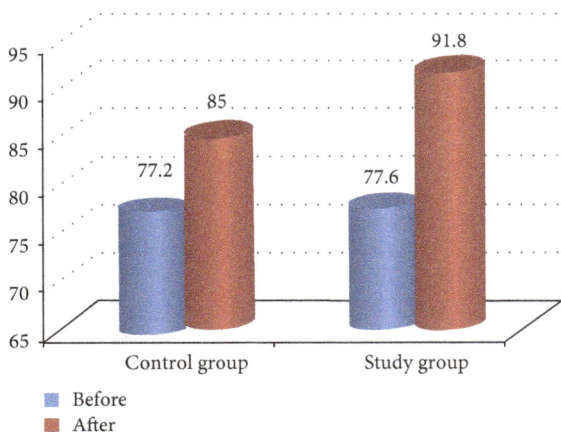

FIGURE 3: Comparison between pre- and posttreatment in popliteal angle for both groups.

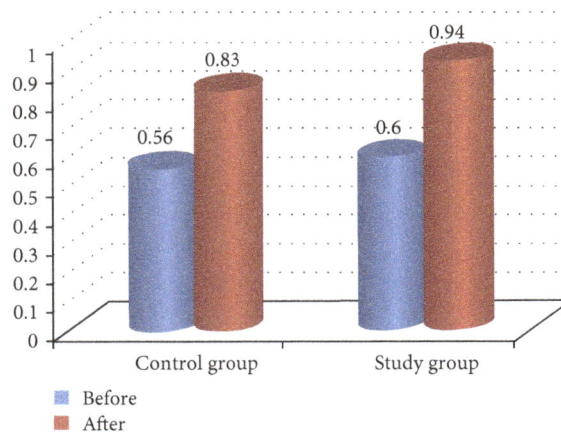

FIGURE 5: Comparison between pre- and posttreatment in stride speed for both groups.

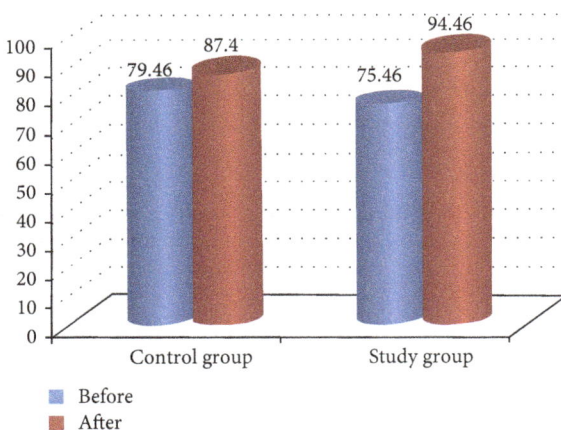

FIGURE 4: Comparison between pre- and posttreatment in stride length for both groups.

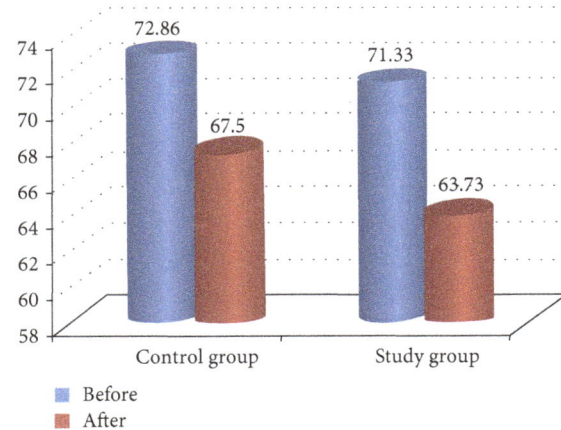

FIGURE 6: Comparison between pre- and posttreatment in stance phase % for both groups.

validity. There was significant improvement in all measured variables for both groups in favor of functional stretching program as the child was functionally trained with correct movement pattern and stretching performed during the whole session, as stretching effect on spasticity lasts for one or two minutes. The result of popliteal angle showed significant improvement after treatment after application of the functional stretching program so it efficiently solved the mechanical problems of the knee joint as hamstring tightness is the main cause of crouch posture.

Walk stand position stretched mainly hamstring muscle in the forward leg and hip flexors and calf muscle of the behind leg, while stride stand position stretched hip adductors muscles. Standing and walking were applied in normal functional pattern that provides a strong proprioceptive stimulation leading to correct body image and Ingram.

The function training exercise was performed with complete knee joint and hip joint abduction and ankle in right angle. Antispastic position applied on hips was abducted at nearly a 45° angle and externally rotated, and the knees were extended and ankles right angle [34]. Antispastic positions prevented muscle contractures and joint limitation in spastic diplegia children [35]. Active movement application during passive stretching improved motor control performance and functional capability [36].

Integration of sensory stimulation during teaching the child function skills with correction of abnormal motor pattern enhanced learning process and acquisition of motor skills, leading to faster transferring of learned skill from the cognitive stage to the autonomous stage which in turn leads to perfect performance of skill and function recovery as motor learning is a set of internal processes associated with practice or experience leading to relatively permanent changes in executive functions and behaviors.

Limitation. A limited number of children participated in the study.

Recommendation. Additional research is recommended to determine the long lasting effect of functional stretching exercises on spasticity and function activities for spastic diplegic children.

6. Conclusion

Functional stretching exercises are effective methods used in rehabilitation of spastic diplegic children; it reduced H\M ratio, increased popliteal angle, and improved gait.

Abbreviations

3D: Three dimensions
CP: Cerebral palsy
EMG: Electromyography
H-reflex: The Hoffmann reflex
ROM: Range of motion
SPSS: Statistical package of social sciences.

Conflict of Interests

The authors declare that there is no conflict of interests regarding the publication of this paper.

Acknowledgment

The authors are grateful and express their sincere gratitude to Dr. Mohamed Farag for statistical analysis.

References

[1] SCPE, "Prevalence and characteristics of children with cerebral palsy in Europe," *Developmental Medicine and Child Neurology*, vol. 44, no. 9, pp. 633–640, 2002.

[2] V. Dietz and T. Sinkjaer, "Spastic movement disorder: impaired reflex function and altered muscle mechanics," *The Lancet Neurology*, vol. 6, no. 8, pp. 725–733, 2007.

[3] N. H. Mayer and A. Esquenazi, "Muscle overactivity and movement dysfunction in the upper motoneuron syndrome," *Physical Medicine and Rehabilitation Clinics of North America*, vol. 14, no. 4, pp. 855–883, 2003.

[4] C. B. Ivanhoe and T. A. Reistetter, "Spasticity: the misunderstood part of the upper motor neuron syndrome," *The American Journal of Physical Medicine and Rehabilitation*, vol. 83, no. 10, p. -S9, 2004.

[5] G. Sheean, "The pathophysiology of spasticity," *European Journal of Neurology*, vol. 9, no. supplement 1, pp. 3–9, 2002.

[6] S. Malhotra, A. D. Pandyan, C. R. Day, P. W. Jones, and H. Hermens, "Spasticity, an impairment that is poorly defined and poorly measured," *Clinical Rehabilitation*, vol. 23, no. 7, pp. 651–658, 2009.

[7] A. B. Ward and M. Kadies, "The management of pain in spasticity," *Disability and Rehabilitation*, vol. 24, no. 8, pp. 443–453, 2002.

[8] L. R. Smith, K. S. Lee, S. R. Ward, H. G. Chambers, and R. L. Lieber, "Hamstring contractures in children with spastic cerebral palsy result from a stiffer extracellular matrix and increased in vivo sarcomere length," *Journal of Physiology*, vol. 589, no. 10, pp. 2625–2639, 2011.

[9] J.-C. Tabary, C. Tardieu, G. Tardieu, and C. Tabary, "Experimental rapid sarcomere loss with concomitant hypoextensibility," *Muscle and Nerve*, vol. 4, no. 3, pp. 198–203, 1981.

[10] A. A. Alhusaini, J. Crosbie, R. B. Shepherd, C. M. Dean, and A. Scheinberg, "Mechanical properties of the plantarflexor musculotendinous unit during passive dorsiflexion in children with cerebral palsy compared with typically developing children," *Developmental Medicine and Child Neurology*, vol. 52, no. 6, pp. e101–e106, 2010.

[11] L. Döderlein and D. Metaxiotis, "Knee bending- and stretching-spastic in infant cerebral palsy. Surgery aimed at functional improvement and its results," *Orthopade*, vol. 33, no. 10, pp. 1138–1151, 2004.

[12] J. R. Gage, "Surgical treatment of knee dysfunction in cerebral palsy," *Clinical Orthopaedics and Related Research*, no. 253, pp. 45–54, 1990.

[13] D. Ganjwala, "Multilevel orthopedic surgery for crouch gait in cerebral palsy: an evaluation using functional mobility and energy cost," *Indian Journal of Orthopaedics*, vol. 45, no. 4, pp. 314–319, 2011.

[14] A. Swierczyńska, K. Renata, and M. Jaworek, "Physical and other methods therapy of the spasticity in children," *Przegląd Lekarski*, vol. 64, no. 11, pp. 974–977, 2007.

[15] Y. N. Wu, M. Hwang, Y. Ren, D. Gaebler-Spira, and L. Q. Zhang, "Combined passive stretching and active movement rehabilitation of lower-limb impairments in children with cerebral palsy using a portable robot," *Neurorehabilitation & Neural Repair*, vol. 25, no. 4, pp. 378–385, 2011.

[16] M. J. Botte, V. L. Nickel, and W. H. Akeson, "Spasticity and contracture. Physiologic aspects of formation," *Clinical Orthopaedics and Related Research*, vol. 233, pp. 7–18, 1988.

[17] R. L. Braddom, *Physical Medicine and Rehabilitation*, WB Saunders, Philadelphia, Pa, USA, 2nd edition, 2000.

[18] H. Moriyama, Y. Tobimatsu, J. Ozawa, N. Kito, and R. Tanaka, "Amount of torque and duration of stretching affects correction of knee contracture in a rat model of spinal cord injury," *Clinical Orthopaedics and Related Research*, vol. 471, no. 11, pp. 3626–3636, 2013.

[19] N. Smania, A. Picelli, D. Munari et al., "Rehabilitation procedures in the management of spasticity," *European Journal of Physical and Rehabilitation Medicine*, vol. 46, no. 3, pp. 423–438, 2010.

[20] K. H. Tsai, C. Y. Yeh, H. Y. Chang, and J. J. Chen, "Effects of a single session of prolonged muscle stretch on spastic muscle of stroke patients," *Proceedings of the National Science Council, Republic of China B*, vol. 25, no. 2, pp. 76–81, 2001.

[21] C. L. Richards, F. Malouin, and F. Dumas, "Effects of a single session of prolonged plantarflexor stretch on muscle activations during gait in spastic cerebral palsy," *Scandinavian Journal of Rehabilitation Medicine*, vol. 23, no. 2, pp. 103–111, 1991.

[22] A. H. Kohan, S. Abootalebi, A. Khoshnevisan, and M. Rahgozar, "Comparison of modified ashworth scale and Hoffmann reflex in study of spasticity," *Acta Medica Iranica*, vol. 48, no. 3, pp. 154–157, 2010.

[23] I. Odeen and E. Knutsson, "Evaluation of the effects of muscle stretch and weight load in patients with spastic paraplegia," *Scandinavian Journal of Rehabilitation Medicine*, vol. 13, no. 4, pp. 117–121, 1981.

[24] H. Zhao, Y. Wu, J. Liu, Y. Ren, D. J. Gaebler-Spira, and L. Zhang, "Changes of calf muscle-tendon properties due to stretching and active movement of children with cerebral palsy—a pilot study," *Conference proceedings: Annual International Conference of the IEEE Engineering in Medicine and Biology Society*, vol. 2009, pp. 5287–5290, 2009.

[25] A. H. Tilton, "Management of spasticity in children with cerebral palsy," *Seminars in Pediatric Neurology*, vol. 11, no. 1, pp. 58–65, 2004.

[26] O. M. Katalinic, L. A. Harvey, R. D. Herbert, A. M. Moseley, N. A. Lannin, and K. Schurr, "Stretch for the treatment and prevention of contractures," *Cochrane Database of Systematic Reviews*, vol. 8, no. 9, p. CD007455, 2010.

[27] R. K. Prabhu, N. Swaminathan, and L. A. Harvey, "Passive movements for the treatment and prevention of contractures," *Cochrane Database of Systematic Reviews*, 2013.

[28] C. Y. Yeh, K. H. Tsai, and J. J. J. Chen, "Effects of prolonged muscle stretch on spasticity by an assessment/treatment system," in *Proceedings of the 23rd Annual International Conference of the IEEE Engineering in Medicine and Biology Society*, pp. 1232–1235, October 2001.

[29] T. Pin, P. Dyke, and M. Chan, "The effectiveness of passive stretching in children with cerebral palsy," *Developmental Medicine and Child Neurology*, vol. 48, no. 10, pp. 855–862, 2006.

[30] O. M. Katalinic, L. A. Harvey, and R. D. Herbert, "Effectiveness of stretch for the treatment and prevention of contractures in people with neurological conditions: a systematic review," *Physical Therapy*, vol. 91, no. 1, pp. 11–24, 2011.

[31] I. Franki, K. Desloovere, J. De Cat et al., "The evidence-base for basic physical therapy techniques targeting lower limb function in children with cerebral palsy: a systematic review using the International Classification of Functioning, Disability and Health as a conceptual framework," *Journal of Rehabilitation Medicine*, vol. 44, no. 5, pp. 385–395, 2012.

[32] L. Wiart, J. Darrah, and G. Kembhavi, "Stretching with children with cerebral palsy: what do we know and where are we going?" *Pediatric Physical Therapy*, vol. 20, no. 2, pp. 173–178, 2008.

[33] G. E. Voerman, J. H. Burridge, R. A. Hitchcock, and H. J. Hermens, "Clinometric properties of a clinical spasticity measurement tool," *Disability and Rehabilitation*, vol. 29, no. 24, pp. 1870–1880, 2007.

[34] M. Kerem, A. Livanelioglu, and M. Topcu, "Effects of Johnstone pressure splints combined with neurodevelopmental therapy on spasticity and cutaneous sensory inputs in spastic cerebral palsy," *Developmental Medicine and Child Neurology*, vol. 43, no. 5, pp. 307–313, 2001.

[35] T. Akbayrak, K. Armutlu, M. K. Gunel, and G. Nurlu, "Assessment of the short-term effect of antispastic positioning on spasticity," *Pediatrics International*, vol. 47, no. 4, pp. 440–445, 2005.

[36] G. E. Nuyens, W. J. De Weerdt, A. J. Spaepen Jr., C. Kiekens, and H. M. Feys, "Reduction of spastic hypertonia during repeated passive knee movements in stroke patients," *Archives of Physical Medicine and Rehabilitation*, vol. 83, no. 7, pp. 930–935, 2002.

22

A Comparison between Two Instruments for Assessing Dependency in Daily Activities: Agreement of the Northwick Park Dependency Score with the Functional Independence Measure

Siv Svensson and Katharina Stibrant Sunnerhagen

Institute of Neuroscience and Physiology/Rehabilitation Medicine, Sahlgrenska Academy, University of Gothenburg, 3rd floor, Per Dubbsgatan 14, 413 45 Gothenburg, Sweden

Correspondence should be addressed to Katharina Stibrant Sunnerhagen, ks.sunnerhagen@neuro.gu.se

Academic Editor: Jeffrey Jutai

Background. There is a need for tools to assess dependency among persons with severe impairments. *Objectives.* The aim was to compare the Functional Independence Measure (FIM) and the Northwick Park Dependency Score (NPDS), in a sample from inpatient rehabilitation. *Material and Methods.* Data from 115 persons (20 to 65 years of age) with neurological impairments was gathered. Analyses were made of sensitivity, specificity, positive predictive, value, and negative predictive value. Agreement of the scales was assessed with kappa and concordance with Goodman-Kruskal's gamma. Scale structures were explored using the Rank-Transformable Pattern of Agreement (RTPA). Content validation was performed. *Results.* The sensitivity of the NPDS as compared to FIM varied between 0.53 (feeding) and 1.0 (mobility) and specificity between 0.64 (mobility) and 1.0 (bladder). The positive predictive value varied from 0.62 (mobility) to 1.0 (bladder), and the negative predictive value varied from 0.48 (bowel) to 1.0 (mobility). Agreement between the scales was moderate to good (four items) and excellent (three items). Concordance was good, with a gamma of $-.856$, an asymptotic error (ase) of .025, and $P < .000$. The parallel reliability between the FIM and the NPDS showed a tendency for NPDS to be more sensitive (having more categories) when dependency is high. *Conclusion.* FIM and NPDS complement each other. NPDS can be used as a measure for severely injured patients who are sensitive when there is a high need of nursing time.

1. Introduction

There is a need for tools to assess dependency among persons with severe impairments. It seems that the number of persons with dependency as a result of acquired brain injuries is increasing or at least more are referred for rehabilitation. This includes not only traditional active rehabilitation aiming at discharge to the home but also for specific treatment of spasticity in persons who are totally dependent. Outcome assessment tools have not only to be valid but also responsive enough to detect changes during rehabilitation [1]. This is a matter of quality of care, for the individual and for the payer.

There are different instruments that aim to describe activities of daily living (ADL) and levels of dependency/independence. Both the Barthel ADL index [2] and the FIM (Functional Independence Measure) [3, 4] can be considered "golden standards" for ADL assessment and both have known floor and ceiling effects. When impairments are severe, the improvements after an intervention are sometimes small, and the feeling of the staff is that achievements are not reflected in the traditional ADL instruments.

The Northwick Park Dependency Score (NPDS) was developed to meet this need [5]. The goal of the NPDS was to assess the nursing time required in the rehabilitation, providing another way to assess dependency and perhaps better reflecting small changes in dependency. Its reliability and validity have been studied [6]. The instrument has been translated into Swedish [7]. Although a very recent review was published [8] that covered five studies, only one study included more than 100 patients [6]. We thus believe that there is a need for further validation studies of the instrument. One way to perform a content validation of an instrument is by linking to the International Classification of Functioning (ICF).

The aim of this study was to compare the assessments of ADL dependency made with two different scales, the FIM and the NPDS, in a sample of persons receiving in-patient rehabilitation. A second aim was to perform a content validation of the scales by using the ICF.

2. Subjects and Methods

Data were gathered from 115 persons, 47 women and 68 men, with a mean age of 50 years (ranging from 20–65 years). Acquired brain injury was the most common cause of the need of in-patient rehabilitation (77% stroke, the most common, 64 persons, and 22 traumatic brain injury). The remaining patients had other neurological diagnoses (multiple sclerosis, Guillain-Barre, or spinal cord injury) requiring rehabilitation.

2.1. Instruments. The FIM instrument [3, 4] was designed to measure the degree of disability experienced, changes over time, and the effectiveness of rehabilitation. It intends to measure severity defined in terms of the need of assistance. The FIM can be used with any rehabilitation client. There is a manual, and the use of FIM requires training. It is designed to be applied in people seven years of age and older. Each item is rated on a seven-point scale, from total assistance to complete independence (13 physical items and five cognitive/social items). Total scores range from 18 to 126, with 126 indicating independence.

NPDS [1] is designed to be used for assessments of the requirement of nursing time in a rehabilitation setting in order to evaluate the full range of dependency. According to the constructer, it seems to be particularly sensitive to small changes in dependency that would not be detected by other instruments. NPDS is divided into two sections: basic care needs (BCNs) and special nursing needs (SNN). A score of 100 indicates dependence in all items (BCH = 65, SNN = 35), and a score of 0 indicates independence in all items. Lower scores thus indicate that the person is more independent, where low dependence is <10, medium dependence is 10–25, and high dependence is >25. NPDS assessments are made by observation. No formal training is said to be needed to use the instrument. A manual is available.

2.2. Data Collection. The raters were trained in the use of FIM and had long experience of working in rehabilitation of neurologically impaired patients. The NPDS does not require formal training; the instrument is meant to be self-explanatory (it does, however, have a manual). This was given to the raters together with a scoring sheet. The FIM assessment was made first (immediately prior to discharge) and this was followed by the NPDS (BCN + SNN sections). The raters also collected descriptive information concerning the patient's age, sex, and diagnoses.

2.3. Comparison of Items of the FIM and NPDS. The procedure for comparison of the FIM and NPDS with the ICF was accomplished by two raters who were experienced in the field of clinical neurorehabilitation and familiar with the ICF. The comparison was carried out independently. The process and the final evaluation of appropriate codes were based on the independent ratings and subsequent discussions between the raters to reach consensus.

The study was approved by the Ethics Committee of the University of Gothenburg. All patients or their next of kin (if the patient could not read or understand) were given a letter containing information about the study. All gave their informed consent to participate.

2.4. Statistical Analysis. The data were analysed using the Statistical Program for the Social Sciences (SPSS) 16.0. Cross-tabulations were made to explore the precision of the instrument in identifying independency/dependency in personal ADL, where the items from the instruments were merged to resemble one another. The items from FIM served as the "golden standard." Sensitivity, specificity, positive predictive values, and negative predictive values are presented. The alpha value was set to ≤0.05.

The agreement on dependency was assessed for the different ADL areas based on Cohen's unweighted kappa as a measure of agreement, *P* values, and values of percentage agreement (PA). Kappa coefficients between 0.40 and 0.80 are considered moderate to good, and those exceeding 0.80 are very good, while values below 0.40 are fair to poor.

Goodman-Kruskal's gamma was calculated to assess concurrent validity between the total score in the FIM and the total score in the BCN section of NPDS. Concordance is defined as a measure of the interchangeability of two scales, which means that, if two scales are concordant, they will produce the same ordering of individuals. Gamma is a measure based on the difference between the numbers of concordant and discordant pairs adjusted for ties on the marginal distribution. Gamma can vary between −1 and 1, where a value of 1 indicates perfect concordance, and the value of 0 indicates a total lack of concordance. If one scale is the reverse of the other, the value of −1 indicates total concordance [9]. The asymptotic standard error (ase) is given in the analysis as a measure of precision for gamma.

The rank-transformable pattern of agreement (RTPA) was used for parallel reliability between the FIM and the NPDS. If scales have different numbers of categories (steps), a strong parallel reliability requires a high level of agreement in the ordering of all individuals involved. Agreement in the ordering of individuals between two scales' assessments is an important condition for scales to be interchangeable. To assess this, observed distribution is compared with the pattern of total agreement in the ordering of all individuals, since the rank ordering of all individuals in the RTPA is independent of the two scales [10]. A change from one scale to another then means a change in categorical labelling but does not mean an alteration in the relative ordering of the individuals. The RTPA is completely defined by the two sets of marginal distributions

TABLE 1: Sensitivity, specificity, positive predictive value, and negative predictive value of the NPDS, with FIM as the golden standard.

	Sensitivity	Specificity	Positive predictive value	Negative predictive value
Feeding	0.53	0.93	0.94	0.69
Toileting	0.83	0.98	0.98	0.87
Dressing	0.89	0.98	0.98	0.88
Bladder	0.72	1.0	1.0	0.55
Bowel	0.74	0.88	0.96	0.48
Mobility	1.0	0.64	0.62	1.0
Showering	0.83	0.98	0.97	0.87

TABLE 2: Agreement between the FIM and the NPDS for different basic ADL areas.

	Kappa value	Ase	Sign
Feeding	0.653	0.068	0.000
Toileting	0.803	0.057	0.000
Dressing	0.860	0.047	0.000
Bladder	0.566	0.071	0.000
Bowel	0.457	0.080	0.000
Mobility	0.570	0.067	0.000
Showering	0.824	0.053	0.000

and is constructed by pairing off the two sets of marginal distribution.

3. Results

The sensitivity of the NPDS as compared to FIM varied between 0.53 (feeding) and 1.0 (mobility) and specificity, between 0.64 (mobility) and 1.0 (bladder). The positive predictive value for NPDS compared to FIM varied from 0.62 (mobility) to 1.0 (bladder) and the negative predictive value varied from 0.48 (bowel) to 1.0 (mobility) (Table 1). Agreement between the scales with kappa analyses was moderate to good (four items) and excellent (three items) (Table 2).

Concordance was good, with a gamma of −.856, an asymptotic error (ase) of .025 and $P < .000$ (Figure 1). The parallel reliability of NPDS and FIM was tested with RTPA. The observed distribution (the total score in the BCN section of NPDS and the total score in FIM) was compared with the total agreement of the total score of each patient (Table 3), where the tendency was for the BCN section of NPDS to have more categories (steps) than FIM when the dependency is high (making it possible to differentiate between persons) and for the FIM to have more categories than NPDS when the dependency is low.

In terms of the total score of the BCN section of NPDS and the total score of FIM in the different items, concordance showed good agreement in all items, with the following distribution: item transfer gamma −.909 and ase .025. The self-care item had a gamma of −.867 and an ase of .030, the

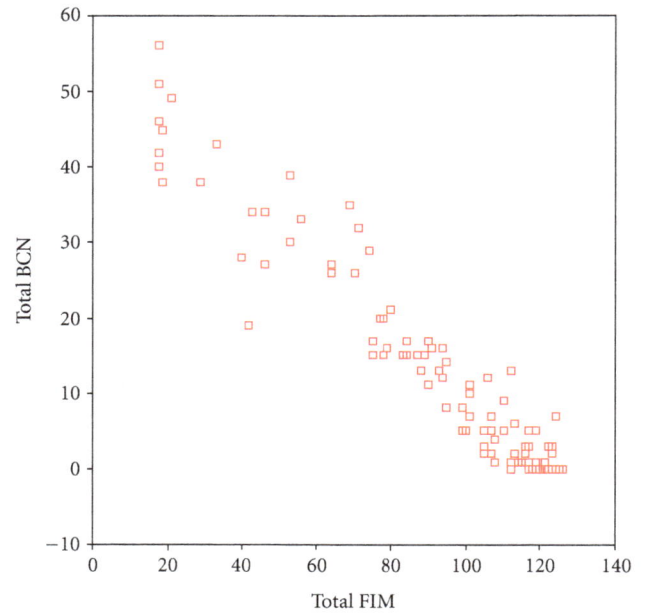

FIGURE 1: Scatterplot showing the distribution of the NPDS total BCN score and the FIM total score.

TABLE 3: The rank-transformable pattern of agreement (RTPA) of the total score of FIM and the BCN section of NPDS.

FIM	NPDS
18	46
29	38
40	35
46	32–28
56–64	27
69	21
75–77	20
78	19–17
79–80	17
84–87	16
88–90	15
91	14
93-94	13
95	11-12
99	8
100-101	7
105-106	5
107	3–5
108-109	3
112–115	2
116–121	1
122–126	0

continence item a gamma of −.833 and an ase of .040, and the cognitive item a gamma of −.790 and an ase of .043.

Corresponding ICF domains could be found for all items in both instruments (Table 4). However, the instruments

TABLE 4: Commonality of items in the FIM and the NPDS.

FIM	NPDS
FIM motor	Basic care needs
Self-care	*Feeding*
Eating	Eating
	Drinking
	Enteral feeding
	Washing, bathing, dressing
Grooming	Washing and grooming
Bathing	
Bathing/showering	
Dressing upper body	Dressing
Dressing lower body	
Toileting	
Continence	*Continence*
Bladder	Toileting-bladder
Bowel	Urinary incontinence
	Toileting-bowels
	Faecal incontinence
Transfers	*Mobility and transfers*
Bed, chair, wheelchair	Mobility
Toilet	Transfers
Tub, shower	
Locomotion	
Walk, wheelchair	
Stairs	
FIM social/cognitive	*Safety, communication, behavior*
	Skin pressure relief
	Safety awareness
Communication	Communication
Comprehension	
Expression	
Social cognition	
Social interaction	Behavior
Problem solving	
Memory	Special nursing needs
	Tracheotomy
	Open wound requiring dressing
	Requires 2 interventions at night
	Requires psychological support
	In isolation (e.g., for MRSA screening)
	Acute medical/surgical intervention
	Needs one-to-one "specializing"

differed when the linking was performed to the fourth level of the ICF (Table 5). The NPDS-BCN section covers items in the sections on sensory functions and pain, which FIM does not. FIM covers items in the areas of learning and applying knowledge, which are not covered in NPDS.

4. Discussion

The key findings of the study are that the NPDS compared with the gold standard FIM had good instrumental qualities. Also NPDS is a good tool of the dependency among severely impaired patients when needs of nursing time are high.

In this work, the convergent validity of the NPDS to FIM was shown to be good. The different areas of basic ADL were good, with high sensitivity and specificity, and there was also good agreement. This confirms the conclusions drawn by Plantinga et al. [6], where a comparison was made with the Barthel index. In that study, however, only a portion of the sample was neurologically impaired (35% of 154), which is different from the present sample.

The diverse qualities of FIM and NPDS for differentiating patients' dependency were shown with the RTPA. One of findings is that the NPDS is more sensitive for change in the more severely disabled patients. However, if the patient is more independent, the FIM is more likely to detect further improvements. This means that, on a ward where the aim is to assess patients' needs, the two instruments are not interchangeable but are complementary since there is usually a variation in patients' functional limitations in any single ward.

Differences and similarities become clearer when two scales are linked to the ICF. This is a way to validate scales by content. The results of the linking give some clues as to why the scales behave differently, that is, why some patients' scores according to the different scales showed that they were more or less dependent. The linking shows that the contents of the items are not the same in spite of the fact that they aim to assess the same area.

One limitation in this study is the relative small sample. However, all patients suffered from neurological disorders, which make the sample representative in that respect. The sample also has a dominance of patients that function quite well and are not highly dependent in many areas. This reflects the selection of patients that receive in-patient rehabilitation in. It is possible that the results would be different in another rehabilitation setting.

5. Conclusion

The correlation between total FIM and the BCN section of the NPDS is high. FIM and NPDS may be used to complement one another. There are potential benefits of using NPDS as a measure of how sensitive the dependency is among severely injured patients when needs of nursing time are high.

Conflict of Interests

The authors declare that they have no conflict of interests.

TABLE 5: Comparing FIM and NPDS to the International Classification of Functioning, Disability, and Health.

ICF	FIM	ICF	NPDS-BCN section
	Self-care	d 560, 445, 440	Drinking
d 550, 560	Eating	d 550	Eating
		b 510	Enteral feeding
d 510, 520	Grooming	d 510, 520	Washing and grooming
d 510	Bathing	d 510, 450, 465	Bathing/showering
d 540	Dressing upper body	d 540	Dressing
d 540	Dressing lower body		
d 530	Toilet	d 530	Toilet bladder
		d 530	Toilet bowels
	Sphincter control		
b 620	Bladder management	b 620	Urinary incontinence
b 525	Bowel management	b 525	Faecal incontinence
	Transfer		Bed transfer
d 420, 410	Bed, chair, wheelchair	d 450, 410, 415	
d 420, 410	Toilet	d 420	requires hoisting
d 420	Tub, shower		
	Locomotion		Mobility
d 450, 455, 465	Walk, wheelchair	d 450	Walk
d 455	Stairs	d 465	With equipment
		b 270	Skin pressure relief
	Communication	d 310, 315	Communication
d 310, 315	Comprehension	d 335	Gestures, contextual cues
d 330, 335	Expression		
	Social, cognition		
d 710	Social interaction	d 720, b 130	Behaviour
d 230, 175	Problem solving	b 114	Safety awareness
b 144	Memory		
			Special nursing needs—SNN
		b 265, 270, 280	
		b 810	

b: Body function.
d: Activity performance.

Acknowledgments

The authors would like to thank the nursing staff and occupational therapists in Göteborg and Borås who collected data for this study. The Swedish Association of Neurologically Disabled (NHR) and the County of Västra Götaland gave financial support for the study.

References

[1] L. Turner-Stokes, S. Paul, and H. Williams, "Efficiency of specialist rehabilitation in reducing dependency and costs of continuing care for adults with complex acquired brain injuries," Journal of Neurology, Neurosurgery and Psychiatry, vol. 77, no. 5, pp. 634–639, 2006.

[2] D. T. Wade and C. Collin, "The Barthel ADL Index: a standard measure of physical disability?" International Disability Studies, vol. 10, no. 2, pp. 64–67, 1988.

[3] G. Grimby, G. Gudjonsson, M. Rodhe, K. S. Sunnerhagen, V. Sundh, and M. L. Östensson, "The functional independence measure in Sweden: experience for outcome measurement in rehabilitation medicine," Scandinavian Journal of Rehabilitation Medicine, vol. 28, no. 2, pp. 51–62, 1996.

[4] B. Hamilton, C. Granger, F. Shervin, F. Zielezny, and J. Tashman, "A uniform national dala system for medical rehabilitation," in Rehabilitation Outcomes: Analysis and Measurements, M. Further, Ed., pp. 137–147, Paul H Brooks, Baltimore, Md, USA, 1987.

[5] L. Turner-Stokes, P. Tonge, K. Nyein, M. Hunter, S. Nielson, and I. Robinson, "The Northwick Park Dependency Score (NPDS): a measure of nursing dependency in rehabilitation," Clinical Rehabilitation, vol. 12, no. 4, pp. 304–318, 1998.

[6] E. Plantinga, L. J. Tiesinga, C. P. Van Der Schans, and B. Middel, "The criterion-related validity of the Northwick Park Dependency Score as a generic nursing dependency instrument for different rehabilitation patient groups," Clinical Rehabilitation, vol. 20, no. 10, pp. 921–926, 2006.

[7] S. Svensson, U. Sonn, and K. Stibrant Sunnerhagen, "Reliability and validity of the Northwick Park Dependency Score (NPDS) Swedish version 6.0," Clinical Rehabilitation, vol. 19, no. 4, pp. 419–425, 2005.

[8] R. J. Siegert and L. Turner-Stokes, "Psychometric evaluation of the Northwick Park Dependency Scale," *Journal of Rehabilitation Medicine*, vol. 42, no. 10, pp. 936–943, 2010.

[9] E. Svensson, "Concordance between ratings using different scales for the same variable," *Statistics in Medicine*, vol. 19, no. 24, pp. 3483–3496, 2000.

[10] E. Svensson and S. Holm, "Separation of systematic and random differences in ordinal rating scales," *Statistics in Medicine*, vol. 13, no. 23-24, pp. 2437–2453, 1994.

23

Effect of Aerobic Exercise Training on Chinese Population with Mild to Moderate Depression in Hong Kong

Cassandra W. H. Ho,[1] **S. C. Chan,**[2] **J. S. Wong,**[2] **W. T. Cheung,**[1]
Dicky W. S. Chung,[2] **and Titanic F. O. Lau**[1]

[1] *Physiotherapy Department, Tai Po Hospital, Wing E, Ground Floor, Tai Po, New Territories, Hong Kong*
[2] *Department of Psychiatry, Tai Po Hospital, Tai Po, New Territories, Hong Kong*

Correspondence should be addressed to Cassandra W. H. Ho; hwh173@ha.org.hk

Academic Editor: Jari P. A. Arokoski

Background. Exercise has been suggested to be a viable treatment for depression. This study investigates the effect of supervised aerobic exercise training on depressive symptoms and physical performance among Chinese patients with mild to moderate depression in early in-patient phase. *Methods.* A randomized repeated measure and assessor-blinded study design was used. Subjects in aerobic exercise group received 30 minutes of aerobic training, five days a week for 3 weeks. Depressive symptoms (MADRS and C-BDI) and domains in physical performance were assessed at baseline and program end. *Results.* Subjects in aerobic exercise group showed a more significant reduction in depressive scores (MADRS) as compared to control (between-group mean difference = 10.08 ± 9.41; P = 0.026) after 3 weeks training. The exercise group also demonstrated a significant improvement in flexibility (between-group mean difference = 4.4 ± 6.13; P = 0.02). *Limitations.* There was lack of longitudinal followup to examine the long-term effect of aerobic exercise on patients with depression. *Conclusions.* Aerobic exercise in addition to pharmacological intervention can have a synergistic effect in reducing depressive symptoms and increasing flexibility among Chinese population with mild to moderate depression. Early introduction of exercise training in in-patient phase can help to bridge the gap of therapeutic latency of antidepressants during its nonresponse period.

1. Introduction

Depression is currently the third leading cause of global disease burden in 2004; it is estimated that it will become the first most common disabling disease by year 2030 [1]. With increasing tightness in healthcare budgets, there has been great interest in the development and evaluation of alternative or augmentation therapies for depression.

Depression is traditionally treated with pharmacological intervention or psychotherapy or a combination of both. However, the effect of treatment is often suboptimal. Despite new development of antidepressants for depression, at least 30% of depressed patients fail to achieve a satisfactory response [2]. Unwanted side effects induced by antidepressants may impair patient's quality of life and reduce compliance [3]. In up to 50% of acute depressive cases, antidepressants require 1 to 4 weeks before showing any therapeutic effect [4].

In recent years, physical activity [5] and exercise therapy have been extensively examined as treatment for depression, both as monotherapy and as augmentation to antidepressants [6]. Results from meta-analyses of exercise for depression have revealed an inverse relationship between exercise and depression [7] while others comment that exercise is as effective as cognitive behavioral therapy [7, 8]. Continuing to exercise following participation also lowers risk of relapse for patients diagnosed with major depressive disorder (MDD) [9].

When comparing aerobic training to no treatment [10] and resistance training versus standard treatment [11], both are equally effective in reducing depressive symptoms. Researchers found the positive effect of exercise training to be intensity related. A moderate exercise dose appears to have greater therapeutic effect for patients with depression when compared with a low exercise dose in adults with MDD of mild to moderate severity [10]. Chu et al. [12] further supported that subjects undergoing high intensity aerobic training reported significantly fewer depressive symptoms than those in low intensity group and stretching group in sedentary women with mild to moderate depressive symptoms.

Depression may present with feeling of tiredness and reduced motivation for physical activity, which ultimately leads to deconditioning and lower physical performance. Depressed mood is associated with increased risk of strength decline leading to disability [13], while handgrip strength has often been used as predictor of functional disability [14]. The behavioral attributes of depressed mood include physical inactivity may worsen the functional mobility which may cause muscle strength decline. Besides, individuals with MDD would experience changes in posture, like increased head flexion and increased thoracic kyphosis, and mild dissatisfaction with their body image during episodes of depression [15]. These changes would further reinforce depressive patients to become physically inactive leading to muscle strength decline. Aerobic exercise produces positive effect on physical performance thus breaking the vicious cycle and subsequently reduces depressive symptoms.

Early introduction of aerobic exercise training during hospitalization may help to supplement the therapeutic latency of antidepressants [16]. Up till now, there has been no reported study on effect of aerobic exercise training among Chinese individuals with depression. Therefore, there is a need to investigate the effect of aerobic exercise training in early in-patient phase among Chinese individuals with depression in local (Hong Kong) setting. This study aimed to assess the effect of a 3-week in-patient aerobic exercise training in addition to pharmacological intervention on depressive symptoms and physical performance among Chinese subjects with mild to moderate depression.

2. Methods

2.1. Study Design.
A randomized, repeated measure, and assessor-blinded design was used.

2.2. Subjects.
Between February 2010 and December 2011, all patients who were admitted to the Psychiatric Unit in Tai Po Hospital were initially screened using 21-item Chinese version of the Beck Depression Inventory (C-BDI). Subjects obtaining a C-BDI score of 9 or above and meeting the International Classification of Disease (ICD-10) criteria for MDD were recruited. Eligibility criteria included (1) males or females aged 18–64 years; (2) sedentariness, as defined by the absence of involvement in any structured or regular exercise activities over the past one month; (3) currently taking an antidepressant. Exclusion criteria were (1) unstable cardiopulmonary disease; (2) major orthopedic or neurological disease that limits exercise capacity; (3) malignancies in the past 5 years; (4) presence of another primary psychiatric disorder; (5) presence of alcohol or substance dependence within the past 6 months; (6) currently receiving psychotherapy or electroconvulsive therapy; (7) high suicide risk.

The objective of the study, possible risks, potential benefits involved, and the contents of the tests were explained to each subject prior to the study. All subjects were given a participant information sheet and written consent was obtained. The study procedures were approved by the Joint Chinese University of Hong Kong and New Territories East Cluster (CUHK-NTEC) Clinical Research Ethics Committee.

2.3. Sample Size Estimation and Randomization.
Based on the meta-analysis by Lawlor and Hopker [7] with weighted mean difference in the Beck Depression Inventory −7.3 when comparing exercise group with no treatment, we calculated the estimated overall sample size of 52 (26 participants in each arm) achieving an 80% power at a two-sided 0.05 significant level.

Subjects were randomly allocated using blocked randomization into one of two groups: aerobic exercise group and control group. A random number list was generated by an investigator with no clinical involvement in the study using online research randomizer.

2.4. Study Protocol.
A physiotherapist who was independent of the recruitment process for allocation consignment would interview all subjects, who were eligible for the study, using the Chinese version of Physical Activity Readiness Questionnaire (PAR-Q) by the Canadian Society for Exercise Physiology as a preparticipation screening. Individuals who had risk factors identified by the PAR-Q should get medical clearance before they participated in the aerobic exercise program. Before participation, a standardized introduction session was delivered to both the aerobic exercise group and control group.

2.4.1. Aerobic Exercise Group.
All subjects in aerobic exercise group attended 5 supervised exercise sessions per week for 3 consecutive weeks. An interval-training exercise regimen was adopted which included both upper extremity and lower extremity aerobic exercise training. Before each interval training, subjects would undergo a 5-minute warm-up with stretching exercise of large muscle group, followed by a 30-minute interval training at an intensity that maintained heart rate within the targeted training zone, and finally concluded with a similar 5-minute cooldown exercise (stretching exercise of large muscle group).

During the 30-minute interval training, subjects were instructed to exercise 3 bouts of 5-minute workout with prescribed training intensity at 40–59% heart rate reserve (HRR) or with modified rate of perceived exertion (RPE) of 4–6 which is a moderate intensity as according to the guideline of the American College of Sports Medicine [17]. Immediately after each 5-minute workout, participants exercised at a reduced intensity of 20–39% HRR or modified RPE of 2-3 for 5 minutes, all together making up a total of 30 minutes of aerobic interval training. Heart rate and RPE were monitored and recorded during each training session by a physiotherapist. In order to enhance the adherence of exercise training, all subjects were requested to record the amount of exercise in an exercise log book.

2.4.2. Control Group. Subjects in control group were reminded to maintain their physical activity level as usual. A 10-minute stretching exercise on large muscle group was given for standardization.

2.5. Outcome Measures. Depression severity rated by clinician using the Montgomery-Asberg Depression Rating Scale (MADRS) was the primary outcome; all other outcomes were secondary. All the outcomes were assessed before and after the program. Demographic data, including age, gender, weight, height, and body mass index, were recorded at baseline to characterize the participants.

2.5.1. Montgomery-Asberg Depression Rating Scale (MADRS). MADRS is a 10-item scale used to measure the severity of depressive symptoms originally designed to be sensitive to the effects of antidepressant medications [18]. A score greater than 35 indicates severe depression, while a final score of 10 or below indicates remission [19]. MADRS has high internal consistency given the high correlation between all test items ($r = 0.95$) [20], interrater reliability ranging from 0.76 to 0.95 [21], and high correlation with the Hamilton Depression Rating Scale (between 0.80 and 0.90) [22]. All subjects were assessed by one of three assessors (2 psychiatrists and one trained physiotherapist) on the Montgomery-Asberg Depression Rating Scale (MADRS), who were blinded to the subjects' allocation throughout the study. In the present study, the interrater reliability among the 3 assessors was established (ICC = 0.95, $n = 10$).

2.5.2. Chinese Version of the Beck Depression Inventory (C-BDI). The Chinese version of the Beck Depression Inventory (C-BDI) is a 21-item self-rating instrument used to measure severity of depression [23]. The scale ranged from 0 to 63; scores between 10 and 18 indicate mild depression, between 19 and 29 indicate moderate depression, and between 30 and 63 indicate severe depression. The C-BDI was found to have good internal consistency (Cronbach's alpha = 0.846) and moderate concurrent validity ($r = 0.566$) when compared with the Chinese version of the Hamilton Depression Rating Scale [23]. It also yielded good sensitivity and acceptable specificity in assessing psychiatric patients with mixed diagnoses [24].

2.5.3. Sit-and-Reach Flexibility Test. Low back and hamstring flexibility are one of the important components of physical performance [25] which strongly affect the posture and body image of a person. A standardized piece of equipment, the specially constructed sit-and-reach box, was used. Subjects sat on the floor with shoes off and placed the bottom of feet against the box with knees straight. Subjects reached forward along the measuring line with the palms facing downwards as far as possible [26]. The test procedure was repeated 3 times and the mean value was recorded. For easy analyses and comparing results, the zero mark was adjusted 23 cm (9 inches) before the feet.

2.5.4. Handgrip Test. Handgrip strength has shown to be predictive of functional limitations and disability [14] and was classically measured by a handheld dynamometer. Subjects were asked to maximally squeeze the handheld dynamometer (JAMAR); test was repeated on both hands 3 times each and mean value was taken.

2.6. Statistical Analysis. For baseline demographics, descriptive statistics with frequency count, percentages, and mean ± standard deviation (SD) would be reported. Intention-to-treat analysis of all randomized subjects was conducted. Missing data were computed by carrying forward the last recorded observation. For the baseline demographics and clinical characteristics, cross tabulations (Chi-squared test or Fisher's exact test, when appropriate) and t-test were used for discrete and continuous variables. Between-group differences comparing mean change and the main effect of treatment were examined using t-test. All data were analyzed using SPSS 16.0 for Windows. All the statistic tests were two-tailed with significant level at $\alpha = 0.05$.

3. Results

3.1. Participants Characteristics. Between February 2010 and December 2011, 96 individuals, admitted to the Psychiatric Unit of Tai Po Hospital (TPH), were screened for eligibility. 44 individuals were excluded from the study; reasons for ineligibility were early discharge from hospital ($n = 10$), BDI score less than 9 ($n = 5$), refusal to join the study ($n = 26$), and having physical problem that limits their exercise capacity ($n = 3$). Of those individuals who met the inclusion criteria, 26 were randomly assigned to exercise group and 26 were to control group. At the end, 40 participants completed the whole program; 12 participants (exercise group = 7, control group = 5) were unable to finish the 3-week training. No adverse side effect was reported in all participants. The major reasons for dropping out were early discharge ($n = 11$) except one who had a change in medical condition ($n = 1$) (Figure 1).

Baseline characteristics of the 52 subjects are shown in Table 1. There were no significant group differences in their demographic characteristics in age, sex, and body mass index. There was also no group significant difference in the 2 depression scores (MADRS and BDI) and physical performance (handgrip strength and sit-and-reach distance) at baseline (Table 1). The mean MADRS scores of the 2 groups range from 18.77 to 19.23, suggesting that participants in both groups were experiencing mild to moderate depressive symptoms.

3.2. Change in Depression Score after Training. At end of the study, both exercise and control groups showed a significant reduction in the 2 depression scores after 3 weeks of training (Table 2). In the exercise group, after intervention mean score reduced was 10.08 ± 9.4 in MADRS and 8.5 ± 11.36 in BDI; both changes were statistically significant (BDI $P = 0.001$ and MADRS $P = 0.000$). In the control group, a less significant decrease in the depression scores was observed; mean change in MADRS was 4.69 ± 7.33 ($P = 0.001$) and mean change in BDI was 4.08 ± 9.14 ($P = 0.031$) (Table 2). However, when examining the between-group differences in the mean

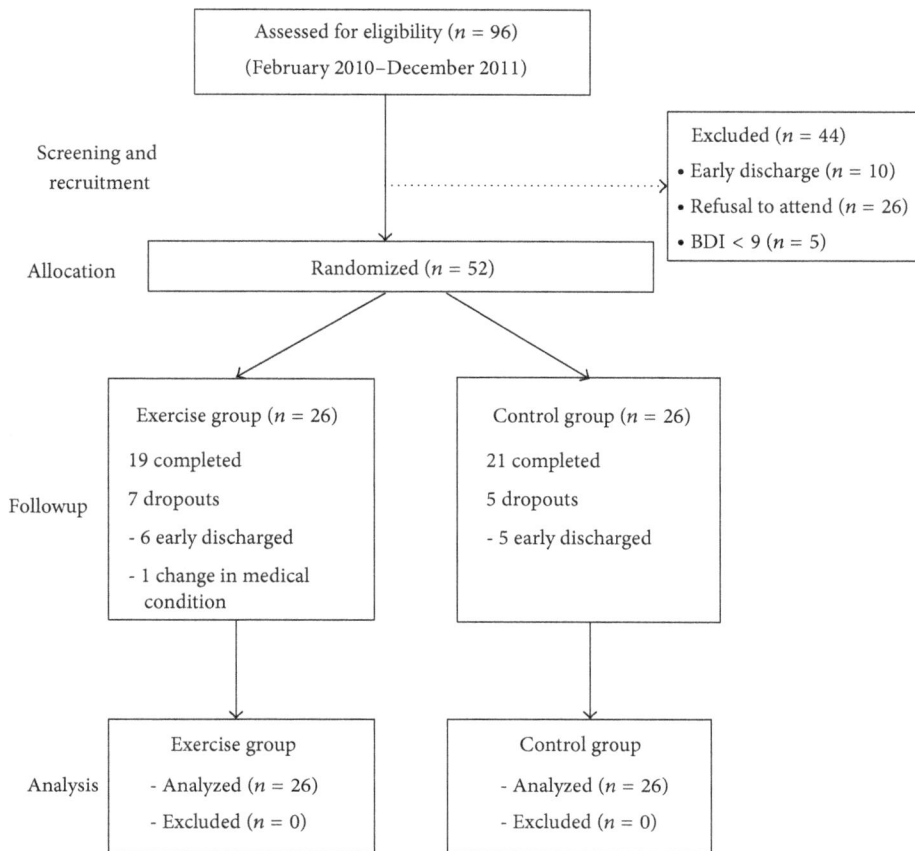

FIGURE 1: CONSORT diagram showing the randomization and subjects flow of the study.

TABLE 1: Demographics, clinical outcomes of subjects collected, P value, and 95% CI of difference between exercise group and control group at baseline.

	Exercise group (n = 26)	Control group (n = 26)	P values	95% CI
Number of females (%)	17 (65%)	18 (69%)	0.77	−0.3–0.23
Age (years)	43.62 ± 13.3	48.81 ± 11.30	0.14	−12.07–1.68
BMI (kgm^{-2})	22.33 ± 3.31	23.22 ± 4.61	0.43	−3.13–1.34
MADRS	19.23 ± 10.48	18.77 ± 10.14	0.87	−5.28–6.20
BDI	26.15 ± 10.63	30.53 ± 11.67	0.16	−10.60–1.83
Handgrip (kg)	34.10 ± 18.70	28.06 ± 18.12	0.24	−4.21–16.30
Sit-and-reach distance (cm)	17.22 ± 10.20	16.45 ± 10.59	0.79	−5.01–6.57

BMI: body mass index; BDI: Beck Depression Inventory; MADRS: Montgomery-Asberg Depression Rating Scale; CI: confidence interval.

change brought about by treatment effect of aerobic training as compared with control, a significantly greater reduction was reported in MADRS only ($P = 0.003$) (Figure 2). Unlike results in MADRS, the reduction of depressive symptoms when comparing effect of treatment to control was found to be not significant in BDI score ($P = 0.103$) (Figure 3). A clinical response (final scores of 10 or below on the MADRS indicate remission) was observed in 14 (54%) patients in the exercise group but in only 7 (27%) patients in the control group ($P = 0.007$).

3.3. Changes in Physical Performance (Handgrip and Flexibility). After 3 weeks of training, exercise group showed a significant improvement in only one physical domain (sit-and-reach flexibility) (Table 2). In exercise group, after intervention mean sit-and-reach distance increased from 17.22±10.2 cm to 21.62±7.89 cm ($P = 0.001$), while in control group, no significant increase in sit-and-reach distance was observed (change in distance was from 16.48±10.59 to 17.25± 11.11; $P = 0.54$). For handgrip strength, both exercise group and control group showed no significant improvement after

TABLE 2: Means and SD for clinical outcomes by group at baseline and program end.

	Exercise group ($n = 26$)		Control group ($n = 26$)		P value (between-group)	95% CI (between-group)
	Baseline	Program end	Baseline	Program end		
MADRS	19.23 ± 10.48	9.15 ± 7.27	18.77 ± 10.14	14.08 ± 9.04		
Mean change	10.08 ± 9.41		4.69 ± 7.33		0.26	-10.08 to -0.69
P value	0.000		0.003			
BDI	26.15 ± 10.63	17.65 ± 11.15	30.54 ± 11.67	26.46 ± 15.05		
Mean change	8.50 ± 11.36		4.08 ± 9.14		0.13	-10.18 to 1.32
P value	0.001		0.032			
Sit-and-reach distance (cm)	17.22 ± 10.2	21.62 ± 7.89	16.45 ± 10.59	17.25 ± 11.11		
Mean change	4.4 ± 6.13		0.8 ± 4.71		0.02	0.55 to 6.64
P value	0.001		0.87			
Handgrip strength (kg)	34.10 ± 18.70	34.41 ± 17.24	28.06 ± 18.12	29.12 ± 16.96		
Mean change	0.31 ± 7.02		1.06 ± 7.51		0.71	-4.8 to 3.3
P value	0.82		0.48			

BDI: Beck Depression Inventory; MADRS: Montgomery-Asberg Depression Rating Scale; CI: confidence interval.

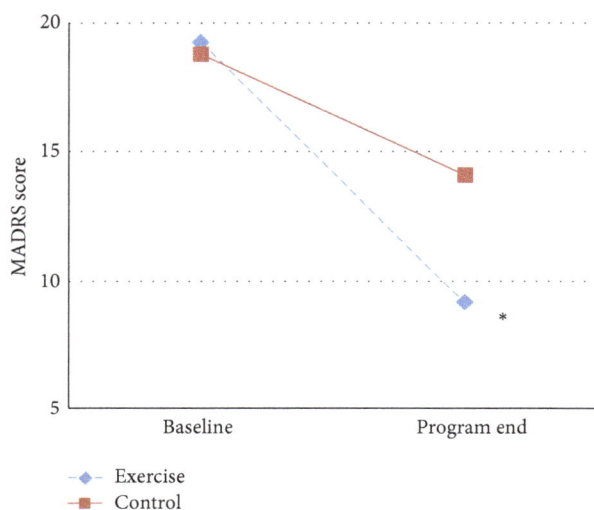

FIGURE 2: Mean change of MADRS score at baseline and program end. MADRS: Montgomery-Asberg Depression Rating Scale; $^*P < 0.05$ versus control group.

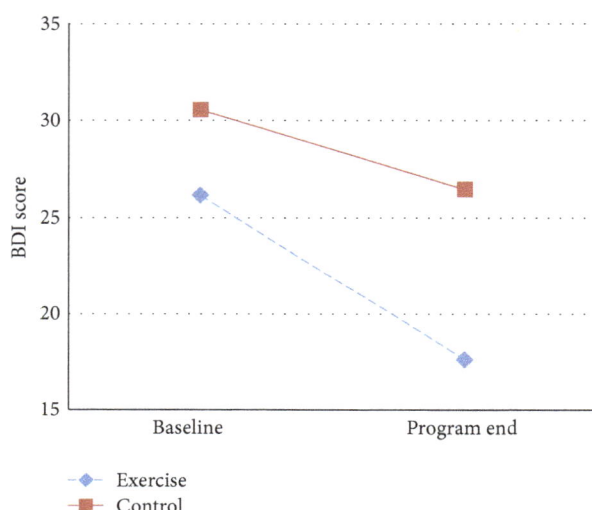

FIGURE 3: Mean change of BDI score at baseline and program end. BDI: Beck Depression Inventory.

3 weeks of training (exercise group: $P = 0.82$; control group: $P = 0.48$).

4. Discussion

The results of our study demonstrated that aerobic exercise in addition to pharmacological intervention is effective in leading to a substantial reduction in depressive symptoms among the Chinese population with mild to moderate depression. In fact, 14 (54%) patients in the exercise group but only 7 (27%) patients in the control group had a MADRS score of 10 or below indicating a remission after completion of 3 weeks of program. In addition, the MADRS scores in exercise group were considerably lower than in the control group at the end

of the study. Thus, the results of our study suggest that aerobic exercise training is effective in reducing depressive symptoms for patients with mild to moderate depression in the first 3 weeks of hospitalization until antidepressants take effect.

Our findings mirror the results of overseas studies that substantial alleviation of depressive symptoms was revealed in patients with major depressive disorder who underwent supervised aerobic training of moderate to high intensity in a short period of time [27, 28]. However, both previous studies had methodological limitations, including small sample [27, 28] and lack of control [27] in the study design. Our results are in contrast with the findings of two previous randomized controlled trials which failed to show significant differences in depressive scores in older depressed patients after exercise training [29, 30]. This may be due to the different clinical conditions of the studied population and intensity of exercise program that patients in previous trials only exercised three times a week. In our study, subjects received moderate intensity of supervised aerobic training five times a week. Thus, it is suggested that it is necessary to reach a certain threshold of energy expenditure to achieve a significant reduction of depression scores in a short time.

It was no surprise that, in both aerobic exercise and control groups, reduction of depressive symptoms was reported simultaneously in BDI and MADRS scores, meaning that the pharmacological treatment was taking effect and was beyond the "zone of uncertainty" [31], the nonresponse period of antidepressants. Nowadays stringent evidence-based guidelines for treating depressive disorders with antidepressants were adopted by clinicians where antidepressants are a first line treatment for major depression in adults [32]. However under a similar regime of pharmacological treatment, depressive symptoms of our subjects in the aerobic exercise group were more significantly reduced than those in control group, meaning that moderate intensity supervised aerobic exercise training is an effective augmentation to antidepressants and especially valuable during the nonresponse period of antidepressants.

In the present study, the between-group treatment effect of the aerobic exercise training as compared with control was demonstrated in MADRS score but not in BDI; this discrepancy may be due to differences in administrative method and the very nature of the tools and of course sensitivity of the measurements. BDI was developed with a structure which reflects the mood, the inner world, and the value of the patient him/herself, which can be subdivided into the somatic and affective domains. It measures attitudes and cognition which are fairly stable over time among depressed patients and therefore may underestimate the degree of improvement during treatment [33]. In the present study, MADRS was not self-administered but assessed by blinded trained personnel. As commented by Svanborg and Asberg [34], the two scales were equivalent with high intercorrelation ($r = 0.869$) only if both were used as a self-assessment instrument. Since MADRS focused on core depressive symptoms, while BDI was demonstrated to tap more maladaptive personality, subjects self-perception of improvement might therefore be less sensitive to change. Furthermore, among some subgroups, like presence of psychosis, lack of insight, and severe hypochondriasis, self-rating scales were associated with smaller effect sizes, thus rendering a smaller improvement in BDI [35].

In the aerobic exercise group, subjects showed significant improvement in body flexibility (sit-and-reach distance) as compared with those in control. Standard stretching exercise of a total of 10 minutes was given to both groups either in one go (control group) or prior to and after the interval training (aerobic group). Hence the improvement in flexibility would not be due to stretching alone but contributed by the 30-minute aerobic training whose positive effect has already been presented in many studies [36–38] not only on flexibility but also on muscle endurance and feeling of fatigue. Canales et al. [39] reported that, during episodes of depression, individuals with major depressive disorder experience changes in posture and mild dissatisfaction with body image; this negative impact might be counterbalanced by the improvement in body flexibility. Unlike flexibility, no improvement was observed in handgrip strength in neither the exercise nor the control group. It might be because no component of strengthening was included in this study and actually there was no obvious decline in handgrip strength as compared with norm data [40].

Intensity of exercise correlates positively with cognitive flexibility and gives feeling of control and fosters social interaction [41, 42]. In fact, both group and individual training are reported to be equally effective in reducing depression [43, 44]. Therefore, effect of social interaction cannot explain results of the present study particularly when the reduction in depression scores was substantially greater in the exercise group indicating an additional effect of aerobic training on depression.

Although the mechanisms accounted for exercise related improvements in depressive symptoms are not known, numerous biological and psychosocial frameworks have been hypothesized to explicate the antidepressant effects of exercise. Exercise may increase serotonin synthesis and reuptake in the brain [45]. Secondly, exercise training can lead to attenuation of the HPA axis response to stress [46]. Thirdly, regular exercise may increase neurogenesis in the hippocampus, a mechanism that has been related to the action of antidepressants [47].

Public healthcare services in Hong Kong are heavily subsidized up to 84% to 98% by the government [48]. The longer the hospitalization is, the more significant the financial impact will be. Early introduction of supervised aerobic training in in-patient phase can have a synergistic effect with pharmacological intervention to reduce depressive symptoms in a short period of time thus minimizing the impact.

There were a few limitations in this study. First of all, this study did not follow up subjects long enough to examine the long-term effect of aerobic exercise on the symptom reduction if the individuals failed to continue the exercise regime. Secondly, the sample size was relatively small as compared to studies of pharmacological treatment and the number of male participants was small. Above all, we detected a lower sensitivity in the BDI which supported the need for a larger sample size to adjust for this smaller one in effect size.

5. Conclusion

There are times when antidepressants have a latency of several weeks until taking effect. During this nonresponse period, both patients and physicians are confronted with a lack of therapeutic options in reducing depressive symptoms in a short period of time. This study demonstrated encouraging results that aerobic exercise training in addition to pharmacological intervention is effective in reducing depressive symptoms and increasing body flexibility among Chinese patients with mild to moderate depression. Early introduction of exercise training in in-patient phase in treating depression can have a synergistic effect with pharmacological intervention in order to ensure the efficacy of rehabilitation.

Conflict of Interests

All authors report no financial interests or potential conflict of interests and no funding sources received.

Acknowledgments

This study was supported by the Physiotherapy Department and the Department of Psychiatry of Tai Po Hospital, Hospital Authority, Hong Kong.

References

[1] World Health Organization, *The Global Burden of Disease: 2004 Updated*, World Health Organization, Geneva, Switzerland, 2008.

[2] S. H. Kennedy, B. S. Eisfeld, J. H. Meyer, and R. M. Bagby, "Antidepressants in clinical practice: limitations of assessment methods and drug response," *Human Psychopharmacology*, vol. 16, no. 1, pp. 105–114, 2001.

[3] P. W. Andrews, J. A. Thomson Jr., A. Amstadter, and M. C. Neale, "Primum non nocere: an evolutionary analysis of whether antidepressants do more harm than good," *Frontiers in Psychology*, vol. 3, no. 117, pp. 1–19, 2012.

[4] I. M. Anderson, D. J. Nutt, and J. F. W. Deakin, "Evidence-based guidelines for treating depressive disorders with antidepressants: a revision of the 1993 British Association for Psychopharmacology guidelines," *Journal of Psychopharmacology*, vol. 14, no. 1, pp. 3–20, 2000.

[5] P. Hassmén, N. Koivula, and A. Uutela, "Physical exercise and psychological well-being: a population study in Finland," *Preventive Medicine*, vol. 30, no. 1, pp. 17–25, 2000.

[6] J. Rimer, K. Dwan, D. A. Lawlor et al., "Exercise for depression," *Cochrane Database of Systematic Reviews*, no. 4, Article ID CD004366, 2008.

[7] D. A. Lawlor and S. W. Hopker, "The effectiveness of exercise as an intervention in the management of depression: systematic review and meta-regression analysis of randomised controlled trials," *British Medical Journal*, vol. 322, no. 7289, pp. 763–767, 2001.

[8] G. Stathopoulou, M. B. Powers, A. C. Berry, J. A. J. Smits, and M. W. Otto, "Exercise interventions for mental health: a quantitative and qualitative review," *Clinical Psychology: Science and Practice*, vol. 13, no. 2, pp. 179–193, 2006.

[9] B. M. Hoffman, M. A. Babyak, W. E. Craighead et al., "Exercise and pharmacotherapy in patients with major depression: one-year Follow-Up of the SMILE study," *Psychosomatic Medicine*, vol. 73, no. 2, pp. 127–133, 2011.

[10] A. L. Dunn, M. H. Trivedi, J. B. Kampert, C. G. Clark, and H. O. Chambliss, "Exercise treatment for depression: efficacy and dose response," *The American Journal of Preventive Medicine*, vol. 28, no. 1, pp. 1–8, 2005.

[11] N. A. Singh, T. M. Stavrinos, Y. Scarbek, G. Galambos, C. Liber, and M. A. F. Singh, "A randomized controlled trial of high versus low intensity weight training versus general practitioner care for clinical depression in older adults," *Journals of Gerontology A*, vol. 60, no. 6, pp. 768–776, 2005.

[12] I.-H. Chu, J. Buckworth, T. E. Kirby, and C. F. Emery, "Effect of exercise intensity on depressive symptoms in women," *Mental Health and Physical Activity*, vol. 2, no. 1, pp. 37–43, 2009.

[13] T. Rantanen, B. W. J. H. Penninx, K. Masaki, T. Lintunen, D. Foley, and J. M. Guralnik, "Depressed mood and body mass index as predictors of muscle strength decline in old men," *Journal of the American Geriatrics Society*, vol. 48, no. 6, pp. 613–617, 2000.

[14] T. Rantanen, J. M. Guralnik, D. Foley et al., "Midlife hand grip strength as a predictor of old age disability," *Journal of the American Medical Association*, vol. 281, no. 6, pp. 558–560, 1999.

[15] J. Z. Canales, T. A. Cordás, J. T. Fiquer, A. F. Cavalcante, and R. A. Moreno, "Posture and body image in individuals with major depressive disorder: a controlled study," *Revista Brasileira de Psiquiatria*, vol. 32, no. 4, pp. 375–380, 2010.

[16] M. Fornaro and P. Giosuè, "Current nosology of treatment resistant depression: a controversy resistant to revision," *Clinical Practice and Epidemiology in Mental Health*, vol. 6, pp. 20–24, 2010.

[17] American College of Sports Medicine, *ACSM's Guidelines for Exercise Testing and Prescription*, Lippincott Williams & Wilkins, Philadelphia, Pa, USA, 2006.

[18] S. A. Montgomery and M. Åsberg, "A new depression scale designed to be sensitive to change," *British Journal of Psychiatry*, vol. 134, no. 4, pp. 382–389, 1979.

[19] C. J. Hawley, T. M. Gale, and T. Sivakumaran, "Defining remission by cut off score on the MADRS: selecting the optimal value," *Journal of Affective Disorders*, vol. 72, no. 2, pp. 177–184, 2002.

[20] A. Galinowski and P. Lehert, "Structural validity of MADRS during antidepressant treatment," *International Clinical Psychopharmacology*, vol. 10, no. 3, pp. 157–161, 1995.

[21] J. Davidson, C. D. Turnbull, R. Strickland, R. Miller, and K. Graves, "The Montgomery-Åsberg depression scale: reliability and validity," *Acta Psychiatrica Scandinavica*, vol. 73, no. 5, pp. 544–548, 1986.

[22] M. J. Müller, H. Himmerich, B. Kienzle, and A. Szegedi, "Differentiating moderate and severe depression using the Montgomery-Åsberg depression rating scale (MADRS)," *Journal of Affective Disorders*, vol. 77, no. 3, pp. 255–260, 2003.

[23] Y. Zheng, L. Wei, L. G. Goa, G. C. Zhang, and C. G. Wong, "Applicability of the Chinese Beck depression inventory," *Comprehensive Psychiatry*, vol. 29, no. 5, pp. 484–489, 1988.

[24] D. W. Chan, "The Beck depression inventory: what difference does the Chinese version make?" *Psychological Assessment*, vol. 3, no. 4, pp. 616–622, 1991.

[25] R. J. Shephard, M. Berridge, and W. Montelpare, "On the generality of the "sit and reach" test: an analysis of flexibility data for an aging population," *Research Quarterly for Exercise and Sport*, vol. 61, no. 4, pp. 326–330, 1990.

[26] K. F. Wells and E. K. Dillon, "The sit and reach. A test of back and leg flexibility," *Research Quarterly for Exercise and Sport*, vol. 23, pp. 115–118, 1952.

[27] F. Dimeo, M. Bauer, I. Varahram, G. Proest, and U. Halter, "Benefits from aerobic exercise in patients with major depression: a pilot study," *British Journal of Sports Medicine*, vol. 35, no. 2, pp. 114–117, 2001.

[28] K. Knubben, F. M. Reischies, M. Adli, P. Schlattmann, M. Bauer, and F. Dimeo, "A randomised, controlled study on the effects of a short-term endurance training programme in patients with major depression," *British Journal of Sports Medicine*, vol. 41, no. 1, pp. 29–33, 2007.

[29] J. Sims, K. Hill, S. Davidson, J. Gunn, and N. Huang, "Exploring the feasibility of a community-based strength training program

for older people with depressive symptoms and its impact on depressive symptoms," *BMC Geriatrics*, vol. 6, article 18, 2006.

[30] N. Kerse, K. J. Hayman, S. A. Moyes et al., "Home-based activity program for older people with depressive symptoms: DeLLITE—a randomized controlled trial," *Annals of Family Medicine*, vol. 8, no. 3, pp. 214–223, 2010.

[31] I. M. Anderson, "Drug treatment of depression: reflections on the evidence," *Advances in Psychiatric Treatment*, vol. 9, no. 1, pp. 11–20, 2003.

[32] I. M. Anderson, I. N. Ferrier, R. C. Baldwin et al., "Evidence-based guidelines for treating depressive disorders with antidepressants: a revision of the 2000 British Association for Psychopharmacology guidelines," *Journal of Psychopharmacology*, vol. 22, no. 4, pp. 343–396, 2008.

[33] C. Cusin, H. Yang, A. Yeung, and M. Fava, "Rating scales for depression," in *Handbook of Clinical Rating Scales and Assessment in Psychiatry and Mental Health*, L. Baer and M. A. Blais, Eds., Human Press, New York, NY, USA, 2012.

[34] P. Svanborg and M. Asberg, "A comparison between the Beck Depression Inventory (BDI) and the self-rating version of the Montgomery Åsberg Depression Rating Scale (MADRS)," *Journal of Affective Disorders*, vol. 64, no. 2-3, pp. 203–216, 2001.

[35] E. Petkova, F. M. Qnitkin, P. J. McGrath, J. W. Stewart, and D. F. Klein, "A method to quantify rater bias in antidepressant trials," *Neuropsychopharmacology*, vol. 22, no. 6, pp. 559–565, 2000.

[36] V. Valim, L. Oliveira, A. Suda et al., "Aerobic fitness effects in fibromyalgia," *Journal of Rheumatology*, vol. 30, no. 5, pp. 1060–1069, 2003.

[37] A. Shahana, U. S. Nair, and S. S. Hasrani, "Effect of aerobic exercise programme on health related physical fitness components of middle aged women," *British Journal of Sports Medicine*, vol. 44, supplement 1, p. i19, 2010.

[38] M. Pazokian, M. Shaban, M. Zakerimoghdam, A. Mehran, and B. Sangelagi, "A comparison between the effect of strtching with aerobic and aerobic exercises on fatigue level in multiple sclerosis patients," *Qom University of Medical Sciences Journal*, vol. 7, no. 1, p. 8, 2013.

[39] J. Z. Canales, T. A. Cordás, J. T. Fiquer, A. F. Cavalcante, and R. A. Moreno, "Posture and body image in individuals with major depressive disorder: a controlled study," *Revista Brasileira de Psiquiatria*, vol. 32, no. 4, pp. 375–380, 2010.

[40] R. C. C. Tsang, "Reference values for 6-minute walk test and hand-grip strength in healthy Hong Kong Chinese adults," *Hong Kong Physiotherapy Journal*, vol. 23, no. 1, pp. 6–12, 2005.

[41] S. Masley, R. Roetzheim, and T. Gualtieri, "Aerobic exercise enhances cognitive flexibility," *Journal of Clinical Psychology in Medical Settings*, vol. 16, no. 2, pp. 186–193, 2009.

[42] B. Resnick, "A seven step approach to starting an exercise program for older adults," *Patient Education and Counseling*, vol. 39, no. 2-3, pp. 243–252, 2000.

[43] J. A. Blumenthal, M. A. Babyak, P. M. Doraiswamy et al., "Exercise and pharmacotherapy in the treatment of major depressive disorder," *Psychosomatic Medicine*, vol. 69, no. 7, pp. 587–596, 2007.

[44] F. Legrand and J. P. Heuze, "Antidepressant effects associated with different exercise conditions in participants with depression: a pilot study," *Journal of Sport & Exercise Psychology*, vol. 29, no. 3, pp. 348–364, 2007.

[45] H. K. Strüder and H. Weicker, "Physiology and pathophysiology of the serotonergic system and its implications on mental and physical performance. Part II," *International Journal of Sports Medicine*, vol. 22, no. 7, pp. 482–497, 2001.

[46] J. Buckworth and R. K. Dishman, *Exercise Psychology*, Human Kinetics, New York, NY, USA, 2002.

[47] C. Ernst, A. K. Olson, J. P. J. Pinel, R. W. Lam, and B. R. Christie, "Antidepressant effects of exercise: evidence for an adult-neurogenesis hypothesis?" *Journal of Psychiatry & Neuroscience*, vol. 31, no. 2, pp. 84–92, 2006.

[48] P. Y. Leung, N. Tse, and D. Yeung, "Sustaining quality, performance and cost-effectiveness in a public hospital system," in *Proceedings of the 37th World Hospital Congress IHF Conference*, Dubai, United Arab Emirates, 2011.

24

Reliability of the Function in Sitting Test (FIST)

Sharon L. Gorman,[1] Monica Rivera,[1] and Lise McCarthy[2]

[1] Department of Physical Therapy, Samuel Merritt University, 450 30th Street, Oakland, CA 94609, USA
[2] McCarthy's Interactive Physical Therapy, 927 Vicente Street, San Francisco, CA 94116, USA

Correspondence should be addressed to Sharon L. Gorman; sgorman@samuelmerritt.edu

Academic Editor: Jeffrey Jutai

The function in sitting test (FIST) is a newly developed, performance-based measure examining deficits in seated postural control. The FIST has been shown to be internally consistent and valid in persons with neurological dysfunction but intra- and interrater reliability and test-retest reliability have not been previously described. Seven patients with chronic neurologic dysfunction were tested and videotaped performing the FIST on two consecutive days. Seventeen acute care and inpatient rehabilitation physical therapist raters scored six of the videotaped performance of the FIST on two occasions at least 2 weeks apart. Intraclass correlation coefficients were used to calculate the test-retest and intra- and interrater reliability of the FIST. ICC of 0.97 (95% CI 0.847–0.995) indicated excellent test-retest reliability of the FIST. Intra- and interrater reliability was also excellent with ICCs of 0.99 (95% CI 0.994–0.997) and 0.99 (95% CI 0.988–0.994), respectively. Physical therapists and other rehabilitation professionals can confidently use the FIST in a variety of clinical practice and research settings due to its favorable reliability characteristics. More studies are needed to describe the responsiveness and minimal clinically important level of change in FIST scores to further enhance clinical usefulness of this measure.

1. Introduction

Research studies indicate that sitting balance ability is a substantial predictor of functional recovery after stroke [1, 2]. There is no universally accepted gold standard measure specific to sitting balance assessment, with many commonly used more global balance measures not specifically isolating sitting balance abilities or examining them at the International Classification of Functioning and Disability (ICF) level of impairment [3–5]. The function in sitting test (FIST) was designed as a concise test of functional sitting balance in patients following acute stroke [3] and another study supports the validity of the FIST in the inpatient rehabilitation population [6]. This test consists of 14 everyday functional tasks, quantifying sitting balance ability and describing sitting balance at the activity level of the ICF. Prior research has shown the FIST to have excellent internal reliability, as well as face, construct, content, and concurrent validity [3, 6]. Studies are underway examining the validity of the FIST in broader clinical populations along with investigating the concurrent and evaluative validity of the FIST in persons undergoing inpatient rehabilitation and the acute care neurological population [6, 7]. Additionally, with the increased emphasis on the use of valid and reliable outcome measures in persons with acute onset of neurologic disorders/diseases, there is need for measures that describe activity limitations in this population [3, 8–11].

Test-retest reliability is an important aspect of a measure, particularly when measuring constructs or performance that is not expected to change over time. In persons with chronic or stable diagnoses, there are limited changes in functional abilities and measures should demonstrate high test-retest reliability. In rehabilitation therapies, where documentation of functional changes is imperative, measures that detect changes during the rehabilitation process are a clear priority for clinical practice and the responsiveness of a measure is valuable. However test-retest reliability is still important as it describes the stability of a measure's score in a stable population. In order to properly examine the test-retest reliability of a measure, the use of a population with stable performance and a one to three day testing window between the two tests are commonly used to mitigate practice effects in the patients being retested [12].

The hallmark of a clinically useful test includes acceptable psychometric qualities related to the inter- and intrarater reliability of the measure [9, 13]. Intrarater reliability describes the ability of the same rater to obtain similar results when testing the same patient, while interrater reliability is related to the ability of multiple raters to arrive at the similar results on a particular measure in the same person. Determination of intra-rater reliability requires that patients to be retested after an interval by the same rater, while interrater reliability requires different raters score the same patient. Both are important in clinical and research settings, with measures that have high or excellent intra- and interrater reliability achieving increased acceptance for wide-spread use. Many design paradigms exist for the investigation of inter- and intratester reliability, but the most clinically applicable one is the partially standardized approach [14]. This methodology is achievable in clinical settings and requires standardized education methods of the raters but is not followed by rigorous checks or further assessment.

It can be difficult for performance-based clinical tests to have multiple raters scoring the same patient performance simultaneously when conducting interrater reliability research, so often these studies employ video recordings of patient performance. Video recording has been used for intertester reliability studies in numerous medical disciplines with acceptable results and can increase the participation of the raters, as it is easier to schedule rating sessions using performance recorded to video [15, 16]. To diminish the effects of recall in the raters, an interval of successive ratings of at least 2 weeks has been recommended [15, 17]. While no specific recommendations regarding the number of raters are prevalent in the literature, multiple studies of other balance tests used in rehabilitation included between seven [17] and ten therapist raters [18]. Additionally, a broad range of patient performance on the videos of the test is required, with the literature specific to other balance tests having between 4 and 20 patients whose performance is scored [17–19].

Currently, it is not known if the FIST has acceptable test-retest, intrarater, or interrater reliability. This study aims to close this gap in understanding of the psychometric qualities of the FIST, furthering its usefulness as a clinical and research measure of sitting balance function. The hypotheses to be tested in this study were that intertester reliability, intratester reliability, and the test-retest reliability of the FIST will fall within the "high" range with intraclass correlation coefficient between 0.70 and 0.89, as defined by Munro [20].

2. Methods

2.1. Participants. This study was approved by the Samuel Merritt University Institutional Review Board. Recruitment of all participants was voluntary and in compliance with the tenants of the Declaration of Helsinki, with all participants (or participants' legal representatives) signing informed consent forms. Participants fell into two categories: balance

participants and therapist rater participants. Balance participants were purposively recruited from the community and included if they met the following criteria: (a) had a diagnosis of central nervous system neurological condition/disorder that was currently stable/chronic (no significant changes in function in the preceding 3 month period), (b) were over 18 years of age, (c) provided written informed consent by the participant or by proxy of a legally authorized representative, (d) scored 3 (moderate disability), 4 (moderately severe disability), or 5 (severe disability) on the Modified Rankin Scale, and (e) were proficient in speaking and reading in English. These balance participants were excluded if (a) medical condition(s) prevented testing procedures, such as but not limited to total hip arthroplasty due to restrictions of hip flexion range of motion, medical status such as subject not cleared for sitting/standing activities by physician, unstable angina, or orthostatic hypotension; (b) severe cognitive deficits limiting ability to follow simple directions; or (c) receiving any physical therapy intervention for balance deficits at the time of the study. Therapist rater participants were included in the study if they had (a) successfully completed the FIST online training module including posttest and/or a one-hour in-service training session, (b) a current license to practice physical therapy, and (c) proficiency speaking and reading in English.

2.2. Test-Retest Procedure. Balance participants were recruited from the community from persons with stable or chronic neurologic conditions; this was to ensure that test-retest data would reflect participants' FIST scores that would be expected to be stable. All balance participants were tested and videotaped performing the FIST twice, one day apart, using the standard FIST testing protocol [3, 21]. Both sessions were videotaped and scored by the same one rater using the standard FIST score sheet (Table 1). A stable sample was purposively recruited inan attempt to control for any changes in FIST scores between the two sessions due to training or intervention effects [13, 14, 22]. Additionally, in an attempt to control the validity threats from maturation or history, the two scoring sessions were held only 1 day apart [13, 14, 22]. To attempt to control the therapist rater recall bias during the 2nd retest session, the therapist rater completed the initial FIST scoring sheets and did not have access to them until after the 2nd retest session was completed (24 hours later). Figure 1 outlines all procedures for this study.

2.3. Intra- and Interrater Reliability Procedure. The videotaped performance of the balance participants' during the test-retest procedure was used for the reliability portion of this study. Balance participant videos were selected based on clear ability to view the administration of the FIST and to obtain a distinctive range of FIST scores. Six FIST test administrations of 6 participants' videos (1 video each) were edited into one longer video, approximately 40 minutes long. One balance participant did not consent to videotaping and could not be used in this portion of the study. The video with the clearest view of the balance participant's performance of the FIST (of the two sessions recorded) was selected. By using

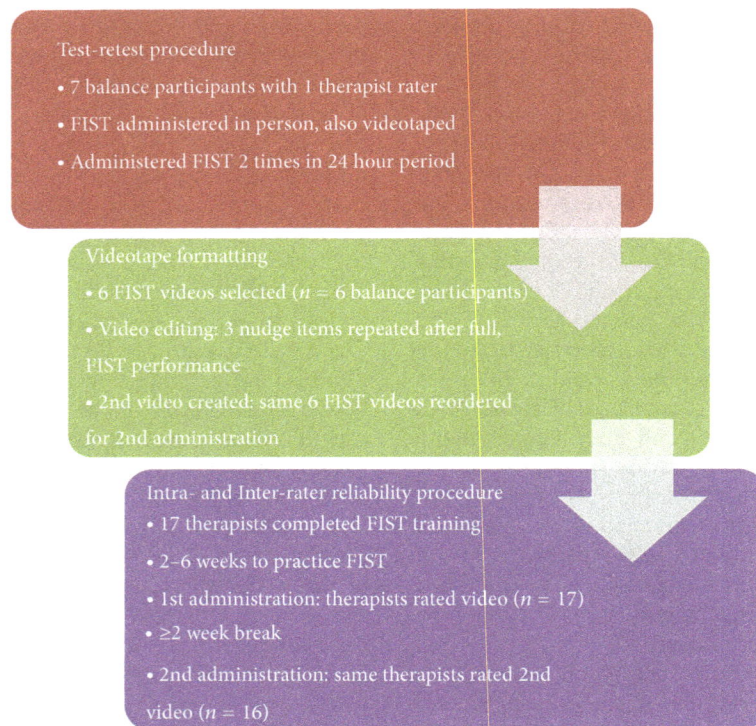

FIST: Function In Sitting Test

FIGURE 1: Study procedures.

6 different videos, a wider range of scores was available in attempt to make the results more generalizable. Videos were edited to replay the 3 nudge items after the full FIST video for each of the 6 balance participants to ensure the therapist raters viewed all 3 nudge FIST test items. This was needed because the 3 randomly performed nudge items on the FIST videos were occasionally missed by the therapist raters (e.g., rater looking down at score sheet during nudge and unable to score nudge) during the pilot testing of the videos being used to score the FIST. To decrease the effect of recall bias by the therapist raters during the second scoring session, these videos were then remixed into a second video package, randomizing the order of the 6 participants' appearance in the video [13–15, 19, 22, 23].

Seventeen therapist raters, purposively recruited from 3 different settings and 3 different facilities, completed the online FIST web-based training [21] or a one-hour training session prior to enrollment in the study and attended an in-service session to answer specific questions about participating in this study, including answering any FIST administration questions. This partial standardized approach to training was selected to allow therapists the opportunity to use the FIST after training with patients within their clinical practice to gain further familiarity with the FIST protocol [14]. Additionally, this training approach closely mimics how training occurs day to day in the clinical setting with regard to the administration of outcome measures. Approximately,

two to six weeks after the introductory training, the first of two therapist rating sessions was held. After obtaining signed informed consent, basic demographic data about the therapist raters was collected. Afterwards, the balance participant videos were viewed by the therapist raters ($n = 17$), who scored the six FIST administrations using a standard FIST score sheet (Table 1). Therapist rater participants did not communicate with one another while scoring and only had the standard FIST score sheet to refer to during the scoring sessions. A second scoring session using the same protocol occurred at least 2 weeks later ($n = 16$) and used the same six balance participant videos but in a different order to further control any recall bias [14, 22]. Figure 1 outlines all procedures for this study.

2.4. Data Analysis. All analyses were conducted using SPSS version 21 [IBM, 2012]. Significance levels of 0.05 were used for all tests, and confidence intervals of 95% were also used. Two-way random model intraclass correlation coefficients ($\text{ICC}_{(2,1)}$) were calculated using absolute agreement definitions. Test-retest reliability used the two scores on the FIST performed one day apart and scored by the same one rater, while intrarater reliability used the first session's FIST item scores (14 FIST items for each of the 6 videos, $n = 16$) and interrater reliability used the first and second scoring sessions FIST item scores (14 FIST items for each of the 6 videos, $n = 17$).

TABLE 1: FIST scoring sheet. Complete details about FIST administration and scoring can be found online at http://www.samuelmerritt.edu/fist.

FIST item	Score
Anterior nudge: light pressure to superior sternum, no warning	
Posterior nudge: light pressure between scapular spines, no warning	
Lateral nudge: to dominant side/strong side, light pressure at acromion, no warning	
Static sitting: 30 seconds	
Sitting, nod "no": left and right	
Sitting, eyes closed: 30 seconds	
Sitting, lift foot: dominant/strong side, lift foot 1 inch twice	
Pick up object from behind: object at midline, hands breadth posterior	
Forward reach: use dominant/strong arm, must complete full motion	
Lateral reach: use dominant/strong arm, lift opposite ischial tuberosity	
Pick object up from floor: from between feet	
Posterior scooting: move backward 2 inches	
Anterior scooting: move forward 2 inches	
Lateral scooting: move to dominant/strong side 2 inches	
Total	

FIST scoring: 4 independent: completes the task independently and successfully; 3 verbal cues or increased time: completes the task independently and successfully but may need verbal cues; 2 upper extremity support: unable to complete task without using upper extremities for support or assistance; 1 needs assistance: unable to complete task successfully without physical assistance; 0 complete assistance: requires complete physical assistance to perform task successfully and is unable to complete task successfully with physical assistance, or dependent.

TABLE 2: Demographics of therapist rater participants ($n = 17$).

Gender	Male 23.5% ($n = 4$)
	Female 76.5% ($n = 13$)
Age (mean)	34.5 years (SD = 10.8, range 24–64 years)
Mean FIST training time	55 minutes (range 45–60 minutes)
Years as licensed physical therapist (mean)	6.6 years (SD = 6.0, range 0–20 years)
Practice setting	Acute care hospital 29.4% ($n = 5$)
	Inpatient rehabilitation 58.8% ($n = 10$)
	Outpatient rehabilitation 5.9% ($n = 1$)
	Academic institution 5.9% ($n = 1$)
Facilities	Facility A 29.4% ($n = 5$)
	Facility B 64.7% ($n = 11$)
	Facility C 5.9% ($n = 1$)
Entry-level physical therapy degree	Bachelors 5.9% ($n = 1$)
	Masters 23.5% ($n = 4$)
	DPT 70.6% ($n = 12$)
Highest degree earned	Ph.D., E.dD., D.Sc. 11.8% ($n = 2$)
	DPT 64.7% ($n = 11$)
	Advanced masters (in PT) 5.9% ($n = 1$)
	Advanced masters (other) 5.9% ($n = 1$)
	None beyond entry-level 11.8% ($n = 2$)

SD: standard deviation; DPT: doctor of physical therapy.

3. Results

Balance participants were primarily female (85.7%, $n = 6$) and had a mean age of 68.7 years. Medical diagnoses of the balance participants included Parkinson's disease ($n = 1$), multiple sclerosis ($n = 1$), and cerebrovascular accident ($n = 5$). Balance participants' performance reflected a variety of scores on the FIST, for individual FIST items as well as total FIST scores. Scores on individual items covered the full scoring range of 0 through 4, using the breadth of the FIST's scoring scale, and the overall FIST scores ranged from 11 to 56, out of the available 0–56.

Therapist rater demographics are presented using summary statistics in Table 2. $ICC_{(2,1)}$ was excellent at 0.97 (95% CI 0.847–0.995) indicating excellent test-retest reliability of the FIST for use with both individuals in a clinical setting and/or groups in a research context [24]. $ICC_{(2,1)}$ for intrarater reliability was calculated for the 16 therapist raters who scored the videos at the two time points and was found to be excellent (ICC = 0.99, 95% CI 0.991–0.995, $n = 16$). $ICC_{(2,1)}$ for interrater reliability was also excellent (ICC = 0.991, 95% CI 0.988–0.994, $n = 17$). The SEM was 3.58 points (out of 56 possible points).

4. Discussion

4.1. Participant Demographics. Balance participants reflected a variety of scores on the FIST, for individual FIST items as well as total FIST scores, and represented neurologic conditions common in the population for which the FIST was created. Because of the small sample size of balance participants ($n = 6$ for inter- and intrarater reliability, $n = 7$ for test-retest reliability), it may be difficult to generalize these results to the broader range of potential patients without further study; however these preliminary results are encouraging.

Therapist rater demographics are presented in Table 2. The 17 therapist raters in this study closely resembled the gender representation for members of the American Physical Therapy Association, but this sample tended to be younger in age and have fewer years as a licensed physical therapist [25]. The therapist raters in this study were more likely to have a DPT degree both as their entry-level degree and as the highest degree earned [25]. However, the therapist raters participating in this study did cover a broad range of education and years in practice. Because the likelihood of using the FIST in clinical practice is higher in acute care and inpatient rehabilitation settings due to the fact that those populations exhibit more problems with sitting balance, and patients in these settings generally demonstrate a higher degree of sitting balance impairment, these therapist groups were purposely oversampled in this study compared to average US distribution, in attempts to make the results more generalizable [25]. While this study represents a small sample size of therapist raters (interrater $n = 17$, intrarater $n = 16$), high levels of reliability were still found even with a potentially underpowered study population.

4.2. Test-Retest Reliability.

An ICC of 0.97 indicates excellent test-retest reliability of the FIST for use with both individuals in a clinical setting and groups in a research context [24]. Using balance participants with chronic histories that included stable neurological conditions and testing each participant twice with a 24-hour period ensured performance stability expectations. If a more acute balance participant population had been used, it would be more difficult to anticipate FIST score stability within the 24-hour testing window, and may have compromised the results of this study.

4.3. Intrarater and Interrater Reliability.

This study demonstrates the excellent intra- and interrater reliability of the FIST. These results, when considered with previous research, indicate that the FIST is a reliable and valid measure of sitting balance function [3, 6]. Clinically, these results are valuable since intrarater reliability and interrater reliability are both in the excellent range; this is important in clinical practice as often the same therapist is not administering follow-up testing. Because many patients with sitting balance dysfunction transition through an episode of rehabilitation across multiple settings seeing multiple therapists, these findings indicate the FIST may be used confidently due to the excellent interrater reliability characteristics. Furthermore, the FIST has the potential to become a vital measure of tracking functional progress in persons who initially possess low function. Often these persons have an extended length of rehabilitation and must undergo serial measurements taken by different therapists in separate care settings. Jette et al. [11] cited common barriers to use of outcome measures by physical therapists, many of which related to the usefulness of the information gained to the specific patients seen: applicability of the measure to direct the plan of care, requirements for training, or costs associated with the use of the measure. All of these are not applicable to the FIST, as it is an activity-based measure appropriate for any patient with sitting balance dysfunction; the FIST test items are everyday functional tasks readily incorporated into the plan of care and are available at no cost [21]. As the results of this study have shown, minimal training is required to obtain excellent inter- and intrarater reliability. Additionally, as a performance-based measure, it addresses additional issues related to administration cited by Jette et al. [11].

These results are further strengthened given the training paradigm used in this study. Therapist raters were trained on FIST administration and scoring using an in-service training session or through a web-based training program. Training was then followed by a period of limited time to practice using the FIST on appropriate patients in their clinical work, followed by the opportunity to ask specific questions and/or to refer to the training website prior to data collection. This type of training most closely reflects the level of most clinical training opportunities in the administration of outcome measures, allowing study results to be more readily generalized to the larger population of therapists who may use the FIST. Additionally, this sequence represents a cost-effective training paradigm which is an important consideration in today's healthcare environment [11].

4.4. Limitations and Future Research.

One limitation of this study was the use of only six balance participants to create the videos scored by the therapist raters. While every effort was made to use participants who demonstrated a wide variety of scores on all 14 FIST items, as well as to have a broad range of overall total FIST scores, not every possible score on each of the 14 items was included in this study. Generalizability was increased by using 17 physical therapist raters from three different settings and three different facilities; however results may not be able to be generalized to all possible raters, especially those from other healthcare professions who may use the FIST. Likewise, by providing training followed by an interval of at least 2 weeks, therapists were given the opportunity to practice administration of the FIST with their patients. However, some therapist raters in this study may have had more or less opportunity to use the FIST in clinical practice during this interval period which might have affected their familiarity when scoring the videos during the two scoring sessions. There was potential that the balance participants experienced a learning effect on the 2 FIST test administrations but is unlikely due to the short duration of the FIST (less than 8 minutes for all participants). Additionally, the test-retest reliability might have been affected by therapist rater recall bias, as the same rater scored all balance participants for these 2 sessions. While this study substantially adds to our understanding of the psychometric properties of the FIST, further psychometric studies of the FIST in different patient populations, determination of responsiveness of the FIST to change with rehabilitation interventions [6], and the ability of the FIST to predict fall risk and discharge disposition are still needed.

5. Conclusions

The FIST is a reliable measure recommended for use in patients with neurological deficits to quantify deficits and/or abilities related to sitting balance. Overall, the FIST demonstrates excellent test-retest, intrarater, and interrater reliability with minimal training in administration. Rehabilitation clinicians and researchers can confidently use the FIST as a reliable and valid tool to measure activity-based deficits and outcomes related to sitting balance in both individual patients and for research purposes.

Conflict of Interests

The authors declare that there is no conflict of interests to disclose. This study was approved by the Institutional Review Board of Samuel Merritt University and all participants and their authorized legal representatives gave written informed consent to participate in this study.

Authors' Contribution

Sharon L. Gorman conceived of the study, participated in its design and coordination, analyzed data, and drafted the paper. Monica Rivera participated in data acquisition, participant recruitment, and data interpretation. Lise McCarthy participated in study design, data acquisition, and participation recruitment. All authors provided critical analysis and paper revision and approved the final version of the paper.

Acknowledgments

The authors would like to thank Rebecca Mustille, PT, and Joan Denzler, PT for their assistance in coordinating the recruitment, training, and scoring sessions for the therapist raters.

References

[1] D. T. Wade, C. E. Skilbeck, R. Langton Hewer, and V. A. Wood, "Therapy after stroke: amounts, determinants and effects," *International Rehabilitation Medicine*, vol. 6, no. 3, pp. 105–110, 1984.

[2] V. Agarwal, M. P. McRae, A. Bhardwaj, and R. W. Teasell, "A model to aid in the prediction of discharge location for stroke rehabilitation patients," *Archives of Physical Medicine and Rehabilitation*, vol. 84, no. 11, pp. 1703–1709, 2003.

[3] S. L. Gorman, S. Radtka, M. E. Melnick, G. M. Abrams, and N. N. Byl, "Development and validation of the function in sitting test in adults with acute stroke," *Journal of Neurologic Physical Therapy*, vol. 34, no. 3, pp. 150–160, 2010.

[4] A. Shumway-Cook and M. H. Wollocott, *Motor Control: Theory and Practical Applications*, Lippencott Williams & Wilkins, New York, NY, USA, 3 edition, 2007.

[5] "International Classification of Functioning, Disability and Health: ICF Short Version," World Health Organization, Geneva, Switzerland, 2001.

[6] S. L. Gorman, C. Harro, and C. Platko, "Responsiveness of the Function In Sitting Test (FIST) in adults in inpatient rehabilitation: preliminary results," *Journal of Rehabilitation Medicine*, vol. 53, p. s99, 2013.

[7] R. Mustille, H. Petersen, J. Abele et al., "A pilot study of the FIST as a functional outcomes measure in a neurological acute care population," *Journal of Acute Care Physical Therapy*, vol. 4, no. 3, pp. 129–130, 2013.

[8] "Neurology Section: Neurology Section Outcome Measures Recommendations StrokEdge," Alexandria, Va, USA, Neurology Section, APTA; c1197-2013, http://www.neuropt.org/special-interest-groups/stroke/strokedge.

[9] K. Potter, G. D. Fulk, Y. Salem, and J. Sullivan, "Outcome measures in neurological physical therapy practice—part I. Making sound decisions," *Journal of Neurologic Physical Therapy*, vol. 35, no. 2, pp. 57–64, 2011.

[10] J. E. Sullivan, A. W. Andrews, D. Lanzino, A. Peron, and K. A. Potter, "Outcome measures in neurological physical therapy practice—part II. A patient-centered process," *Journal of Neurologic Physical Therapy*, vol. 35, no. 2, pp. 65–74, 2011.

[11] D. U. Jette, J. Halbert, C. Iverson, E. Miceli, and P. Shah, "Use of standardized outcome measures in physical therapist practice: perceptions and applications," *Physical Therapy*, vol. 89, no. 2, pp. 125–135, 2009.

[12] A. B. Sorsdahl, R. Moe-Nilssen, and L. I. Strand, "Observer reliability of the gross motor performance measure and the quality of upper extremity skills test, based on video recordings," *Developmental Medicine and Child Neurology*, vol. 50, no. 2, pp. 146–151, 2008.

[13] W. R. Shadish, T. D. Cook, and D. T. Campbell, *Experimental and Quasi-Experimental Designs for Generalized Causal Inference*, Houghton Mifflin, Boston, Mass, USA, 2002.

[14] E. Domholdt, "Methodological research," in *Rehabilitation Research: Principles and Applications*, Elsevier, St. Louis, Mo, USA, 4th edition, 2011.

[15] J. Nunnally and I. Bernstein, *Psychometric Theory*, McGraw-Hill, New York, NY, USA, 3rd edition, 1994.

[16] N. F. Horgan, A. M. Finn, M. O'Regan, and C. J. Cunningham, "A new stroke activity scale—results of a reliability study," *Disability and Rehabilitation*, vol. 25, no. 6, pp. 277–285, 2003.

[17] L. de Wit, H. Kamsteegt, B. Yadav, G. Verheyden, H. Feys, and W. De Weerdt, "Defining the content of individual physiotherapy and occupational therapy sessions for stroke patients in an inpatient rehabilitation setting. Development, validation and inter-rater reliability of a scoring list," *Clinical Rehabilitation*, vol. 21, no. 5, pp. 450–459, 2007.

[18] S. F. Tyson and L. H. DeSouza, "Reliability and validity of functional balance tests post stroke," *Clinical Rehabilitation*, vol. 18, no. 8, pp. 916–923, 2004.

[19] A.-M. Keenan and T. M. Bach, "Video assessment of rearfoot movements during walking: a reliability study," *Archives of Physical Medicine and Rehabilitation*, vol. 77, no. 7, pp. 651–655, 1996.

[20] B. Munro, *Statistical Methods of Health Care Research*, J. B. Lippincott, Philadelphia, Pa, USA, 4th edition, 2000.

[21] Function In Sitting Test, Samuel Merritt University, Oakland, Calif, USA, 2013, http://www.samuelmerritt.edu/fist.

[22] L. G. Portney and M. P. Watkins, *Foundations of Clinical Research: Applications to Practice*, Prentice Hall, Upper Saddle River, NJ, USA, 3rd edition, 2008.

[23] J. Simondson, P. Goldie, K. Brock, and J. Nosworthy, "The mobility scale for acute stroke patients: intra-rater and inter-rater reliability," *Clinical Rehabilitation*, vol. 10, no. 4, pp. 295–300, 1996.

[24] Rehabilitation Measures Database Statistics Review, Rehabilitation Institute of Chicago, Chicago, Ill, USA, 2013, http://www.rehabmeasures.org/rehabweb/rhstats.aspx.

[25] Physical Therapist Member Demographic Profile 2010, American Physical Therapy Association, Alexandria, Va, USA, 2010–2013, http://www.apta.org/WorkforceData.

25

Preoperative Predictors of Ambulation Ability at Different Time Points after Total Hip Arthroplasty in Patients with Osteoarthritis

Akiko Kamimura,[1,2,3] Harutoshi Sakakima,[1] Fumio Tsutsumi,[4] and Nobuhiko Sunahara[3]

[1] *Course of Physical Therapy, School of Health Sciences, Faculty of Medicine, Kagoshima University, 8-35-1 Sakuragaoka, Kagoshima 890-8544, Japan*
[2] *Kagoshima Physical Therapy Association, Kagoshima 897-0132, Japan*
[3] *Red Cross Kagoshima Hospital, Kagoshima 891-0133, Japan*
[4] *Department of Physical Therapy, Kyushu Nutrition Welfare University, Fukuoka 800-0298, Japan*

Correspondence should be addressed to Harutoshi Sakakima; sakaki@health.nop.kagoshima-u.ac.jp

Academic Editor: Velio Macellari

The aims of this study were to identify the preoperative factors influencing ambulation ability at different postoperative time points after total hip arthroplasty (THA) and to examine the cutoff values of predictive preoperative factors by receiver operating characteristic (ROC) curves. Forty-eight women with unilateral THA were measured for hip extensor, hip abductor, and knee extensor muscle strength in both legs; hip pain (visual analog scale, VAS); and the Timed Up and Go (TUG) test pre- and postoperatively. Multiple regression analysis indicated that preoperative knee extensor strength ($\beta = -0.379, R^2 = 0.409$) at 3 weeks, hip abductor strength ($\beta = -0.572, R^2 = 0.570$) at 4 months, and age ($\beta = 0.758, R^2 = 0.561$) at 7 months were strongly associated with postoperative ambulation, measured using the TUG test. Optimal preoperative cutoff values for ambulation ability were 0.56 Nm/kg for knee extensor strength, 0.24 Nm/kg for hip abductor strength, and 73 years of age. Our results suggest that preoperative factors predicting ambulation ability vary by postoperative time point. Preoperative knee extensor strength, hip abductor strength, and age were useful predictors of ambulation ability at the early, middle, and late time points, respectively, after THA.

1. Introduction

Total hip arthroplasty (THA) is commonly performed in patients with hip osteoarthritis (OA). THA is effective in decreasing pain, increasing range of motion of the hip joint, increasing muscle strength and stability, and enabling patients with hip OA to return to their normal daily activities. The greatest amount of functional improvement is observed within 6 months postoperatively, with further improvements occurring for up to 2 years [1, 2]. The number of patients undergoing THA has increased due to rapid advancements in surgical techniques and other developments by healthcare professionals to achieve excellent outcomes, with early functional recovery and short hospital stays [3]. However, not all patients obtain the same amount of benefits from THA, and preoperative functional status appears to be an important predictor of the postoperative outcome [4–7].

As postoperative ambulation ability is an important factor for living an active life and independently performing daily activities, many patients wish to improve their postoperative ambulation ability. Several studies suggest that poor preoperative functional status is associated with poorer outcome after THA [4, 8]. Several parameters have been considered as possible preoperative predictors of ambulation outcome after THA in patients with OA. Preoperative factors associated with functional outcome include age, gender, physical function, level of pain, comorbid conditions, Medical Outcomes Study 36-Item Short Form Health Survey (SF-36) score,

Western Ontario and McMaster Universities Osteoarthritis (WOMAC) score, and perception of self-efficacy [2, 4, 5, 9–13]. Based on these studies, we hypothesized that certain preoperative factors would influence changes in ambulation ability at different postoperative time points after THA.

Muscle atrophy occasionally occurs in patients with hip OA due to preoperative inactivity and may persist after THA; this muscle atrophy contributes to reduced ambulatory capacity and hip and knee muscle strength deficits [14, 15]. Hip abductor weakness on the operated side is reportedly a major risk factor for complications of THA surgery, such as joint instability or loosening [1, 16]. Greater preoperative knee extensor strength on the operated side is associated with better physical function at 12 weeks after THA [6]. However, the relationship between preoperative lower extremity muscle strength and postoperative ambulation ability at different postoperative time points after surgery is unclear.

In the present study, we investigated the recovery of lower extremity muscle strength, pain, and the Timed Up and Go (TUG) test results as indicators of ambulation ability at 3 weeks, 4 months, and 7 months after THA. Furthermore, we identified which preoperative factors were most likely to predict improvement in ambulation ability at each postoperative time point and examined the cutoff values for these factors by receiver operating characteristic (ROC) curves.

2. Materials and Methods

2.1. Participants. We performed a prospective observational study involving a preoperative inception cohort. A total of 74 patients underwent THA at Kagoshima Red Cross Hospital between August 2010 and November 2012. Our inclusion criteria were primary THA for unilateral hip OA, no symptoms in the contralateral hip joint, and informed consent to participate in this study. Patients undergoing arthroplasty for neoplastic disease or articular rheumatism were excluded. Forty-eight female patients who consented to participation were included in this study. The patient characteristics were mean age, 67.6 years (standard deviation [SD]: 10.2, range: 43–85); mean height, 150.4 cm (SD: 7.9, range: 134–170); mean body weight, 57.0 kg (SD: 9.6, range: 39–86); and mean body mass index, 25.2 kg/m^2 (SD: 3.8, range: 18.6–37.5). All patients had undergone primary THA using a posterolateral approach with noncemented prostheses. For walking ability, all patients had a limp before surgery, including 5 with a mild limp, 21 with a severe limp, 20 with walking difficulty, and 2 who could not walk, indicating that the patients had severe hip OA. Most patients were only able to maintain an indoor walking speed and, if able to walk, required assistance device support.

All patients participated in a prescribed 3-week conventional rehabilitation program during hospitalization, according to the protocol of the Kagoshima Red Cross Hospital. This program consisted of joint range of motion, muscle strength, and functional exercises. Range of motion exercise of the knee or hip joint consisted of passive flexion, extension, abduction, and external rotation performed manually by a physical therapist. Muscle strength exercises were single-joint exercises for hip abduction/adduction, hip flexion/extension, and knee

flexion/extension. Initially, active assisted and then active exercises without resistance were used. Later, exercises against progressive resistance were introduced, which was applied manually by a physical therapist. For hip abduction, resistance was applied by a Thera-Band fixed to the ankle with the patients in supine position. Partial weight bearing was initiated from the third postoperative day. Full weight bearing was initiated from postoperative day 14. Gait training started from the third postoperative day using a parallel bar, dependent on muscle pain. The walking distance on a level surface was increased gradually. All patients could walk independently with or without any device support at 3 weeks after surgery. Calf raise exercises, squatting, and single-leg standing exercises were performed to increase muscle strength and improve balance capacity. Physical therapy sessions lasted 1 hour per day. Outcome measurements were assessed at 3 weeks (at discharge) and at 4 and 7 months postoperatively. After discharge, participants presented as outpatients, at which time the measurements were recorded. All measurements were recorded by the same physical therapist. Informed consent was obtained from all patients, and this study was approved by the Ethics Committee of Kagoshima Red Cross Hospital.

2.2. Clinical Parameters. Leg muscle strength on the operated and nonoperated sides was measured using a hand-held dynamometer (HHD, Anima Co., μ-TasF1, Japan) during isometric contraction for 3 s with manual resistance. The HHD is a widely used, reliable, and valid instrument for measuring isometric peak force in studies of elderly patients or THA [6, 16, 17]. Positions chosen for testing were based on the previous literature [18–20] and considered patient safety for adherence to postoperative precautions after THA. To measure hip abductor strength, the subject lay in the supine position, with the hip and knee in neutral flexion/extension and the hips in neutral abduction/adduction. A force sensor was placed 5 cm proximal to the lateral epicondyle of the femur, and a dynamometer stabilizing belt passing around a bar secured the contralateral leg. During measurement of hip extensor strength, the subject was laid in the supine position, with the hip in 30° flexion, the knee in 50° flexion with a triangle stand under the knee, and the hip in neutral abduction/adduction. The force sensor was placed 5 cm proximal to the lateral epicondyle of the femur. During the measurement of knee extensor strength, the subject sat on the bed with the hip and knee at angles of 90°, the force sensor was placed 5 cm above the lateral malleolus, and a dynamometer stabilizing belt passing around a bar was secured behind the back legs of the bed. Successive measurements were performed 3 times, and the average score was used for analysis. Torque was calculated by multiplying strength by the lever arm and was expressed as a percentage of body weight (Nm/kg).

We evaluated hip pain using the visual analogue scale (VAS). The VAS score reflects the subjective degree of pain. Patients place a mark on a 100 mm line—complete absence of pain is indicated by a mark placed at the left edge at 0 mm, while maximum pain is indicated by a mark placed at the right edge at 100 mm.

TABLE 1: Descriptive statistics for clinical measurements obtained pre- and postoperatively.

	Preoperative	3 weeks	4 months	7 months
Hip extensors (Nm/kg)				
Operated side	$0.30 \pm 0.12^{\dagger}$	$0.38 \pm 0.13^{*\dagger}$	$0.59 \pm 0.13^{*\dagger}$	$0.59 \pm 0.30^{*\dagger}$
Nonoperated side	0.38 ± 0.13	0.46 ± 0.15	$0.62 \pm 0.12^{*}$	$0.63 \pm 0.04^{*}$
Hip abductors (Nm/kg)				
Operated side	$0.24 \pm 0.11^{\dagger}$	$0.32 \pm 0.1^{*\dagger}$	$0.50 \pm 0.10^{*\dagger}$	$0.51 \pm 0.12^{*\dagger}$
Nonoperated side	0.34 ± 0.12	0.39 ± 0.10	$0.54 \pm 0.09^{*}$	$0.57 \pm 0.15^{*}$
Knee extensors (Nm/kg)				
Operated side	$0.54 \pm 0.28^{\dagger}$	$0.51 \pm 0.22^{\dagger}$	$0.76 \pm 0.17^{*\dagger}$	$0.80 \pm 0.08^{*\dagger}$
Nonoperated side	0.64 ± 0.24	0.64 ± 0.23	$0.85 \pm 0.21^{*}$	$0.93 \pm 0.13^{*}$
VAS score (mm)	48.1 ± 24.4	$7.5 \pm 10.6^{*}$	0^{*}	0^{*}
TUG test score (s)	23.2 ± 15.4	19.5 ± 7.8	$11.9 \pm 3.4^{*}$	$10.7 \pm 2.3^{*}$

Values are presented as mean ± SD. VAS: visual analog scale. TUG test: Timed Up and Go test. $^{*}P < 0.05$, for comparisons with preoperative values. $^{\dagger}P < 0.05$ for comparisons with the nonoperated side.

To assess ambulation ability, we used the TUG test, including balancing and walking. The TUG test consists of standing up from an armless chair (seat height: 45 cm), walking in a straight line for 3 m, returning to the chair, and sitting down. Patients performed the test while wearing their own shoes and at a self-selected speed. We measured the TUG test performance time in seconds.

2.3. Patient Classification. Patients with a TUG test score > 13.5 seconds were classified as fallers in community-dwelling older adults [19]. Mean patient age was relatively elderly. Therefore, based on TUG test times, the patients were divided into the good (less than 13.5 s) and nongood (over 13.5 s) ambulation groups at 3 weeks, 4 months, and 7 months after THA.

2.4. Statistical Analysis. One-way analysis of variance (ANOVA) was used to compare clinical measurements. If significance was achieved, the Bonferroni test was performed to determine where the significant differences occurred. Student's t-test was used to determine differences in lower extremity muscle strength between the operated and nonoperated sides. The levels of association between the TUG test score and clinical parameters were examined using Pearson's rank correlation coefficients. When significant correlation coefficients were observed, stepwise multiple regression analysis was used to investigate the effect of the physical variables (preoperative hip abductor and extensor strength, knee extensor strength, VAS, TUG, age, and BMI), while using the TUG test results at different postoperative time points as the dependent variable. Mann-Whitney's U test was used to determine differences in preoperative parameters between the good and nongood ambulation groups. Subsequently, the discriminative properties of preoperative knee extensor strength, hip abductor strength, and age for ambulation ability were investigated by applying a receiver operating characteristic (ROC) curve. For this purpose, the area under the curve (AUC), sensitivity, and specificity were calculated. Statistical analyses were performed using SPSS (Version 20.0, SPSS Inc., Chicago, IL). For all tests, a P value

of < 0.05 was considered statistically significant. All data are shown as mean ± standard deviation.

3. Results

3.1. Recovery of Clinical Parameters. Descriptive statistics of the pre- and postoperative values for lower extremity muscle strength, VAS, and TUG test score are indicated in Table 1. Hip extensor and abductor strength on the operated side improved significantly at 3 weeks postoperatively compared to the preoperative value. However, knee extensor strength at 3 weeks postoperatively was not significantly improved compared to the preoperative value. Hip and knee muscle strength on the operated side was significantly lower compared to that on the nonoperated side, both pre- and postoperatively. The VAS score significantly decreased at 3 weeks postoperatively (approximately 84%) compared with the preoperative value, and none of the patients reported hip pain at 4 and 7 months. The TUG test score significantly improved at 4 and 7 months postoperatively, compared to the preoperative value.

3.2. Preoperative Factors as Predictors of Ambulatory Ability. The results of Pearson's rank correlation analysis to assess the effect of preoperative factors on the postoperative TUG test score are shown in Table 2. At 3 weeks postoperatively (i.e., at discharge), the TUG test score was significantly correlated with all examined preoperative clinical parameters, except for hip extensor strength and VAS score. At 4 months postoperatively, the TUG test score was significantly correlated with all examined preoperative clinical parameters, except for VAS score. At 7 months postoperatively, the TUG test score was significantly correlated with preoperative knee extensor strength, TUG test score, age, and BMI.

These significant variables were entered into a stepwise multiple regression model as dependent variables, using the TUG test score for each postoperative phase as the dependent variable (Table 3). At 3 weeks postoperatively (at discharge), knee extensor strength, age, and BMI were significantly associated with the TUG test score. At 4 months postoperatively, hip abductor strength and age were significantly associated with

TABLE 2: Pearson's rank correlation coefficients between clinical parameters and ambulation ability (measured using the TUG test) after THA.

	3 weeks postoperatively	4 months postoperatively	7 months postoperatively
Hip			
Extensors	−0.292	−0.476**	−0.437
Abductors	−0.382*	−0.612**	−0.131
Knee extensors	−0.483**	−0.579**	−0.598**
VAS score	−0.002	0.006	0.281
TUG test score	0.480**	0.492**	0.668**
Age	0.436**	0.638**	0.612**
BMI	0.393**	0.404*	0.390*

Values are correlation coefficients. VAS: visual analog scale. TUG: Timed Up and Go test. BMI: body mass index. $^*P < 0.05$, $^{**}P < 0.01$.

TABLE 3: Multiple regression analysis using the TUG test score for ambulation ability at 3 weeks, 4 months, and 7 months after THA.

	3 weeks postoperatively	4 months postoperatively	7 months postoperatively
Hip			
Extensors		ns	
Abductors	ns	$\beta = -0.572^{**}$	
Knee extensors	$\beta = -0.379^{**}$	ns	ns
TUG test score	ns	ns	ns
Age	$\beta = 0.334^{**}$	$\beta = 0.444^{**}$	$\beta = 0.758^{**}$
BMI	$\beta = 0.314^{**}$	ns	$\beta = 0.363^*$
	$R^2 = 0.409$	$R^2 = 0.570$	$R^2 = 0.561$
Model fit	$F = 9.31$	$F = 23.7$	$F = 11.9$
	$P < 0.001$	$P < 0.001$	$P < 0.001$

β is the standardization coefficient. R^2 is the coefficient of determination. VAS: visual analog scale. TUG: Timed Up and Go test. BMI: body mass index. $^*P < 0.05$, $^{**}P < 0.01$.

with the TUG test score. At 7 months postoperatively, age and BMI were significantly associated with the TUG test score.

Furthermore, the patients were divided into good and nongood ambulation groups to determine the cutoff values of these preoperative factors. Table 4 shows age, BMI, and the clinical parameters of the 2 patient groups at different postoperative time points. Some preoperative clinical parameters were significantly decreased in the nongood ambulation group compared to the good ambulation group. ROC curves were then determined for the 3 associated preoperative factors for ambulation ability at 3 weeks and 4 and 7 months: preoperative knee extensor strength, hip abductor strength, and age, respectively. The ROC curve of each model was graphically displayed (Figure 1). Optimal preoperative cutoff values for ambulation ability of 0.56 Nm/kg knee extensor strength, 0.24 Nm/kg hip abductor strength, and 73 years of age were found, with area under the ROC curve (AUC) of 0.848 (95% confidence interval (CI): 0.715–0.981), 0.778 (95% CI: 0.637–0.919), and 0.749 (95% CI: 0.568–0.929), respectively. Sensitivity was 1.00 (95% CI: 1.000–1.000) for preoperative knee extensor strength, 0.667 (95% CI: 0.419–0.913) for preoperative hip abductor strength, and 0.711 (95% CI: 0.008–0.570) for preoperative age. Specificity was 0.69 (95% CI: 0.241–1.015) for preoperative knee extensor strength, 0.875 (95% CI: 0.725–0.989) for preoperative hip abductor strength, and 0.778 (95% CI: 0.072–0.327) for preoperative age.

4. Discussion

In this study, we identified that preoperative knee extensor strength, but not hip muscle strength, was strongly associated with ambulation ability, as measured by the TUG test, at 3 weeks postoperatively. Hip muscle strength is influenced by hip pain in patients with OA. Our results showed that hip muscle strength increased with decreasing hip pain but that knee extensor strength did not significantly increase at 3 weeks postoperatively. Knee extensor strength decreased in patients with hip OA and was associated with motor performance [21, 22]. Most patients with THA undergo a short rehabilitation program and are discharged immediately after regaining minimal ambulatory ability, such as walking with a cane. Therefore, preoperative knee extensor strength may be considered as a predictor of ambulation ability at an early phase after surgery. This study suggests that preoperative knee extensor strength may be useful as a predictor of ambulation ability at approximately the first month after THA.

Our analysis showed that preoperative hip abductor strength, but not knee and hip extensor strength, was strongly associated with ambulation ability at 4 months postoperatively. Our patients did not experience hip pain at this time and showed progressive improvement in clinical parameters from 3 weeks to 4 and 7 months postoperatively. The TUG test score is influenced by the degree of hip function, as well as pain, leg muscle strength, and range of motion. Loss of

TABLE 4: Preoperative clinical parameters of patients with good and nongood ambulation ability at 3 weeks, 4 months, and 7 months after THA.

| | 3 weeks postoperatively | | 4 months postoperatively | | 7 months postoperatively | |
	Good ($n = 7$)	Nongood ($n = 41$)	Good ($n = 31$)	Nongood ($n = 17$)	Good ($n = 39$)	Nongood ($n = 9$)
Hip						
Extensors (Nm/kg)	0.41 ± 0.12*	0.28 ± 0.11	0.33 ± 0.12*	0.24 ± 0.11	0.30 ± 0.11	0.28 ± 0.16
Abductors (Nm/kg)	0.34 ± 0.09	0.22 ± 0.10	0.28 ± 0.10*	0.17 ± 0.08	0.25 ± 0.10	0.18 ± 0.13
Knee extensors (Nm/kg)	0.84 ± 0.24*	0.49 ± 0.25	0.62 ± 0.27*	0.40 ± 0.23	0.55 ± 0.25	0.53 ± 0.42
VAS score (mm)	34.0 ± 29.4	50.5 ± 23.6	48.0 ± 24.5	48.3 ± 26.4	46.6 ± 24.4	62.1 ± 17.3
TUG test score (s)	13.1 ± 2.6*	25.2 ± 16.1	19.6 ± 12.1*	30.7 ± 19.0	21.8 ± 12.2	31.0 ± 27.1
Age (years)	59.6 ± 6.4*	69.0 ± 10.1	64.5 ± 10.3*	73.3 ± 7.2	65.9 ± 10.0*	73.8 ± 8.7
BMI (kg/m^2)	24.1 ± 1.3	25.4 ± 4.1	25.0 ± 3.9	25.4 ± 3.8	25.0 ± 4.0	25.9 ± 3.5

Values are presented as mean ± SD. VAS: visual analog scale. TUG test: Timed Up and Go test. *$P < 0.05$ for comparisons with nongood values.

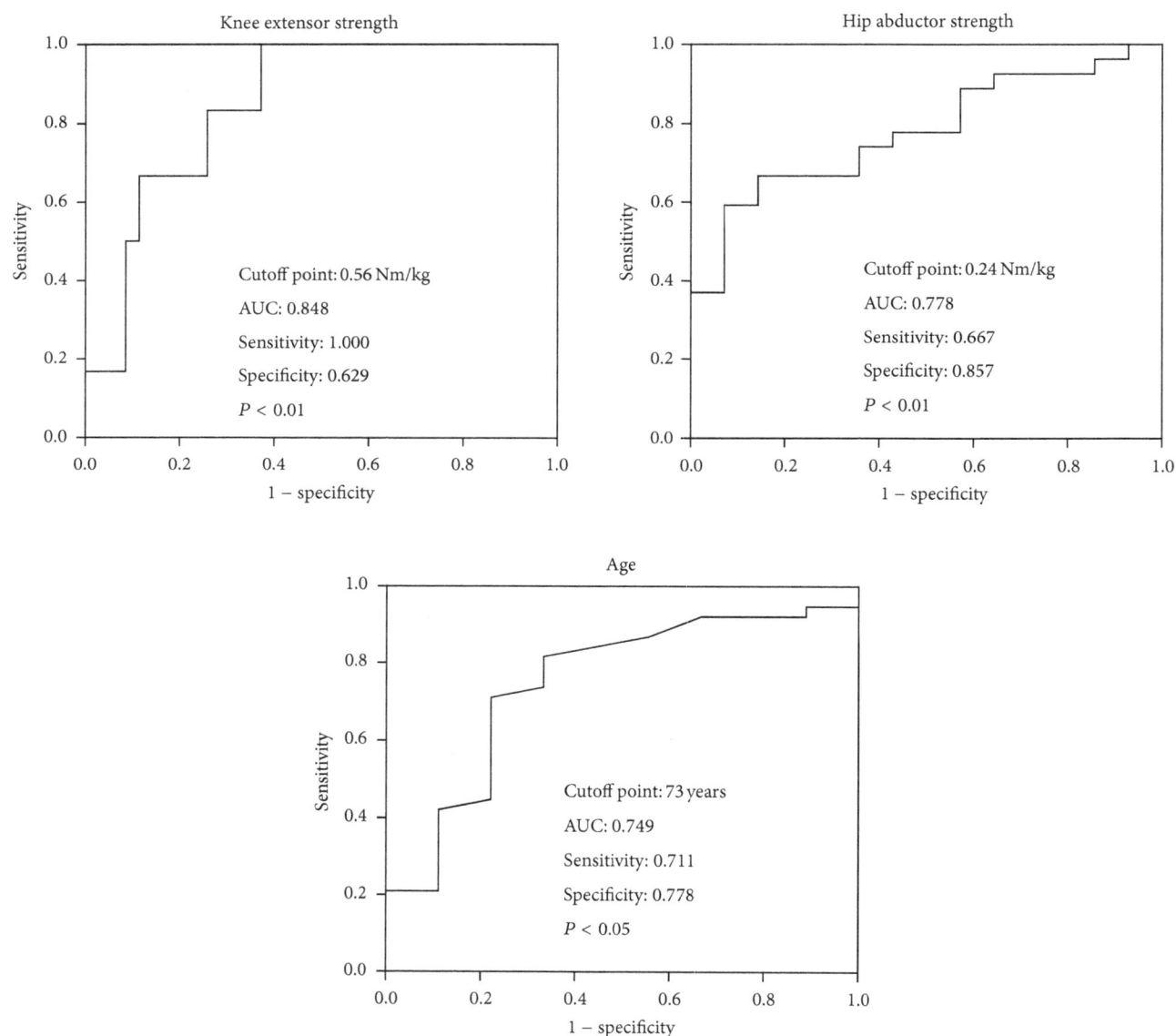

FIGURE 1: Receiver operating characteristic (ROC) curve of assessment of ambulation ability at 3 weeks, 4 months, and 7 months postoperatively, with preoperative knee extensor strength, hip abductor strength, and age, respectively.

abduction power is a common problem for patients with OA and is a major risk factor for complications of THA surgery. Weaker hip muscles, especially hip abductor muscles, on the affected site in patients with THA may also contribute to poor trunk control while walking [16]. Hip abductor strength may have a long-term effect on gait function. Therefore, preoperative hip abductor muscle strength can be used as a predictor of ambulation ability at 4 months after THA, in conjunction with decreased pain and increased hip function. However, our analysis revealed that preoperative age, but not hip and knee muscle strength, was significantly associated with ambulation ability at 7 months postoperatively. Our analysis showed that age and BMI were associated with the TUG test score at all postoperative time points. It is possible to identify patients with THA who are at risk of an unsuccessful outcome by using variables such as BMI, age, and sex [13]. Our findings suggest that age may also be an important predictor of ambulation ability when muscle strength and leg function had almost improved after THA.

The TUG test is widely used to assess functional mobility in elderly people. Preoperative lower extremity muscle strength and the TUG test scores have been found to be sensitive to functional changes in patients following THA [6, 23]. Therefore, we used the TUG test to assess ambulation ability. Nankaku et al. [23] reported that patients with a preoperative TUG test score of less than 10 seconds are likely to walk without an assistive device at 6 months after THA. In this study, few patients had a preoperative TUG test score less than 10 seconds because of severe hip pain. Our patients with end-stage OA had a lower TUG test score than patients in other studies [19, 23]. Therefore, we used the TUG test score classification for elderly people.

Individuals with hip OA are less physically active than their healthy peers [19]. Lower level of physical activities in individuals with hip OA was evident in diminished functional ability and was a risk factor for future physical limitation [24, 25]. Because our patients had less physical activity and activity of daily life preoperatively, they may have had severe disuse atrophy of leg muscles as well as severe hip pain. Therefore, the values of preoperative hip and knee muscle strength were low compared with other studies on Japanese women undergoing THA. Our patients might have had not only severe hip pain, but also a sense of fear during the leg muscle strength test. Due to the hip pain, we did not give positive verbal encouragement during the muscle strength test. However, all patients had improved clinical parameters after surgery, including decreased hip pain. The improved clinical parameters may be reflected because of the low preoperative values in the patients with less physical activity and disuse leg muscle atrophy.

The present study further suggests that preoperative knee extensor strength, hip abductor strength, and age, with cutoff points of 0.56 Nm/kg, 0.24 Nm/kg, and 73 years, may be a good predictive factor for ambulation ability at 3 weeks and 4 and 7 months after THA. Most patients with THA are anxious about the postoperative recovery of their ability to walk before surgery. It is thus very helpful for them to be able to predict their ambulation ability after THA from preoperative lower extremity muscle strength even if this study included

severe OA patients with less preoperative physical activity. The TUG test scores were not significantly correlated with the preoperative VAS scores in the present study. Therefore, other parameters may be needed to investigate ambulation ability, such as 6 min walking distance or biomechanical analysis, in patients with THA.

Preoperative exercise programs are feasible and effective in improving early recovery of physical function after THA [7]. Gait speed is affected by knee extension and hip abduction muscle strength [26]. In this study, preoperative knee extensor and hip abductor strength were correlated with ambulation ability at 3 weeks and 4 months postoperatively. Therefore, preoperative exercise programs should target not only hip abductor muscle strengthening, but also knee muscle strengthening to improve ambulation ability. Generally, knee extension and hip abduction muscle strength are very important for ambulation ability following THA. It is important for physical therapists to know that preoperative predictors for ambulation ability vary by postoperative time points. Intensive preoperative exercise programs and instruction of physical therapy after surgery may be necessary for the patients who are below cutoff values in the present study.

The present study has certain limitations. First, we used a small sample size. Second, we measured only 3 muscle groups: hip abductor and extensor muscles and knee extensor muscles. The hip extensor, flexor, and abductor muscle strength as well as the knee extensor muscle strength have been found to be sensitive to OA, rather than the hip adductor and knee flexor strength [27]. In addition, as our subjects were operated on using the posterolateral approach, this surgery may cause a greater decrease in hip extensor strength than hip flexor strength. Therefore, we selected the hip abductor and extensor and knee extensor muscles to assess patients who underwent THA in the present study. Third, no long-term followup measurements were recorded. Most of the patients with THA are discharged within 3-4 weeks postoperatively, and the greatest amount of functional improvement after THA is observed within 6 months postoperatively [16, 17, 27]. Therefore, the final measurement in our study was performed at 7 months postoperatively. Despite these limitations, this study yields valuable findings that will help predict ambulation ability after THA in patients with hip OA.

5. Conclusion

This study suggests that preoperative factors predicting ambulation ability vary from early to late postoperative time points, and preoperative cutoff values of 0.56 Nm/kg for knee extensor strength, 0.24 Nm/kg for hip abductor strength, and 73 years of age were reliable predictors of ambulation ability at 3 weeks, 4 months, and 7 months, respectively, after THA in patients with OA.

Conflict of Interests

The authors have no competing financial interest to declare.

Authors' Contribution

Akiko Kamimura and Harutoshi Sakakima contributed equally to this study.

References

[1] W. T. Long, L. D. Dorr, B. Healy, and J. Perry, "Functional recovery of noncemented total hip arthroplasty," *Clinical Orthopaedics and Related Research*, no. 288, pp. 73–77, 1993.

[2] D. M. Kennedy, S. E. Hanna, P. W. Stratford, J. Wessel, and J. D. Gollish, "Preoperative function and gender predict pattern of functional recovery after hip and knee arthroplasty," *The Journal of Arthroplasty*, vol. 21, no. 4, pp. 559–566, 2006.

[3] M. S. Ibrahim, M. A. Khan, I. Nizam, and F. S. Haddad, "Perioperative interventions producing better functional outcomes and enhanced recovery following total hip and knee arthroplasty: an evidence-based review," *BMC Medicine*, vol. 11, no. 1, article 37, 2013.

[4] P. R. Fortin, A. E. Clarke, L. Joseph et al., "Outcomes of total hip and knee replacement: preoperative functional status predicts outcomes at six months after surgery," *Arthritis and Rheumatism*, vol. 42, no. 8, pp. 1722–1728, 1999.

[5] A.-K. Nilsdotter, I. F. Petersson, E. M. Roos, and L. S. Lohmander, "Predictors of patient relevant outcome after total hip replacement for osteoarthritis: a prospective study," *Annals of the Rheumatic Diseases*, vol. 62, no. 10, pp. 923–930, 2003.

[6] M. S. Holstege, R. Lindeboom, and C. Lucas, "Preoperative quadriceps strength as a predictor for short-term functional outcome after total hip replacement," *Archives of Physical Medicine and Rehabilitation*, vol. 92, no. 2, pp. 236–241, 2011.

[7] E. Oosting, M. P. Jans, J. J. Dronkers et al., "Preoperative home-based physical therapy versus usual care to improve functional health of frail older adults scheduled for elective total hip arthroplasty: a pilot randomized controlled trial," *Archives of Physical Medicine and Rehabilitation*, vol. 93, no. 4, pp. 610–616, 2012.

[8] J. Holtzman, K. Saleh, and R. Kane, "Effect of baseline functional status and pain on outcomes of total hip arthroplasty," *Journal of Bone and Joint Surgery A*, vol. 84, no. 11, pp. 1942–1948, 2002.

[9] B. Dohnke, B. Knäuper, and W. Müller-Fahrnow, "Perceived self-efficacy gained from, and health effects of, a rehabilitation program after hip joint replacement," *Arthritis and Rheumatism*, vol. 53, no. 4, pp. 585–592, 2005.

[10] C. Röder, L. P. Staub, S. Eggli, D. Dietrich, A. Busato, and U. Müller, "Influence of preoperative functional status on outcome after total hip arthroplasty," *The Journal of Bone and Joint Surgery A*, vol. 89, no. 1, pp. 11–17, 2007.

[11] J. M. Quintana, A. Escobar, U. Aguirre, I. Lafuente, and J. C. Arenaza, "Predictors of health-related quality-of-life change after total hip arthroplasty," *Clinical Orthopaedics and Related Research*, vol. 467, no. 11, pp. 2886–2896, 2009.

[12] N. D. Clement, D. MacDonald, C. R. Howie, and L. C. Biant, "The outcome of primary total hip and knee arthroplasty in patients aged 80 years or more," *Journal of Bone and Joint Surgery B*, vol. 93, no. 9, pp. 1265–1270, 2011.

[13] E. J. Slaven, "Prediction of functional outcome at six months following total hip arthroplasty," *Physical Therapy*, vol. 92, no. 11, pp. 1386–1394, 2012.

[14] A. Rasch, A. H. Byström, N. Dalen, and H. E. Berg, "Reduced muscle radiological density, cross-sectional area, and strength of major hip and knee muscles in 22 patients with hip osteoarthritis," *Acta Orthopaedica*, vol. 78, no. 4, pp. 505–510, 2007.

[15] A. Rasch, A. H. Byström, N. Dalén, N. Martinez-Carranza, and H. E. Berg, "Persisting muscle atrophy two years after replacement of the hip," *The Journal of Bone and Joint Surgery B*, vol. 91, no. 5, pp. 583–588, 2009.

[16] M. Nankaku, T. Tsuboyama, R. Kakinoki, H. Akiyama, and T. Nakamura, "Prediction of ambulation ability following total hip arthroplasty," *Journal of Orthopaedic Science*, vol. 16, no. 4, pp. 359–363, 2011.

[17] A. Kamimura, H. Sakakima, M. Miyazaki et al., "Pelvic inclination angle and hip abductor muscle strength after total hip arthroplasty," *Journal of Physical Therapy Science*, vol. 25, no. 2, pp. 215–219, 2013.

[18] K. Thorborg, T. Bandholm, and P. Hölmich, "Hip- and knee-strength assessments using a hand-held dynamometer with external belt-fixation are inter-tester reliable," *Knee Surgery, Sports Traumatology, Arthroscopy*, vol. 21, no. 3, pp. 550–555, 2013.

[19] D. L. Judd, A. C. Thomas, M. R. Dayton, and J. E. Stevens-Lapsley, "Strength and functional deficits in individuals with hip osteoarthritis compared to healthy, older adults," *Disability and Rehabilitation*, vol. 36, no. 4, pp. 307–312, 2014.

[20] R. W. Bohannon, D. J. Bubela, Y. C. Wang, S. R. Magasi, and R. C. Gershon, "Adequacy of belt-stabilized testing of knee extension strength," *Journal of Strength and Conditioning Research*, vol. 25, no. 7, pp. 1963–1967, 2011.

[21] Y.-. Lin, R. C. Davey, and T. Cochrane, "Tests for physical function of the elderly with knee and hip osteoarthritis," *Scandinavian Journal of Medicine and Science in Sports*, vol. 11, no. 5, pp. 280–286, 2001.

[22] C. Suetta, P. Aagaard, S. P. Magnusson et al., "Muscle size, neuromuscular activation, and rapid force characteristics in elderly men and women: effects of unilateral long-term disuse due to hip-osteoarthritis," *Journal of Applied Physiology*, vol. 102, no. 3, pp. 942–948, 2007.

[23] M. Nankaku, T. Tsuboyama, H. Akiyama et al., "Preoperative prediction of ambulatory status at 6 months after total hip arthroplasty," *Physical Therapy*, vol. 93, no. 1, pp. 88–93, 2013.

[24] C. Veenhof, P. A. Huisman, J. A. Barten, T. Takken, and M. F. Pisters, "Factors associated with physical activity in patients with osteoarthritis of the hip or knee: a systematic review," *Osteoarthritis and Cartilage*, vol. 20, no. 1, pp. 6–12, 2012.

[25] M. F. Pisters, C. Veenhof, G. M. van Dijk, M. W. Heymans, J. W. R. Twisk, and J. Dekker, "The course of limitations in activities over 5 years in patients with knee and hip osteoarthritis with moderate functional limitations: Risk factors for future functional decline," *Osteoarthritis and Cartilage*, vol. 20, no. 6, pp. 503–510, 2012.

[26] R. W. Bohannon, "Comfortable and maximum walking speed of adults aged 20-79 years: reference values and determinants," *Age and Ageing*, vol. 26, no. 1, pp. 15–19, 1997.

[27] A. Rasch, N. Dalén, and H. E. Berg, "Muscle strength, gait, and balance in 20 patients with hip osteoarthritis followed for 2 years after THA," *Acta Orthopaedica*, vol. 81, no. 2, pp. 183–188, 2010.

26

Can Morning Rise in Salivary Cortisol Be a Biological Parameter in an Occupational Rehabilitation Clinic? A Feasibility Study

Kari Storetvedt[1,2] and Anne Helene Garde[3]

[1] *The Occupational Rehabilitation Centre in Rauland (AiR), 3864 Rauland, Norway*
[2] *Department for Physical and Rehabilitation Medicine, University Hospital of Northern Norway (UNN), 9038 Tromsø, Norway*
[3] *National Research Center for the Working Environment, Lersø Parkalle 105, 2100 København Ø, Denmark*

Correspondence should be addressed to Kari Storetvedt; kstoretv@online.no

Academic Editor: Francesco Giallauria

Objective. To test the feasibility of measuring salivary cortisol in an inpatient clinic for occupational rehabilitation, and cortisol as a biological parameter. *Methods.* In 17 patients in vocational rehabilitation, cortisol in saliva was measured at awakening, 30 min after and before bedtime. The cortisol measures were taken on day 2 and day 22 of the rehabilitation period. Cortisol awakening response was estimated in absolute value and as percent rise of the value at awakening. *Results.* The cortisol awakening response in absolute value was 6.7 (SD = 4.9) nmol/L on day 2 and 2.7 (SD = 5.6) nmol/L on day 22. The change was not statistically significant. The mean value for cortisol morning rise calculated in percent was 186% on day 2 and 51% on day 22. *Conclusion.* It is possible to conduct a clinical study including salivary cortisol in a rehabilitation clinic. This study indicates that cortisol morning rise may be a useful biological parameter for effect of intervention in a rehabilitation clinic; this remains to be tested in a larger population.

1. Introduction

Patients in occupational rehabilitation clinics often present with long lasting musculoskeletal pain and depression, with perceived job stress and general life stress. Musculoskeletal pain and psychiatric diagnosis are among the most frequent causes for sick leave and disability pension in Norway; see Brage et al. [1] and Knudsen et al. [2]. Through the last forty years the role of cortisol in stress regulation and as a potential factor in development of chronic pain and stress related disease has been explored but is still sparsely understood. The pattern of cortisol activity has been shown to vary with both psychological and biological factors in several studies; some of them are referred below. The possibility to measure cortisol in saliva has given new options for using cortisol as a biological parameter in clinical studies.

The rise in free cortisol measured in saliva from the time of awakening and to the peak value or through the first hour after awakening has been termed the cortisol awakening response (CAR). The CAR has been found useful as a measure of reactivity of the hypothalamic-pituitary-adrenal (HPA) axis as described by Pruessner et al. [3] and Wilhelm et al. [4].

In their literature review of saliva cortisol studies, M. Kristenson et al. [5] address both the great interest in using saliva cortisol measurement in research on health, disease, work stress, and social differences and also the frustrations in opposing and ambiguous results.

Several studies have addressed the effect of work related stressors on the CAR. Experienced chronic stress, self-perceived work overload, depressive symptoms, and worrying were associated with higher CAR in studies by Pruessner et al. [6] and Schlotz et al. [7]. Morning cortisol has been related to recovery from work in a study by Gustafsson et al. [8], and Harris et al. [9] found CAR related to reestablishing of normal diurnal rhythm after shift work.

In a meta-analysis, Chida and Steptoe [10] found that CAR was positively associated with job stress and general life stress but negatively associated with fatigue, burnout, and exhaustion. In major depression (MDD) Hsiao et al. [11] found that a higher level of self-reported depression correlated with lower cortisol at awakening time and higher evening value. In fibromyalgia low cortisol on awakening was found by Riva et al. [12]. Cortisol concentration in the first hour after awakening was inversely related with level of posttraumatic stress disorder (PTSD) symptoms in a study by Neylan et al. [13], and Roberts et al. [14] found a lower cortisol during 60 min postawakening, in 56 patients diagnosed with chronic fatigue syndrome (CFS).

A vulnerability to chronic muscle pain could have a background in genes involved in adrenergic control and reaction to stress, as shown by Skouen et al. [15]. A recent study from Canada by Vachon-Presseau et al. [16], including 16 patients, found that patients with chronic back pain had higher levels of cortisol on five measures during the day, including time of awakening and 30 min thereafter.

A prospective study from England by McBeth et al. [17] showed that high cortisol after Dexamethasone 0,25 mg could predict development of chronic widespread pain (CWP). This was also true for low cortisol in the morning and high cortisol in the evening, indicating a role of cortisol regulation in development of chronic widespread pain. Geiss et al. [18] looked at cortisol in the morning in a group of patients suffering from persistent sciatic pain 8 weeks after discectomy. They found a lower cortisol immediately after awakening but a higher rise 30 min thereafter (CAR) compared with control group. The high CAR was associated with elevated interleukin 6 (IL-6). There is a close relationship between the stress system components regulated by the HPA-axis, the sympathetic nervous system (SNS), and the immune system as described by Chrousos [19], Glaser and Kiecolt-Glaser [20], and Segerstrom and Miller [21].

Pathophysiology and psychological factors behind chronic widespread pain, leading to disability are items of great importance. Such conditions lead to individual suffering and society costs; see Brage et al. [1] and Knudsen et al. [2]. Searching for interventions that could reduce work disability risk will be of great importance. There is a great need for studies aimed at better understanding of the physiology and psychological factors behind chronic pain conditions. Likewise a biological measurable parameter indicating effect of an intervention could be of great interest to the rehabilitation field. Could cortisol, with its widespread and complex biological influence be such a measurable biological parameter?

This feasibility study aimed to see if it would be possible to use salivary cortisol measures in a 24-hour-based occupational rehabilitation clinic, in a distant rural region.

These questions were asked: would patients in this occupational rehabilitation clinic, with different diagnoses and often with overlapping symptoms, as measured with the Subjective Health Complaint (SHC) inventory, described by Eriksen et al. [22], have disturbed cortisol diurnal rhythm at a group level? And if so, could any change in cortisol rythm be detected after the twenty days rehabilitation periode (time between cortisol measures)?

In spite of a small number of participants, the authors and coworkers would also look for correlations between cortisol measures and health complaints in the SHC, perceived memory and attention, sleep parameters, duration of sick leave, number of pain sites, and body mass index (BMI).

2. Method

2.1. Participants.
A total of 17 patients (51% of the patients invited) at the rehabilitation clinic, 12 women and 5 men, participated in the study. The mean age was 45, ranging from 32 to 60 years. Two groups of patients who arrived in summer and early autumn in 2012 were invited to participate. One patient had ischias with discectomy, four had only psychiatric diagnoses, and 12 had combined somatic and psychiatric diagnoses, including one with CFS and one with fibromyalgia. The most common psychiatric diagnosis was depression ($n = 11/17$), mild ($n = 9$) or moderate ($n = 2$). Informed consent was obtained from all participants prior to taking part in the study. All data were obtained according to the Helsinki Declaration. The Medical Ethics Committee, Region South-East in Norway, approved this study.

2.2. Procedure.
Saliva cortisol rhythm was measured on days 2 and day 22, of a 4-week rehabilitation program in a patient group with compound health problems and health complaints. Test days 2 and 22 were chosen for practical reasons and were days without a very challenging program. Patients were invited to participate on the first day of arrival to the clinic. Those who agreed to participate were given a questionnaire together with 6 small plastic tubes (without a swab, delivered to the clinic from our collaborating laboratory) for salivary sampling. Oral and written information was given, about how to collect saliva samples for cortisol analyses. Questionnaires were handed in to the first author along with the first three test tubes on the third day at the clinic. Diagnosis at arrival, diagnosis given at end of the stay, duration of sick leave, and medication used during the stay were obtained from the patient journal at the clinic.

2.3. Saliva Cortisol Sampling.
Sampling of cortisol was done on a Friday, the second day after arrival, and on the twenty-second day, a Thursday, 6 days before leaving the clinic. Patients were instructed to refrain from eating, drinking, smoking, and tooth brushing the last 30 min before sampling. The three samples were collected immediately after waking up in the morning (I), 30 minutes thereafter (II), and before going to sleep at night (III). The exact time for sampling was written on a schema and on the labeled test tube. The tubes with saliva were kept in the participant's room until next morning. Then samples were gathered and placed in a freezer ($-20°C$) for one or four weeks, or in a refrigerator for two or three days, before they were transported to the laboratory under cooling conditions. Salivary cortisol has been shown by Garde and Hansen [23] to have great stability under storing conditions.

2.4. Questionnaire.
Background variables, including gender, age, BMI, smoking and menstrual data for women, and presence of hypertension, hypothyreosis, airway allergy, food intolerance, and frequent infections were registered from questionnaires.

Health complaints were measured with the subjective health complaints (SHC) inventory that cover 29 questions concerning common health complaints experienced during the last 30 days; see Eriksen et al. [22]. In addition to the SHC questionnaire we asked for perceived cognitive function as problem with attention and memory and about pain in hands, hips, knees, legs, or feet during the last months. All items were answered on a four-point scale (1: not at all, 2: a little, 3: some, and 4: severe). We counted pain sites according to the study of Kamaleri et al. [24], where a number of pain sites were correlated with later disability pension, in a strong way. On the same day when participants collected saliva samples, they registered wakeup time, exact time for collecting saliva, the last nights total sleep time, numbers of wakeups during the night and time before falling asleep.

2.5. Multidisciplinary Occupational Rehabilitation Program.
This study was conducted at a national occupational rehabilitation centre offering a four-week inpatient multidisciplinary rehabilitation program. The rehabilitation team is made up of physician, nurse, physiotherapist, vocational social worker, and sports educator. The program is tailored to improve the patients' level of functioning and work ability with an emphasis on physical activity, counseling psychology, mindfulness, and cognitive behavioral modifications. The main aim is to improve the person's self-efficacy, self-esteem, and coping and resilience related to family and working life along with strengthening physical fitness. Balancing physical training with rest and restitution is an important theme.

2.6. Cortisol Analyses.
After arrival in the laboratory, all saliva samples were stored at $-20°C$ until analysed. At the day of analysis, the samples were left to thaw at room temperature for approximately 45 min and centrifuged at 3500 g for 10 min. Liquid-liquid extraction of 200 μL saliva with 1 mL ethyl acetate, evaporated to dryness under nitrogen flow and redissolved in 200 μL 10% methanol (MeOH), was carried out as described by Jensen et al. [25]. D-4-cortisol was used as internal standard. The calibration range was 0.5–90.0 nmol/L.

2.7. Determination of Cortisol.
A volume of 25 μL was injected into an Agilent 1200 HPLC (Agilent technologies, Santa Clara, CA, USA) equipped with a C18 2.1 × 50 mm 2.6 μm Kinetex column and a Krud-katcher ultrafilter (Phenomenex, Torrance, CA). The mobile phase consisted of a 2 mM aquatic solution of ammonium acetate with 0.1% (v/v) formic acid (A) and MeOH with 2 mM ammonium acetate and 0.1% (v/v) formic acid (B). A linear gradient was run over 3 min from 10% to 100% B and maintained at 100% MeOH for 1.5 min, followed by 2 min of equilibration at 10% MeOH resulting in a total run time of 6.5 min. The flow rate was 0.5 mL/min and the temperatures of the autosampler and column oven were 8°C and 40°C, respectively. Detection of cortisol was performed by a mass spectrometer: an Agilent 6460 QQQ (Agilent technologies, Santa Clara, CA) equipped with a jet stream ESI ion source was operated in the positive ion mode as described by Jensen et al. [25]. The transitions were m/z 363.2 → m/z 121.1 for cortisol; m/z 367.2 → m/z 121.2 for D-4-cortisol.

To show equivalence between different runs, natural saliva samples (1.96 nmol/L and 8.08 nmol/L) were used as control materials and analyzed together with the samples. Westgard control charts (see Westgard et al. [26]) were used to document that the analytical method remained under analytical and statistical control—in other words, that the trueness and the precision of the analytical methods remained stable.

2.8. Statistical Procedures and Data Analysis.
Absolute cortisol values in nmol/L were used in statistical analyses, without a logarithmic transformation.

CAR was estimated as the difference between the cortisol value measured 30 minutes after awakening and the value immediately after wakeup, in absolute value (CARi).

At a group level CAR% was defined as the mean value of CARi in percent of the mean cortisol value at wakeup and estimated from the mean cortisol values, according to Pruessner et al. [3] and Wust et al. [27]. The cortisol slope during the day was estimated in two different ways; the low slope defined as the difference between the cortisol value on awakening and the evening sample, and the high slope, defined as the difference between 30 minutes after wakeup and the evening sample. SPSS (version 20) was used for statistical analyses. Differences in cortisol levels before and after the rehabilitation program were analyzed using paired sample t-test. Correlations between health-related factors, attention, memory, pain and cortisol variables at baseline were investigated using Pearson product—moment correlation analyses.

3. Results

3.1. Background Variables.
The mean BMI was 30 kg/m^2 with a range from 21 kg/m^2 to 41 kg/m^2. Less than 20% reported to be smokers (19%), to have hypertension (12%), hypothyreosis (12%), food intolerance (12%), airway allergy (18%) or frequent infections (18%).

3.2. Saliva Cortisol Measures.
All 17 participants delivered the 6 saliva samples as planned. Mean time of awakening was 06.30 (range 04.25–07.30) in the start, and 06.55 (range 05.30–07.40) in the end of the stay. The mean CARi on day 2 was 6.7 nmol/L (sd = 4.9) and on day 22 mean CARi was 2.7 nmol/L (sd = 5.6) (Table 1). This difference or other differences found between cortisol variables in the beginning and at the end of the rehabilitation period, were not statistic significant.

The mean calculated CAR% changed from 186% at the start to 51% at the end of the stay (Figure 1).

3.3. Recording of Symptom Load/Questionnaires.
On the subjective health complaints (SCH) inventory, almost all (94%) reported musculoskeletal complaints and 76% reported gastrointestinal complaints, during the last 30 days. In the SHC category called pseudoneurology, this patient group also have high scores, 90% with tiredness, 75% with depression and 65% with sleep problems. This patient group shows,

TABLE 1: Saliva cortisol nmol/L (mean value and standard deviation) in the beginning and end of a rehabilitation program.

	Start	End	Sig.
At awakening	3.58 (2.21)	5.33 (4.53)	0.07
30 minutes after wakeup	10.29 (5.81)	8.07 (4.35)	0.25
Evening	0.75 (.48)	1.46 (2.23)	0.19
CARi	6.71 (4.86)	2.74 (5.61)	0.09
Slope high	9.54 (5.51)	6.60 (5.58)	0.18
Slope low	2.84 (2.11)	3.86 (4.65)	0.32

CARi: cortisol awakening response, increase from awakening time to 30 min after.

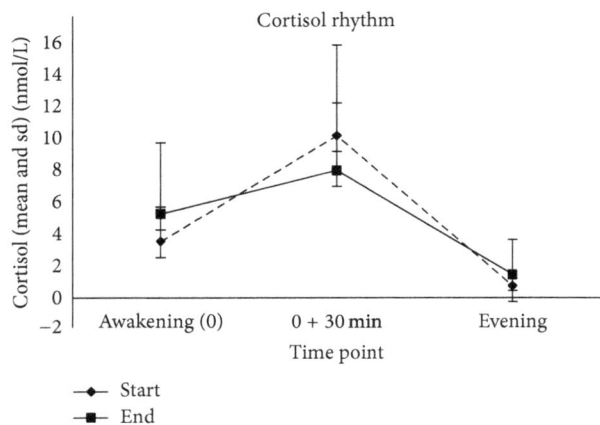

FIGURE 1: The figure shows that the mean rise in cortisol in the morning (CARi) changed from 6.71 nmol/L (sd = 4.86) in the start of the intervention to 2.74 nmol/L (sd = 5.61) at the end of the stay, and the mean rise in percent of the value at awakening (CAR%) changed from 186% in the beginning to 51% in the end of the stay.

according to SHC answers, a great symptom load compared to the general population in Norway. (The SHC inventory was filled in only once, in the beginning of the stay. This questionnaire, measuring complaints during the last 30 days, is not suitable for repeated measures in the beginning and end of a three week period). Perceived cognitive problems were common, with attention problems in 90% and problem with memory in 75%.

Pain sites were counted according to Kamaleri et al. [24]. Of the ten pain sites chosen, head, neck, shoulders, arms, hands, upper back, lower back, hips, knees, and feet, 10 patients (59%) reported 5–10 pain sites and 7 patients (41%) reported 0–4 pain sites.

There were no statistical significant correlations between symptoms in SHC, number of pain sites, attention, memory, or time on sick leave, and cortisol variables as measured in this study group. Neither recorded time of awakening or other sleep variables were correlated with cortisol values in this study.

4. Discussion

This study was carried out as a pilot study in a clinic for occupational rehabilitation with a small number ($n = 17$)

of subjects participating. The study was accomplished without unforeseen problems and with little personal resources required.

Two days after arrival to the clinic, the mean rise in cortisol following awakening (CAR) in percent of the value at wakeup was high, 186% (Figure 1). Pruessner et al. [3] found in their studies of 152 subjects that cortisol increased by 50–75% within the first 30 minutes after awakening. Wust et al. [27] confirm this result in their study of 509 subjects, finding a mean cortisol increase of about 50% within the first 30 minutes. They mention a great interindividual variation in CAR.

In their review Chida and Steptoe [10] found that CAR was positively correlated with job stress and general life stress. This could explain the high CAR on arrival in our patient group, attending vocational rehabilitation due to problems coping with work, health problems, and general life problems. A high CAR has been found in persistent sciatic pain by Geiss et al. [18], while a group with cronic back pain studied by Vachon-Presseau et al. [16] showed high cortisol as well at wake up as after 30 min. In this actual study 65% reported lower back pain the last month. This could possibly contribute to the high CAR in our patient group.

A possible confounder for high cortisol values at arrival could be an activation of HPA axis with high CAR, as described by Kirschbaum and Hellhammer [28] and Kudielka et al. [29], due to the actual situation, including newly arrival at the clinic, new environments with expectations, and anxiety about the rehabilitation program and also included in this study.

Chida and Steptoe [10] found that CAR is negatively related to fatigue, burnout or exhaustion. In syndromes as fibromyalgia, CFS and PTSD Riva et al. [12], Roberts et al. [14] and Neylan et al. [13] found low cortisol response to awakening. Possibly such an expected negative influence on the CAR in this patient group could be overshadowed by a great patient number with a high CAR.

Results two days after admission also show a low cortisol value at wakeup (Figure 1). Low cortisol at wakeup has been found in patients with persistent sciatic pain after discectomy by Geiss et al. [18], in fibromyalgia by Riva et al. [12], and also in primary insomnia by Backhaus et al. [30]. Pain conditions and sleep problems could possibly contribute to the low cortisol value at awakening in the actual patient group two days after admission.

As a confounder, the time or hour of awakening could have an impact on the cortisol values measured at wakeup. Patients on sick leave recently admitted to the clinic could be used to a later wakeup time at home and after adapting to the clinics schedule they maybe wake up on an earlier stage of the natural rising cortisol curve during the late night, as described by Williams et al. [31].

Throughout the last decade many authors have strained the high grade of comorbidity and overlap of symptoms in patients suffering from symptom based conditions as chronic muscelosceletal pain, fibromyalgia, other chronic pain, depressive disorder, post traumatic stress disorder and irritable bowle syndrome, see Kato et al. [32], Cohen et al. [33], and Croft et al. [34]. Such overlap of symptoms was confirmed in this patient group from occupational rehabilitation, with high symptom score on the SHC inventory and supplying questionnaire.

It has been proposed that these sparsely understood conditions with different diagnoses can have common causes and common pathophysiologic pathways. Such mechanisms can according to Getz et al. [35] involve as well biological as cognitive and emotional factors. Kirkengen and Ulvestad [36] discuss if the reason why the pathophysiological mechanisms and disease processes in such conditions are still sparsely understood could be a lack in coherence with "the biomedical paradigm of understanding". Such thoughts resulted in the idea to study these patients at a group level and not divided due to different diagnoses.

Long lasting stress load can influence the immune system. Cortisol is assumed to take part in regulation of immune processes and can be a link between stress and the immune system; see Segerstrom and Miller [21] and Glaser and Kiecolt-Glaser [20]. This can possibly be a pathway for disease in pain conditions, with low grade of inflammation in muscle, tendons, and joints. Cortisol can have an inhibiting as well as an activating effect on inflammation. High cortisol due to long lasting stress can activate inflammation processes. This effect exists in peripheral tissues but especially in the central nervous system (CNS). Cortisol can influence cognitive processes in the hippocampal area and also inhibit glucose entrance to nerve cells according to Sorrells and Sapolsky [37]. These mechanisms can possibly be of importance to cognitive problems, as problem with attention and memory, often experienced by patients in the occupational rehabilitation clinic.

Chrousos [19] suggests that symptoms in pain and fatigue syndromes (as fibromyalgia and CFS) could be due to unbalance between the immune reactions and the stress response, resulting in a "sickness syndrome" with fatigue, depression, social withdrawal, hyperalgesia, and "sickness behavior".

In this pilot study, the mean diurnal cortisol curve in the end of the rehabilitation program, on day 22, shows a CAR close to previously reported normal value for CAR, 51% rise in cortisol in the first 30 minutes, as described by Pruessner et al. [3] and Wust et al. [27]. In contrast, a 186% rise in cortisol (CAR) was observed on the second day of the stay (Figure 1), which indicates a more dysregulated HPA axis function. Although not statistically significant it may be speculated that this change in the morning CAR could be related to the intervention. The lack of statistical significance could be due to the small number of participants in this pilot study, and the results could come out differently in a larger patient group.

It remains to be further explored in an extended study with a greater number of patients if a high CAR in a patient group like this is common in the start of rehabilitation, possibly due to high stress load and if a more normal value will be found after the rehabilitation program. If significant results are found, it could indicate an effect of the rehabilitation intervention on HPA axis regulation, cortisol diurnal curve, and morning rise in cortisol (CAR).

An extended study could possibly contribute to a better understanding of the pathophysiology of complex and stress related disease as here addressed. In an extended study with a greater number of patients, it would be of importance to supply the study with measure of the diurnal cortisol rhythm some days or a week before arrival to the clinic, to avoid the possible confounding effect of HPA axis activation shortly after arrival. A control group with cortisol measures a few days before and after a 4-week vacation could be of interest, to compare cortisol rhythm in the patient group, with a group from the working population, and to compare effect of the rehabilitation program with a possible effect of ordinary vacation.

This study shows that it is fully possible to conduct a clinical study including cortisol measures in a rehabilitation clinic, even in a distant area. If change in cortisol morning rise (CAR) may be a useful parameter for effect of intervention in a rehabilitation clinic, remains to be tested in a larger population.

Conflict of Interests

The first author was employed at The Occupational Rehabilitation Centre in Rauland (AiR) as a chief physician at the time of the study.

Funding

This study was funded by means from The Occupational Rehabilitation Centre in Rauland (AiR), including wedges to the author and laboratory costs. The National Centre for Occupational Rehabilitation, a part of the Centre, contributed with costs to the research collaboration with Uni Helse Bergen.

Acknowledgments

Thanks are due to Holger Ursin, Uni Helse Bergen, for supporting the first idea to this study and thereby making it possible to be carried out. Thanks are due to Anette Harris, Uni Helse Bergen, for great help and support in planning the study and the design, with practical advice and statistical analysis. Thanks are due to the staff at the National Research Centre for the Working Environment, Copenhagen, Denmark, who has been responsible for chemical analysis of cortisol in saliva. Thanks are due to leaders and members of the staff at The Occupational Rehabilitation Centre in Rauland for their support to make this study possible. Thanks are due to Dag Bruusgaard and Bård Natvig, University of Oslo, who read an earlier version of this paper and encouraged our attempts to have it published. At last, thanks are due to patients at the rehabilitation centre for dedicated participation and for making it all right.

References

[1] S. Brage, C. Ihlebæk, B. Natvig, and D. Bruusgaard, "Musculoskeletal disorders as causes of sick leave and disability benefits," *Tidsskr Nor Laegeforen*, vol. 130, pp. 2369–2370, 2010.

[2] A. K. Knudsen, S. B. Harvey, A. Mykletun, and S. Øverland, "Common mental disorders and long-term sickness absence in general working population. The Hordaland Health Study," *Acta Psychiatrica Scandinavica*, vol. 127, pp. 287–297, 2012.

[3] J. C. Pruessner, O. T. Wolf, D. H. Hellhammer et al., "Free cortisol levels after awakening: a reliable biological marker for the assessment of adrenocortical activity," *Life Sciences*, vol. 61, no. 26, pp. 2539–2549, 1997.

[4] I. Wilhelm, J. Born, B. M. Kudielka, W. Schlotz, and S. Wüst, "Is the cortisol awakening rise a response to awakening?" *Psychoneuroendocrinology*, vol. 32, no. 4, pp. 358–366, 2007.

[5] M. Kristenson, P. Garvin, and U. Lundberg, *The Role of Saliva Cortisol Measurement in Health and Disease*, Bentham Science Publishers, Sharjah, United Arab Emirates, 2011.

[6] M. Pruessner, D. H. Hellhammer, J. C. Pruessner, and S. J. Lupien, "Self-reported depressive symptoms and stress levels in healthy young men: associations with the cortisol response to awakening," *Psychosomatic Medicine*, vol. 65, no. 1, pp. 92–99, 2003.

[7] W. Schlotz, J. Hellhammer, P. Schulz, and A. A. Stone, "Perceived work overload and chronic worrying predict weekend-weekday differences in the cortisol awakening response," *Psychosomatic Medicine*, vol. 66, no. 2, pp. 207–214, 2004.

[8] K. Gustafsson, P. Lindfors, G. Aronsson, and U. Lundberg, "Relationships between self-rating of recovery from work and morning salivary cortisol," *Journal of Occupational Health*, vol. 50, no. 1, pp. 24–30, 2008.

[9] A. Harris, S. Waage, H. Ursin, Å. M. Hansen, B. Bjorvatn, and H. R. Eriksen, "Cortisol, reaction time test and health among offshore shift workers," *Psychoneuroendocrinology*, vol. 35, no. 9, pp. 1339–1347, 2010.

[10] Y. Chida and A. Steptoe, "Cortisol awakening response and psychosocial factors: a systematic review and meta-analysis," *Biological Psychology*, vol. 80, no. 3, pp. 265–278, 2009.

[11] F. H. Hsiao, T. T. Yang, R. T. H. Ho et al., "The self-perceived symptom distress and health-related conditions associated with morning to evening diurnal cortisol patterns in outpatients with major depressive disorder," *Psychoneuroendocrinology*, vol. 35, no. 4, pp. 503–515, 2010.

[12] R. Riva, P. J. Mork, R. H. Westgaard, M. Rø, and U. Lundberg, "Fibromyalgia syndrome is associated with hypocortisolism," *International Journal of Behavioral Medicine*, vol. 17, no. 3, pp. 223–233, 2010.

[13] T. C. Neylan, A. Brunet, N. Pole et al., "PTSD symptoms predict waking salivary cortisol levels in police officers," *Psychoneuroendocrinology*, vol. 30, no. 4, pp. 373–381, 2005.

[14] A. D. L. Roberts, S. Wessely, T. Chalder, A. Papadopoulos, and A. J. Cleare, "Salivary cortisol response to awakening in chronic fatigue syndrome," *British Journal of Psychiatry*, vol. 184, pp. 136–141, 2004.

[15] J. S. Skouen, A. J. Smith, N. M. Warrington et al., "Genetic variation in the beta-2 adrenergic receptor is assosiated with chronic musculoskeletal complaints in adolescents," *European Journal of Pain*, vol. 16, pp. 1232–1242, 2012.

[16] E. Vachon-Presseau, M. Roy, M. O. Martel et al., "The stress model of chronic pain: evidence from basal cortisol and hippocampal structure and function in humans," *Brain*, vol. 136, pp. 815–827, 2013.

[17] J. McBeth, A. J. Silman, A. Gupta et al., "Moderation of psychosocial risk factors through dysfunction of the hypothalamic-pituitary-adrenal stress axis in the onset of chronic widespread musculoskeletal pain: findings of a population-based prospective cohort study," *Arthritis and Rheumatism*, vol. 56, no. 1, pp. 360–371, 2007.

[18] A. Geiss, E. Varadi, K. Steinbach, H. W. Bauer, and F. Anton, "Psychoneuroimmunological correlates of persisting sciatic pain in patients who underwent discectomy," *Neuroscience Letters*, vol. 237, no. 2-3, pp. 65–68, 1997.

[19] G. P. Chrousos, "Stress, chronic inflammation, and emotional and physical well-being: concurrent effects and chronic sequelae," *Journal of Allergy and Clinical Immunology*, vol. 106, supplement 5, pp. S275–S291, 2000.

[20] R. Glaser and J. K. Kiecolt-Glaser, "Stress-induced immune dysfunction: Implications for health," *Nature Reviews Immunology*, vol. 5, no. 3, pp. 243–251, 2005.

[21] S. C. Segerstrom and G. E. Miller, "Psychological stress and the human immune system: a meta-analytic study of 30 years of inquiry," *Psychological Bulletin*, vol. 130, no. 4, pp. 601–630, 2004.

[22] H. R. Eriksen, C. Ihlebæk, and H. Ursin, "A scoring system for subjective health complaints (SHC)," *Scandinavian Journal of Public Health*, vol. 27, no. 1, pp. 63–72, 1999.

[23] A. H. Garde and Å. M. Hansen, "Long-term stability of salivary cortisol," *Scandinavian Journal of Clinical and Laboratory Investigation*, pp. 1–4, 2005.

[24] Y. Kamaleri, B. Natvig, C. M. Ihlebaek, and D. Bruusgaard, "Does the number of musculoskeletal pain sites predict work disability? A 14-year prospective study," *European Journal of Pain*, vol. 13, no. 4, pp. 426–430, 2009.

[25] M. A. Jensen, Å. M. Hansen, P. Abrahamsson, and A. W. Nørgaard, "Development and evaluation of a liquid chromatography tandem mass spectrometry method for simultaneous determination of salivary melatonin, cortisol and testosterone," *Journal of Chromatography B*, vol. 879, no. 25, pp. 2527–2532, 2011.

[26] J. O. Westgard, P. L. Barry, M. R. Hunt, and T. Groth, "A multirule Shewhart chart for quality control in clinical chemistry," *Clinical Chemistry*, vol. 27, pp. 493–501, 1981.

[27] S. Wust, J. Wolf, D. H. Hellhammer, I. Federenko, N. Schommer, and C. Kirschbaum, "The cortisol awakening response—normal values and confounds," *Noise & Health*, vol. 7, pp. 79–88, 2000.

[28] C. Kirschbaum and D. H. Hellhammer, "Salivary cortisol in psychobiological research: an overview," *Neuropsychobiology*, vol. 22, no. 3, pp. 150–169, 1989.

[29] B. M. Kudielka, D. H. Hellhammer, and S. Wüst, "Why do we respond so differently? Reviewing determinants of human salivary cortisol responses to challenge," *Psychoneuroendocrinology*, vol. 34, no. 1, pp. 2–18, 2009.

[30] J. Backhaus, K. Junghanns, and F. Hohagen, "Sleep disturbances are correlated with decreased morning awakening salivary cortisol," *Psychoneuroendocrinology*, vol. 29, no. 9, pp. 1184–1191, 2004.

[31] E. Williams, K. Magid, and A. Steptoe, "The impact of time of waking and concurrent subjective stress on the cortisol response to awakening," *Psychoneuroendocrinology*, vol. 30, no. 2, pp. 139–148, 2005.

[32] K. Kato, P. F. Sullivan, B. Evengård, and N. L. Pedersen, "Chronic widespread pain and its comorbidities: a population-based study," *Archives of Internal Medicine*, vol. 166, no. 15, pp. 1649–1654, 2006.

[33] H. Cohen, L. Neumann, Y. Haiman, M. A. Matar, J. Press, and D. Buskila, "Prevalence of post-traumatic stress disorder in fibromyalgia patients: overlapping syndromes or post-traumatic fibromyalgia syndrome?" *Seminars in Arthritis and Rheumatism*, vol. 32, no. 1, pp. 38–50, 2002.

[34] P. Croft, K. M. Dunn, and M. von Korff, "Chronic pain syndromes: you can't have one without another," *Pain*, vol. 131, no. 3, pp. 237–238, 2007.

[35] L. Getz, A. L. Kirkengen, and E. Ulvestad, "The human biology—saturated with experience," *Tidskr Nor Legeforen*, vol. 131, pp. 683–687, 2011.

[36] A. L. Kirkengen and E. Ulvestad, "Heavy burdens and complex disease—an integrated perspective," *Tidsskrift for den Norske Laegeforening*, vol. 24, pp. 3228–3231, 2007.

[37] S. F. Sorrells and R. M. Sapolsky, "An inflammatory review of glucocorticoid actions in the CNS," *Brain, Behavior, and Immunity*, vol. 21, no. 3, pp. 259–272, 2007.

27

The Use of NeuroAiD (MLC601) in Postischemic Stroke Patients

Jose C. Navarro, Mark C. Molina, Alejandro C. Baroque II, and Johnny K. Lokin

Stroke Unit, Department of Neurology and Psychiatry, University of Santo Tomas Hospital, España Boulevard, San Vicente Ferrer Ward, 1008 Manila, Philippines

Correspondence should be addressed to Jose C. Navarro, josecnavarromd@gmail.com

Academic Editor: K. S. Sunnerhagen

Aim. We aimed to assess the efficacy of MLC601 on functional recovery in patients given MLC601 after an ischemic stroke. *Methods.* This is a retrospective cohort study comparing poststroke patients given open-label MLC601 ($n = 30$; 9 female) for three months and matching patients who did not receive MLC601 from our Stroke Data Bank. Outcome assessed was modified Rankin Scale (mRS) at three months and analyzed according to: (1) achieving a score of 0-2, (2) achieving a score of 0-1, and (3) mean change in scores from baseline. *Results.* At three months, 21 patients on MLC601 became independent as compared to 17 patients not on MLC601 (OR 1.79; 95% CI 0.62–5.2; $P = 0.29$). There were twice as many patients ($n = 16$) on MLC601 who attained mRS scores similar to their prestroke state than in the non-MLC601 group ($n = 8$) (OR 3.14; 95% CI 1.1–9.27; $P = 0.038$). Mean improvement in mRS from baseline was better in the MLC601 group than in the non-MLC601 group (-1.7 versus -0.9; mean difference -0.73; 95% CI -1.09 to -0.38; $P < 0.001$). *Conclusion.* MLC601 improves functional recovery at 3 months postischemic stroke. An ongoing large randomized control trial of MLC601 will help validate these results.

1. Introduction

There are currently few therapeutic options for acute ischemic strokes which are mainly limited to revascularization, antithrombotic agents and admission to a stroke unit [1–4]. Neuroprotection trials in acute ischemic stroke have consistently failed [5–7]. Furthermore, aside from rehabilitation, postacute stage long-term options for improving poststroke disabilities have not generated enough interest to be adequately addressed by pharmacological interventions.

Recently, many studies have been published on the efficacy and safety of MLC601 (NeuroAiD) in improving functional and neurological outcomes among nonacute poststroke patients [8–15]. MLC601 has been registered in the Philippines since 2006. For several years now, we have had the opportunity to use MLC 601 in patients with ischemic stroke. Practitioners prescribe it to poststroke patients at a dose used in an ongoing large randomized controlled trial, that is, four capsules three times daily for 3 months [16].

It is the aim of this study to present our experience on the usefulness of MLC601 in ischemic stroke by assessing its efficacy on recovery from functional disability.

2. Methods

2.1. Study Design. This is a nested retrospective cohort study of patients in our Stroke Data Bank who were diagnosed with acute ischemic stroke confirmed by cranial computed tomography (CT) scan or magnetic resonance imaging (MRI). The Stroke Data Bank was duly approved by the institution for research and data analysis purposes and follows the Helsinki declaration on the rights of the patients. For this particular analysis, patients who received NeuroAiD (MLC601) during the course of their medical care from 2008 to 2011 were included and individually matched based on age and gender with an equal number of stroke patients who did not receive MLC601.

2.2. Patients. In this analysis, patients were identified and included in the MLC601 group if they were 18 years old or older, had a prestroke modified Rankin Scale (mRS) score of less than or equal to 1, presented with cerebral infarction with compatible cranial CT scan or MRI findings, started on MLC601 within 6 months of stroke onset and completed treatment of 3 months at the standard recommended dosage

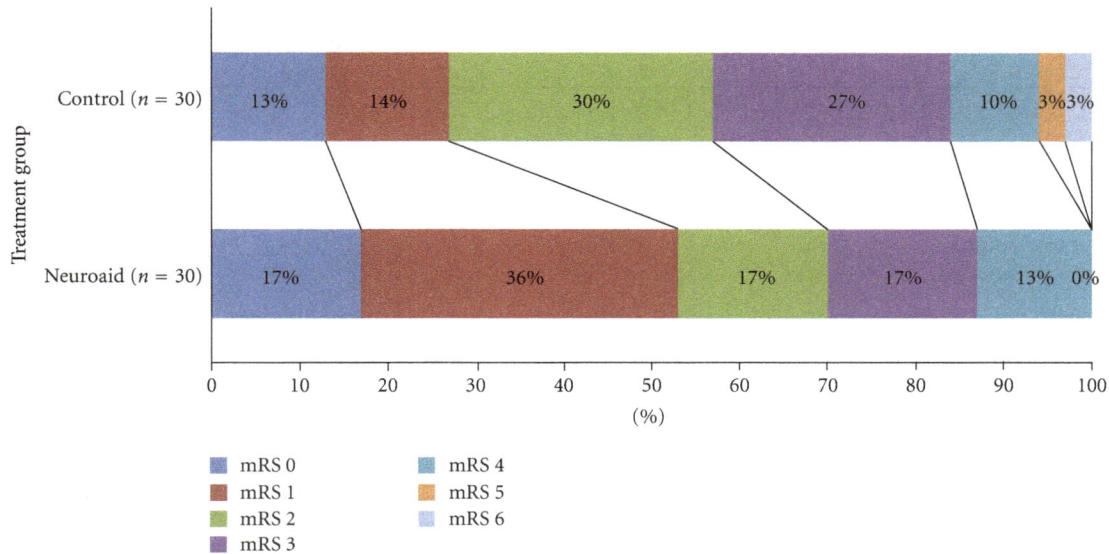

FIGURE 1: Distribution of mRS scores at 3 months.

of 4 capsules 3 times a day, and had data available on mRS scores at baseline and after 3 months of treatment.

In addition to age- and gender-matching, comparison stroke patients were consecutively identified from the same Stroke Data Bank if they met the same criteria above, but did not receive MLC601 yet had mRS assessments at the same time from stroke as the matching MLC601 patient (Figure 1).

All patients received standard stroke treatment as necessary and prescribed by the treating physician, including the use of antiplatelets, antihypertensives, hypoglycemic drugs, statins, and rehabilitation.

The average number of day to initiation of treatment with the MLC601 regimen was 43 days from the time of stroke onset.

2.3. Statistical Analysis. Baseline characteristics collected were age, gender, medical history and vascular risk factors, prestroke and baseline mRS scores, and details of the index stroke including vascular distribution and the classification of the index stroke based on the Trial of Org 10172 in Acute Stroke Treatment (TOAST). The mRS scores at 3 months were obtained by reviewing the patient's outpatient records and via phone interview.

Baseline characteristics of the two groups were compared using Fisher's exact test for categorical variables and Student's t-test for quantitative data. The mRS scores at 3 months were analysed in three manners: by dichotomizing the mRS to either independent (mRS 0–2) or dependent (mRS 3–6), by dichotomizing mRS to either having returned back the prestroke mRS of 0-1 or not (mRS 2–6), and by comparison of mean mRS change from baseline to month 3.

The Mantel-Haenszel test was used to compare the proportion of patients who were independent 3 months after treatment and to compare the proportion of patients who achieved an outcome similar to prestroke mRS. Inverse variance method was used to assess the mean change of mRS score from baseline to 3 months. SPSS statistics version 17.0 (SPSS, Chicago, IL, USA) software was utilized for statistical analysis with a level of significance set at $P < 0.05$.

3. Results

Thirty MLC601-treated patients and 30 correspondingly matched non-MLC601 patients were identified using the criteria and were included in this analysis. Baseline characteristics including age, gender, mRS score at baseline, vascular distribution of strokes, classification based on the TOAST, and risk factors were similar between the two groups (Table 1).

The distributions of the mRS at 3 months for the MLC601 and non-MLC601 groups are shown in Figure 1. None of the MLC601 patients reported any serious adverse event during the 3-month course of treatment.

Among the MLC601-treated patients, 21 (70%) achieved functional independence defined as mRS 0–2 by the third month as compared to 17 (57%) in the non-MLC601 group although the difference did not reach statistical significance (OR 1.79; 95% CI 0.62–5.2; $P = 0.29$) (Table 2). However, there were twice as many patients who were able to achieve an mRS score of 0-1, which is similar to their prestroke conditions, in the MLC601 group ($n = 16$, 53%) as compared to the non-MLC601 group ($n = 8$, 27%) (OR 3.14; 95% CI 1.1–9.27; $P = 0.038$) (Table 2). While both groups showed statistically significant improvement in mRS scores from baseline to 3 months: by −1.7 (95% CI −1.35 to −1.98; $P < 0.001$) in the MLC601 group and −0.9 (95% CI −0.62 to −1.8; $P < 0.001$) in the non-MLC601 group (Table 3), the improvement was significantly better among the MLC601-treated patients with mean difference of −0.73, 95% CI −1.09 to −0.38; $P < 0.001$) (Table 4).

TABLE 1: Baseline characteristics of MLC601-treated and -nontreated patients.

	MLC601 $N = 30$	Non-MLC601 $N = 30$	P value
Age, years	66 ± 11	65 ± 12	0.71
Female, n (%)	9 (30)	9 (30)	—
Baseline mRS score	3.4 ± 1.04	3.2 ± 1.3	0.083
Vascular distribution n (%)			
Left anterior circulation	14 (47)	15 (50)	0.99
Right anterior circulation	13 (43)	12 (40)	0.99
Posterior circulation	3 (10)	3 (10)	—
Classification of the Index Stroke Based on the TOAST Criteria n (%)			
Large artery atherosclerosis	18 (60)	19 (63)	0.99
Cardioembolism	5 (17)	4 (13)	0.99
Small vessel occlusion	7 (23)	7 (23)	—
Stroke of other determined etiology	0	0	—
Stroke of undetermined etiology	0	0	—
Risk factors n (%)			
Hypertension	25 (83)	27 (90)	0.70
Diabetes	9 (30)	9 (30)	—
Coronary artery disease	8 (27)	6 (20)	0.76
Dyslipidemia	18 (60)	18 (60)	—
Atrial fibrillation	5 (17)	4 (13)	0.99
Prior stroke	4 (13)	6 (20)	0.73
Average days to initiation of MLC601	44 days	—	—

TABLE 2: Results of statistical comparisons of mRS score at 3 months between MLC601 and non-MLC601 patients.

	MLC601 ($n = 30$)	Non-MLC601 ($n = 30$)	Odds ratio (95% CI)	P value
	n (%)	n (%)		
At 3 months				
mRS 0 to 2	21 (70%)	17 (57%)	1.79 (0.62 to 5.2)	0.29
mRS 0 to 1	16 (53%)	8 (27%)	3.14 (1.1 to 9.27)	0.038

TABLE 3: Mean difference (95% CI) in mRS score from baseline to 3 months.

	MLC601 ($n = 30$)	Non-MLC601 ($n = 30$)
Mean baseline mRS	3.4 ± 1.04	3.2 ± 1.3
Mean mRS at 3 months	1.7 ± 1.3	2.3 ± 1.5
Mean difference in mRS from baseline to 3 months (95% CI)	−1.7 (−1.35 to −1.98)	−0.9 (−0.62 to −1.8)
P value	<0.001	<0.001

4. Discussion

In Asia, many poststroke patients seek alternative therapies due to dissatisfaction with their degree of recovery [17]. The utilization of traditional medicines has been part of stroke treatment in Asian countries such as in India and China [18].

Numerous articles in Chinese medical literatures regarding the usefulness and safety of traditional Chinese medicine (TCM) have been published [19]. However, most of these clinical trials have been of poor methodological quality [20].

MLC601 consists of 9 herbal (*Radix astragali, Radix salviae miltiorrhizae, Radix paeoniae rubra, Rhizoma chuanxiong, Radix angelicae sinensis, Carthamus tinctorius, Prunus persica, Radix polygalae,* and *Rhizoma acori tatarinowii*) and 5 animal (*Hirudo, Eupolyphaga seu steleophaga, Calculus bovisartifactus, Buthus martensii,* and *Cornu saigae tataricae*) components. Recent publications have shown benefit in the use of MLC601 in postischemic stroke patients. Many patients in these studies were nonacute and were included from within 1 week to up to 6 months since their stroke onset [8–15]. These studies offer an opportunity to intervene and improve functional and neurological outcomes further even if started in the recovery phase.

Our study looked at the same population of nonacute patients, but specifically using a well-established and most

TABLE 4: Comparison of the mean difference mRS between MC601 and non-MLC60 patients.

	MLC601 ($n = 30$)	Non-MLC601 ($n = 30$)	Odds ratio (95% CI)	P value
Mean difference in mRS between MC601 and Non-MLC601	-1.7 (-1.35 to -1.98)	-0.9 (-0.62 to -1.8)	-0.73 (-1.09 to -0.38)	<0.001

often used measurement tool for functional disability in stroke, the modified Rankin Scale [21]. We found that stroke patients given MLC601 in addition to standard treatment were more likely to attain better functional outcome without serious adverse effect after 3 months of treatment.

We are very much aware of the limitations of this study. Outcome assessment bias may be reduced to a certain extent in our study since patients' information were systematically collected at the time they were included in the Stroke Data Bank, before the hypothesis being tested in this study was defined. However, it is difficult to avoid biases in an open-label, nonrandomized, nonblinded study, hence the large double-blind placebo-controlled randomized study will help confirm and validate the results observed in our small cohort.

The exact mechanisms of MLC601 is yet unknown and MLC601 may very well act on many different pathways. However, the neuroprotective and, more importantly, neuroproliferative effects of MLC601 in animal models of focal and global ischemia [22, 23] is consistent with our clinical observation and that of other studies, and further strengthens the concept that intervention to reduce disabilities even long after the acute phase of a stroke may be feasible by enhancing neuroplasticity and neurogenesis.

Acknowledgments

These data were presented in abstract form at the 21st European Stroke Conference in Lisbon, Portugal on May 22–25, 2012. The authors are grateful to the consultant staff of the Department of Neurology and Psychiatry, University of Santo Tomas Hospital, for allowing us to include their patients in this study. J. C. Navarro has received speaker honoraria from Moleac.

References

[1] J. R. Marler, "Tissue plasminogen activator for acute ischemic stroke," *The New England Journal of Medicine*, vol. 333, no. 24, pp. 1581–1587, 1995.

[2] P. A. G. Sandercock, "The international stroke trial (IST): a randomised trial of aspirin, subcutaneous heparin, both, or neither among 19 435 patients with acute ischaemic stroke," *The Lancet*, vol. 349, no. 9065, pp. 1569–1581, 1997.

[3] Z.-M. Chen, "CAST: randomised placebo-controlled trial of early aspirin use in 20,000 patients with acute ischaemic stroke," *The Lancet*, vol. 349, no. 9066, pp. 1641–1649, 1997.

[4] Stroke Unit Trialists' Collaboration, "Organised inpatient (stroke unit) care for stroke," *Cochrane Database of Systematic Reviews*, no. 3, 2001.

[5] B. A. Sutherland, J. Minnerup, J. S. Balami, F. Arbal, A. M. Buchan, and C. Kleinschnitz, "Neuroprotection for ischaemic stroke: translation from the bench to the bedside," *International Journal of Stroke*, vol. 7, pp. 407–418, 2012.

[6] V. E. O'Collins, M. R. Macleod, G. A. Donnan, L. L. Horky, B. H. Van Der Worp, and D. W. Howells, "1,026 Experimental treatments in acute stroke," *Annals of Neurology*, vol. 59, no. 3, pp. 467–477, 2006.

[7] M. D. Ginsberg, "Current status of neuroprotection for cerebral ischemia synoptic overview," *Stroke*, vol. 40, supplement 1, pp. S111–S114, 2009.

[8] C. Chen, N. Venketasubramanian, R. N. Gan et al., "Danqi Piantang Jiaonang (DJ), a traditional Chinese medicine, in poststroke recovery," *Stroke*, vol. 40, no. 3, pp. 859–863, 2009.

[9] A. A. Harandi, R. Abolfazli, A. Hatemian et al., "Safety and efficacy of MLC601 in Iranian patients after stroke: a double-blind, placebo-controlled clinical trial," *Stroke Research and Treatment*, vol. 2011, Article ID 721613, 5 pages, 2011.

[10] S. H. Y. Young, Y. Zhao, A. Koh et al., "Safety profile of MLC601 (Neuroaid) in acute ischemic stroke patients: a Singaporean substudy of the chinese medicine neuroaid efficacy on stroke recovery study," *Cerebrovascular Diseases*, vol. 30, no. 1, pp. 1–6, 2010.

[11] R. Gan, C. Lambert, J. Lianting et al., "Danqi Piantan Jiaonang does not modify hemostasis, hematology, and biochemistry in normal subjects and stroke patients," *Cerebrovascular Diseases*, vol. 25, no. 5, pp. 450–456, 2008.

[12] R. Bavarsad Shahripour, G. Shamsaei, H. Pakdaman et al., "The effect of NeuroAiD (MLC601) on cerebral blood flow velocity in subjects' post brain infarct in the middle cerebral artery territory," *European Journal of Internal Medicine*, vol. 22, pp. 509–513, 2011.

[13] K. H. Kong, S. K. Wee, C. Y. Ng et al., "A double-blind, placebo-controlled, randomized phase II pilot study to investigate the potential efficacy of the traditional Chinese medicine neuroaid (MLC 601) in enhancing recovery after stroke (TIERS)," *Cerebrovascular Diseases*, vol. 28, no. 5, pp. 514–521, 2009.

[14] K. Ghandehari, Z. I. Mood, S. Ebrahimzadeh, D. Picard, and Y. Zhang, "NeuroAid (MLC601) versus piracetam in the recovery of post-infarct homonymous hemianopsia," *Neural Regeneration Research*, vol. 6, no. 6, pp. 418–422, 2011.

[15] C. H. C. Siow, "Neuroaid in stroke recovery," *European Neurology*, vol. 60, no. 5, pp. 264–266, 2008.

[16] N. Venketasubramanian, C. L. H. Chen, R. N. Gan et al., "A double-blind, placebo-controlled, randomized, multicentre study to investigate Chinese Medicine Neuroaid Efficacy on Stroke recovery (CHIMES Study)," *International Journal of Stroke*, vol. 4, no. 1, pp. 54–60, 2009.

[17] G. B. W. Lee, T. C. Charn, Z. H. Chew, and T. P. Ng, "Complementary and alternative medicine use in patients with chronic diseases in primary care is associated with perceived quality of care and cultural beliefs," *Family Practice*, vol. 21, no. 6, pp. 654–660, 2004.

[18] S. S. Hasan, S. I. Ahmed, N. I. Bukhari, and W. C. W. Loon, "Use of complementary and alternative medicine among patients with chronic diseases at outpatient clinics,"

Complementary Therapies in Clinical Practice, vol. 15, no. 3, pp. 152–157, 2009.

[19] Z. Junhua, F. Menniti-Ippolito, G. Xiumei et al., "Complex traditional chinese medicine for poststroke motor dysfunction: a systematic review," *Stroke*, vol. 40, no. 8, pp. 2797–2804, 2009.

[20] B. Wu, M. Liu, H. Liu et al., "Meta-analysis of traditional Chinese patent medicine for ischemic stroke," *Stroke*, vol. 38, no. 6, pp. 1973–1979, 2007.

[21] R. Bonita and R. Beaglehole, "Recovery of motor function after stroke," *Stroke*, vol. 19, no. 12, pp. 1497–1500, 1988.

[22] C. Heurteaux, C. Gandin, M. Borsotto et al., "Neuroprotective and neuroproliferative activities of NeuroAid (MLC601, MLC901), a Chinese medicine, in vitro and in vivo," *Neuropharmacology*, vol. 58, no. 7, pp. 987–1001, 2010.

[23] H. Quintard, M. Borsotto, J. Veyssiere et al., "MLC901, a Traditional Chinese Medicine protects the brain against global ischemia," *Neuropharmacology*, vol. 61, no. 4, pp. 622–631, 2011.

28

How Important Are Social Support, Expectations and Coping Patterns during Cardiac Rehabilitation

Maria J. C. Blikman,[1] **Hege R. Jacobsen,**[1] **Geir Egil Eide,**[2,3] **and Eivind Meland**[1]

[1] Department of Global Public Health and Primary Care, Research Group of General Practice, University of Bergen, Kalfarveien 31, 5018 Bergen, Norway
[2] Centre for Clinical Research, Haukeland University Hospital, Armauer Hansen's House, Bergen, Norway
[3] Department of Global Public Health and Primary Care, Research Group of Lifestyle Epidemiology, University of Bergen, Bergen, Norway

Correspondence should be addressed to Maria J. C. Blikman; mjcblikman@hotmail.com

Academic Editor: Francesco Giallauria

Purpose. To investigate the predictive role of relevant social and psychosocial determinants on emotional distress among patients after cardiac rehabilitation. *Methods.* A longitudinal prospective study examined short-term (6 months) and long-term (2 years) impact of predictors on anxiety and depression complaints in 183 patients with 6-months follow-up data attending a four-week rehabilitation stay at the Krokeide Centre in Bergen, Norway. The patients mainly suffered from coronary heart disease. Emotional distress, coping, social support, socioeconomic status, and negative expectations were measured by means of internationally validated questionnaires. A composite score of anxiety and depression complaints was used as the outcome measure in the study. *Results.* This study revealed that task-oriented coping improved emotional status in long-term followup, and negative expectations were associated with emotional distress in short-term followup. A higher socioeconomic status and more social support predicted improved emotional status in short- as well as long-term followup. *Conclusions.* Fewer negative expectations and functional coping along with social support are important factors for the prevention of emotional distress after cardiac disease. Such elements should be addressed and encouraged in patients during cardiac rehabilitation.

1. Introduction

Coronary heart disease (CHD) is a common disease in the western world, including Norway [1]. CHD can be regarded as a traumatic event with concomitant emotional distress for the patients afflicted [2], and patients commonly develop psychological problems after experiencing CHD, including depression [3, 4]. A large amount of evidence shows a clear association between psychological health (including anxiety and depression) and the pathogenesis of cardiovascular disease in the sense that poor psychological health is a risk factor for developing CHD including recurrent CHD [5–9]. A broader understanding of factors influencing a healthy adaptation and coping is needed, not only to improve the quality of life, but also to limit future risk for CHD. The clinicians engaged in cardiac rehabilitation play a pivotal role in promoting a healthy adaptation.

Coping is assessable by means of self-report inventories and measures [10]. Lazarus and Folkman [11] originally distinguished two major functions of coping: problem-focused and emotion-focused. Later work suggested that three broad coping strategies are important: task, emotion, and avoidance strategies, which formed the basis for the more well-known General Coping Questionnaire [12]. Studies that pertain to this dimension during cardiac rehabilitation (CR) are sparse. Although the research literature is mostly focused on domain specific self-efficacy beliefs, general efficacy beliefs and expectations seem relevant, also among cardiac patients [13].

We wanted to identify other social and psychosocial factors influencing healthy adaptation and thereby psychological health after a coronary event. Low socioeconomic status (SES) is related to poor health including a higher risk of CHD [14]. This association can be explained by more environmental challenges and fewer psychosocial resources, which leads to the expectation of negative outcomes, loss of coping ability, strain, hopelessness, and chronic stress [14, 15]. In addition, a higher amount of experienced social support leads to less anxiety and depression in a group of patients who underwent coronary bypass grafting [16]. Furthermore, negative expectations are associated with depression in a group of heart failure patients [17]. We therefore hypothesized that expectancy beliefs, experienced social support, SES, and coping patterns were important factors influencing psychological health for patients after cardiac disease.

The objective of the present study was, accordingly, to examine the impact of social and psychosocial factors on emotional status at short- and long-term followup.

2. Patients and Methods

Two hundred and sixty-six patients attending a four-week CR programme at Krokeide Rehabilitation Centre (outside Bergen, Norway) were invited to participate in a clinical controlled trial during the years 2000 to 2002. Followup data were recorded until 2004. Recruitment, enrolment, and dropouts are described in a former study [18]. Sixty-one per cent had suffered a myocardial infarction (MI). Most of the others suffered from angina pectoris. We obtained followup data for 183 and 176 patients who were eligible for six months and two-year followup analyses, respectively. The baseline data of our patient group are presented in Table 1. In this observational study we combined the cohorts of the randomized controlled trial (RCT) and did not compare the two groups. The intervention in the RCT aimed primarily at lifestyle improvements and did not lead to significant group differences concerning emotional status (t-test P: 0.4 at both short- and long-term followup). Dropout rates were highest among young participants and people with high level of emotional distress [18].

An Anxiety-Depression-Irritability questionnaire measured emotional status/distress. The questionnaire is a 12-item semantic differential scale, exploring the present emotional status with pairs of words like "frightened"—"courageous" (anxiety) and "unhappy"—"happy" (depression), rated with a seven-point Likert scale. In studies of Norwegian CHD patients the questionnaire has shown good reliability and validity [4]. The anxiety and depression dimensions were strongly correlated (Pearson correlation: 0.77) and were therefore combined as a measure of emotional status. Due to low reliability the irritability dimension was left out, leaving an eight-item combined Cronbach's alpha of 0.88 for the anxiety and depressive complaints (Table 1). The combined score was used as the emotional status dependent variable. Increasing values indicated increasing emotional distress.

The questionnaires used for the independent variables in our study were composed of various internationally used and validated measures. Coping styles, health expectations, amount of received social support, and a variety of demographic factors were measured at inclusion. We evaluated the corresponding reliabilities by means of Cronbach's alphas

(Table 1). The different coping styles were evaluated by means of the General Coping Questionnaire (GCQ-30), measuring task-focused, emotion-focused, and avoidance-focused coping strategies, which was developed on a conceptual basis by Joseph et al. [12]. This questionnaire rates each item on a four-point Likert scale from "never" to "very often."

Self-reported household income was chosen as the SES predictor. Five different income categories were presented for the participants. Negative expectations were measured by means of a General Expectancy (GE) Questionnaire, adapted from the seven-item Positive Expectation Subscale [13]. The descriptive data, the reliability, and the construct validity of the current GE measure have previously been presented and established [18]. The amount of experienced social support was measured by five questions pertaining to the experience of being understood, closeness in relations with family members, closeness with friends, emotional acceptance in relations, and support from others. The items pertain to the functional aspects of social support and are adapted from a questionnaire used in research among breast cancer and heart transplant patients [19]. Each question was rated on a seven-point Likert scale and the overall mean was computed for each participant. The reliability of the measure is satisfactory (Table 1).

2.1. Statistical Analyses. We used Cronbach's alpha to measure the internal consistency and thereby the reliability of our survey instruments (Table 1). In our study the GCQ-30 showed suboptimal Cronbach's alphas for the task (0.69), emotion (0.60), and avoidance (0.62) questions. These are the values obtained after optimization by means of leaving out one and two questions that showed low internal consistency, for these two constructs. The suboptimal reliability of the Norwegian translation of the GCQ-30 questionnaire has also been demonstrated in a former study [20].

We explored to what extent coping patterns, SES, and other social and psychosocial factors influenced psychological health at short- (six months) and long-term (24 months) followup. For this, multiple linear regression analysis was used. Firstly, regression of emotional status on each predictor at six and 24 months, respectively, was done adjusting for gender and age by including these in the models. Secondly, all the predictors, including gender and age, were included in the multiple regression model, and a backward stepwise selection of predictors was performed excluding the least significant predictor with $P > 0.05$ at each step until a final model with only significant predictors was obtained. Gender and age were forced into all models. We performed the full model analyses in order to control the interrelations between the independent variables. The results were reported with estimated regression coefficients (B), 95% confidence intervals (CI), and P values. Preconditions for linear regression analyses were satisfactory. Analyses of residuals from the regression analyses showed no serious deviations from normality. The intercorrelations between the independent variables showed absolute values <0.51 (Pearson's correlation −0.50 between social support and negative expectations). Accordingly, multicollinearity can hardly invalidate

TABLE 1: Baseline data on 183 patients with valid six-month data participating in a four-week cardiac rehabilitation programme at Krokeide Rehabilitation Centre, Bergen, Norway, from 2000 to 2002.

Variables	Total	Missing	Cronbach's α
Males, % (n)	80.3 (146)	0 (0)	
Age in years, mean (SD)	55.1 (9.2)	0 (0)	
Married/cohabiting			
Yes, % (n)	83.8 (151)	1.6 (3)	
No, % (n)	16.2 (29)		
Household income, mean (SD)	3.5[a] (1.3)	14.2 (26)[b]	
Social support[c], mean (SD)	5.4 (0.9)	0 (0)	0.74
Emotional status[d], mean (SD)	3.0 (1.2)	0 (0)	0.88
Coping[e]			
Task, mean (SD)	2.5 (0.4)	0 (0)	0.69
Emotion, mean (SD)	2.2 (0.3)	0 (0)	0.60
Avoid, mean (SD)	2.0 (0.4)	0 (0)	0.62
Negative expectations[d], mean (SD)	2.2 (1.0)	0 (0)	0.73

n: subsample size; SD: standard deviation.
[a]$3.5 \approx 400,000$ NOK (70.000 USD) (scales 1–5: 3 = 301,000–400,000 NOK, 4 = 401,000–500,000 NOK).
[b]Household income data were obtained after conclusion of the study (at 24 months) and were completed for all participants with valid followup data.
[c]Total mean score social support (scales 1–7).
[d]Total mean score of anxiety and depression complaints (scales 1–7).
[e]Total mean score coping style (scales 1–4).

the results from the multivariable analyses. P values ≤ 0.05 were considered as statistically significant. SPSS (version 18.0) was used for all statistical analyses with the GLM procedure for linear regression.

2.2. Ethics. The Regional Committee for Medical Research Ethics, Health Region III, and the Norwegian Data Inspectorate approved the study.

3. Results

In total, 80% of the participants were men. The mean age was 55 years for both genders. The average household income was about 400.000 NOK (70.000 USD) yearly.

Table 2 reports the short-term (six months) prognostic influence of both psychological and social factors on emotional status. The first columns demonstrate the impact of each predictor variable adjusted for gender and age. Regarding the psychological predictors, a task-oriented coping style was related to a lower level of emotional distress ($B = -0.58$, $P = 0.010$). An avoidant coping style predicted a higher degree of emotional distress ($B = 0.57$, $P = 0.01$). An emotional-oriented coping style showed no significant association with emotional distress. Negative expectations were related to impaired emotional status: $B = 0.50$, $P < 0.001$. In the final, full model, negative expectations ($B = 0.25$, $P = 0.01$) maintained significant prognostic associations with emotional distress.

Table 2 also shows that among the social determinants a higher degree of experienced social support predicted an improved emotional status at short-term followup ($B = -0.59$, $P < 0.001$). A higher household income was related to improved emotional status ($B = -0.34$, $P < 0.001$). Marital

or cohabiting status predicted less emotional distress ($B = -0.82$, $P = 0.001$). In the final, full model, social support and household income remained significantly associated with emotional distress ($B = -0.53$, $P < 0.001$; $B = -0.21$, $P = 0.001$, resp.). Male gender was associated with impaired emotional status in short-term followup ($B = 0.41$, $P = 0.04$),

Table 3 demonstrates that a task-oriented coping style predicts less emotional distress at 24 months of followup ($B = -0.97$, $P < 0.001$). An avoidant coping style, although significantly related to short-term prognosis of emotional status, was only borderline significant at long-term followup ($B = 0.38$, $P < 0.10$). An emotional-oriented coping style showed no significant association with emotional distress either at short- or long-term followup. Negative expectations were also at long-term followup strongly associated with emotional distress ($B = 0.36$, $P < 0.001$) but in the full model analysis only proved borderline significant ($P = 0.07$). However, a task-oriented coping style remained significantly associated with improved emotional status at long-term followup ($B = -0.79$, $P < 0.001$) in the model with all independent variables entered.

Table 3 also reports that among the social factors, social support and household income are strongly related with improved emotional status at long-term followup ($B = -0.46$, $P < 0.001$ and $B = -0.35$, $P < 0.001$, resp.). Marital and cohabiting status predicted less emotional distress at 24 months of followup ($B = -0.59$, $P = 0.01$). We also observe from Table 3 that in the final, full model, social support and household income remain significantly associated with emotional distress at long-term followup ($B = -0.33$, $P = 0.001$; $B = -0.23$, $P < 0.001$). Emotional status improved with increasing age ($B = -0.029$, $P = 0.001$) at two years of followup.

TABLE 2: Multiple linear regression of coping styles and other predictive factors on emotional status (anxiety and depression complaints) measured at short-term followup (6 months) at Krokeide Rehabilitation Centre, Bergen, Norway, included from 2000 to 2002.

Variables	n	Adjusted models[a]			Final model (n = 182)[b]		
		B	95% CI	P value	B	95% CI	P value[c]
Age (in years)							0.26
Gender (male/female)					0.41	(0.01, 0.82)	0.04
Employed (yes/no)	161	0.10	(−0.36, 0.55)	0.68			0.84
Cohabiting (yes/no)	180	−0.82	(−1.28, −0.36)	0.001			0.31
Household income	157	−0.34	(−0.49, −0.20)	<0.001	−0.21	(−0.33, −0.08)	0.001
Coping style							
Task	183	−0.58	(−1.01, −0.14)	0.01			0.16
Emotion	183	0.01	(−0.41, 0.44)	0.96			0.75
Avoid	183	0.57	(0.14, 1.01)	0.01			0.91
Social support	183	−0.59	(−0.76, −0.43)	<0.001	−0.53	(−0.72, −0.33)	<0.001
Negative expectations	183	0.50	(0.33, 0.66)	<0.001	0.25	(0.1, 0.4)	0.01
Intercept					5.13	(3.7, 6.6)	<0.001
Explained variance[d] (R^2)							
Nonadjusted						0.36	
Adjusted						0.34	

n: subsample size; B: estimated regression coefficient; CI: confidence interval.
[a]Eight models adjusted for age and gender.
[b]Obtained by backward stepwise selection.
[c]The nonsignificant P values were retrieved from the excluded variables table of the backward stepwise selection analysis.
[d]R^2 for final model.

4. Discussion

This study revealed that task-oriented coping improved emotional status in long-term followup, and negative expectations predicted emotional distress in short-term followup when we controlled the other variables. Increasing SES and social support improved emotional status in short- and long-term followup. The study confirmed that a lower household income and lack of social support are independent prognostic factors also when we controlled differences in coping styles, expectations, and other factors. Only a slight attenuating effect was observed in the multiple regression analyses with all variables entered in the model.

4.1. Psychological Predictors. Previous research has indicated that avoidant coping strategies lead to more emotional distress and that a task-focused coping style is negatively related or unrelated to anxiety and depression [17, 21, 22]. However, these studies also found that an emotional coping style associates with more psychological problems. We were unable to confirm this. Although our measure of emotional coping showed unsatisfactory reliability with concomitant danger of type II error, we observed regression coefficients close to zero. Unlike the present study, Endler and coworkers found that an avoidant coping style was not related to more psychological distress [10]. These inconsistencies may be explained by different characteristics of the patient groups included in the respective studies, the use of diverse coping scales, the fact that most coping scales have psychometric limitations, and differences in followup time [10, 17].

In former studies from this project specific expectancy beliefs (self-efficacy) concerning future lifestyle changes predicted health behavior changes more reliably than general expectancy. The influence of general expectancy also in these studies decreased significantly with time [23, 24]. It seems from the current results that general expectancy beliefs are important, but first and foremost in short-term followup.

In spite of some inconsistencies in the research literature, our study confirms that task-focused coping improves emotional status, whereas avoidant coping hampers psychological adaptation at least in short-term followup. Likewise, negative expectations strongly hamper emotional adaptation in CR patients. This is inline with a previous study including a population of heart failure patients [17]. Furthermore, negative expectations have been associated with long-term mortality in CHD patients [25].

4.2. Social Predictors. The association between low SES and poor health, including CHD, is well established [14, 26–29]. Psychosocial factors are suggested as important mediators for these effects [15]. However, such factors do not account for all of the SES impact on cardiovascular health [27]. Our study confirms that psychosocial factors, although important for emotional adaptation, do not account for the impact of SES on emotional health. In the present study coping, expectations, and social support only had a slightly attenuating effect on the relations between SES and emotional adaptation during followup.

The amount and quality of experienced social support also contributed to emotional health, as shown by our finding

TABLE 3: Multiple linear regression of coping styles and other predictive factors on emotional status (anxiety and depression complaints) measured at long-term followup (24 months) at Krokeide Rehabilitation Centre, Bergen, Norway, included from 2002–2004.

Variables	n	Adjusted models[a]			Final model (n = 173)[b]		
		B	95% CI	P value	B	95% CI	P value[c]
Age (in years)					−0.03	(0.05, 0.01)	0.001
Gender (male/female)					0.32	(−0.06, 0.70)	0.10
Employed (yes/no)	173	−0.02	(−0.45, 0.41)	0.92			0.17
Cohabiting (yes/no)	170	−0.59	(−1.05, −0.13)	0.01			0.51
Household income	168	−0.35	(−0.48, −0.21)	<0.001	−0.23	(−0.36, −0.11)	<0.001
Coping style							
Task	174	−0.97	(−1.40, −0.54)	<0.001	−0.79	(−1.22, −0.36)	<0.001
Emotion	174	−0.16	(−0.61, 0.28)	0.47			0.23
Avoid	174	0.38	(−0.07, 0.83)	<0.10			0.18
Social support	174	−0.46	(−0.64, −0.29)	<0.001	−0.33	(−0.52, −0.15)	0.001
Negative expectations	174	0.36	(0.19, 0.53)	<0.001	0.17	(−0.01, 0.36)	0.07
Intercept					7.95	(6.02, 9.87)	<0.001
Explained variance[d] (R^2)							
Nonadjusted						0.36	
Adjusted						0.34	

n: subsample size; B: estimated regression coefficient; CI: confidence interval.
[a]Eight models adjusted for age and gender.
[b]Obtained by backward stepwise selection.
[c]The nonsignificant P values were retrieved from the excluded variables table of the backward stepwise selection analysis.
[d]R^2 for final model.

that social support predicts less emotional distress at both short- and long-term followup. This concurs with earlier studies among patients after coronary artery bypass grafting [16, 30]. However, a recent review article reported more conflicting results concerning the relationship between social support and emotional distress [31]. The absence of social or marital support is nevertheless a significant risk factor for poor prognoses in cardiac patients [32].

Some researchers claim that material and income differences are the main explanation for health inequality among people with different SES [33]. An increasing number of studies indicate, however, that psychosocial factors such as lack of control, anxiety, insecurity, depression, and lack of social affiliations are more relevant than the actual income difference [34]. General expectancy, social support, and adequate coping are important factors also in the present study, but SES seems to impact the emotional health significantly even when we adjust for these factors.

4.3. Clinical Relevance. Although the ENRICHD trial intervention did not improve the cardiovascular prognosis for depressed patients with CHD, cognitive behaviour therapy significantly improved emotional status [35] and quality of life [36] as compared with standard treatment. These effects are important rehabilitation measures that challenge clinicians also to attend to patients' cognitive interpretations in order to achieve beneficial psychosocial functioning. Emotional distress limits vitality and impairs the ability to return to work after cardiac disease [37]. Recent development

in cognitive treatment methodology emphasizes functional coping in order to help patients develop alternatives to avoidant behaviour and strengthen their commitment to important values and goals in life [38]. The findings of the present study may support that this is relevant also in CR.

4.4. Limitations and Strengths of This Study. The low reliability particularly of emotional and avoidant coping styles introduces measurement "noise" for these constructs, especially for emotional coping style. The study is based on self-reported data and is prone to self-report bias. The strength of our study is that it concerns an important and prevalent clinical problem where knowledge is sparse concerning coping and its prognostic impact on health during CR. Explained variances are high and demonstrate that we have included relevant measures.

5. Conclusion

Fewer negative expectations and functional coping along with social support are associated with improved emotional health after cardiac disease. Such elements should be addressed and encouraged in patients during cardiac rehabilitation.

Conflict of Interests

The authors declare that there is no conflict of interests regarding the publication of this paper.

Acknowledgments

This project was supported by The Association of Heart and Lung Disease, University of Bergen, and The Norwegian Medical Association (AFU-Grant 2010).

References

[1] "Death Certificate Register," Statistisk sentralbyrå, Oslo, Norway, 2007, http://www.ssb.no/emner/03/01/10/dodsarsak/arkiv/tab-2009-/4-/7-01.html.

[2] R. S. Lazarus, "Coping with the stress of illness," *WHO Regional Publications. European Series*, vol. 44, pp. 11–31, 1992.

[3] K. K. Larsen, M. Vestergaard, J. Sondergaard, and B. Christensen, "Screening for depression in patients with myocardial infarction by general practitioners," *European Journal of Preventive Cardiology*, vol. 20, no. 5, pp. 800–806, 2012.

[4] O. E. Havik and J. G. Maelands, "Patterns of emotional reactions after a myocardial infarction," *Journal of Psychosomatic Research*, vol. 34, no. 3, pp. 271–285, 1990.

[5] K. van der Kooy, H. van Hout, H. Marwijk, H. Marten, C. Stehouwer, and A. Beekman, "Depression and the risk for cardiovascular diseases: systematic review and meta analysis," *International Journal of Geriatric Psychiatry*, vol. 22, no. 7, pp. 613–626, 2007.

[6] M. Hamer, G. J. Molloy, and E. Stamatakis, "Psychological distress as a risk factor for cardiovascular events: pathophysiological and behavioral mechanisms," *Journal of the American College of Cardiology*, vol. 52, no. 25, pp. 2156–2162, 2008.

[7] A. L. Kirkengen, L. Getz, and I. Hetlevik, "A different cardiovascular epidemiology," *Tidsskrift for den Norske Laegeforening*, vol. 128, no. 19, pp. 2181–2184, 2008.

[8] M. Zuidersma, H. J. Conradi, J. P. van Melle, J. Ormel, and P. de Jonge, "Self-reported depressive symptoms, diagnosed clinical depression and cardiac morbidity and mortality after myocardial infarction," *International Journal of Cardiology*, 2013.

[9] A. Compare, E. Germani, R. Proietti, and D. Janeway, "Clinical psychology and cardiovascular disease: an up-to-date clinical practice review for assessment and treatment of anxiety and depression," *Clinical Practice and Epidemiology in Mental Health*, vol. 7, pp. 148–156, 2011.

[10] N. S. Endler, J. D. Parker, and J. N. Butcher, "A factor analytic study of coping styles and the MMPI-2 content scales," *Journal of Clinical Psychology*, vol. 59, no. 10, pp. 1049–1054, 2003.

[11] R. S. F. S. Lazarus, *Stress, Appraisal, and Coping*, Springer, New York, NY, USA, 1984.

[12] S. Joseph, R. Williams, and W. Yule, "Crisis support, attributional style, coping style, and post-traumatic symptoms," *Personality and Individual Differences*, vol. 13, no. 11, pp. 1249–1251, 1992.

[13] B. Leedham, B. E. Meyerowitz, J. Muirhead, and W. H. Frist, "Positive expectations predict health after heart transplantation," *Health Psychology*, vol. 14, no. 1, pp. 74–79, 1995.

[14] G. Rose and M. G. Marmot, "Social class and coronary heart disease," *The British Heart Journal*, vol. 45, no. 1, pp. 13–19, 1981.

[15] M. Kristenson, H. R. Eriksen, J. K. Sluiter, D. Starke, and H. Ursin, "Psychobiological mechanisms of socioeconomic differences in health," *Social Science and Medicine*, vol. 58, no. 8, pp. 1511–1522, 2004.

[16] M. Koivula, K. Hautamäki-Lamminen, and P. Åstedt-Kurki, "Predictors of fear and anxiety nine years after coronary artery bypass grafting," *Journal of Advanced Nursing*, vol. 66, no. 3, pp. 595–606, 2010.

[17] R. B. Trivedi, J. A. Blumenthal, C. O'Connor et al., "Coping styles in heart failure patients with depressive symptoms," *Journal of Psychosomatic Research*, vol. 67, no. 4, pp. 339–346, 2009.

[18] T. Mildestvedt and E. Meland, "Examining the "Matthew Effect" on the motivation and ability to make lifestyle changes in 217 heart rehabilitation patients," *Scandinavian Journal of Public Health*, vol. 35, no. 2, pp. 140–147, 2007.

[19] J. Muirhead, B. E. Meyerowitz, B. Leedham, T. E. Eastburn, W. H. Merrill, and W. H. Frist, "Quality of life and coping in patients awaiting heart transplantation," *Journal of Heart and Lung Transplantation*, vol. 11, no. 2 I, pp. 265–272, 1992.

[20] J. Eid, J. F. Thayer, and B. H. Johnsen, "Measuring post-traumatic stress: a psychometric evaluation of symptom- and coping questionnaires based on a Norwegian sample," *Scandinavian Journal of Psychology*, vol. 40, no. 2, pp. 101–108, 1999.

[21] N. S. Endler, "Coping Inventory for Stressful Situations (CISS): Manual," Multi-Health Systems, Toronto, Canada, 1990.

[22] J. Suls and B. Fletcher, "The relative efficacy of avoidant and nonavoidant coping strategies: a meta-analysis," *Health Psychology*, vol. 4, no. 3, pp. 249–288, 1985.

[23] T. Mildestvedt, E. Meland, and G. E. Eide, "No difference in lifestyle changes by adding individual counselling to group-based rehabilitation RCT among coronary heart disease patients," *Scandinavian Journal of Public Health*, vol. 35, no. 6, pp. 591–598, 2007.

[24] T. Mildestvedt, E. Meland, and E. G. Eide, "How important are individual counselling, expectancy beliefs and autonomy for the maintenance of exercise after cardiac rehabilitation?" *Scandinavian Journal of Public Health*, vol. 36, no. 8, pp. 832–840, 2008.

[25] J. C. Barefoot, B. H. Brummett, R. B. Williams et al., "Recovery expectations and long-term prognosis of patients with coronary heart disease," *Archives of Internal Medicine*, vol. 171, no. 10, pp. 929–935, 2011.

[26] A. Rosengren, S. Hawken, S. Ôunpuu et al., "Association of psychosocial risk factors with risk of acute myocardial infarction in 11 119 cases and 13 648 controls from 52 countries (the INTERHEART study): case-control study," *The Lancet*, vol. 364, no. 9438, pp. 953–962, 2004.

[27] G. A. Kaplan and J. E. Keil, "Socioeconomic factors and cardiovascular disease: a review of the literature," *Circulation*, vol. 88, no. 4 I, pp. 1973–1998, 1993.

[28] M. Kristenson, Z. Kucinskiene, B. Bergdahl, H. Calkauskas, V. Urmonas, and K. Orth-Gomer, "Increased psychosocial strain in Lithuanian versus Swedish men: the LiVicordia study," *Psychosomatic Medicine*, vol. 60, no. 3, pp. 277–282, 1998.

[29] A. Rozanski, J. A. Blumenthal, K. W. Davidson, P. G. Saab, and L. Kubzansky, "The epidemiology, pathophysiology, and management of psychosocial risk factors in cardiac practice: the emerging field of behavioral cardiology," *Journal of the American College of Cardiology*, vol. 45, no. 5, pp. 637–651, 2005.

[30] E. Okkonen and H. Vanhanen, "Family support, living alone, and subjective health of a patient in connection with a coronary artery bypass surgery," *Heart and Lung: Journal of Acute and Critical Care*, vol. 35, no. 4, pp. 234–244, 2006.

[31] C. Zarbo, A. Compare, E. Baldassari, A. Bonardi, and C. Romagnoni, "In sickness and in health: a literature review about

function of social support within anxiety and heart disease association," *Clinical Practice and Epidemiology in Mental Health*, vol. 9, pp. 255–262, 2013.

[32] A. Compare, C. Zarbo, G. M. Manzoni et al., "Social support, depression, and heart disease: a ten year literature review," *Frontiers in Psychology*, vol. 4, p. 384, 2013.

[33] J. W. Lynch, G. A. Kaplan, and J. T. Salonen, "Why do poor people behave poorly? Variation in adult health behaviours and psychosocial characteristics by stages of the socioeconomic lifecourse," *Social Science and Medicine*, vol. 44, no. 6, pp. 809–819, 1997.

[34] M. Marmot and R. G. Wilkinson, "Psychosocial and material pathways in the relation between income and health: a response to Lynch et al," *British Medical Journal*, vol. 322, no. 7296, pp. 1233–1236, 2001.

[35] Writing Committee for the ENRICHD Investigators, "Effects of treating depression and low perceived social support on clinical events after myocardial infarction: the enhancing recovery in coronary heart disease patients (ENRICHD) randomized trial," *Journal of the American Medical Association*, vol. 289, no. 23, pp. 3106–3116, 2003.

[36] C. F. Mendes de Leon, S. M. Czajkowski, K. E. Freedland et al., "The effect of a psychosocial intervention and quality of life after acute myocardial infarction: the Enhancing Recovery in Coronary Heart Disease (ENRICHD) clinical trial," *Journal of Cardiopulmonary Rehabilitation*, vol. 26, no. 1, pp. 9–13, 2006.

[37] E. Meland, S. Grønhaug, K. Øystese, and T. Mildestvedt, "Examining the Matthew effect on the motivation and ability to stay at work after heart disease," *Scandinavian Journal of Public Health*, vol. 39, no. 5, pp. 517–524, 2011.

[38] S. C. Hayes, J. B. Luoma, F. W. Bond, A. Masuda, and J. Lillis, "Acceptance and commitment therapy: model, processes and outcomes," *Behaviour Research and Therapy*, vol. 44, no. 1, pp. 1–25, 2006.

29

Association between Functional Severity and Amputation Type with Rehabilitation Outcomes in Patients with Lower Limb Amputation

Amol M. Karmarkar,[1] **James E. Graham,**[1] **Timothy A. Reistetter,**[2] **Amit Kumar,**[1]
Jacqueline M. Mix,[3] **Paulette Niewczyk,**[3] **Carl V. Granger,**[3] **and Kenneth J. Ottenbacher**[1]

[1] Division of Rehabilitation Sciences, University of Texas Medical Branch, 301 University Boulevard,
  Mail Route No. 1137, Galveston, TX 77555, USA
[2] Occupational Therapy Department, University of Texas Medical Branch, Galveston, TX, USA
[3] Uniform Data System for Medical Rehabilitation, A Division of UB Foundation Activities Inc. and Department of
  Rehabilitation Medicine, University at Buffalo, Buffalo, NY, USA

Correspondence should be addressed to Amol M. Karmarkar; amkarmar@utmb.edu

Academic Editor: Stephen Sprigle

The purpose of this study was to determine independent influences of functional level and lower limb amputation type on inpatient rehabilitation outcomes. We conducted a secondary data analysis for patients with lower limb amputation who received inpatient medical rehabilitation ($N = 26,501$). The study outcomes included length of stay, discharge functional status, and community discharge. Predictors included the 3-level case mix group variable and a 4-category amputation variable. Age of the sample was 64.5 years (13.4) and 64% were male. More than 75% of patients had a dysvascular-related amputation. Patients with bilateral transfemoral amputations and higher functional severity experienced longest lengths of stay (average 13.7 days) and lowest functional rating at discharge (average 79.4). Likelihood of community discharge was significantly lower for those in more functionally severe patients but did not differ between amputation categories. Functional levels and amputation type are associated with rehabilitation outcomes in inpatient rehabilitation settings. Patients with transfemoral amputations and those in case mix group 1003 (admission motor score less than 36.25) generally experience poorer outcomes than those in other case mix groups. These relationships may be associated with other demographic and/or health factors, which should be explored in future research.

1. Introduction

Comprehensive medical rehabilitation in inpatient rehabilitation facilities (IRFs) that involve several clinicians (e.g., physiatrists, rehabilitation nurses, physical therapist, occupational therapist, clinical psychologists, and social workers) is an effective component in the continuum of care for patients following amputation. Postacute inpatient rehabilitation is associated with reduced mortality, decreased chances of reamputation, improved functional independence, increased procurement of prosthetic devices, and increased probability for discharge to community settings [1–4]. The IRF setting is also reported to be a cost-effective option for caring for patients following dysvascular amputations relative to skilled nursing facilities [3]. However, there is limited evidence regarding the overall effectiveness and/or efficiency of inpatient rehabilitation for patients with amputation [2, 4]. Prior research suggests that inpatient rehabilitation is underutilized by patients receiving dysvascular-related amputations; less than 10% of patients are admitted to an IRF, with the majority being discharged home or to a skilled nursing facility [5].

Amputation is one of the 13 eligible medical conditions for IRFs to meet the current "60%-rule" criteria (which mandates that 60% of patients admitting to IRF to have one or more of the 13 eligible medical conditions) under the IRF prospective payment system developed by the Centers for Medicare and Medicaid Services [6]. The basis for reimbursement under the IRF prospective payment system is a patient's impairment-specific case mix group (CMG). CMGs were developed to account for resource utilization requirements of patients with similar functional deficits and rehabilitation needs [6] and are often used as a proxy for patient functional severity. Amputation-related CMGs are derived from admission motor functional independence measure (FIM) instrument ratings within the inpatient rehabilitation facility patient assessment instrument [6]. There are three CMGs for amputation (CMG 1001 (FIM admission motor score greater than 47.65), CMG 1002 (FIM admission motor score greater than 36.25 and less than 47.65), and CMG 1003 (FIM admission motor score less than 36.25)). Neither the number (unilateral versus bilateral) nor the level (transtibial versus transfemoral) of the amputation(s) is directly factored into the prospective payment equation (CMG calculations). There is a lack of published information regarding the potential benefits of including definitive amputation characteristics along with CMG in models designed to predict the rehabilitation experiences and outcomes of patients following amputation [5].

The purpose of this study was to determine the impact of the type of lower limb amputation and functional level (CMGs) at admission on rehabilitation outcomes in patients receiving inpatient medical rehabilitation in a nationally representative sample of IRF patients in the United States. The primary objective of this study was to test utility of clinical characteristics (amputation levels) that can be observed by clinicians and case mix groups that are defined by the payers, which classify patients based on the admission motor scores and prospectively allocate resources (utilization of services and length of stay) at inpatient rehabilitation facilities. These adjustments might be helpful in refining case mix and prospective payment system for patients with lower limb amputation seeking inpatient rehabilitative services.

2. Methods

2.1. Study Design. The study was a secondary analysis of medical records from 901 IRFs that subscribe to the Uniform Data System for Medical Rehabilitation (UDS$_{MR}$). The UDS$_{MR}$ database is the world's largest nongovernmental registry for IRF data and accounts for over 70% of the market share in the United States. For this study, we extracted data related to patient demographics, health characteristics, and rehabilitation. The study was approved by the institutional review board (IRB) at primary author's institution.

2.2. Study Sample. Patients aged 18 years and older who received inpatient medical rehabilitation for lower limb amputation from October 2005 to December 2007 were included in our study sample.

The total eligible sample using amputation rehabilitation impairment group codes (05.3, 05.4, 05.5, 05.6, and 05.7) was 102,049 cases. We included only those cases admitted for initial rehabilitation, admitted directly from acute hospitals,

those without rehabilitation program interruption, and those living in the community prior to their acute admissions.

We excluded cases with missing information on the type of lower limb amputation and those died during rehabilitation stay. The final sample contained 26,501 patients with lower limb amputations.

2.3. Independent Variables. Lower limb amputation category was assigned according to four impairment codes for lower limb amputation: unilateral transtibial (05.4), unilateral transfemoral (05.3), bilateral transtibial (05.7), and bilateral transfemoral (05.5). Transtibial amputation of one side and transfemoral amputation of the other side (05.6) were included in the bilateral transfemoral group. Such classification was made, as the clinical characteristics of cases with transfemoral and transtibial amputation were similar to that of bilateral transfemoral group compared to bilateral transtibial group.

Case mix groups (CMGs) are used to group patients with similar clinical characteristics in order to estimate resources that will be utilized in the IRF. The basis for calculating CMGs in lower limb amputation patients is from weighted motor FIM ratings calculated at admission. The weighted motor FIM rating methodology was created by CMS as a way of accounting for the impact of each FIM motor item on the cost of providing care in the IRF. Patients with lower limb amputation are categorized into three CMGs: CMG 1001 (FIM motor greater than 47.65), CMG 1002 (FIM motor greater than 36.25 and less than 47.65), and CMG 1003 (FIM motor less than 36.25).

2.4. Rehabilitation Outcome Variables. Length of stay is the total number of days spent in IRF. For patients who were transferred to an acute-care setting and returned to IRF within three days, the days spent in acute-care were not included in computing the length of stay variable. Functional status was assessed by the FIM instrument items within the inpatient rehabilitation facility patient assessment instrument. The functional items of the inpatient rehabilitation facility patient assessment instrument are administered within three days of admission to IRF and again within three days of discharge [7]. The FIM instrument includes a total of 18 items which span two domains (motor and cognitive) and six subdomains (self-care, sphincter control, transfers, mobility, communication, and social integration). Ratings for each item range from 1 (total assistance) to 7 (complete independence). Total FIM ratings are derived by summing all 18 individual items to come up with a composite score which ranges from 18 to 126 [8]. The FIM instrument has been demonstrated to be a valid and reliable measure of functional status in a variety of IRF patient populations [9].

Discharge setting was dichotomized as community discharge (home, board and care, and transitional or assisted living) versus not community discharge (intermediate care, skilled nursing facility, acute unit own facility, acute unit another facility, chronic hospital, rehabilitation facility, alternate level of care, subacute setting, and others).

2.5. Covariates. Demographic factors included age, gender, race/ethnicity (non-Hispanic white, black, Hispanic, and others), and marital status (married versus unmarried). Health characteristics included etiology for amputation (dysvascular versus nondysvascular, trauma-related, cancer-related, or any other etiology), which was computed using International Classification of Disease, Clinical Modification codes (ICD9-CM) associated with amputation [1], diabetes status (yes versus no, also identified through ICD9-CM codes), and a summed score for the total number of other nondiabetes comorbidities (range: 0–10).

2.6. Data Analyses. Patient demographic characteristics, health characteristics, and outcomes were stratified by amputation type. Univariate analyses were used to test for differences between amputation categories, using one-way ANOVA for continuous variables and chi-square tests for categorical variables. This screening was done in order to select the variables that are associated with the proposed outcomes of the study. Covariates with a significant association with the outcomes were included in the regression models. Two multiple linear regression models were constructed to determine the impact of independent variables (CMG and amputation level) on predicting rehabilitation outcomes (LOS and discharge functional rating) while controlling for other demographic and health characteristics (covariates). Similarly, a logistic model was constructed to determine the association between CMG and amputation type on likelihood for community discharge. We also tested for interaction between CMGs and amputation levels in the model. The six interaction terms controlled for in all regression models were CMG 1002 by bilateral transtibial, CMG 1002 by unilateral transfemoral, CMG 1002 by unilateral transtibial, CMG 1001 by bilateral transtibial, CMG 1001 by unilateral transfemoral, and CMG 1002 by unilateral transtibial. All statistical analyses were computed using PASW v18.0 (SPSS IBM) software.

3. Results

A total of 26,501 records of patients with lower limb amputation were identified. The mean age of the sample was 64.5 years (sd = 13.4), and nearly two-thirds (64%) were male. Unilateral transtibial amputation was the single largest amputation category: approximately 60% of the total sample. Approximately 80% of both bilateral and unilateral transtibial amputations were dysvascular-related. Diabetes is more frequently reported in patients with bilateral (77%) and unilateral (73%) transtibial amputations. Table 1 shows patient characteristics and rehabilitation outcomes for the entire sample and is stratified by amputation category.

Without adjusting for other covariates, patients with bilateral transfemoral level of amputation under CMG 1003 had the highest LOS (13.7 days) as compared to patients with other levels of amputation and CMG. Those with unilateral transtibial level of amputation under CMG 1001 had the lowest LOS in IRF (7.2 days) (Figure 1). Discharge functional rating was lowest for those with bilateral transfemoral level of amputation under CMG 1003 (79.4) and highest for

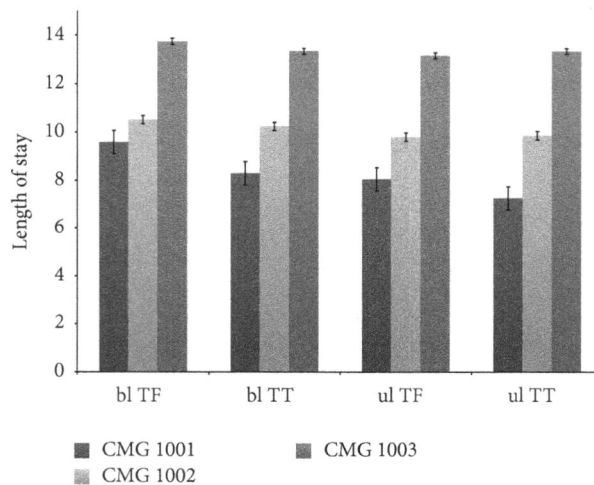

FIGURE 1: Length of stay by amputation levels for case mix group after adjustment of function. ul = unilateral, bl = bilateral, TF = transfemoral, and TT = transtibial.

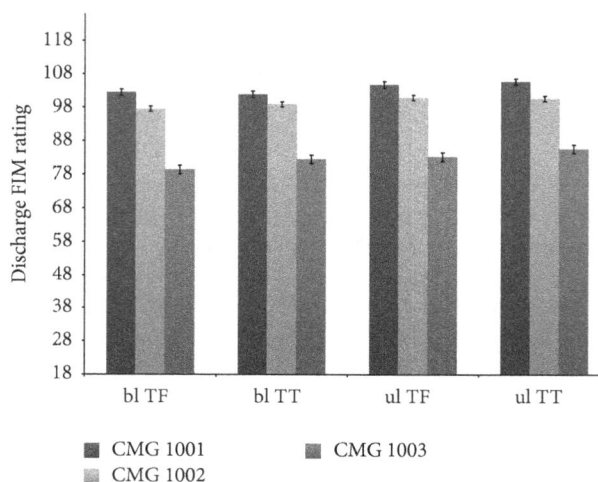

FIGURE 2: Discharge FIM rating by amputation levels for case mix group after adjustment of function. ul = unilateral, bl = bilateral, TF = transfemoral, and TT = transtibial.

those with unilateral transtibial level of amputation under CMG 1001 (105.6) (Figure 2). Proportion of discharge to community was lowest among patients categorized into CMG 1003 compared to those under either 1002 or 1001, irrespective of amputation levels. This proportion was also lower for those patients under CMG 1002 than CMG 1001 for all except bilateral transtibial amputation level (Figure 3).

Tables 2 and 3 show the results of the linear and logistic regression analysis. CMG was strongly associated with all three outcomes; significant differences were observed between each CMG level. As expected, patients in CMG 1003 demonstrated the longest lengths of stay and lowest functional ratings at discharge and were least likely to be discharged home, as compared to both CMG 1001 and CMG 1002. Amputation category was also associated with all three

TABLE 1: Demographic characteristics and rehabilitation outcomes by amputation levels.

	Total	ul TT	ul TF	bl TT	bl TF
N	26,501	15,798	7,495	1,610	1,598
Demographics					
Age*	64.5 ± 13.4	63.8 ± 13.2	66.3 ± 13.6	62.6 ± 13.5	64.2 ± 13.1
Men (%)*	64.0	65.7	59.9	68.5	62.5
Race/ethnicity*%					
Non-Hispanic white	63.5	63	66.7	57.5	58.3
Black	21.0	20.4	20.2	25.8	26
Hispanic	7.6	8.5	6.2	7.1	6.7
Other	7.9	8.1	6.9	9.6	8.9
Married (%)*	50.4	50.7	50.1	52.9	47.6
Etiology-dysvascular (%)*	76.5	79.8	68.7	80.4	76.8
Diabetes (%)*	66.0	72.8	50.3	76.6	62.1
Comorbidities (sum)*	2.2 ± 1.4	2.3 ± 1.4	1.9 ± 1.3	2.7 ± 1.5	2.3 ± 1.5
Case mix group*(%)					
CMG1001	8.3	8.5	8.4	8.1	6.7
CMG1002	29.3	31.6	27.1	24.8	21.7
CMG1003	62.3	59.9	64.5	67.1	71.6
Admission functional rating					
FIM motor admission*	38.8 ± 11.4	39.6 ± 11.1	37.9 ± 11.8	37.6 ± 11.6	35.5 ± 11.8
FIM cog admission*	27.3 ± 6.4	27.5 ± 6.2	26.9 ± 6.6	26.9 ± 6.3	26.7 ± 6.7
FIM total admission*	67.9 ± 16.4	69 ± 15.9	66.7 ± 17	66.2 ± 16.5	63.8 ± 17
Rehabilitation outcomes					
FIM motor discharge*	55 ± 14.1	56.1 ± 13.5	54.2 ± 14.7	53.2 ± 14.1	50.4 ± 15.2
FIM cog discharge*	29.5 ± 5.7	29.9 ± 5.5	29.2 ± 6	29.3 ± 5.8	28.6 ± 6.4
FIM total discharge*	88 ± 19.4	89.5 ± 18.6	86.8 ± 20.2	85.7 ± 19.4	82 ± 21.2
Length of stay (days)*	13.3 ± 6.5	13.2 ± 6.4	13.2 ± 6.5	13.6 ± 6.9	14.2 ± 6.8
Discharged home (%)	72.4	72.6	72.4	71.8	70.7

ul = unilateral, bl = bilateral, TF = transfemoral, and TT = transtibial.
*A significant relationship between amputation category and denoted variable at $P < .05$.
Case mix groups (CMGs) are calculated from weighted admission FIM motor ratings: CMG 1001 (FIM motor greater than 47.65), CMG 1002 (FIM motor greater than 36.25 and less than 47.65), and CMG 1003 (FIM motor less than 36.25).

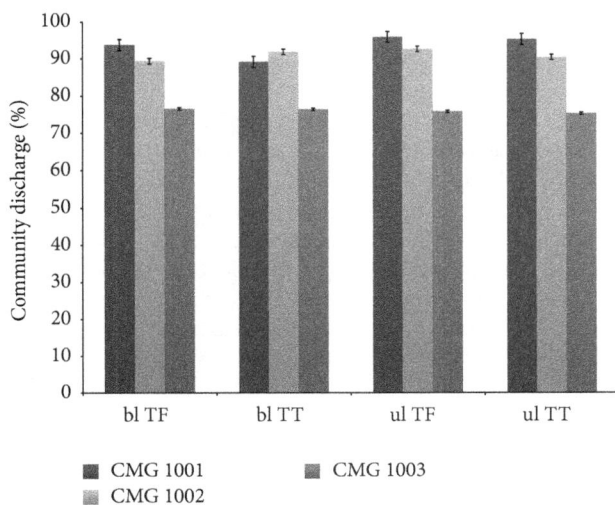

FIGURE 3: Community discharge by amputation levels for CMG after adjustment of function. ul = unilateral, bl = bilateral, TF = transfemoral, and TT = transtibial.

outcomes. Patients with bilateral transfemoral amputations demonstrated the longest lengths of stay and lowest functional ratings at discharge. However, there was no significant association between amputation level and discharge to home in our sample. For LOS we found interaction between CMG 1001 and unilateral transtibial amputation category ($P < .05$). For discharge functional rating an interaction was significant for CMG 1002 and unilateral transtibial level of amputation ($P < .05$). For discharge to home interaction was only significant between CMG 1002 and unilateral transfemoral amputation level ($P < .05$) (Figure 3).

4. Discussion

Our study investigated the impact of case mix group and lower limb amputation type on inpatient rehabilitation outcomes. We analyzed data from 901 inpatient rehabilitation facilities in USA for the years 2005–2007. More than 75% of the patients had amputation due to dysvascular and/or peripheral vascular disorder conditions. The prevalence of

TABLE 2: Coefficient estimates from multiple linear regression models: predictors for length of stay and discharge FIM rating, source UDSMR database.

Variables	Length of stay		Discharge FIM rating	
	Coefficient estimate	Confidence interval (95%)	Coefficient estimate	Confidence interval (95%)
Age, yrs	0.03*	0.02 to 0.032	−0.29*	−0.31 to −0.27
Male	0.27*	0.12 to 0.432	−1.27*	−1.69 to −0.85
White	−0.24*	−0.40 to −0.088	2.32*	1.90 to 2.73
Married	−0.78*	−0.93 to −0.63	−0.22	−0.62 to 0.18
Dysvascular	0.11	−0.06 to 0.29	−1.14*	−1.61 to −0.66
Diabetes	0.35*	0.18 to 0.52	−0.014	−0.45 to 0.43
Comorbid, sum	0.26*	0.22 to 0.29	−0.53*	−0.62 to −0.45
CMG 1003 (Ref)				
CMG 1002	−3.22*	−3.96 to −2.5	18.17*	16.23 to 20.11
CMG 1001	−4.16*	−5.37 to −2.9	23.02*	19.79 to 26.25
bl TF (Ref)				
bl TT	−0.41	−0.91 to 0.10	3.08*	1.74 to 4.42
ul TF	−0.59*	−0.98 to −0.19	3.76*	2.72 to 4.81
ul TT	−0.42*	−0.79 to −0.04	6.17*	5.18 to 7.16
CMG 1002 × bl TT	0.13	−0.88 to 1.1	−1.76	−4.44 to .92
CMG 1002 × ul TF	−0.14	−0.93 to 0.66	−0.45	−2.56 to 1.66
CMG 1002 × ul TT	−0.25	−1.01 to 0.51	−3.15*	−5.16 to −1.13
CMG 1001 × bl TT	−0.89	−2.53 to 0.76	−3.65	−8.01 to 0.70
CMG 1001 × ul TF	−0.95	−2.27 to 0.36	−1.46	−4.94 to 2.03
CMG 1001 × ul TT	−1.92*	−3.18 to −0.65	−2.97	−6.32 to 0.38

ul = unilateral, bl = bilateral, TF = transfemoral, and TT = transtibial.
*Significance at $P < .05$.
× = interaction term.

diabetes alone was 66%. Presence of diabetes associated with foot ulcers or other dysvascular conditions is a common reason for lower limb amputation in patients over the age of 40 [3, 5, 10, 11]. Lifetime risk of lower limb amputation among patients with diabetes is approximately 15% [12]. As the incidence rate of dysvascular conditions continues to increase, so will the number of lower limb amputations. Older adults are significantly more likely to experience dysvascular-related amputations compared to younger patients, who experience relatively more trauma-related amputations [13]. Higher mortality, increased numbers of reamputation, and greater cost are associated with dysvascular-related amputations compared with other causes (e.g., trauma or cancer) [2, 3].

In our study, patients who were assigned to lower level CMGs at admission showed better outcomes related to LOS and discharge functional rating, as compared to those assigned to higher level CMGs. These findings are of no surprise, as CMGs are used to estimate use of resources by patients, and higher CMG categories are expected to have higher utilization compared to patients assigned lower CMGs. In addition, we also found that patients with bilateral transfemoral amputations were more likely to stay longer in IRFs compared to those with unilateral amputations. Others have shown higher utilization in terms of longer lengths of stay and increased costs associated with higher levels of amputation (e.g., transfemoral), compared to lower

levels of amputation (e.g., transtibial or foot) [2, 3]. Our results of a positive association between age and LOS also support previous findings demonstrating the increased risk of amputation with age resulting in higher resources use. We also found a significant association between presence of diabetes and longer LOS in our sample.

Regarding discharge functional rating, patients with higher level bilateral amputations had significantly lower FIM discharge ratings compared to those with lower level and/or unilateral amputations. A study by Pezzin and colleagues reported lower physical rating (on SF-36) associated with higher amputation levels for their sample from a trauma center [14]. Findings from the current study are important as FIM items are a core component of functional assessment in IRF, and discharge FIM ratings are associated with long-term recovery in various impairment categories [15]. In our study, age was negatively associated with discharge FIM rating, which supports previous conclusions regarding poor outcomes associated with higher age in patients with lower limb amputation [14]. Additionally, we found that diabetes was negatively associated with discharge FIM rating.

Higher CMG assignment (1003) was also associated with lower probabilities of discharge to the community compared to patients assigned to lower CMGs (1001 and 1002). However, we did not find an association between amputation level and community discharge in our sample. Patients with unilateral transtibial, unilateral transfemoral, and bilateral transtibial

TABLE 3: Odds ratios from multiple logistic regression model.

Variables	Community discharge	
	Odds ratio	Confidence interval (95%)
Age, yrs	0.98	0.98 to 0.99
Male	1.13	1.06 to 1.20
White	0.97	0.91 to 1.03
Married	1.51*	1.42 to 1.60
Dysvascular	0.94	0.88 to 1.01
Diabetes	1.06	0.99 to 1.13
Comorbid, sum	0.95	0.93 to 0.96
CMG 1003 (Ref)		
CMG 1002	2.56*	1.86 to 3.52
CMG 1001	4.54*	2.26 to 9.12
bl TF (Ref)		
bl TT	0.99	0.82 to 1.18
ul TF	0.96	0.83 to 1.10
ul TT	0.93	0.82 to 1.06
CMG 1002 × bl TT	1.36	0.86 to 1.68
CMG 1002 × ul TF	1.56*	1.10 to 1.33
CMG 1002 × ul TT	1.20	0.86 to 1.67
CMG 1001 × bl TT	0.56	0.23 to 1.33
CMG 1001 × ul TF	1.60	0.73 to 3.47
CMG 1001 × ul TT	1.43	0.69 to 2.97

ul = unilateral, bl = bilateral, TF = transfemoral, and TT = transtibial.
*Significance at $P < .05$.
× = interaction term.

had higher likelihood of being discharged to community settings compared to those with bilateral transfemoral amputations. Age did not have a significant impact on discharge destination in our sample. Among other covariates, being married versus unmarried was strongly associated with community discharge. This finding is consistent with previous reports showing a strong relationship between the availability of caregiving support and likelihood of home (community) discharge for patients with stroke [16].

There are limitations to consider in the current study. First, we did not include health insurance status in the regression models. Availability and type of health insurance could have a direct impact on rehabilitation processes (access and utilization of services) and certain outcomes such as length of rehabilitation stay and discharge setting (community versus other settings). Secondly, the data were limited to the years following substantial changes in the way CMGs for amputation being determined. In October 2005, the Centers for Medicare and Medicaid Services introduced the weighted motor index and reduced the number of amputation-related CMGs from five to three. Future research is needed to examine the impact which changes in CMG classification for amputation had on rehabilitation outcomes. This study did not use a standardized comorbidity index; instead we summed all comorbidities and presented them as numbers. This was done in order to separate all diabetes comorbidities

from others. Also, CMGs were developed by the Centers for Medicare and Medicaid Services as a way to allocate resources prospectively for rehabilitation impairment categories. Therefore we could only assume that the prospective resources allocation would also be pertinent to patients in our sample under the age of 65 and those who were non-Medicare enrollees. It is also important to note that we did not look at date of functional assessment, which could have been later than admission dates and earlier than discharge date. A key strength of this study is that it includes a large cohort of patients with lower limb amputation undergoing inpatient medical rehabilitation. Other strengths include use of case mix groups, which is an understudied area of research in medical rehabilitation.

5. Conclusion

Both CMG and amputation categories were significant predictors of rehabilitation outcomes: rehabilitation length of stay and discharge functional rating. CMG and amputation levels were associated with discharge to home, along with being married. Clinicians (e.g., physiatrist, rehabilitation nurses, physical therapist, and occupational therapist) are involved in provision of rehabilitation services for individuals with lower limb amputation at inpatient rehabilitation settings. This investigation indicates that use of amputation categories is important in projecting outcomes associated with provision of rehabilitation services for patients with lower limb amputation. Including something as easily observable as amputation category along with the standard CMG level may help clinicians, researchers, and policymakers better understand and predict the unique rehabilitation needs and experiences of different patients with lower limb amputations.

Acknowledgments

This work was funded in part by the National Institutes of Health, National Center for Medical Rehabilitation Research in the National Institute of Child Health and Human Development and the National Institute of Neurological Disorders and Stroke (Grant nos. K12-HD055929, R24-HD065702, and K01-HD068513), and National Institutes of Health Clinical and Translational Science Award (UL1TR000071). No commercial party having a direct financial interest in the results of the research supporting this paper has or will confer a benefit on the authors or on any organization with which the authors are associated. Dr. Granger is employed by the State University of New York at Buffalo, which is affiliated with the Uniform Data System for Medical Rehabilitation. The Uniform Data System for Medical Rehabilitation owns the copyright and trademark for the FIM instrument.

Conflict of Interests

The authors declare that there is no conflict of interests regarding the publication of this paper.

References

[1] T. R. Dillingham and L. E. Pezzin, "Rehabilitation setting and associated mortality and medical stability among persons with amputations," *Archives of Physical Medicine and Rehabilitation*, vol. 89, no. 6, pp. 1038–1045, 2008.

[2] T. R. Dillingham, L. E. Pezzin, and E. J. MacKenzie, "Incidence, acute care length of stay, and discharge to rehabilitation of traumatic amputee patients: an epidemiologic study," *Archives of Physical Medicine and Rehabilitation*, vol. 79, no. 3, pp. 279–287, 1998.

[3] T. R. Dillingham, L. E. Pezzin, and A. D. Shore, "Reamputation, mortality, and health care costs among persons with dysvascular lower-limb amputations," *Archives of Physical Medicine and Rehabilitation*, vol. 86, no. 3, pp. 480–486, 2005.

[4] M. G. Stineman, P. L. Kwong, J. E. Kurichi et al., "The effectiveness of inpatient rehabilitation in the acute postoperative phase of care after transtibial or transfemoral amputation: study of an integrated health care delivery system," *Archives of Physical Medicine and Rehabilitation*, vol. 89, no. 10, pp. 1863–1872, 2008.

[5] T. R. Dillingham, L. E. Pezzin, and E. J. MacKenzie, "Discharge destination after dysvascular lower-limb amputations," *Archives of Physical Medicine and Rehabilitation*, vol. 84, no. 11, pp. 1662–1668, 2003.

[6] Department of Health and Human Services Centers for Medicare & Medicaid Services, *Medicare Program; Inpatient Rehabilitation Facility Prospective Payment System for Federal Fiscal Year 2010 Final Rule, in Federal Register*, Department of Health and Human Services Centers for Medicare & Medicaid Services, Washington, DC, USA, 2010.

[7] UB Foundation Activities Inc, *Uniform Data Systems for Medical Rehabilitation (UDS$_{MR}$), IRF-PAI Training Manual*, UB Foundation Activities Inc, Buffalo, NY, USA, 2004.

[8] K. J. Ottenbacher, Y. Hsu, C. V. Granger, and R. C. Fiedler, "The reliability of the functional independence measure: a quantitative review," *Archives of Physical Medicine and Rehabilitation*, vol. 77, no. 12, pp. 1226–1232, 1996.

[9] M. G. Stineman, J. A. Shea, A. Jette et al., "The functional independence measure: tests of scaling assumptions, structure, and reliability across 20 diverse impairment categories," *Archives of Physical Medicine and Rehabilitation*, vol. 77, no. 11, pp. 1101–1108, 1996.

[10] T. R. Dillingham, L. E. Pezzin, and E. J. MacKenzie, "Limb amputation and limb deficiency: epidemiology and recent trends in the United States," *Southern Medical Journal*, vol. 95, no. 8, pp. 875–883, 2002.

[11] N. Singh, D. G. Armstrong, and B. A. Lipsky, "Preventing foot ulcers in patients with diabetes," *Journal of the American Medical Association*, vol. 293, no. 2, pp. 217–228, 2005.

[12] Department of Health Human Services: Agency for Healthcare Research Quality, *Guide to Prevention Quality Indicators: Hospital Admission for Ambulatory Care Sensitive Conditions*, 2007.

[13] T. R. Dillingham, L. E. Pezzin, and E. J. MacKenzie, "Racial differences in the incidence of limb loss secondary to peripheral vascular disease: a population-based study," *Archives of Physical Medicine and Rehabilitation*, vol. 83, no. 9, pp. 1252–1257, 2002.

[14] L. E. Pezzin, T. R. Dillingham, and E. J. MacKenzie, "Rehabilitation and the long-term outcomes of persons with trauma-related amputations," *Archives of Physical Medicine and Rehabilitation*, vol. 81, no. 3, pp. 292–300, 2000.

[15] T. A. Dodds, D. P. Martin, W. C. Stolov, and R. A. Deyo, "A validation of the Functional Independence Measurement and its performance among rehabilitation inpatients," *Archives of Physical Medicine and Rehabilitation*, vol. 74, no. 5, pp. 531–536, 1993.

[16] T.-A. Nguyen, A. Page, A. Aggarwal, and P. Henke, "Social determinants of discharge destination for patients after stroke with low admission FIM instrument scores," *Archives of Physical Medicine and Rehabilitation*, vol. 88, no. 6, pp. 740–744, 2007.

30

A Pilot Project of Early Integrated Traumatic Brain Injury Rehabilitation in Singapore

Siew Kwaon Lui,[1] **Yee Sien Ng,**[1,2] **Annie Jane Nalanga,**[1]
Yeow Leng Tan,[1] **and Chek Wai Bok**[1,2]

[1] *Department of Rehabilitation Medicine, Singapore General Hospital, 20 College Road, Academia Level 4, Singapore 169856*
[2] *Duke-National University of Singapore (NUS) Graduate Medical School, 8 College Road, Singapore 169857*

Correspondence should be addressed to Siew Kwaon Lui; lui.siew.kwaon@sgh.com.sg

Academic Editor: Sarah Blanton

Objective. Document acute neurosurgical and rehabilitation parameters of patients of all traumatic brain injury (TBI) severities and determine whether early screening along with very early integrated TBI rehabilitation changes functional outcomes. *Methods.* Prospective study involving all patients with TBI admitted to a neurosurgical department of a tertiary hospital. They were assessed within 72 hours of admission by the rehabilitation team and received twice weekly rehabilitation reviews. Patients with further rehabilitation needs were then transferred to the attached acute inpatient TBI rehabilitation unit (TREATS) and their functional outcomes were compared against a historical group of patients. Demographic variables, acute neurosurgical characteristics, medical complications, and rehabilitation outcomes were recorded. *Results.* There were 298 patients screened with an average age of 61.8 ± 19.1 years. The most common etiology was falls (77.5%). Most patients were discharged home directly (67.4%) and 22.8% of patients were in TREATS. The TREATS group functionally improved ($P < 0.001$). Regression analysis showed by the intervention of TREATS, that there was a statistically significant FIM functional gain of 18.445 points (95% CI -30.388 to -0.6502, $P = 0.03$). *Conclusion.* Our study demonstrated important epidemiological data on an unselected cohort of patients with TBI in Singapore and functional improvement in patients who further received inpatient rehabilitation.

1. Introduction

Traumatic brain injury (TBI) is a significant medical, social, and public healthcare problem worldwide [1]. More than 1.7 million people sustain TBI annually in the United States [2].

Trauma was the fifth leading cause of death locally in 2011, and it was the leading cause of deaths in persons under 45 years which contributed more than a third of deaths in this group [3].

Traumatic brain injury results in high mortality and morbidity with large numbers of patients sustaining permanent disability [4].

The economic cost of TBI is tremendous with the annual economic burden of TBI in the United States approximated at US $76.5 billion [5, 6]. A local study of 91 TBI selected admissions to rehabilitation over a 2-year period indicates a total median rehabilitation charge per episode [7] of S $7845.50.

Although health-care costs associated with TBI are substantial, studies have shown that rehabilitation of TBI patients is cost-effective [8] with reduction of mortality by approximately 3607 lives annually [9].

Very early rehabilitation is characterized by rehabilitation in acute medical units commencing as soon as patients are medically stable. In a very early rehabilitation trial for stroke (AVERT), it seems to be safe to start ambulatory therapy in patients who satisfied physiologic safety criteria within 24 hours of stroke [10]. This optimizes early neuroplastic changes leading to better recovery [11–13]. Very early rehabilitation also has benefits of faster improvement in independence and better reported quality of life [14, 15].

Although there are benefits associated with very early rehabilitation, there is often a paucity of a coordinated effort to address the rehabilitation needs early in the acute medical units where the primary focus is to manage the acute medical problems.

There are datasets of TBI demographics in several national databases, but most of the patient cohorts are generally of moderate or severe TBI which do not represent the entire TBI spectrum [16–18]. There are also acute neurosurgical TBI databases, but these mainly contain acute surgical data and provide limited information on rehabilitation characteristics and functional outcomes [19].

Hence the objectives of the study are as follows:

(i) document both acute neurosurgical clinical characteristics and rehabilitation data of patients of all TBI severities admitted into the acute hospital;

(ii) determine whether early screening and provision of very early integrated TBI rehabilitation service changes functional outcomes in the group who received further inpatient rehabilitation.

2. Methods

2.1. Study Design, Setting, and Participants. This prospective study involved patients of all TBI severities presenting through Department of Neurosurgery (NES) of Singapore General Hospital (SGH) between November 1, 2010, and February 15, 2012.

The patients were screened within 72 hours of admission. Patients were included in our study if they had a diagnosis of TBI. The diagnosis of TBI was made through an appropriate clinical history and examination by the admitting team and supported with computed tomography or magnetic resonance imaging brain scans.

2.2. Very Early Integrated TBI Rehabilitation. All patients with TBI received regular twice weekly multidisciplinary reviews from the physiatrist-led rehabilitation team. This team included a nurse, physiotherapist, occupational therapist, speech therapist, dietician, and medical social worker. The aims of the review included verifying data accuracy and formulating rehabilitation plans. Our definition of very early integrated TBI rehabilitation consisted of TBI rehabilitation, while the patients were still in the acute NES unit and it served as a coordinated effort by the rehabilitation team to manage the rehabilitation issues early and facilitate functional recovery. Depending on individual needs and the medical condition of the patient, patients received approximately half an hour to two hours of therapy per day, 5 days of the week. In consultation with the multidisciplinary team, all patients received an individual specific discharge plan. Patients who were medically stable and required further inpatient rehabilitation were then further transferred to the acute inpatient rehabilitation unit of the Department of Rehabilitation Medicine, SGH, or to subacute rehabilitation facilities at the local community hospitals. The need for further inpatient rehabilitation was determined by the physiatrist-led team at the twice weekly reviews and examples of such needs included management of disorders of consciousness, motor, sensory, and cognitive deficits, language impairments, and neurobehavioral problems. The parameters collected were determined based on (1) the best available literature on known factors predicting recovery after TBI, (2) country,

social, and cultural specific data, and (3) multidisciplinary team consensus meetings.

2.3. Clinical Variables and Outcome Measures. The data of the acute admissions with TBI were categorized into the following categories:

(1) demographic variables including age, gender, and race;

(2) acute neurosurgical characteristics including etiology, severity measured via Glasgow Coma Scale (GCS) upon admission, neuroimaging findings, and neurosurgical interventions;

(3) comorbidities and complications including nosocomial infections and need for tracheostomy;

(4) acute inpatient stay data including the acute length of stay (ALOS) and the discharge disposition;

(5) rehabilitation outcomes including the Functional Independence Measure (FIM), Ranchos Los Amigos Score (RLA), and the Westmead Post-Traumatic Amnesia Score (PTA).

In order to evaluate whether early screening and provision of very early integrated TBI rehabilitation service changes functional outcomes, we compared functional outcomes of the TREATS group of patients against the historical group.

The definition of the TREATS group was patients with TBI who underwent early screening and received further inpatient rehabilitation at the SGH Department of Rehabilitation Medicine.

The definition of the historical group was patients with TBI who received inpatient rehabilitation in the same acute rehabilitation unit prior to the implementation of the early "reach-in" screening program and these patients were usually referred to by the primary department, that is, Department of NES. Data of the historical group of patients were obtained from the Rehabilitation Database of the Department of Rehabilitation Medicine, SGH.

The difference in outcomes between the TREATS and the historical groups was measured by comparison of the FIM gain, the acute length of stay (ALOS), and the rehabilitation length of stay (RLOS) of the 2 groups.

Patients aged 65 or more were defined as geriatric patients [20].

The etiologies of TBI were listed as falls, road traffic accidents, sports, assault, and others. For the patients who fell, the mechanisms of falls were further classified into mechanical falls (e.g., slipped and fell on wet surface), nonmechanical falls (e.g., fell as a result of muscle weakness), and unwitnessed falls. This distinction is important as patients will require further investigations for falls in the presence of medical stressors [21]. The GCS was documented on admission and used to classify the severity of TBI into mild (GCS 13–15), moderate (9–12), and severe (GCS 3–8) categories.

The main types of TBI were based on predominant neuroimaging findings. These were categorized into subdural hematoma, subarachnoid hemorrhage, contusion, intracerebral hemorrhage, and extradural hemorrhage. Patients were defined as having a concussion if there were no structural abnormalities on neuroimaging but with presence of "physical, cognitive, emotional, and/or sleep-related symptoms that may or may not involve a loss of consciousness" [22]. All neurosurgical interventions were recorded. Comorbidities and complications such as nosocomial infections, deep venous thrombosis, and seizures were documented.

The ALOS was recorded for all patients who were acutely screened and was defined as the time from admission to the hospital to discharge to home, an acute/subacute rehabilitation unit or a nursing home. The RLOS was defined as the time from admission to the SGH inpatient rehabilitation unit to discharge to home, subacute rehabilitation facility, or a nursing home.

The main functional outcome measure is the Functional Independence Measure (FIM) which is a widely used standardized functional outcome measure in medical rehabilitation [23]. It consists of 13 motor and 5 cognitive items, with established content and construct validity, sensitivity, and interrater reliability for the measurement of general functional ability across a wide range of rehabilitation conditions. Scores range from 1 (totally dependent) to 7 (totally independent) for each of the 18 items, with a maximum score of 126 indicating total functional independence. The FIM was recorded during the first assessment of all the patients within 72 hours of admission.

The FIM gain which is the difference between rehabilitation discharge and admission FIM were recorded for the TREATS and historical groups as it is a measure of functional improvement. The FIM gain of the 2 groups was compared against one another to determine whether functional outcomes were different between the 2 groups.

Posttraumatic amnesia (PTA) was documented as it is a strong predictor of recovery after TBI. The Westmead PTA Scale is used in our study to determine the severity of memory and cognitive impairment in TBI in addition to the commonly used GCS [24, 25]. The PTA scale was administered when patients were alert and able to communicate intelligibly. Daily scores were obtained by the rehabilitation team until the patient emerged from PTA or was discharged from the acute admission. The total duration of PTA included the time from TBI to the first day the patient achieved 3 consecutive full scores of 12/12 prior to discharge.

The Rancho Los Amigos Levels of Cognitive Function Scale (RLA) is used to assess cognitive functioning in postcoma patients for the planning of treatment, tracking of recovery, and classifying outcome levels [26, 27]. This scale comprises of levels from I to VIII. The RLA scale was recorded for patients who were out of general sedation upon first assessment.

Further data on patient stay in the subacute rehabilitation facilities at the community hospitals were unobtainable.

2.4. Statistical Analysis. Data was recorded on Microsoft Excel 97–2003 and was analyzed with SPSS Statistics for Windows, version 17.0. Chicago: SPSS Inc. We conducted descriptive analyses on the demographics of the patients who were acutely screened, their acute neurosurgical characteristics, comorbidities and complications, and rehabilitation outcomes.

Spearman's rank correlation coefficient was used to evaluate the association between ALOS and variables such as age, GCS, and total FIM in the total cohort of screened patients with TBI.

Differences between groups such as men and women in the total cohort of patients with TBI and between the TREATS and historical subgroups were analyzed using nonparametric tests when they were not of normal distributions.

Regression analysis was carried out to evaluate for clinical variables associated with FIM gain in the TREATS group.

A P value less than 0.05 was considered to be statistically significant.

This study was approved by the hospital institutional review board.

3. Results

3.1. Demographics, Acute Neurosurgical, and Rehabilitation Data. There were 298 patients with TBI during the study period from November 1, 2010, and February 15, 2012.

The average age of the cohort was 61.8 ± 19.1 years (range 15–99) with a significant difference of the women being older than the men in the cohort ($P < 0.001$) (Table 1). Almost half of the cohort (49.0%) was geriatric patients (Table 2). There were almost twice as many males who sustained a TBI (male/female ratio 1.9 : 1).

The most common etiology of the TBI was falls (77.5%), followed by road traffic accidents (10.0%) (Table 1). Less common etiologies were assault and sports. There was a statistically significant difference between genders when compared for the etiologies of TBI ($P = 0.03$) (Table 1).

Within the fall category, 61.9% were males and almost half (48.7%) of the falls were of nonmechanical origin. These included patients who fell due to syncope or other neurological symptoms. Thirty one percent of falls were mechanical in origin, while unwitnessed suspected falls constituted 20.2% of the fall cohort. Among those who fell, 57.8% were aged 65 and above ($P = 0.018$) and the most number of falls happened in the age group 70–79 years (Table 2) with a high significance of falls in the geriatric age group (91.8% versus 63.8%, $P < 0.001$).

The admission GCS scores indicated that the majority of patients (83.2%) sustained mild TBI (Table 1) and there seemed to be an increase in frequency of mild TBI with increasing age with the highest number in patients aged 70–79 years old (Figure 1). There was no significant difference between the 195 men and 103 women regarding severity of injury based on GCS scores on admission ($P = 0.37$) (Table 1). The majority of patients (67.3%) sustained subdural hematoma (SDH) or subarachnoid hemorrhage (SAH) or both SDH and SAH (Table 3).

Sixty-two patients (20.8%) received various neurosurgical interventions such as burr hole drainage, craniectomy, and external ventricular drain insertion. Six patients (2%) required tracheostomy.

Forty-eight patients (16.1%) had nosocomial infections with the 2 most common infections being pneumonia and urinary tract infection (Table 3).

TABLE 1: Age, injury severity, etiology, and FIM scores in 298 men and women.

	Total ($n = 298$)	Men ($n = 195$)	Women ($n = 103$)	P value
Age (years)				
Mean (SD)	61.8 (19.1)	58.8 (19.2)	67.6 (17.5)	<0.001
Range	15–99	15–99	16–97	
Severity categories				
Mild (GCS 13–15)	248 (83.2%)	158 (81.0%)	90 (87.4%)	
Moderate (GCS 9–12)	24 (8.1%)	18 (9.2%)	6 (5.8%)	0.37
Severe (GCS 3–8)	26 (8.7%)	19 (9.8%)	7 (6.8%)	
GCS				
Mean	13.6 (2.8)	13.4 (3.0)	13.9 (2.3)	0.17
Median	15	15	15	
Motor FIM				
Mean (SD)	48.3 (29.7)	49.4 (30.2)	46.1 (28.5)	
Median	52.0	55.0	48.0	0.28
Range	13–91	13–91	13–91	
Cognitive FIM				
Mean (SD)	23.3 (12.2)	23.5 (12.1)	23.1 (12.4)	
Median	30.0	30.0	30.0	0.64
Range	5–35	5–35	5–35	
Total FIM				
Mean (SD)	71.6 (40.0)	72.9 (40.5)	69.2 (39.0)	
Median	76.5	83.0	73.0	0.30
Range	18–126	18–126	18–126	
ALOS (days)				
Mean (SD)	19.9 (28.7)	21.0 (29.7)	17.6 (26.6)	
Median	9.0	10.0	8.0	0.25
Range	1–199	1–199	1–176	
TBI Etiology				
Assault	14 (4.7%)	13 (4.4%)	1 (0.3%)	
Fall	231 (77.5%)	143 (48.0%)	88 (29.5%)	
Road traffic accidents (RTA)	30 (10.1%)	19 (6.4%)	11 (3.7%)	0.03
Sports	7 (2.3%)	6 (2.0%)	1 (0.3%)	
Others	16 (5.4%)	14 (4.7%)	2 (0.7%)	

TABLE 2: Distribution of etiology of TBI according to age groups (years) in 298 patients.

TBI etiology	Age group (years)								
	0–19	20–29	30–39	40–49	50–59	60–69	70–79	80–89	≥90
Assault	0	1	7	1	2	2	1	0	0
Fall	2	9	13	17	31	44	59	46	10
RTA	1	3	5	6	4	7	3	1	0
Sports	2	3	0	2	0	0	0	0	0
Others	0	0	2	4	1	4	4	1	0
Total	5	16	27	30	38	57	67	48	10

About half of the TBI patients (50.7%) were in the RLA VIII category (Table 4).

More than half of the TBI patients (63.8%) were in PTA during assessment.

Most of the patients (67.4%) from the acute neurosurgical ward were discharged home. About a quarter of the patients (25.8%) required further inpatient rehabilitation in a rehabilitation facility and majority of these patients (88.3%) were transferred to the Department of Rehabilitation Medicine of SGH (TREATS). The remaining 9 patients were transferred to subacute rehabilitation facilities at the community hospitals. There was a statistically significant difference between the TREATS group of patients and the directly discharged group of patients in the admission GCS scores (13 versus 14, resp.; $P < 0.001$) and admission total FIM (51.1 versus 85.7, resp.; $P < 0.001$). Seven (2.3%) patients were discharged to

TABLE 3: Demographics and clinical variables of patients with TBI (N = 298).

Variable	Frequency n (%)
Age groups	
<50 years old	78 (26.2%)
50–64 years old	74 (24.8%)
≥65 years old	146 (49.0%)
Race	
Chinese	223 (74.8%)
Malay	25 (8.4%)
Indian	25 (8.4%)
Others	25 (8.4%)
Main radiological findings	
Subdural hematoma (SDH)	108 (36.2%)
Subarachnoid hemorrhage (SAH)	53 (17.7%)
SDH and SAH	40 (13.4%)
Concussion	38 (12.8%)
Contusion	19 (6.4%)
Extradural hematoma (EDH)	18 (6.0%)
Intracerebral hemorrhage (ICH)	22 (7.4%)
Types of neurosurgical interventions	
None	236 (79.2%)
Craniectomy	26 (8.7%)
Burr hole surgery	34 (11.4%)
Burr hole surgery and craniectomy	1 (0.3%)
External ventricular drain insertion	1 (0.3%)
Types of infections	
None	250 (83.9%)
Pneumonia	21 (7.0%)
Urinary tract infections (UTI)	17 (5.7%)
Pneumonia and UTI	7 (2.3%)
Others	3 (1.0%)

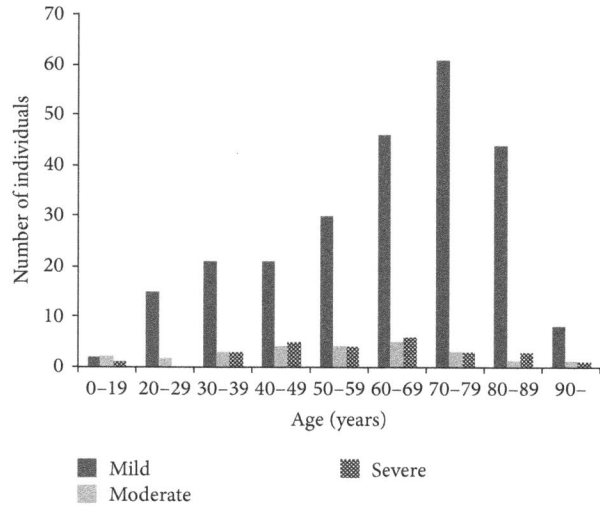

FIGURE 1: Distribution of severity of brain injury according to age groups.

a nursing home facility. Eight men (mean age 61.6, range 38–84) and 5 women (mean age 74.8, range 54–97) died. Out of these 13 patients, 5 sustained a severe TBI, 1 a moderate TBI, and 7 a mild TBI.

The mean total FIM of the 298 patients on admission was 71.6 ± 40.0 (range 18–126). The median FIM score was 76.5. The mean motor FIM score was 48.3 ± 29.7 (range 13–91) and the mean cognitive FIM score was 23.3 ± 12.2 (range 5–35). There was no significant difference in the FIM scores on admission between men and women (Table 1).

The average ALOS in the cohort of 298 patients with TBI was 19.9 ± 28.7 days (range 1–199). The ALOS was shown to have a moderately negative correlation with GCS on admission (r = −0.387, P < 0.001) and total FIM (r = −0.517, P < 0.001). However, the relationship between ALOS and age was poor (r = −0.140, P = 0.015).

3.2. Outcome and Subgroup Analyses of TREATS Group.
Sixty-eight patients were in the TREATS group. This was compared against a group of 51 historical patients.

The mean age of TREATS was 66.2 ± 17.0 (range 15–92), whereas the mean age of the historicals was 47.8 ± 20.1 (range 14–81) (P < 0.001).

Patients in the TREATS group showed functional improvement during the inpatient rehabilitation stay as demonstrated by statistically significant changes in FIM (P < 0.001) (Table 5).

There was no statistically significant difference between the TREATS and historical groups regarding the total FIM on admission and upon discharge (Table 5). There was also no difference in the total FIM gain, motor FIM gain, and cognitive FIM gain in both groups (Table 5).

The total LOS of TREATS was longer than historicals (47.2 days ± 36.8 versus 44.7 days ± 52.8, P = 0.329). The ALOS of TREATS was shorter (20.5 days ± 20.8) compared against historicals (24.3 days ± 45.9) (P = 0.929) and the RLOS of TREATS was longer (26.7 days ± 22.0) compared against historicals (20.4 days ± 16.9) (P = 0.089) (Table 5).

The rate of medical complications was 39.7% in the TREATS group and was similar to that of the historical group (37.3%).

The rate of neurosurgical interventions was 35.3% in the TREATS group compared against 43.1% in the historical group.

3.3. Regression Analyses.
The regression analysis on total FIM gain in TREATS and historicals demonstrated with the intervention of TREATS, there was a statistically significant functional gain of 18.445 points in FIM (95% CI −30.388 to −0.6502) (P = 0.03).

The regression model on total FIM gain in the TREATS group estimated about two-thirds of the variance in this variable (adjusted R^2 = 0.67) (Table 6). Factors associated with a higher FIM gain were shorter RLOS and younger age. Factors associated with a lower FIM gain were higher admission FIM scores. Gender, neurosurgical interventions, and medical complications such as infections, deep venous thrombosis, and seizures were not significantly associated with FIM gain.

TABLE 4: RLA in 298 patients with TBI.

RLA Level	Total ($n = 298$)	Men ($n = 195$)	Women ($n = 103$)
(i) No response	12 (4.0%)	9 (3.0%)	3 (1.0%)
(ii) Generalised response	6 (2.0%)	3 (1.0%)	3 (1.0%)
(iii) Localised response	13 (4.4%)	10 (3.4%)	3 (1.0%)
(iv) Confused and agitated	14 (4.7%)	13 (4.4%)	1 (0.3%)
(v) Confused and inappropriate	22 (7.4%)	12 (4.0%)	10 (3.4%)
(vi) Confused and appropriate	38 (12.8%)	29 (9.7%)	9 (3.0%)
(vii) Automatic and appropriate	42 (14.1%)	22 (7.4%)	20 (6.7%)
(viii) Purposeful and appropriate	151 (50.7%)	97 (32.6%)	54 (18.1%)

TABLE 5: Demographics and functional outcomes of TREATS versus historicals.

	TREATS ($n = 68$)	Historicals ($n = 51$)	P value
Age (years)			
Mean (SD)	66.2 (17.0)	47.8 (20.1)	<0.001
Range	15–92	14–81	
Total FIM on admission			
Mean (SD)	51.2 (32.4)	59.2 (27.2)	
Median	50.5	60.0	0.064
Range	18–126	18–122	
Total FIM on discharge			
Mean (SD)	80.4 (26.7)[*]	79.2 (27.8)	
Median	89.0	83.0	0.697
Range	18–126	18–123	
FIM gain			
Mean (SD)	29.3 (34.9)	20.0 (23.1)	0.201
Motor FIM gain			
Mean (SD)	22.9 (25.6)	17.5 (19.4)	0.222
Cognitive FIM gain			
Mean (SD)	6.4 (11.7)	2.5 (5.1)	0.216
ALOS (days)			
Mean (SD)	20.5 (20.8)	24.3 (45.9)	
Median	14.0	14.0	0.929
Range	2–115	0–320	
RLOS (days)			
Mean (SD)	26.7 (22.0)	20.4 (16.9)	
Median	20.5	16.0	0.089
Range	2–118	3–105	
Total LOS (days)			
Mean (SD)	47.2 (36.8)	44.7 (52.8)	
Median	32.0	30.0	0.329
Range	13–199	14–348	
TBI etiology			
Assault	3 (4.4%)	3 (5.9%)	
RTA	5 (7.4%)	17 (33.3%)	
Sports	1 (1.5%)	0 (0%)	
Falls	55 (80.9%)	26 (51.0%)	
Others	4 (5.9%)	4 (7.8%)	
Unknown	0 (0%)	1 (2.0%)	
GCS	13.0	11.1	0.005

[*]$P < 0.001$.

TABLE 6: Multiple linear regression analysis model on FIM Gain in TREATS group.

Variable	B^*	SE	B	P
Female	−5.11	6.45	−0.64	0.431
Age	−0.60	0.167	−0.29	0.001
Admission cognitive FIM scores	−0.87	0.39	−2.22	0.031
Admission motor FIM scores	−0.81	0.20	−0.52	<0.001
RLOS	−0.38	0.13	−0.24	0.006
Surgical interventions	−4.68	5.82	−0.07	0.424
Complications	−9.41	6.36	−0.13	0.144

B^*: unstandardized coefficient; SE: standard error; B: standardized coefficient.
Adjusted $R^2 = 0.67$.

4. Discussion

Our aims of this study were firstly to prospectively look at the demographics, clinical characteristics of patients of all TBI severities admitted into the acute hospital, and secondly to determine whether early screening and provision of very early integrated TBI rehabilitation service changes functional outcomes in the group who received further inpatient rehabilitation.

There are very few studies that looked at early "reach-in" service of patients with TBI within 72 hours of neurosurgical admission and these studies mainly looked at selected cohorts of patients with TBI especially severe TBI [28–30]. Our study looked at early rehabilitation of patients of all TBI severities. We are not aware of any studies similar to ours locally.

The most common etiology of TBI in our total cohort of 298 screened patients was falls followed by road traffic accidents. This could be due to our cohort that was generally older with an average age of 61.8 years and the elderly are at risk of falls due to age-related physical frailty, immobility, and reduced functional capacity. It seems like our elderly are very susceptible to falls with 91.8% of the geriatric age group sustained a fall leading to TBI. This trend was also seen in the United States with falls attributing to 61% of TBI among adults aged 65 and above [31]. This further emphasizes the need to look into fall prevention strategies and prioritize health-care resources for the elderly as our local population is rapidly ageing. By the year 2030, the number of estimated residents in Singapore aged 65 and above will reach about 20% of the total population [32].

The statistically significant difference in age between the TREATS and historical groups could reflect more comprehensive patient screening and identification processes inherent in the early "reach-in" screening program.

In our study, males are almost twice as likely as females to sustain a TBI and this is consistent with the general TBI cohort in both overseas and local settings [7, 33]. This is in spite of our cohort having more falls than road traffic accidents, but the reasons for more males were predisposed to falls is unclear. This observation is different from that seen in some of the local studies which had shown that females tend to fall more than males [34, 35], but the different observations could be related to different cohorts of patients that were selected from different settings.

Although the LOS of the TREATS and historical groups were not statistically different, the observation of the ALOS of the TREATS group was shorter than that of the historical group and the RLOS of the TREATS group was longer than that of the historical group supported the fact that early "reach-in" screening picked up patients with rehabilitation needs earlier. By provision of early screening and integrated TBI rehabilitation, the TREATS group functionally improved.

Both of the ALOS of our total cohort of 298 screened patients with TBI (19.9 days) as well as ALOS of the TREATS group (20.5 days) were shorter compared with a local study on a selected group of patients undergoing TBI rehabilitation in a dedicated facility (34.9 days) [7]. This may be explained by, firstly, average time from injury to admission to TBI rehabilitation unit was shortened with early screening of all patients with TBI admitted into the neurosurgical unit. Secondly, most of our screened cohort and the TREATS group sustained mild TBI with higher average admission GCS scores (GCS 13.6 and 13.0, resp., versus 8.3) which also reflected most of our patients that were discharged home directly.

Mammi et al. carried out a similar study which involved the early participation of a physiatrist in ICU and neurosurgery rounds 3 times a week with the aim to start comprehensive rehabilitation as soon as possible [28]. In their study, 88 patients with TBI were accepted for inpatient rehabilitation after the early screening during the 4-year study period. Their mean ALOS was 18 days which was similar to that of our TREATS group (20.5 days). However, their mean RLOS was longer than our TREATS group (37.0 days versus 26.7 days). This difference could possibly be explained by their group of patients having more severe injuries as reflected by the lower mean GCS (7.01 versus 13.0). Their demographics were also different from our group. The cause of TBI in their cohort was mostly due to motor vehicle accidents (85%), whereas the cause in our TREATS group was mostly related to falls (80.9%). Their patients were younger (35.12 years versus 66.2 years) than our patients in the TREATS group. Both their study and our study also showed a statistically significant gain in FIM after inpatient rehabilitation.

Our study showed a poor relationship between ALOS and age. Frankel et al. also reported that ALOS did not differ between older (age > 44 years) and younger (age ≤ 44) patients [36]. This indicated that although age was one of the prognostic indicators of TBI recovery [37], there could be other more significant factors that impacted ALOS such as the initial GCS and the total FIM on admission.

5. Conclusion

In conclusion, our study provided important country and culture specific epidemiological data on an unselected cohort of patients with TBI in Singapore. It was noted that the leading cause of TBI was falls and our patients were generally elderly. This data may serve as an important reference when planning for a national database and could help prioritize limited health-care resources in our local setting. It emphasizes the need for a comprehensive country wide falls prevention initiative especially in the elderly population.

By providing very early integrated TBI rehabilitation within the acute hospital setting, patients with TBI were seen by the rehabilitation team earlier and those with further rehabilitation needs were sent to the dedicated TBI rehabilitation unit earlier. Our results showed that there are functional improvements in the subset of patients who further received inpatient rehabilitation. Our study has shown that it is feasible to provide such an early integrated TBI rehabilitation service within an acute level I trauma center.

As several overseas studies have shown that early rehabilitation improves functional outcomes [8, 9] during the acute hospitalization which in turn leads to significant reduction in economic costs [38, 39], we have plans to continue this program with the aims to collect more data especially assessment of long-term functional outcomes to further determine the long-term benefits and cost effectiveness of such a very early integrated TBI rehabilitation program.

Study Limitations

Our study looked at screening patients with TBI of all severities for early acute rehabilitation. This is a heterogeneous group where functional outcomes are widely different.

Although we attempted to collect data on duration of PTA, much of the data was incomplete so we were not able to report PTA duration in the results.

We were not able to carry out a randomized controlled trial because it did not seem ethical to deny patients with TBI early screening and provision of early integrated TBI rehabilitation. Instead, we carried out subgroup analysis of the TREATS group who received further inpatient rehabilitation in a dedicated TBI rehabilitation unit and compared against the historical group who did not undergo early screening.

We recognized that the TREATS group may not be exactly comparable against the historical group as these 2 groups of patients were heterogeneous with a wide spectrum of injury severities and clinical variables. Nevertheless, it provided valuable information regarding functional outcomes of early screening followed by early provision of TBI rehabilitation during acute hospitalization in patients of all TBI severities.

Conflict of Interests

The authors declare that there is no conflict of interests regarding the publication of this paper.

Acknowledgment

The authors would like to thank the Department of Neurosurgery of Singapore General Hospital for its support in this study and Ms. Hung Chew Wong, Biostatistics Unit, Yong Loo Lin School of Medicine Dean's office, National University of Singapore, for her help in statistical analysis. Selected findings from this study have been presented at the International Brain Injury Association Ninth Annual World Congress March 2012.

References

[1] I. Baguley, S. Slewa-Younan, R. Lazarus, and A. Green, "Long-term mortality trends in patients with traumatic brain injury," *Brain Injury*, vol. 14, no. 6, pp. 505–512, 2000.

[2] Centers for Disease Control and Prevention. Injury Prevention and Control: Traumatic Brain Injury, 2011, http://www.cdc.gov/TraumaticBrainInjury.

[3] Speech by Director of Medical Services, Prof K. Satkunanantham, at the Opening Ceremony of the 7th Singapore Trauma Conference, 2013, http://www.moh.gov.sg/content/moh_web/home/pressRoom/speeches_d/2013/speech-by-director-of-medical-services–prof-k–satkunanantham–.html.

[4] K. K. Lee, W. T. Seow, and I. Ng, "Demographic profiles of adult severe traumatic brain injury patients: implications for healthcare planning," *Singapore Medical Journal*, vol. 47, no. 1, pp. 31–36, 2006.

[5] E. Finkelstein, P. Corso, and T. R. Miller, *The Incidence and Economic Burden of Injuries in the United States*, Oxford University Press, New York, NY, USA, 2006.

[6] V. G. Coronado, L. C. McGuire, M. Faul et al., "Traumatic brain injury epidemiology and public health issues," in *Brain Injury Medicine: Principles and Practice*, N. D. Zasler, D. I. Katz, R. D. Zafonte, and D. B. Arciniegas, Eds., p. 93, Demos Medical Publishing, New York, NY, USA, 2012.

[7] K. S. G. Chua, A. Earnest, Y. Chiong, and K.-H. Kong, "Characteristics and correlates of rehabilitation charges during inpatient traumatic brain injury rehabilitation in Singapore," *Journal of Rehabilitation Medicine*, vol. 42, no. 1, pp. 27–34, 2010.

[8] N. Cope, "Traumatic brain injury rehabilitation outcome studies in the United States," in *Brain Injury & Neuropsychological Rehabilitation: International Perspectives*, A. L. Christensen and B. P. Uzzell, Eds., Lawrence Earlbaum Associates, Hillsdale, NJ, USA, 1994.

[9] M. Faul, M. M. Wald, W. Rutland-Brown, E. E. Sullivent, and R. W. Sattin, "Using a cost-benefit analysis to estimate outcomes of a clinical treatment guideline: testing the Brain Trauma Foundation guidelines for the treatment of severe traumatic brain injury," *The Journal of Trauma*, vol. 63, no. 6, pp. 1271–1278, 2007.

[10] T. B. Cumming, A. G. Thrift, J. M. Collier et al., "Very early mobilization after stroke fast-tracks return to walking: further results from the phase II AVERT randomized controlled trial," *Stroke*, vol. 42, no. 1, pp. 153–158, 2011.

[11] S. G. Lomber and J. J. Eggermont, *Reprogramming the Cerebral Cortex: Plasticity Following Central and Peripheral Lesions*, Oxford University Press, Oxford, UK, 2006.

[12] J. Biernaskie, G. Chernenko, and D. Corbett, "Efficacy of rehabilitative experience declines with time after focal ischemic

brain injury," *Journal of Neuroscience*, vol. 24, no. 5, pp. 1245–1254, 2004.

[13] M. Lippert-Grüner, M. Maegele, J. Pokorný et al., "Early rehabilitation model shows positive effects on neural degeneration and recovery from neuromotor deficits following traumatic brain injury," *Physiological Research*, vol. 56, no. 3, pp. 359–368, 2007.

[14] L. E. Craig, J. Bernhardt, P. Langhorne, and O. Wu, "Early mobilization after stroke: an example of an individual patient data meta-analysis of a complex intervention," *Stroke*, vol. 41, no. 11, pp. 2632–2636, 2010.

[15] K. Tyedin, T. B. Cumming, and J. Bernhardt, "Quality of life: an important outcome measure in a trial of very early mobilisation after stroke," *Disability and Rehabilitation*, vol. 32, no. 11, pp. 875–884, 2010.

[16] The Traumatic Brain Injury Model Systems of Care and National Database Update Complied by the Traumatic Brain Injury Model Systems National Data and Statistical Center, 2012, https://www.tbindsc.org/.

[17] G. D. Murray, G. M. Teasdale, R. Braakman et al., "The European Brain Injury Consortium survey of head injuries," *Acta Neurochirurgica*, vol. 141, no. 3, pp. 223–236, 1999.

[18] C. Jourdan, E. Bayen, V. Bosserelle et al., "Referral to rehabilitation after severe traumatic brain injury: results from the PariS-TBI study," *Neurorehabilitation and Neural Repair*, no. 1, pp. 2735–2744, 2013.

[19] A. Rudehill, B.-M. Bellander, E. Weitzberg, S. Bredbacka, M. Backheden, and E. Gordon, "Outcome of traumatic brain injuries in 1,508 patients: Impact of prehospital care," *Journal of Neurotrauma*, vol. 19, no. 7, pp. 855–868, 2002.

[20] W. He, M. Sengupta, V. A. Velkoff et al., *65+ in the United States: 2005*, U.S. Census Bureau, Washington, DC, USA, 2005.

[21] K. Simon, "A breakdown on falls in the elderly," The Canadian Journal of CME, 2005, http://www.stacommunications.com/journals/cme/2005/April/PDF/059.pdf.

[22] 2013, Centers for Disease Control and Prevention. National Center for Injury Prevention and Control. Heads up: Facts for Physicans about Mild Traumatic Brain Injury (MTBI), 2013, http://www.cdc.gov/concussion/headsup/pdf/Facts_for_Physicians_booklet-a.pdf.

[23] C. V. Granger, B. B. Hamilton, J. M. Linacre, A. W. Heinemann, and B. D. Wright, "Performance profiles of the functional independence measure," *The American Journal of Physical Medicine and Rehabilitation*, vol. 72, no. 2, pp. 84–89, 1993.

[24] E. A. Shores, J. E. Marosszeky, J. Sandanam, and J. Batchelor, "Preliminary validation of a clinical scale for measuring the duration of post-traumatic amnesia," *Medical Journal of Australia*, vol. 144, no. 11, pp. 569–572, 1986.

[25] N. E. V. Marosszeky, L. Ryan, E. A. Shores et al., *The PTA Protocol: Guidelines for Using the Westmead Post-Traumatic Amnesia (PTA) Scale*, Wild & Wooley, Sydney, Australia, 1998.

[26] D. X. Cifu, J. S. Kreutzer, J. H. Marwitz et al., "Functional outcomes of older adults with traumatic brain injury: a prospective, multicenter analysis," *Archives of Physical Medicine and Rehabilitation*, vol. 77, no. 9, pp. 883–888, 1996.

[27] S. M. Fakhry, A. L. Trask, M. A. Waller, D. D. Watts, A. Chendrasekhar, and J. S. Hammond, "Management of brain-injured patients by an evidence-based medicine protocol improves outcomes and decreases hospital charges," *Journal of Trauma*, vol. 56, no. 3, pp. 492–500, 2004.

[28] P. Mammi, B. Zaccaria, and M. Franceschini, "Early rehabilitative treatment in patients with traumatic brain injuries: outcome at one-year follow-up," *Europa Medicophysica*, vol. 42, no. 1, pp. 17–22, 2006.

[29] M. Lippert-Grüner, "Early rehabilitation of comatose patients after traumatic brain injury," *Neurologia i Neurochirurgia Polska*, vol. 44, no. 5, pp. 475–480, 2010.

[30] N. Andelic, E. Bautz-Holter, P. Ronning et al., "Does an early onset and continuous chain of rehabilitation improve the long-term functional outcome of patients with severe traumatic brain injury?" *Journal of Neurotrauma*, vol. 29, no. 1, pp. 66–74, 2012.

[31] M. Faul, L. Xu, M. M. Wald et al., *Traumatic Brain Injury in the United States: Emergency Department Visits, Hospitalizations, and Deaths*, Centers for Disease Control and Prevention, National Center for Injury Prevention and Control, Atlanta, Ga, USA, 2010.

[32] Ministry of Community Development, Youth and Sports. Committee on Ageing Issues: Report on the Ageing Population, 2012, http://app.msf.gov.sg/Portals/0/Summary/research/CAI_report.pdf.

[33] J. A. Langlois, W. Rutland-Brown, and K. E. Thomas, *Traumatic Brain Injury in the United States: Emergency Department Visits, Hospitalizations, and Deaths*, Centers for Disease Control and Prevention, Atlanta, Ga, USA, 2006.

[34] Y. Y. C. Yeo, S. K. Lee, C. Y. Lim, L. S. Quek, and S. B. S. Ooi, "A review of elderly injuries seen in a Singapore emergency department," *Singapore Medical Journal*, vol. 50, no. 3, pp. 278–283, 2009.

[35] K. M. Chan, W. S. Pang, C. H. Ee et al., "Epidemiology of falls among the elderly community dwellers in Singapore," *Singapore Medical Journal*, vol. 38, no. 10, pp. 427–431, 1997.

[36] J. E. Frankel, J. H. Marwitz, D. X. Cifu, J. S. Kreutzer, J. Englander, and M. Rosenthal, "A follow-up study of older adults with traumatic brain injury: taking into account decreasing length of stay," *Archives of Physical Medicine and Rehabilitation*, vol. 87, no. 1, pp. 57–62, 2006.

[37] S. Kothari, "Prognosis after severe TBI: a practical, evidence based approach," in *Brain Injury Medicine: Principles and Practice*, N. D. Zasler, D. I. Katz, and R. D. Zafonte, Eds., pp. 169–199, Demos, New York, USA, 2007.

[38] A. K. Wagner, T. Fabio, R. D. Zafonte, G. Goldberg, D. W. Marion, and A. B. Peitzman, "Physical medicine and rehabilitation consultation: relationships with acute functional outcome, length of stay, and discharge planning after traumatic brain injury," *The American Journal of Physical Medicine and Rehabilitation*, vol. 82, no. 7, pp. 526–536, 2003.

[39] M. J. Sirois, A. Lavoie, and C. E. Dionne, "Impact of transfer delays to rehabilitation in patients with severe trauma," *Archives of Physical Medicine and Rehabilitation*, vol. 85, no. 2, pp. 184–191, 2004.

31

Evaluation of a Community Reintegration Outpatient Program Service for Community-Dwelling Persons with Spinal Cord Injury

Alana Zinman,[1] Nicole Digout,[1] Patricia Bain,[2] Sylvia Haycock,[1] Debbie Hébert,[1,3] and Sander L. Hitzig[4]

[1]Department of Occupational Science and Occupational Therapy, Faculty of Medicine, University of Toronto, Toronto, ON, Canada M5G 1V7

[2]Lyndhurst Centre, Toronto Rehabilitation Institute, University Health Network, Toronto, ON, Canada M4G 3V9

[3]Toronto Rehabilitation Institute, University Health Network, Toronto, ON, Canada M5G 2A2

[4]Institute for Life Course and Aging, Faculty of Medicine, University of Toronto, 263 McCaul Street, Suite 328, Toronto, ON, Canada M5T 1W7

Correspondence should be addressed to Sander L. Hitzig; sander.hitzig@utoronto.ca

Academic Editor: Eva Widerström-Noga

Objective. To evaluate the effectiveness of a community reintegration outpatient (CROP) service for promoting well-being and community participation following spinal cord injury (SCI). *Participants.* Community-dwelling adults ($N = 14$) with traumatic and nontraumatic SCI. *Interventions.* The CROP service is a 12-week (1 × week; 120 minutes) interprofessional closed therapeutic education service. *Main Outcome Measure(s).* Moorong Self-Efficacy Scale (MSES); Impact on Participation and Autonomy (IPA); Positive Affect and Negative Affect Scale (PANAS); Coping Inventory of Stressful Situations (CISS); World Health Organization Quality of Life (WHOQOL-BREF); semistructured qualitative interviews. *Methods.* Twenty-one participants were recruited from two subsequent CROP services, with only 14 persons completing all data assessments. Data were collected at baseline (week 0), at exit (week 12), and at a three-month follow-up. Semistructured interviews were conducted at exit. *Results.* Self-efficacy (MSES) and positive affect (PANAS) improved from baseline to exit ($P < .05$), but the changes were not maintained at follow-up. Qualitative analysis identified four major themes related to therapeutic benefits: (1) role of self; (2) knowledge acquisition; (3) skill application; and (4) group processes. *Conclusions.* Participation in a therapeutic education service has the potential to improve well-being in persons with SCI, but there is a need to identify strategies to maintain long-term gains.

1. Introduction

After sustaining a spinal cord injury (SCI), individuals must often cope with various physical, psychological, and social issues that occur as a result of their injuries [1]. The primary impairment of paralysis, along with the host of associated secondary health conditions (i.e., pain, depression, and bowel and bladder dysfunction) [2], causes significant burden to the individual and incurs substantial costs to the healthcare system. Recent data estimating the direct medical costs associated with traumatic SCI reported that the lifetime economic burden per individual ranges from $1.5 million for persons with incomplete paraplegia to $3.0 million for persons with complete tetraplegia [3]. Furthermore, SCI and associated conditions cause significant challenges for maintaining well-being in the community [4].

To mitigate the impact of the injury, people with SCI need to learn to adjust and accommodate to the resulting lifestyle changes [5]. The ability to adjust after SCI is often independent of the level and/or severity of injury; rather it is dependent on the coping strategies employed by the individual [6]. If an individual copes poorly with difficulties encountered during the reintegration process after SCI, then there is a greater likelihood of that person experiencing high levels of emotional distress, anxiety, and/or a depressive disorder [7, 8]. Thus, having a good repertoire of positive coping strategies can serve to manage common stressors associated with living with an SCI, which can contribute to better community participation and quality of life (QoL) [9].

There is a growing body of work on the use of self-management programs to help people with SCI address the challenges associated with living their injuries [10]. Self-management programs can serve to minimize the occurrence or impact of secondary health conditions by providing knowledge and skills related to risk and protective factors [11], while fostering appropriate coping mechanisms for a variety of life situations impacted by an SCI (e.g., employment, family relations, etc.) [10]. Although there are a variety of existing programs, such as the Stanford Chronic Disease Self-Management Program, it has been suggested that there is a need for more programs that are specifically tailored for people with SCI [12, 13]. For instance, programs need to provide information that is relevant to persons who have limited mobility or who are dependent on a wheelchair [13]. There is also a need for programs that can serve to enhance self-efficacy (one's belief in his/her ability to succeed and manage challenging situations and accomplish goals [14]) and psychosocial care after SCI [15] given that self-confidence or self-efficacy to manage one's SCI has been found to be suboptimal in this population [16].

The high costs associated with living with SCI and its impacts on physical and mental health indicate there is a need for more research on the effectiveness of self-management programs to promote well-being in persons with SCI. Thus, the primary objective of this study was to investigate the efficacy of the community reintegration outpatient (CROP) service for community-dwelling individuals with an SCI. The CROP is a closed therapeutic education service that imparts self-management strategies by offering education on various aspects of coping with an SCI (i.e., pain management, stress management, self-care, etc.), with the goal of enhancing community participation. It was hypothesized that persons who participated in the CROP service would demonstrate improvements in psychological, emotional, and social well-being. The findings from this study can serve to inform the development and implementation of SCI-specific self-management programs at other rehabilitation settings.

2. Methods

2.1. The Community Reintegration Outpatient (CROP) Service.
The CROP service is a 12-week (1 × week) closed therapeutic education service, cofacilitated by an occupational therapist and social worker at a tertiary SCI rehabilitation hospital, where clients with SCI are provided with opportunities (1) to learn and understand the role of the "self" in the recovery process; (2) to share experiences and learn from one another; and (3) to identify and develop a visual roadmap for improving coping, well-being, and overall self-management skills while reintegrating back into the community.

The development of the CROP was initiated by an interprofessional group of clinicians providing SCI outpatient rehabilitation services in response to an identified gap in clinical practice related to community integration support after discharge from initial SCI rehabilitation. The clinicians noted that some clients with SCI were having difficulty reintegrating back into their communities and hypothesized that these challenges were partly attributable to low self-efficacy and limited opportunities for meaningful social participation (e.g., employment, leisure, etc.). To address these issues, the interprofessional team initiated the development of a specialized service to help persons with SCI successfully participate in their physical and psychosocial environment. Specifically, the service would provide a structured platform to enable people with SCI to reflect on their experiences living with the injury and acquire the necessary skills and knowledge to engage (or resume) in appropriate social roles, statuses, activities, and productive behaviours in "natural" community settings [17, 18]. With support from the organization, in-kind contributions (e.g., provision of space, clinical release time to develop the service, etc.) were provided to staff to establish and deliver a time-specific pilot project to promote better outcomes in the community for outpatients with SCI. The development of the CROP occurred through a series of systematic steps, which included (1) literature review; (2) development of a model of care; and (3) iterative service planning and quality improvement processes.

2.2. Literature Review.
The first step towards developing the CROP was a review of the literature to identify barriers and facilitators influencing community participation following SCI. The review was focused on identifying physical, environmental, emotional, and social stressors associated with SCI. For instance, poorer health as a result of the injury [19], reduced employment opportunities [9, 20], limited social support and family role functioning [21, 22], limited access to recreational and leisure activities [23, 24], and a lack of accessible transportation [25, 26] were all noted to affect participation. There are also invisible and conceptual barriers that arise from the attitudes and beliefs of the individual with the SCI and from society as a whole. For example, a poor locus of control and the belief that a person is not capable of accomplishing the same things that he/she could do before injury can lead to him/her not being proactive in community life [1]. Successful integration back to the community following SCI requires new learning, problem solving, adaptation to lifestyle changes, and effective coping skills [9]. Along with the clinical experience of the interprofessional team, the review of the literature provided a working model on which topics needed to be addressed to support optimal community engagement after SCI.

2.3. Model of Care.
With regard to client selection and delivery approach, existing clinical models and services were reviewed to identify best practices for the implementation of the CROP. In terms of finding appropriate clients interested and willing to attend the service, the clinicians working to develop the CROP service were providing SCI outpatient rehabilitation services within a therapeutic day program (TDP) to persons who were recently discharged from the inpatient rehab program. Although the TDP was initially

identified as relevant source for recruitment to the first iteration of the CROP, there were drawbacks to this targeted recruitment strategy. Due to a limited number of patients in the TDP, staggered starting dates, and a high dropout rate due to other attended services' ending, it was decided to make the CROP service available to all patients accessing outpatient services.

With regard to service delivery, a group work approach was deemed as a clinically efficient way of providing the service. Group work processes help promote individual identity and enhance personal strengths, increase motivation and optimism, create sources of support, and provide an environment for constructive growth and problem solving [27]. In order to foster perceived control and self-discovery in participants, it was decided to use guided facilitation to manage the group process. Thus, a closed group model under the guidance of consistent facilitators was adopted for the planned therapeutic group service.

2.4. Service Planning and Quality Improvement. Service planning and quality improvement were an evolutionary process and served to further refine the CROP service. The use of outcome measures, group process facilitation skills, and the development of topic themes emerged through clinical observations and a formal client feedback process. A program logic model was used to provide a framework for developing the structure of the service. For instance, the group facilitation process was driven by the concept of the role of self, each patient's commitment to the group, and readiness for change and for self-management within the community.

Central to the development of the written content and take-home assignments were the barriers and success factors identified in the community participation literature review (described above). Each weekly session focused on active involvement in learning by incorporating education/lectures, reflections, and interactive discussions and activities. The group structure, process, and content were founded on multiple theoretical models including cognitive behavioural therapy [28], the Canadian Model of Occupational Performance [29], principles of adult learning [30, 31], group process theory [32], goal setting [33], and client-centered care.

The first iteration of the CROP was evaluated using the Reintegration to Normal Living Index (RNL) [34], a measure reflective of community participation, and through patient feedback surveys developed by the interprofessional team. Using feedback from the initial group of CROP service participants, the service developed a stronger emphasis on goal setting, self-efficacy, self-identity, and life roles. Unfortunately, the findings from the RNL indicated no improvements in community participation from baseline to program exit for CROP participants. Although the RNL is validated for use with SCI [35], the tool may not have been sensitive enough to detect changes over a relative short time since the version used employed a three-point numeric scale. Another potential limitation of the RNL is that it was not designed to assess changes in all of the targeted domains (e.g., coping, self-efficacy) deemed amenable by the CROP. Thus, it was determined that a more robust evaluation of the service

was required, which included the use of more standardized measures that would be more appropriate for assessing the efficacy of the service (see *"instruments"* description below).

2.5. CROP Service. The revised CROP service and formal program evaluation framework was initiated in May 2011 (Session 1), with a subsequent session held in May 2012 (Session 2). The CROP service was held over a 12-week period, with each weekly session lasting approximately 120 minutes. The CROP was cofacilitated by a social worker and occupational therapist and was provided at no-cost to the participants. A different topic relevant to managing an SCI in the community was covered each week (see Figure 1). The selected topics for discussion were based on earlier feedback from the participants of the initial CROP session (described above) and were reflective of the issues noted in the SCI literature and the clinical problems being reported by the patients attending the outpatient services at the rehabilitation centre (e.g., pain, stress, etc.).

A key feature for facilitating personal growth and group discussion was a goal setting process. At the initial CROP session (week 1), participants established a specific goal they wanted to accomplish over the 12-week service (see Figure 1), which was formulated by using a S.M.A.R.T. approach (specific, measureable, attainable, realistic, and time-sensitive). Strategies for accomplishing the selected goals of the participants were discussed by the group on a rotating basis, with each member having an opportunity to discuss their progress and to receive feedback from the group at regular intervals on how to overcome any challenges or obstacles they were encountering. To facilitate the weekly discussions and to support the goal attainment process, a teaching manual designed by the social worker and occupational therapist who implemented the service was provided to each participant on the different topics (see Figure 2). The teaching manual contained information sheets about a variety of topics, which included self-care, stress management, energy conservation, emotional adjustment, and coping strategies (see Figure 1). The components of the manual were informed by the literature review and existing clinical materials and were subsequently vetted by several clinical staff members of the SCI outpatient service team. Each session also assigned weekly homework tasks, which consisted of simple and more in-depth reflection exercises (see Figure 2). An example of a simple homework task was to write down and complete a "Do One Thing" cue card, which encouraged participants to undertake an action step related to the topic of the week (e.g., making a phone call to a friend). An example of an in-depth reflection assignment was a "Stop, Think, and Reflect" question related to each session's content. For example, the "Session 2—Self Care" questions included "What are the top 5 things I value in life? Is maintaining good health and well-being on this list? If not, why?" and "What do I focus the majority of my time and energy on?" Although regularly assigned, completion of the homework was not mandatory. Different visual and learning aids were also used throughout the CROP services (see Figure 2). In order to provide a "real-world" opportunity to implement skills and knowledge gained from the CROP, one session took place in

S.M.A.R.T. goal setting

CROP topics

| S | Specific
What do I want to accomplish? |

| M | Measurable
How will I know when I achieve my goal? |

| A | Achievable
Is my goal within my capabilities? |

| R | Relevant
Is my goal meaningful to me? |

| T | Timely
Do I have time to complete the
tasks necessary to achieve my goals? |

Self-care and you
Identifying individual and societal roles in self-care

Adjustment and transition
Role transition. Grieving styles. Doing, being, and belonging

Stress management
The nature of stress, signs, and triggers

Problem solving
The role of cognitive executive function in the coping process

Emotions
Affect, feeling, and emotions

Self-talk
The relationship between cognition, emotion, and behaviour

Communication
Communication styles

Energy management
The principles of energy conservation

Pain management
Understanding pain. Body/mind connection

Community outing
Application of learning

Hope and happiness
Social, emotional, and physical well-being. Looking forward

Resources/visual roadmap
Individual presentations. Next steps

Setting S.M.A.R.T. goals is a foundational principle of the group
Intertwined throughout the group process is education and practice for setting goals

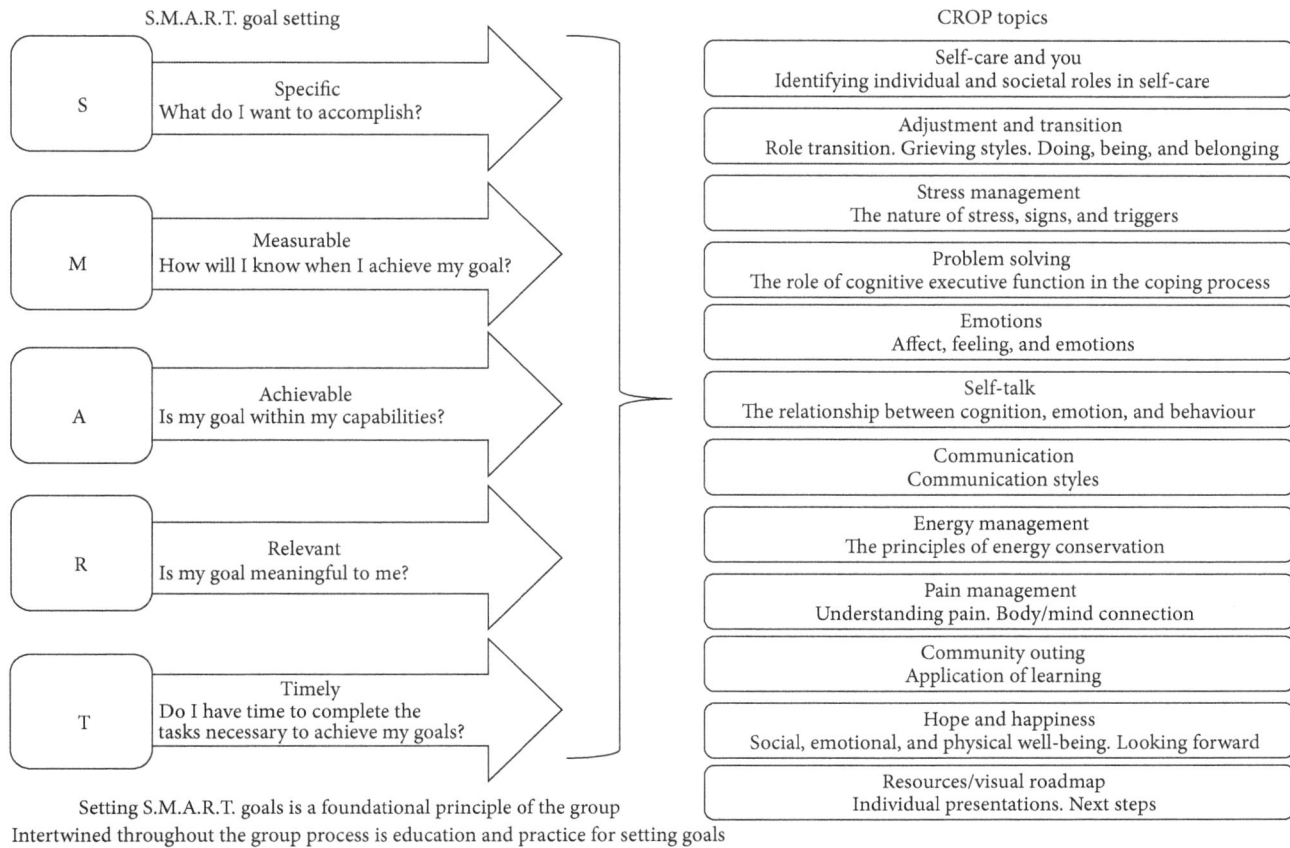

FIGURE 1: CROP S.M.A.R.T. goals and topics.

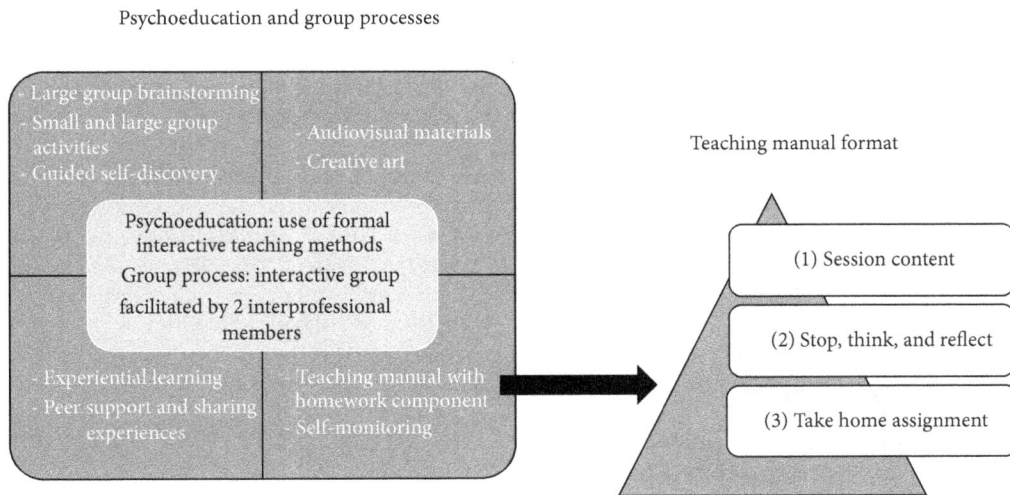

Psychoeducation and group processes

- Large group brainstorming
- Small and large group activities
- Guided self-discovery

- Audiovisual materials
- Creative art

Psychoeducation: use of formal interactive teaching methods
Group process: interactive group facilitated by 2 interprofessional members

- Experiential learning
- Peer support and sharing experiences

- Teaching manual with homework component
- Self-monitoring

Teaching manual format

(1) Session content

(2) Stop, think, and reflect

(3) Take home assignment

FIGURE 2: CROP processes and materials.

a community setting towards the end of the service. Overall the selected topics for discussion, the goal setting exercises, minihomework assignments, learning aids, and community outing were all designed to increase participant motivation to acquire skills and knowledge for community living from the interprofessional team while facilitating opportunities for the group to share their experiences of managing their SCI with one another. It should be noted that the CROP services were implemented on a trial basis and not part of standard clinical care at the SCI rehabilitation centre.

2.6. Participants. A convenience sample of twenty-one adults (10 men; 11 women) with traumatic and nontraumatic SCI was recruited from two subsequent CROP services (Session 1: May 2011 to July 2011; and Session 2: May 2012–July 2012). Inclusion criteria were community-dwelling adults (18 years or older) with traumatic or nontraumatic SCI, who were less than 3 years after injury/onset, who were fluent in English, and could attend the 12 weekly sessions of the CROP service. The exclusion criteria were persons who were not medically stable, who were not fluent in English (to the extent it would create a barrier for participation), or who had a cognitive impairment.

2.7. Instruments

2.7.1. World Health Organization Quality of Life (WHOQOL-BREF). The WHOQOL-BREF is a measure of QoL, grouped into four domains: physical capacity, psychological well-being, social relationships, and environment [36]. Higher scores on each subscale indicate better QoL. It has demonstrated excellent responsiveness with SCI and for program evaluation in rehabilitation [37]. Cronbach's alpha coefficients for the physical, psychological, social, and environment factors were computed to be 0.82, 0.82, 0.74, and 0.80, respectively [37].

2.7.2. Coping Inventory for Stressful Situations (CISS). The CISS measures three main coping strategies that people may use in stressful situations: task-oriented, emotion-oriented, and avoidance-oriented approach (distraction and social diversion) [38]. Studies evaluating the tool have concluded it has good predictive validity [39]. Cronbach alpha coefficients for the Problem, Emotion, and Avoidance scales for the CISS were found to be 0.91, 0.89, and 0.84, respectively. Test-retest reliability ranges from 0.76 to 0.90 [38].

2.7.3. Positive Affect and Negative Affect Schedule (PANAS). The PANAS measures positive and negative constructs as both states and traits [40]. A positive affect and negative affect subscale are calculated. The PANAS has demonstrated reliability among a sample of patients who have received inpatient medical rehabilitation, with a test-retest ICC of 0.79 for positive affect and 0.93 for negative affect [40]. In the general adult population, Cronbach's alpha has been demonstrated to be 0.89 and 0.85 for positive affect and negative affect, respectively [41, 42].

2.7.4. Moorong Self-Efficacy Scale (MSES). The MSES is a 16-item SCI self-efficacy scale, scored on a Likert scale from 1 to 7 [43]. Higher scores indicate higher levels of self-efficacy. The scale has good internal consistency and a test-retest reliability of 0.74 [44]. Significant correlations with self-concept measures, emotional distress scales, and functional independence measures demonstrate the validity of the MSES [44].

2.7.5. Impact on Participation and Autonomy (IPA). The IPA quantifies limitations in participation and autonomy via five subscales: autonomy indoors, family role, autonomy outdoors, social life and relationships, and work and education [45]. Higher scores represent poorer participation and autonomy. Test-retest reliability from a cross-disability sample, including SCI, ranges from 0.56 to 0.90 [46]. In one SCI study, the IPA had high internal consistency and ICCs, with all values greater than 0.70 [47]. In the same study [47], the minimal detectable change by IPA domain was found to be 0.70 for autonomy indoors, 1.18 for autonomy outdoors, 0.83 for family life, 0.76 for social life and relationships, and 0.86 for work and education.

2.7.6. Qualitative Interviews. Semistructured interviews with participants were conducted at the end of the CROP service (week 12) to gain their insights about their participation and to gain feedback on how the service could be improved. The interview guide is described in the Appendix.

2.8. Procedure. A nonrandomized single arm study design was employed. Survey data were collected prior to participation (baseline), at completion (exit), and at 3 months after intervention (follow-up) by members of the research team. Participants also underwent semistructured interviews, which asked about their perceptions of the CROP service.

As noted, participants were recruited from two CROP services (Sessions 1 and 2). Twelve participants were recruited at Session 1 and 9 participants were recruited at Session 2. Sixteen participants completed baseline and exit assessments; 14 of them completed baseline, exit, and follow-up assessments (see Figure 3 with flow diagram). Twelve participants took part in the semistructured interview at exit. Each interview lasted approximately 30 minutes. All interviews were audiotaped and transcribed for data analysis.

This study was approved by the Research Ethics Board of the Toronto Rehabilitation Institute and the University of Toronto, and we certify that all applicable institutional and governmental regulations concerning the ethical use of human volunteers were followed.

2.9. Analysis. Descriptive statistics and frequencies were used to describe the sample and scores on the outcome measures. For participants who only completed the baseline and exit assessments ($n = 16$), the data met the assumptions for normality, and thus paired t-tests were conducted. Effect sizes were calculated following the procedures described by Lakens [48]. This included providing common language (CL) effect sizes, which converts effect sizes into percentages, and

> "expresses the probability that a randomly sampled person from one group will have a higher observed measurement than a randomly sampled person from the other group (for between-designs) or (for within-designs) the probability that an individual has a higher value on one measurement than the other." [48, page 4].

For those who completed baseline, exit, and follow-up assessments ($n = 14$), Friedman tests were used to analyze the data given the small sample size and because not all of the data met the assumptions of normality. Post hoc comparisons were conducted using Wilcoxon t-tests with a bonferroni

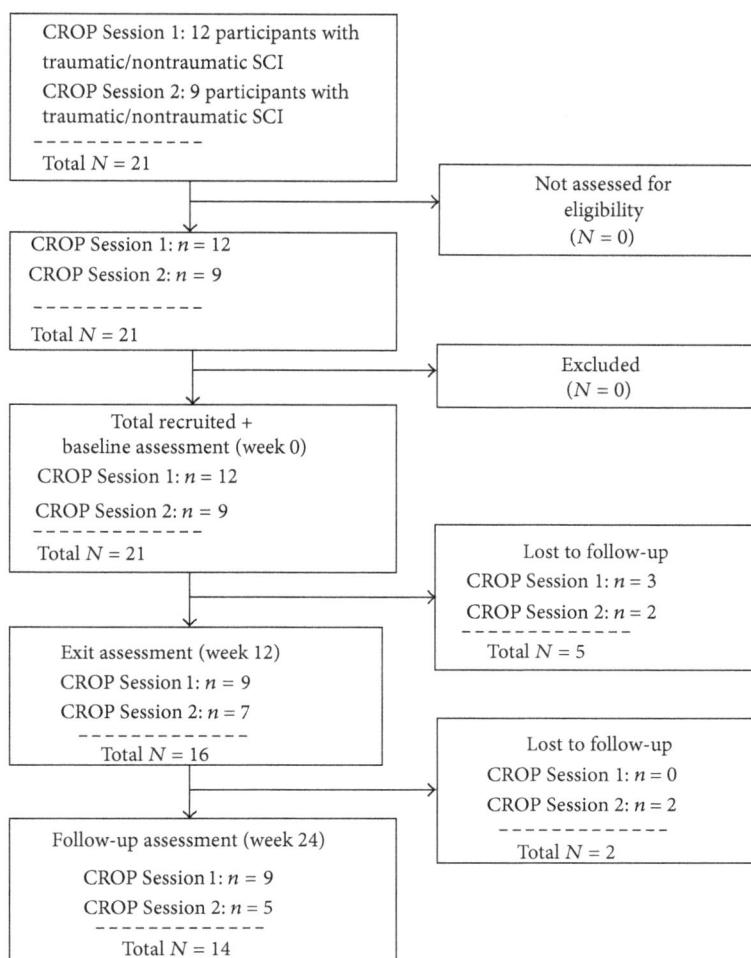

FIGURE 3: CROP service participant recruitment and assessment flow diagram.

correction. Effect sizes for these analyses were calculated using the formula $r = Z/\sqrt{n}$.

For the qualitative data, an inductive content analysis was conducted [49–52]. This process involved using open-coding and creating categories that emerged from the participant transcripts [52]. Two investigators independently coded each transcript and regularly met to corroborate their findings in order to form a decision of what aspects of the interview belonged under the same category. Points of disagreement were resolved through discussion and documented through an audit trail. The technique of "code-recode" was conducted to verify content validity, and major themes and associated subthemes were identified. Investigator triangulation was used at each stage of the analysis process to ensure trustworthiness of the data [51]. This included involving a third investigator who confirmed the subsequent coding frameworks served to resolve points of disagreement between the two main coders. The end-goal of the data analysis process was to achieve saturation, in which no new information emerges from the transcripts [50].

3. Results

3.1. Quantitative Analysis. Table 1 presents the sociodemographic and injury profiles of persons who completed baseline and exit ($n = 16$) and the sample characteristics of those who completed the baseline, exit, and follow-up assessments ($n = 14$). It should be noted that no differences emerged between persons from CROP Session 1 and CROP Session 2 in terms of sociodemographics (age, gender) or impairment (etiology, level of injury, severity of injury, and months after onset).

3.2. Changes between CROP Baseline and Exit Scores. For persons who completed both baseline and exit assessments ($n = 16$; Table 2), there was a significant increase in self-efficacy from baseline ($M = 68.6$, SD $= 15.6$) to exit ($M = 77.6$, SD $= 16.1$), $t(15) = 3.90$, $P = 0.001$, 95% CI [4.05, 13.82], and Hedges's grm $= 0.55$. The common language (CL) effect size indicates that after controlling for individual differences, the likelihood that a person would score higher on self-efficacy at exit than at baseline is 83%. With regard to

TABLE 1: Sample characteristics.

	Baseline $n = 21$	Baseline and exit $n = 16$	Baseline, exit, and follow-up $n = 14$
Gender (%)			
Male	10 (47.6%)	8 (50.0%)	8 (57.1%)
Female	11 (52.4%)	8 (50.0%)	6 (42.9%)
Age (M; SD)	46.0 (11.4)	46.3 (10.1)	46.6 (10.1)
Months after injury (M; SD)	44.6 (64.5)	52.2 (70.4)	41.4 (61.8)
Education (%)			
Less than postsecondary	3 (14.3%)	3 (18.8%)	3 (21.4%)
Postsecondary	18 (85.7%)	13 (81.3%)	11 (78.6%)
Employment (%)			
Employed	3 (14.0%)	2 (12.5%)	2 (14%)
Unemployed/LTD	18 (86.0%)	14 (87.5%)	12 (86%)
Trauma (%)			
Traumatic	14 (66.7%)	11 (68.8%)	10 (71.4%)
Nontraumatic	7 (33.3%)	5 (31.3%)	4 (28.6%)
Level (%)			
Paraplegia	7 (33.3%)	5 (31.3%)	4 (28.6%)
Tetraplegia	12 (57.1%)	9 (56.3%)	9 (64.3%)
N/A	2 (9.5%)	2 (12.5%)	1 (7.1%)
Severity (%)			
Complete	4 (19.0%)	2 (12.5%)	2 (14.3%)
Incomplete	15 (71.4%)	12 (75.0%)	11 (78.6%)
N/A	2 (9.5%)	2 (12.5%)	1 (7.1%)

M: mean; SD: standard deviation; %: percent.

TABLE 2: CROP scores: baseline and exit ($n = 16$).

Scale	Baseline M (SD)	Exit M (SD)	$\overline{X_D}$ (SD)	95% CI	P
CISS: task-oriented	56.1 (7.1)	64.3 (8.1)	8.1 (10.6)	[2.5, 13.8]	0.008
CISS: emotion-oriented	48.1 (11.2)	42.8 (11.8)	−5.3 (10.2)	[−10.7, 0.2]	0.057
CISS: avoidance	42.2 (10.7)	48.6 (11.0)	6.4 (9.9)	[1.2, 11.7]	0.020
CISS: distraction	20.4 (5.9)	22.6 (5.5)	2.3 (6.4)	[−1.2, 5.7]	0.180
CISS: social diversion	14.6 (4.4)	16.9 (5.2)	2.3 (3.4)	[0.5, 4.1]	0.015
IPA: autonomy indoors	7.7 (7.9)	6.9 (6.5)	−0.8 (4.2)	[−3.0, 1.5]	0.483
IPA: autonomy outdoors	11.4 (5.2)	9.3 (4.5)	−2.2 (3.2)	[−3.9, −0.5]	0.015
IPA: family role	14.7 (7.9)	12.1 (6.3)	−2.6 (5.5)	[−5.5, 0.4]	0.084
IPA: social life	7.1 (5.8)	8.4 (5.6)	1.3 (5.0)	[−1.3, 4.0]	0.307
IPA: work and education[a]	7.9 (6.1)	5.9 (4.7)	−2.0 (6.0)	[−5.8, 1.8]	0.275
MSES	68.6 (15.6)	77.6 (16.1)	8.9 (9.2)	[4.1, 13.8]	0.001
PANAS PA	30.8 (7.4)	38.3 (8.0)	7.5 (7.6)	[3.5, 11.5]	0.001
PANAS NA	26.2 (10.6)	22.3 (8.3)	−4.1 (7.5)	[−8.1, −0.1]	0.047
WHOQOL: physical	20.7 (2.8)	20.9 (3.6)	0.3 (2.5)	[−1.1, 1.6]	0.697
WHOQOL: psychological	18.4 (3.6)	20.0 (3.8)	1.4 (2.3)	[0.1, 2.6]	0.031
WHOQOL: social	9.4 (2.6)	9.6 (2.5)	0.1 (2.0)	[−1.0, 1.2]	0.809
WHOQOL: environment	26.9 (5.2)	28.2 (5.6)	1.2 (4.8)	[−1.3, 3.8]	0.315

CISS: Coping Inventory for Stressful Situations; IPA: Impact on Participation and Autonomy; MSES: Moorong Self-Efficacy Scale; PANAS PA: Positive and Negative Affect Scale; PA: positive affect; NA: negative affect; WHOQOL-BREF: World Health Organization Quality of Life.
[a]$n = 13$; $\overline{X_D}$: mean difference; 95% CI: 95% confidence interval of the mean difference; SD: standard deviation; P: P value.

TABLE 3: CROP baseline, exit, and follow-up scores ($n = 14$).

Scale	Baseline M (IQR)	Exit M (IQR)	Follow-up M (IQR)	P
CISS: task-oriented	57.0 (13.0)	66.0 (9.0)	60.5 (17.0)	0.223
CISS: emotion-oriented	50.0 (18.0)	45.5 (20.0)	44.0 (22.0)	0.166
CISS: avoidance	41.5 (14.0)	48.0 (21.0)	43.0 (11.0)	0.089
CISS: distraction	22.0 (9.0)	22.5 (9.0)	16.5 (12.0)	0.102
CISS: social diversion	14.5 (6.0)	16.0 (10.0)	17.0 (6.0)	0.074
IPA: autonomy indoors	6.5 (11.0)	7.0 (11.0)	4.0 (11.0)	0.247
IPA: autonomy outdoors	12.5 (6.0)	10.0 (7.0)	12.0 (9.0)	0.199
IPA: family role	17.0 (13.0)	12.5 (10.0)	9.5 (14.0)	0.083
IPA: social life	7.9 (10.0)	7.5 (10.0)	7.5 (7.0)	0.945
IPA: work and educational[a]	7.0 (11.0)	4.0 (6.0)	4.0 (12.0)	0.559
MSES	68.5 (19.0)	77.5 (26.0)	77.0 (17.0)	0.027
PANAS PA	31.5 (15.0)	39.0 (11.0)	33.5 (14.0)	0.027
PANAS NA	26.0 (21.0)	19.0 (10.0)	24.0 (16.0)	0.584
WHOQOL: physical	21.0 (3.0)	21.0 (6.0)	22.5 (5.0)	0.020
WHOQOL: psychological	18.5 (6.0)	19.5 (7.0)	19.0 (6.0)	0.247
WHOQOL: social	10.0 (6.0)	10.0 (7.0)	9.0 (5.0)	0.472
WHOQOL: environment	25.0 (6.0)	29.0 (9.0)	27.5 (10.0)	0.410

CISS: Coping Inventory for Stressful Situations; IPA: Impact on Participation and Autonomy; MSES: Moorong Self-Efficacy Scale; PANAS PA: Positive and Negative Affect Scale; PA: positive affect; NA: negative affect; WHOQOL-BREF: World Health Organization Quality of Life.
[a]$n = 12$; M: median; IQR: interquartile range; P = P value.

positive affect, there was an increase in scores from baseline ($M = 30.75$, SD = 7.4) to exit ($M = 38.3$, SD = 8.0), $t(15) = 3.97$, $P = 0.001$, 95% CI [3.48, 11.53], and Hedges's grm = 0.95. The CL effect size indicates that after controlling for individual differences, the likelihood that a person would score higher on positive affect at exit than at baseline is 84%. Conversely, scores on negative affect decreased from baseline ($M = 26.19$, SD = 10.6) to exit ($M = 22.1$, SD = 8.3), $t(15) = -2.17$, $P = 0.047$, 95% CI [−8.06, −0.06], and Hedges's grm = 0.40. The CL effect size indicates that after controlling for individual differences, the likelihood that a person would score lower on negative affect at exit than at baseline is 71%.

With regard to task-oriented coping style as measured by the CISS, the mean score at exit ($M = 64.3$, SD = 8.1) was significantly higher than the mean score at baseline ($M = 56.1$, SD = 7.1), $t(15) = 3.05$, $P = 0.008$, 95% CI [2.45, 13.80], and Hedges's grm = 1.04. The CL effect size indicates that after controlling for individual differences, the likelihood that a person would score higher on CISS task-orientation at exit than on baseline is 77%. In terms of CISS avoidance-oriented coping, the mean score at exit ($M = 48.6$, SD = 11.0) was significantly higher than the mean score at baseline ($M = 42.2$, SD = 10.7), $t(15) = 2.61$, $P = 0.020$, 95% CI [1.17, 11.70], and Hedges's grm = 0.58. The CL size indicates that after controlling for individual differences, the likelihood that a person would score higher on CISS avoidance-oriented coping at exit than at baseline is 74%. Similarly, scores on CISS social diversion were significantly higher at exit ($M = 16.9$, SD = 5.2) than at baseline ($M = 14.6$, SD = 4.4), $t(15) = 2.74$, $P = 0.015$, 95% CI [0.511, 4.11], and Hedges's grm = 0.46. The CL effect size indicates that after controlling for individual

differences, the likelihood that a person would score higher on CISS social diversion at exit than at baseline is 75%.

In terms of QoL, there was an increase in psychological QoL (WHOQOL-BREF) from baseline ($M = 18.38$, SD = 3.6) to exit ($M = 19.75$, SD = 3.8), $t(15) = 2.39$, $P = 0.031$, 95% CI [0.15, 2.60], and Hedges's grm = 0.36. The CL effect size indicates that after controlling for individual differences, the likelihood that a person would score higher on psychological QoL at exit than at baseline is 72%. With regard to community participation, there was a significant decrease in the perceived barriers to autonomy in the outdoors (IPA) from baseline to exit, with scores decreasing from ($M = 11.4$, SD = 5.2) to ($M = 9.3$, SD = 4.5), $t(15) = -2.75$, $P = 0.015$, 95% CI [−3.89, −0.49], and Hedges's grm = 0.43. The CL effect size indicates that after controlling for individual differences, the likelihood that a person would have a better score on perceived outdoor autonomy at exit than at baseline is 75%.

3.3. Changes across CROP Baseline, Exit, and Follow-Up Scores. For persons who completed all the assessments ($n = 14$; Table 3), Friedman test indicated a significant difference for self-efficacy scores across time (MSES; $x^2 = 7.259$, $P = 0.027$). Post hoc comparisons revealed that self-efficacy scores at exit (median = 77.5) were significantly higher ($P = 0.003$) than baseline scores (median = 68.5) and that the increase was moderate in size ($r = 0.56$). However, no differences emerged between baseline and follow-up (median = 77.5) scores nor between exit and follow-up self-efficacy scores. Positive affect improved over time (PANAS; $x^2 = 7.259$, $P = 0.027$), with the difference ($P = 0.009$) only emerging between baseline (median = 31.5) and exit (median = 39.0) scores, and the size of this increase was moderate ($r = 0.50$).

TABLE 4: Themes and subthemes related to CROP service participation.

Theme	Role of self	Knowledge acquisition	Skill application	Group processes
	Gaining insight	Learning about SCI	Specific skill set	Group dynamics
	Assertiveness		Community participation	Share knowledge
Subtheme	Self-confidence	Skill acquisition		Learn from others
	Self-development	Tools		
	Timing of service	Topics		Supportive environment

Although there was a significant difference detected for physical QoL (WHOQOL-BREF; $x^2 = 7.840$, $P = 0.020$), post hoc comparisons negated this effect.

3.4. Qualitative Analysis. Four major themes (Table 4) related to therapeutic benefits emerged from the semistructured interviews: (1) role of self, (2) knowledge acquisition, (3) skill application, and (4) group processes. In addition, satisfaction with the CROP service was identified as a theme and subcategorized into positive and negative perceptions of the service, as well as a subcategory describing suggestions for CROP service improvement.

3.4.1. Role of Self. Participants spoke about finding themselves and their "post-SCI identity" through their participation in the program. The therapeutic benefits gained with regard to "role of self" included improved self-esteem, self-confidence, and a better understanding of their limitations associated with SCI.

The need to be assertive and advocate for necessary care to achieve important goals was also expressed by the sample. Some participants spoke of the importance of self-advocacy, specifically as it related to communicating their needs and limitations to caregivers, friends, and/or family. Participants expressed that their participation in the service enabled them to better assert themselves, which was related to their gains in self-confidence and a better understanding of their needs:

> "Suddenly I'll vocalize limitations, so they're like, are you wimping out on us... cause before I was like strong and I'm still strong, but now... I want a more balanced life... I respect my body a lot more." (ID number 115)

> "... it's also helped me deal with, like being more assertive, that was always an issue for me... like being able to say what I want to say instead of being quiet." (ID number 1209)

They were also better able to communicate this lifestyle change to their family:

> "... I've got the language." (ID number 115)

Timing of the service was also critical for some participants who recently were transitioned from inpatient to outpatient rehabilitation and were readjusting to community living. Gaining insight was frequently expressed and was a salient theme that emerged across interviews. For instance, participants gained not only insight into the limitations and

challenges associated with an SCI but also the ability to accept the limitations and move forward with a positive outlook:

> "It was a combination of learning about myself and you know how my situation relates to other people's situations." (ID number 119)

> "And I think it was [social worker] who said that sometime we're not even aware of emotions that are really kind of bogging us down, and I wasn't, and I think that as hard as it was at times facing those emotions, like the sadness and the loss that I feel... actually having faced them... the thing is that I feel lighter... like I can see myself opening up more in terms of accepting my limitations, I'm so much better." (ID number 115)

> "I mean you can always throw your towel in and surrender... or you can you know just smarten up and say-okay yes you know come to the realization of your present circumstances and deal with it." (ID number 120)

> "It (the CROP program) just changed my whole outlook on life and it's made a lot of positive changes." (ID number 1203)

> "... it helped me kind of realize I can, you know, do stuff on my own and, you know, everything would be okay, and how to deal with different things, emotions and all that kind of stuff that you're going through." (ID number 1209)

Most importantly, the CROP service instilled hope in many of the participants, and they expressed that the program opened up possibilities for the future:

> "It has widened my horizon as to the possibilities. Things could get better and you know... you know other things will come in." (ID number 120)

> "Psychologically, intellectually it's really... It changed my life... In the way that I think... and there is still some light." (ID number 121)

> "And in going through this program slowly got me to turn around and look more at what I still could do and why I should feel lucky rather than depressed." (ID number 1203)

> "It just helped to show us that there's still a hell of a lot that we can be thankful for." (ID number 1203)

3.4.2. Knowledge Acquisition. Participants spoke about how they acquired knowledge by participating in the program. Specifically, they described how they gained knowledge related to their SCI, which included self-management strategies. The knowledge and strategies were derived from the educational materials and from their "interactions with the group." Many of the participants were first interested in participating in the CROP service to acquire skills for community participation:

> "So life after SCI, if there's anymore... Like anything I can gain to help me integrate back into society." (ID number 116)

The CROP service allowed them to acquire specific skill sets and tools to assist them in the community:

> "I mean just like learning about the different issues and how not to just live with them, how to live well with them." (ID number 115)

> "It was really good... especially the resources that they can provide you... like readings and different materials... cause now you have all this information so, you know, if I need to look at something if I'm dealing with stress or something emotional, sometimes I just go and kind of look back at what we did and it's like oh yeah, I can deal with it, things in a different or better way." (ID number 1209)

3.4.3. Skill Application. Participants spoke about the opportunity the service provided them on being able to implement the skills gained in the community setting. Comments related to this were specifically related to the community outing undertaken by the group, which was done with support by the clinical facilitators. The community outing challenged them to use the skills that were taught throughout the group, such as energy conservation:

> "The outing was really useful... it was a good application of what we learned and talked about for all those weeks. Because like before you heard pace yourself, take breaks when you need to... then you go there and you do the exact opposite, you know? Until it starts taking its toll and then you realize-oh no I'm supposed to stop and rest. You know and you sort of reflect back at all those things were taught." (ID number 119)

Participants also spoke about how they applied the specific skills they learned (i.e., stress management) to their everyday lives:

> "For me it was just coping you know... you know the caregivers... and the course taught me how to take control, you know of my care and with the realization that nobody's gonna look after you like you." (ID number 116)

Many participants also expressed the desire to participate more actively in their community post-CROP service by setting short- and long-term goals, with a number of them relating specifically to work and leisure activities:

> "I've been doing the computer classes at the spinal cord resource centre... maybe I might end up being able to go back to work. But when I started out I had a grade 8 education, drove (a) truck all my life. I can't go back to that... I had nothing to offer anybody. Now I'm getting these courses... and we'll see what happens." (ID number 1203)

> "One of the sessions was... make a goal and do it... like trying, you know, different new sports. Like I'm going into a marathon, which I would have never done before... I'm just gonna do it. And I don't think I would have done that before without some of the issues that we discussed and having that confidence..." (ID number 1209)

3.4.4. Group Processes. Participants spoke about the group dynamics and supportive environment facilitating their learning and experiences in the CROP service. They were able to share their own knowledge and experiences of SCI and also learn from the experiences of others. Involvement in a group provided participants with an opportunity to reflect on how their condition was similar or different from other patients:

> "You know cause I felt like as someone who was once an able bodied person and now facing this new challenge of mobility and... I just wanted to get other people's take on it and see if I can benefit and if I can share any of my experiences with them also." (ID number 119)

The same participant also mentioned that

> "The group dynamic that I participated in was just phenomenal in the sense that everyone... participated, everyone gave some input... Like it was a real sharing." (ID number 119)

Group dynamics appeared to be an important factor of the group since they were able to relate to one another and discuss their struggles managing their SCI.

3.4.5. Program Satisfaction. The group was highly satisfied with the CROP service, particularly among the following areas: (1) supportive environment/facilitators, (2) format/topics, (3) resources, and (4) community outing. However, a majority of the group members felt that more time was needed for each session. They also felt that the program could have been longer overall (e.g., more sessions). Many of the participants spoke about how a follow-up service or additional resources after CROP completion would be beneficial for helping them to maintain their perceived gains in well-being.

4. Discussion

The aim of this project was to evaluate a therapeutic education service, namely, the CROP service, for improving well-being in community-dwelling persons with SCI. The findings indicate that there were a number of therapeutic benefits at the end of the service, with the gains in self-efficacy and positive affect having the most robust effect. However, the changes in these domains were not maintained over time (3 months later). Similarly, the patterns of scores for the other targeted domains, albeit nonsignificant, were in the expected direction but also returned towards baseline values at the 3-month follow-up. It is important to note that managing an SCI is a lifelong process due to the many secondary conditions that can occur [53] and not uncommon for someone to experience three to eight health conditions at any given time [2, 22]. Experiencing even one moderate or severe health condition (e.g., pressure ulcer) can have a significant impact on physical, psychological, and social well-being [4, 6, 8, 11]. Hence, the lack of significant findings at the follow-up assessment might be attributable to some of our participants having a "flare-up" of health conditions that impacted their well-being across a number of areas. Overall, our hypotheses were only partially confirmed, but the moderate and reliable effect sizes related to improved mood and self-efficacy provide important evidence for the clinical utility of the CROP service.

The qualitative analysis revealed that participants experienced therapeutic gains and were highly satisfied with the service, which provides additional evidence on the perceived value of the CROP service. Many of the participants felt they gained relevant knowledge and coping skills for community participation and valued the opportunity for sharing their insights with peers. The comments provided by the participants also suggest that the domains the outcome measures assessed were appropriate (e.g., gains in self-confidence). The lack of significant findings on the standardized outcome measures may have been due to the need for a follow-up service or additional resources after CROP completion to sustain the positive effects of the program over time. This issue was highlighted by the participants, who felt that having an additional or "booster" session following the service would be helpful. Although the service was held over an intense three-month period (12 weeks × 1 session per week for 120 minutes each session), the need for more time was a salient theme, which suggests either the weekly sessions could have been extended or perhaps the intensity of the program could be delivered in wider intervals (e.g., every two weeks). There is some evidence on the effectiveness of self-management programs after SCI that are implemented across wider time periods (e.g., bimonthly) and that have longer sessions (e.g., half-day) [54].

The findings regarding self-efficacy are particularly noteworthy since it is a key construct associated with positive outcomes after SCI [16, 54]. Several other self-management programs also strive to improve self-efficacy in their clients [13, 54, 55]. For instance, in "Project Shake-It-Up," which is a health promotion and capacity building program for people with SCI, multiple sclerosis, and related neurological impairments, it was found that self-efficacy increased in participants compared to nonparticipants and that these gains were maintained over a 12-month period [54]. The maintained increases in self-efficacy might be attributable to the program incorporating leisure-based activities and taking

place entirely in the community. For instance, participants were provided with opportunities to engage in a variety of indoor and outdoor physical recreational activities (e.g., strength training, sailing, sea kayaking, hand cycling, etc.) each afternoon of the program, while the morning seminar sessions took place in different community-based settings (e.g., libraries, university campuses, state parks, etc.). As such, the opportunity to "learn" in the community and to engage in "physical/recreational" activities may have provided an additional boost towards elevating and maintaining self-efficacy in the "Project Shake-It-Up" participants. Engagement in physically active recreational activities has been shown to elevate both mood and self-efficacy in people with SCI [56]. Although the CROP service did provide a community outing, there might be a need for more opportunities for the group to practice the skills and knowledge learned in a variety of community settings.

Based on the findings from other self-management programs [13, 54, 55], along with the demonstrated increases in mood and self-efficacy in the present sample, it appears that the tools, resources, and support provided by the CROP service provided participants with the perception that they have the skills to manage challenges and achieve their goals for community living. Participants expressed that the group processes within a supportive environment facilitated their learning and promoted therapeutic gains. Engaging in group sessions may have contributed to a significant increase in self-efficacy since social comparison is an important mechanism for self-efficacy [13].

The themes that emerged from the interviews are closely related to the phenomenon of "posttraumatic growth." This describes individuals who have experienced a traumatic event and have come to view the event as an avenue for personal development and growth [57]. This perception tends to lead to positive outcomes, such as (1) improved interpersonal relationships, (2) positive change in the perception of the self, and (3) an emerging or developing philosophy of life [57]. Themes such as gaining insight, group dynamics, and self-development suggest that participants may have been describing their experience of posttraumatic growth. Although further work is required to explore this construct, participation in the CROP service may serve to foster posttraumatic growth for this population.

The evaluation of the CROP service was done to provide information on its impact for helping people with SCI maintain health and well-being in the community. At this time, the CROP service is only being provided on a pilot basis, and data supporting its efficacy will serve to determine its value for including it as part of standard clinical care. The evaluation also provided important information related to decision making on the CROP service implementation since there is a need to further refine strategies on how initial gains can be maintained over time. Relatedly, program evaluation should be an on-going process to ensure that clinical programs are effectively meeting the needs of their clients. The present evaluation was framed within a research perspective but future evaluations will work to refine the selection and use of outcome measures in order to provide information that is clinically meaningful to both clinicians and patients to aid in evaluating the CROP service's efficacy at the individual level [58]. Doing so may better provide insight to what processes promote immediate gains after service in the participant and what additional supports they can access to maintain their long-term gains.

4.1. Study Limitations. A limitation of the current study is the small size of our sample, which may have accounted for our lack of significant findings. Further work using a larger sample size may conclusively demonstrate the effectiveness of the CROP service. However, the findings from the qualitative component achieved saturation, which indicates a number of positive outcomes associated with participating in the service. A second limitation is that participant interviews were conducted at completion of the service. A follow-up interview at the three-month follow-up may have provided additional insight on why the gains in self-efficacy and positive affect were not maintained over time. It is also possible that the group did undergo some actual changes in the ability to cope with living with an SCI in the community, but our long-term follow-up surveys may not have been suited or sensitive enough to capture these changes. The use of a "waiting list" control group may have also helped to demonstrate if the changes in scores were directly attributable to participation in the CROP. Another limitation was the inability to follow-up with our entire sample on all of the planned assessments. Only 16 of the initial 21 persons completed the baseline and exit assessments and only 14 completed all three assessments. The loss of participants across assessment intervals may have affected our outcomes.

5. Conclusion

There is a need for effective interventions for improving community participation and QoL after SCI, and the CROP service is a promising intervention for helping people with SCI to achieve this goal. Further work is required to help participants maintain the long-term therapeutic gains in the community but is an important service that provides skills and knowledge to people with SCI on how to better manage the emotional, environmental, and social stressors that challenge community participation.

Clinical Messages

(i) Sustaining a spinal cord injury (SCI) creates a number of challenges for maintaining health and well-being in the community. Self-management programs, such as the community reintegration outpatient (CROP) service, are promising for helping people to offset regular stressors associated with SCI.

(ii) Self-management programs using a group approach might contribute to gains in self-efficacy and positive affect, but follow-up sessions or additional resources might be required to sustain therapeutic gains over time.

Appendix

The purpose of this interview is to get an understanding of your experiences from participating in the CROP service.

Question 1: what were your expectations of the CROP service?

Question 2: what aspects of the program did you find enjoyable?

Question 3: what aspects of the program did you not like or thought could be improved?

Question 4: what were some of the changes (emotional, physical, etc.), if any, you noticed about yourself during or after the CROP service?

Question 5: what types of community-based activities, if any, do you think you may pursue after participating in the program that you were not pursuing before attending?

Question 6: overall, how satisfied were you with the program?

Conflict of Interests

Alana Zinman, Nicole Digout, Debbie Hébert, and Sander L. Hitzig have no conflict of interests regarding the publication of this paper. Patricia Bain and Sylvia Haycock designed and implemented the CROP program.

Acknowledgments

Salary support to Dr. Sander L. Hitzig was provided by the Ontario Neurotrauma Foundation and the Rick Hansen Institute (Grant no. 2010-RHI-MTNI-836). Support was provided by the Toronto Rehabilitation Institute, which receives funding under the Provincial Rehabilitation Research Program from the Ministry of Health and Long-Term Care in Ontario. The views expressed do not necessarily reflect those of the Ministry.

References

[1] K. A. Boschen, M. Tonack, and J. Gargaro, "Long-term adjustment and community reintegration following spinal cord injury," *International Journal of Rehabilitation Research*, vol. 26, no. 3, pp. 157–164, 2003.

[2] S. L. Hitzig, M. Tonack, K. A. Campbell et al., "Secondary health complications in an aging canadian spinal cord injury sample," *American Journal of Physical Medicine and Rehabilitation*, vol. 87, no. 7, pp. 545–555, 2008.

[3] H. Krueger, V. K. Noonan, L. M. Trenaman, P. Joshi, and C. S. Rivers, "The economic burden of traumatic spinal cord injury in Canada," *Chronic Diseases and Injuries in Canada*, vol. 33, no. 3, pp. 113–122, 2013.

[4] M. Tonack, S. L. Hitzig, B. C. Craven, K. A. Campbell, K. A. Boschen, and C. F. McGillivray, "Predicting life satisfaction after spinal cord injury in a Canadian sample," *Spinal Cord*, vol. 46, no. 5, pp. 380–385, 2008.

[5] P. Kennedy, P. Lude, and N. Taylor, "Quality of life, social participation, appraisals and coping post spinal cord injury: a review of four community samples," *Spinal Cord*, vol. 44, no. 2, pp. 95–105, 2006.

[6] E. Martz, H. Livneh, M. Priebe, L. A. Wuermser, and L. Ottomanelli, "Predictors of psychosocial adaptation among people with spinal cord injury or disorder," *Archives of Physical Medicine and Rehabilitation*, vol. 86, no. 6, pp. 1182–1192, 2005.

[7] S. Mehta, S. Orenczuk, K. T. Hansen et al., "An evidence-based review of the effectiveness of cognitive behavioral therapy for psychosocial issues post-spinal cord injury," *Rehabilitation Psychology*, vol. 56, no. 1, pp. 15–25, 2011.

[8] H.-Y. Song, "Modeling social reintegration in persons with spinal cord injury," *Disability and Rehabilitation*, vol. 27, no. 3, pp. 131–141, 2005.

[9] P. Kennedy, P. Lude, M. L. Elfström, and E. Smithson, "Appraisals, coping and adjustment pre and post SCI rehabilitation: a 2-year follow-up study," *Spinal Cord*, vol. 50, no. 2, pp. 112–118, 2012.

[10] A. Gélis, A. Stéfan, D. Colin et al., "Therapeutic education in persons with spinal cord injury: a review of the literature," *Annals of Physical and Rehabilitation Medicine*, vol. 54, no. 3, pp. 189–210, 2011.

[11] T. Kroll, M. T. Neri, and P.-S. Ho, "Secondary conditions in spinal cord injury: results from a prospective survey," *Disability and Rehabilitation*, vol. 29, no. 15, pp. 1229–1237, 2007.

[12] S. E. P. Munce, F. Webster, M. G. Fehlings, S. E. Straus, E. Jang, and S. B. Jaglal, "Perceived facilitators and barriers to self-management in individuals with traumatic spinal cord injury: a qualitative descriptive study," *BMC Neurology*, vol. 14, article 48, 2014.

[13] R. C. Hirsche, B. Williams, A. Jones, and P. Manns, "Chronic disease self-management for individuals with stroke, multiple sclerosis and spinal cord injury," *Disability and Rehabilitation*, vol. 33, no. 13-14, pp. 1136–1146, 2011.

[14] A. Bandura, *Social Foundations of Thought and Actions: A Social Cognitive Theory*, Prentice Hall, Englewood Cliffs, NJ, USA, 1986.

[15] M. A. van Loo, M. W. M. Post, J. H. A. Bloemen, and F. W. A. van Asbeck, "Care needs of persons with long-term spinal cord injury living at home in the Netherlands," *Spinal Cord*, vol. 48, no. 5, pp. 423–428, 2010.

[16] M. Y. C. Pang, J. J. Eng, K.-H. Lin, P.-F. Tang, C. Hung, and Y.-H. Wang, "Association of depression and pain interference with disease-management self-efficacy in community-dwelling individuals with spinal cord injury," *Journal of Rehabilitation Medicine*, vol. 41, no. 13, pp. 1068–1073, 2009.

[17] J. D. Corrigan, "Community integration following traumatic brain injury," *NeuroRehabilitation*, vol. 4, no. 2, pp. 109–121, 1994.

[18] M. Dijkers, "Community integration: conceptual issues and measurement approaches in rehabilitation research," *Topics in Spinal Cord Injury Rehabilitation*, vol. 4, no. 1, pp. 1–15, 1998.

[19] I. B. Lidal, M. Veenstra, N. Hjeltnes, and F. Biering-Sørensen, "Health-related quality of life in persons with long-standing spinal cord injury," *Spinal Cord*, vol. 46, no. 11, pp. 710–715, 2008.

[20] C. Carpenter, S. J. Forwell, L. E. Jongbloed, and C. L. Backman, "Community participation after spinal cord injury," *Archives of Physical Medicine and Rehabilitation*, vol. 88, no. 4, pp. 427–433, 2007.

[21] *2006 Annual Statistical Report*, National Spinal Cord Injury Statistical Center, University of Alabama at Birmingham, 2006.

[22] L. Noreau, P. Proulx, L. Gagnon, M. Drolet, and M.-T. Laramée, "Secondary impairments after spinal cord injury: a population-based study," *American Journal of Physical Medicine & Rehabilitation*, vol. 79, no. 6, pp. 526–535, 2000.

[23] C. Pollard and P. Kennedy, "A longitudinal analysis of emotional impact, coping strategies and post-traumatic psychological growth following spinal cord injury: a 10-year review," *British Journal of Health Psychology*, vol. 12, no. 3, pp. 347–362, 2007.

[24] M. Vissers, R. van den Berg-Emons, T. Sluis, M. Bergen, H. Stam, and H. Bussmann, "Barriers to and facilitators of everyday physical activity in persons with a spinal cord injury after discharge from the rehabilitation centre," *Journal of Rehabilitation Medicine*, vol. 40, no. 6, pp. 461–467, 2008.

[25] R. J. Cox, D. I. Amsters, and K. J. Pershouse, "The need for a multidisciplinary outreach service for people with spinal cord injury living in the community," *Clinical Rehabilitation*, vol. 15, no. 6, pp. 600–606, 2001.

[26] G. Whiteneck, M. A. Meade, M. Dijkers, D. G. Tate, T. Bushnik, and M. B. Forchheimer, "Environmental factors and their role in participation and life satisfaction after spinal cord injury," *Archives of Physical Medicine and Rehabilitation*, vol. 85, no. 11, pp. 1793–1803, 2004.

[27] G. Whitfield, "Group cognitive-behavioural therapy for anxiety and depression," *Advances in Psychiatric Treatment*, vol. 16, no. 3, pp. 219–227, 2010.

[28] A. T. Beck, A. J. Rush, B. F. Shaw et al., *Cognitive Therapy of Depression*, Guilford Press, 1979.

[29] C. Dedding, M. Cardol, I. C. J. M. Eyssen, J. Dekker, and A. Beelen, "Validity of the Canadian occupational performance measure: a client-centred outcome measurement," *Clinical Rehabilitation*, vol. 18, no. 6, pp. 660–667, 2004.

[30] D. Kolb, *Experiential Learning: Experience as the Source of Learning and Development*, Prentice Hall, Englewood Cliffs, NJ, USA, 1984.

[31] M. J. Knowles, *The Adult Learner: A Neglected Species*, Gulf Publishing, Houston, Tex, USA, 3rd edition, 1994.

[32] I. Yalom, *The Theory and Practice of Group Psychotherapy*, Basic Books, 4th edition, 1995.

[33] J. R. White and A. Freeman, Eds., *Cognitive-Behavioral Group Therapy for Specific Problems and Populations*, American Psychological Association, 2000.

[34] S. L. Wood-Dauphinee, M. A. Opzoomer, J. I. Williams, B. Marchand, and W. O. Spitzer, "Assessment of global function: the reintegration to normal living index," *Archives of Physical Medicine and Rehabilitation*, vol. 69, no. 8, pp. 583–590, 1988.

[35] S. L. Hitzig, E. M. Romero Escobar, L. Noreau, and B. C. Craven, "Validation of the reintegration to normal living index for community-dwelling persons with chronic spinal cord injury," *Archives of Physical Medicine and Rehabilitation*, vol. 93, no. 1, pp. 108–114, 2012.

[36] S. M. Skevington, M. Lotfy, and K. A. O'Connell, "The World Health Organization's WHOQOL-BREF quality of life assessment: psychometric properties and results of the international field trial. A report from the WHOQOL Group," *Quality of Life Research*, vol. 13, no. 2, pp. 299–310, 2004.

[37] S. M. Miller, F. Chan, J. M. Ferrin, C.-P. Lin, and J. Y. C. Chan, "Confirmatory factor analysis of the World Health Organization quality of life questionnaire: brief version for individuals with spinal cord injury," *Rehabilitation Counseling Bulletin*, vol. 51, no. 4, pp. 221–228, 2008.

[38] N. S. Endler and J. D. A. Parker, "Assessment of multidimensional coping: task, emotion, and avoidance strategies," *Psychological Assessment*, vol. 6, no. 1, pp. 50–60, 1994.

[39] D. A. Groomes and M. J. Leahy, "The relationships among the stress appraisal process, coping disposition, and level of acceptance of disability," *Rehabilitation Counseling Bulletin*, vol. 46, no. 1, pp. 12–23, 2002.

[40] D. Watson, L. A. Clark, and A. Tellegen, "Development and validation of brief measures of positive and negative affect: The PANAS scale," *Journal of Personality and Social Psychology*, vol. 54, no. 6, pp. 1063–1070, 1988.

[41] G. V. Ostir, P. M. Smith, D. Smith, and K. J. Ottenbacher, "Reliability of the positive and negative affect schedule (PANAS) in medical rehabilitation," *Clinical Rehabilitation*, vol. 19, no. 7, pp. 767–769, 2005.

[42] J. R. Crawford and J. D. Henry, "The Positive and Negative Affect Schedule (PANAS): construct validity, measurement properties and normative data in a large non-clinical sample," *British Journal of Clinical Psychology*, vol. 43, no. 3, pp. 245–265, 2004.

[43] J. W. Middleton, R. L. Tate, and T. J. Geraghty, "Self-efficacy and spinal cord injury psychometric properties of a new scale," *Rehabilitation Psychology*, vol. 48, no. 4, pp. 281–288, 2003.

[44] S. M. Miller, "The measurement of self-efficacy in persons with spinal cord injury: psychometric validation of the moorong self-efficacy scale," *Disability and Rehabilitation*, vol. 31, no. 12, pp. 988–993, 2009.

[45] M. Cardol, R. J. de Haan, G. A. M. van den Bos, B. A. de Jong, and I. J. M. de Groot, "The development of a handicap assessment questionnaire: the Impact on Participation and Autonomy (IPA)," *Clinical Rehabilitation*, vol. 13, no. 5, pp. 411–419, 1999.

[46] S. R. Magasi, A. W. Heinemann, and G. G. Whiteneck, "Participation following traumatic spinal cord injury: an evidence-based review for research," *The Journal of Spinal Cord Medicine*, vol. 31, no. 2, pp. 145–156, 2008.

[47] V. K. Noonan, J. A. Kopec, L. Noreau et al., "Measuring participation among persons with spinal cord injury: comparison of three instruments," *Topics in Spinal Cord Injury Rehabilitation*, vol. 15, no. 4, pp. 49–62, 2010.

[48] D. Lakens, "Calculating and reporting effect sizes to facilitate cumulative science: a practical primer for t-tests and ANOVAs," *Frontiers in Psychology*, vol. 4, article 863, 2013.

[49] M. Sandelowski, "Whatever happened to qualitative description?" *Research in Nursing & Health*, vol. 23, no. 4, pp. 334–340, 2000.

[50] J. W. Creswell, *Research Design: Qualitative, Quantitative, and Mixed Methods Approaches*, Sage, Thousand Oaks, Calif, USA, 2nd edition, 2003.

[51] U. H. Graneheim and B. Lundman, "Qualitative content analysis in nursing research: concepts, procedures and measures to achieve trustworthiness," *Nurse Education Today*, vol. 24, no. 2, pp. 105–112, 2004.

[52] P. Burnard, "A method of analysing interview transcripts in qualitative research," *Nurse Education Today*, vol. 11, no. 6, pp. 461–466, 1991.

[53] S. L. Hitzig, J. J. Eng, W. C. Miller, and B. M. Sakakibara, "An evidence-based review of aging of the body systems following spinal cord injury," *Spinal Cord*, vol. 49, no. 6, pp. 684–701, 2011.

[54] P. Block, E. A. Vanner, C. B. Keys, J. H. Rimmer, and S. E. Skeels, "Project shake-it-up: using health promotion, capacity building and a disability studies framework to increase self efficacy," *Disability and Rehabilitation*, vol. 32, no. 9, pp. 741–754, 2010.

[55] P. Block, S. E. Skeels, C. B. Keys, and J. H. Rimmer, "Shake-It-Up: health promotion and capacity building for people with spinal cord injuries and related neurological disabilities," *Disability and Rehabilitation*, vol. 27, no. 4, pp. 185–190, 2005.

[56] S. L. Hitzig, C. Alton, N. Leong, and K. Gatt, "The evolution and evaluation of a therapeutic recreation cottage program for persons with spinal cord injury," *Therapeutic Recreation Journal*, vol. 46, no. 3, pp. 218–233, 2012.

[57] R. G. Tedeschi and L. G. Calhoun, "The posttraumatic growth inventory: measuring the positive legacy of trauma," *Journal of Traumatic Stress*, vol. 9, no. 3, pp. 455–471, 1996.

[58] D. A. Revicki, D. Cella, R. D. Hays, J. A. Sloan, W. R. Lenderking, and N. K. Aaronson, "Responsiveness and minimal important differences for patient reported outcomes," *Health and Quality of Life Outcomes*, vol. 4, article 70, 2006.

Permissions

List of Contributors

Lampros Samartzis
Department of Neurology, General Hospital of the Greek Red Cross "Korgialeneio-Benakeio", Athens, Greece
Department of Psychiatry, Athalassa Mental Health Hospital, Nicosia, Cyprus
St. George's University of London Medical School, University of Nicosia, Nicosia, Cyprus

Efthymia Gavala, Achilleas Aspiotis and Thomas Thomaides
Department of Neurology, General Hospital of the Greek Red Cross "Korgialeneio-Benakeio", Athens, Greece

Yiannis Zoukos
Department of Neurology, St. Bartholomew's Royal London and Broomfield Hospitals, London, UK

Rozina Bhimani
Department of Nursing, St. Catherine University, St. Paul, MN 55105, USA

Lisa Anderson
Department of Integrative Biology and Physiology, University of Minnesota, Minneapolis, MN 55455, USA

Annick Champagne, François Prince and Vicky Bouffard
Department of Kinesiology, University of Montreal, Montreal, QC, Canada H3T 1J4

Danik Lafond
Department of Kinesiology, University of Montreal, Montreal, QC, Canada H3T 1J4
Department of Physical Activity Sciences, University of Quebec, Trois-Rivi`eres, QC, Canada G9A 5H7

Giuseppe Caminiti, Francesca Ranghi, Sara De Benedetti, Daniela Battaglia, Arianna Arisi, Alessio Franchini, Fabiana Facchini, Veronica Cioffi, and Maurizio Volterrani
Cardiovascular Research Unit, Department of Medical Sciences, IRCCS San Raffaele, Via della Pisana 235, 00163 Rome, Italy

David A. Barclay
Department of Social Work, Gallaudet University, 800 Florida Avenue NE, Washington, DC 20008, USA

Yvonne Severinsson
Department of Stomatognathic Physiology, Institute of Odontology, The Sahlgrenska Academy, University of Gothenburg, Gothenburg, Sweden

Lena Elisson and Olle Bunketorp
Department of Orthopaedics, The Institute of Clinical Sciences, The Sahlgrenska Academy, University of Gothenburg, Gothenburg, Sweden

D. M. van Leeuwen and A. de Haan
MOVE Research Institute Amsterdam, Faculty of Human Movement Sciences, VU University Amsterdam, Van der Boechorststraat 9, 1081 BT, Amsterdam, The Netherlands
Institute for Biomedical Research into Human Movement and Health, Manchester Metropolitan University, Manchester M1 5GD, UK

C. J. de Ruiter
MOVE Research Institute Amsterdam, Faculty of Human Movement Sciences, VU University Amsterdam, Van der Boechorststraat 9, 1081 BT, Amsterdam, The Netherlands

P. A. Nolte
Department of Orthopedics, Spaarne Hospital, Spaarnepoort 1, 2134 TM Hoofddorp, The Netherlands

Natasha Layton
School of Health and Social Development, Deakin University, 221 Burwood Highway, Burwood, VIC 3125, Australia

Kamal Narayan Arya, Shanta Pandian, C. R. Abhilasha and Ashutosh Verma
Pandit Deendayal Upadhyaya Institute for the Physically Handicapped (University of Delhi), Ministry of Social Justice and Empowerment, Government of India, 4 VD Marg, New Delhi 110002, India

Kirsten Fonager
Department of Social Medicine, Center for Cardiovascular Research, Aalborg University Hospital, 9100 Aalborg, Denmark
Department of Health Science and Technology, Faculty of Medicine, Aalborg University, 9220 Aalborg, Denmark

Søren Lundbye-Christensen
Department of Social Medicine, Center for Cardiovascular Research, Aalborg University Hospital, 9100 Aalborg, Denmark

Jan Jesper Andreasen
Department of Cardiothoracic Surgery, Center for Cardiovascular Research, Aalborg University Hospital, 9100 Aalborg, Denmark
Department of Clinical Medicine, Aalborg University, 9100 Aalborg, Denmark

Mikkel Futtrup, Anette Luther Christensen, Khalil Ahmad and Martin Agge Nørgaard
Department of Cardiothoracic Surgery, Center for Cardiovascular Research, Aalborg University Hospital, 9100 Aalborg, Denmark

Emil Sundstrup, Markus D. Jakobsen and Kenneth Jay
National Research Centre for the Working Environment, Lersø Parkalle 105, 2100 Copenhagen O, Denmark
Institute for Sports Science and Clinical Biomechanics, University of Southern Denmark, 5230 Odense M, Denmark

Juan Carlos Colado
Laboratory of Physical Activity and Health, Research Group in Sport and Health, Department of Physical Education and Sports, University of Valencia, 46010 Valencia, Spain

Yuling Wang
Department of Rehabilitation Medicine, The Sixth Affiliated Hospital of Sun Yat-sen University, No. 26 Yuancun 2nd Cross Road, Guangzhou 510655, China

Lars L. Andersen and Mikkel Brandt
National Research Centre for the Working Environment, Lersø Parkalle 105, 2100 Copenhagen O, Denmark

M.-N. Levaux
Cognitive Psychopathology Unit, Department of Psychology: Cognition and Behavior, University of Liége, 4000 Liége, Belgium
Psychiatry Service I, Inserm 666 Unit, 67091 Strasbourg, France

B. Fonteneau and F. Larøi
Cognitive Psychopathology Unit, Department of Psychology: Cognition and Behavior, University of Liége, 4000 Liége, Belgium

I. Offerlin-Meyer and J.-M. Danion
Psychiatry Service I, Inserm 666 Unit, 67091 Strasbourg, France

M. Van der Linden
Cognitive Psychopathology Unit, Department of Psychology: Cognition and Behavior, University of Liége, 4000 Liége, Belgium
Cognitive Psychopathology and Neuropsychology Unit, University of Geneva, 1211 Geneva, Switzerland

Michel Silva Reis
Department of Physical Therapy, School of Medicine, Federal University of Rio de Janeiro, 8° Floor 3 (8E-03), Prof Rodolpho Paulo Rocco Street, 21941-913 Rio de Janeiro, RJ, Brazil

João Luiz Quagliotti Durigan
Physical Therapy Division, University of Brasília, QNN 14 Área Especial, Ceilândia Sul, 72220-140 Brasília, DF, Brazil

Ross Arena
Department of Physical Therapy and Integrative Physiology Laboratory, College of Applied Health Sciences, University of Illinois, 1919W. Taylor Street (MC 898), Chicago, IL 60612, USA

Bruno Rafael Orsini Rossi
Healthy-School Unit, Federal University of Sao Carlos, 235 Km. Washington Luis Rodovia, 13565-905 Sao Carlos, SP, Brazil

Renata Gonçalves Mendes and Audrey Borghi-Silva
Laboratory of Cardiopulmonary Physiotherapy, Federal University of Sao Carlos, 235 Km. Washington Luis Rodovia, 13565-905 Sao Carlos, SP, Brazil

Michael O. Harris-Love
Research Service/Geriatrics and Extended Care, Washington, DC Veterans Affairs Medical Center, 50 Irving Street, NW, Room 11G, Washington, DC 20422, USA
School of Public Health and Health Services, George Washington University, 2033 K Street, NW, Suite 210, Washington, DC 20006, USA
Rehabilitation Medicine Department, Clinical Center, Department of Health and Human Services (DHHS), National Institutes of Health (NIH), 10 Center Drive, Bethesda, MD 20892, USA

Lindsay Fernandez-Rhodes
National Institute of Neurological Disorders and Stroke (NINDS), Neurogenetics Branch, Department of Health and Human Services (DHHS), National Institutes of Health (NIH), Building 35, Room 2A-1000, 35 Convent Drive, MSC 3705, Bethesda, MD 20892, USA
Department of Epidemiology, University of North Carolina at Chapel Hill Gillings, School of Global Public Health, 170 Rosenau Hall, Campus Box 7400, 135Dauer Drive, Chapel Hill, NC 27599,USA

Ellen Levy, Galen Joe and Joseph A. Shrader
Rehabilitation Medicine Department, Clinical Center, Department of Health and Human Services (DHHS), National Institutes of Health (NIH), 10 Center Drive, Bethesda, MD 20892, USA

Alison La Pean Kirschner
National Institute of Neurological Disorders and Stroke (NINDS), Neurogenetics Branch, Department of Health and Human Services (DHHS), National Institutes of Health (NIH), Building 35, Room 2A-1000, 35 Convent Drive, MSC 3705, Bethesda, MD 20892, USA
Center for Patient Care and Outcomes Research, Medical College of Wisconsin, 8701Watertown Plank Road, Milwaukee ,WI 53226, USA

Sungyoung Auh
ClinicalNeurosciences Program, NINDS, NIH, 10 Center Drive, Room 5N230, Bethesda, MD20814, USA

Cheunju Chen
National Institute of Neurological Disorders and Stroke (NINDS), Neurogenetics Branch, Department of Health and Human Services (DHHS), National Institutes of Health (NIH), Building 35, Room 2A-1000, 35 Convent Drive, MSC 3705, Bethesda, MD 20892, USA
Neurology Department, University of Maryland, 110 South Paca Street, Baltimore, MD 21201, USA

Li Li
Rehabilitation Medicine Department, Clinical Center, Department of Health and Human Services (DHHS), National Institutes of Health (NIH), 10 Center Drive, Bethesda, MD 20892, USA
Physical Medicine and Rehabilitation Service, Veterans Affairs Medical Center, 650 East Indian School Road, Phoenix AZ 85012, USA

Todd E. Davenport
Department of Physical Therapy, Thomas J. Long School of Pharmacy & Health Sciences, University of the Pacific, 3601 Pacific Avenue, Stockton, CA 95211, USA

Angela Kokkinis, Nicholas A. Di Prospero and Kenneth H. Fischbeck
National Institute of Neurological Disorders and Stroke (NINDS), Neurogenetics Branch, Department of Health and Human Services (DHHS), National Institutes of Health (NIH), Building 35, Room 2A-1000, 35 Convent Drive, MSC 3705, Bethesda, MD 20892, USA

Chinonso Igwesi-Chidobe
Department of Medical Rehabilitation, Faculty of Health Sciences and Technology, College of Medicine, University of Nigeria, Enugu Campus, 400006 Enugu, Nigeria

Kazuhiro Yasuda and Yuki Sato
Global Robot Academia Laboratory, Green Computing Systems Research Organization, Waseda University, 27Waseda-cho, Shinjuku-ku, Tokyo 162-0042, Japan

Naoyuki Iimura and Hiroyasu Iwata
Graduate School of Creative Science and Engineering, Waseda University, 3-4-1 Okubo, Shinjuku-ku, Tokyo 169-8555, Japan

Yu-ping Chen
Department of Physical Therapy, Georgia State University, P.O. Box 4019, Atlanta, GA 30302-4019, USA
Center for Pediatric Locomotion Sciences, Georgia State University, Atlanta, GA 30302-3975, USA

Michelle Caldwell, Erica Dickerhoof, Anastasia Hall, Bryan Odakura and Kimberly Morelli
Department of Physical Therapy, Georgia State University, P.O. Box 4019, Atlanta, GA 30302-4019, USA

Hsin-Chen Fanchiang
Center for Pediatric Locomotion Sciences, Georgia State University, Atlanta, GA 30302-3975, USA

Noel Rao, Gnanapradeep Priyan Perera, Padma Srigiriraju and Gnanapragasam
Marianjoy Rehabilitation Hospital, 26W171 Roosevelt Road, Wheaton, IL 60187, USA

JasonWening and Daniel Hasso
Scheck & Siress, 1551 Bond Street, Naperville, IL 60563, USA

Alexander S. Aruin
Marianjoy Rehabilitation Hospital, 26W171 Roosevelt Road, Wheaton, IL 60187, USA
Department of Physical Therapy (MC 898), University of Illinois at Chicago, 1919West Taylor Street, Chicago, IL 60612, USA

Takashi Fukaya
Department of Physical Therapy, Faculty of Health Sciences, Tsukuba International University, 6-8-33 Manabe, Ibaraki, Tsuchiura 300-0051, Japan

HirotakaMutsuzaki and YasuyoshiWadano
Department of Orthopedic Surgery, Ibaraki Prefectural University of Health Sciences, 4669-2 Ami, Ibaraki, Ami-machi 300-0394, Japan

Hirofumi Ida
Department of Human System Science, Tokyo Institute of Technology, 2-12-1 Oh-okayama, Meguro, Tokyo 152-8550, Japan

Luciana Bahia Gontijo and Ana Paula Santos
Physical Therapy Department, Federal University of the Valleys of Jequitinhonha and Mucuri, 39100-000 Diamantina, MG, Brazil

Polianna Delfino Pereira
Department of Neuroscience and Behavioral Sciences, School of Medicine of Ribeirão Preto, University of São Paulo, 14049-900 Ribeirão Preto, SP, Brazil

Camila Danielle Cunha Neves
Multicenter Post Graduation Program in Physiological Sciences, Federal University of the Valleys of Jequitinhonha and Mucuri, 39100-000 Diamantina, MG, Brazil

Dionis de Castro DutraMachado
Physical Therapy Department, Brain Mapping Lab & Functionality, Federal University of Piauí, 64202-020 Parnaíba, PI, Brazil

Victor Hugo do Vale Bastos
Physical Therapy Department, Brain Mapping Lab & Functionality, Federal University of Piauí, 64202-020 Parnaíba, PI, Brazil
CNPq, 71605-001 Brasília, DF, Brazil

Mohamed Ali Elshafey
Department of Physical Therapy for Growth and Developmental Disorder in Children and Its Surgery,Faculty of Physical Therapy, Cairo University, Egypt

Adel Abd-Elaziem
Faculty of Medicine, Zagazig University, Egypt

Rana Elmarzouki Gouda
Physical Therapy Department, General Hospital of Mit Ghamr, Egypt

Siv Svensson and Katharina Stibrant Sunnerhagen
Institute of Neuroscience and Physiology/Rehabilitation Medicine, Sahlgrenska Academy, University of Gothenburg, 3rd floor, Per Dubbsgatan 14, 413 45 Gothenburg, Sweden

Cassandra W. H. Ho, W. T. Cheung and Titanic F. O. Lau
Physiotherapy Department, Tai Po Hospital, Wing E, Ground Floor, Tai Po, New Territories, Hong Kong

S. C. Chan, J. S. Wong, Dicky and W. S. Chung
Department of Psychiatry, Tai Po Hospital, Tai Po, New Territories, Hong Kong

Sharon L. Gorman and Monica Rivera
Department of Physical Therapy, Samuel Merritt University, 450 30th Street, Oakland, CA 94609, USA

Lise McCarthy
McCarthy's Interactive PhysicalTherapy, 927 Vicente Street, San Francisco, CA 94116, USA

Akiko Kamimura
Course of Physical Therapy, School of Health Sciences, Faculty of Medicine, Kagoshima University, 8-35-1 Sakuragaoka, Kagoshima 890-8544, Japan
Kagoshima Physical Therapy Association, Kagoshima 897-0132, Japan
Red Cross Kagoshima Hospital, Kagoshima 891-0133, Japan

Harutoshi Sakakima
Course of Physical Therapy, School of Health Sciences, Faculty of Medicine, Kagoshima University, 8-35-1 Sakuragaoka, Kagoshima 890-8544, Japan

Fumio Tsutsumi
Department of Physical Therapy, Kyushu Nutrition Welfare University, Fukuoka 800-0298, Japan

Nobuhiko Sunahara
Red Cross Kagoshima Hospital, Kagoshima 891-0133, Japan

Kari Storetvedt
The Occupational Rehabilitation Centre in Rauland (AiR), 3864 Rauland, Norway
Department for Physical and Rehabilitation Medicine, University Hospital of Northern Norway (UNN), 9038 Tromsø, Norway

Anne Helene Garde
National Research Center for theWorking Environment, Lersø Parkalle 105, 2100 København Ø, Denmark

Jose C. Navarro, Mark C. Molina, Alejandro C. Baroque II and Johnny K. Lokin
Stroke Unit, Department of Neurology and Psychiatry, University of Santo Tomas Hospital, España Boulevard, San Vicente Ferrer Ward, 1008 Manila, Philippines

Maria J. C. Blikman, Hege R. Jacobsen and Eivind Meland
Department of Global Public Health and Primary Care, Research Group of General Practice, University of Bergen, Kalfarveien 31, 5018 Bergen, Norway

Geir Egil Eide
Centre for Clinical Research, Haukeland University Hospital, Armauer Hansen's House, Bergen, Norway
Department of Global Public Health and Primary Care, Research Group of Lifestyle Epidemiology, University of Bergen, Bergen, Norway

Amol M. Karmarkar, James E. Graham, Amit Kumar and Kenneth J. Ottenbacher
Division of Rehabilitation Sciences, University of Texas Medical Branch, 301 University Boulevard, Mail Route No. 1137, Galveston, TX 77555, USA

Timothy A. Reistetter
Occupational Therapy Department, University of Texas Medical Branch, Galveston, TX, USA

JacquelineM.Mix, Paulette Niewczyk and Carl V. Granger
Uniform Data System for Medical Rehabilitation, A Division of UB Foundation Activities Inc. and Department of Rehabilitation Medicine, University at Buffalo, Buffalo, NY, USA

Siew Kwaon Lui, Annie Jane Nalanga and Yeow Leng Tan
Department of Rehabilitation Medicine, Singapore General Hospital, 20 College Road, Academia Level 4, Singapore 169856

Yee Sien Ng and ChekWaiBok
Department of Rehabilitation Medicine, Singapore General Hospital, 20 College Road, Academia Level 4, Singapore 169856
Duke-National University of Singapore (NUS) Graduate Medical School, 8 College Road, Singapore 169857

Alana Zinman, Nicole Digout and Sylvia Haycock
Department of Occupational Science and Occupational Therapy, Faculty of Medicine, University of Toronto, Toronto, ON, Canada M5G 1V7

Patricia Bain
Lyndhurst Centre, Toronto Rehabilitation Institute, University Health Network, Toronto, ON, Canada M4G 3V9

Debbie Hébert
Department of Occupational Science and Occupational Therapy, Faculty of Medicine, University of Toronto, Toronto, ON, Canada M5G 1V7
Toronto Rehabilitation Institute, University Health Network, Toronto, ON, Canada M5G 2A2

Sander L. Hitzig
Institute for Life Course and Aging, Faculty of Medicine, University of Toronto, 263 McCaul Street, Suite 328, Toronto, ON, Canada M5T 1W7

www.ingramcontent.com/pod-product-compliance
Lightning Source LLC
Chambersburg PA
CBHW080503200326
41458CB00012B/4073